Textbook of
Practical
Laparoscopic Surgery

2nd Edition

RK Mishra MRCS, MMAS (UK)
Director, Laparoscopy Hospital, New Delhi
Professor and Head of Minimal Access Surgery, TGO University

Member Society of American Gastrointestinal and Endoscopic Surgeons (SAGES)
Member World Association of Laparoscopic Surgeon (WALS)
Member European Association for Transluminal Surgery (EATS)
Member Indian Association of Gastrointestinal Endosurgeons (IAGES)

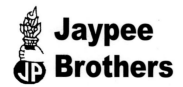

Jaypee Brothers

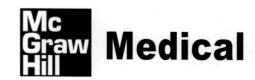

Mc Graw Hill Medical

© 2009, Jaypee Brothers Medical Publishers
First published in India in 2009 by

Jaypee Brothers Medical Publishers (P) Ltd.

Corporate Office
4838/24 Ansari Road, Daryaganj, **New Delhi** - 110002, India, +91-11-43574357

Registered Office
B-3 EMCA House, 23/23B Ansari Road, Daryaganj, **New Delhi** 110 002, India
Phones: +91-11-23272143, +91-11-23272703, +91-11-23282021,
+91-11-23245672, Rel: +91-11-32558559 Fax: +91-11-23276490, +91-11-23245683
e-mail: jaypee@jaypeebrothers.com, Website: www.jaypeebrothers.com

First published in USA by The McGraw-Hill Companies, 2 Penn Plaza, New York, NY 10121.
Exclusively worldwide distributor except South Asia (India, Nepal, Sri Lanka, Bhutan, Pakistan, Bangladesh, Malaysia).

ISBN-13: 978-0-07-163449-6
ISBN-10: 0-07-163449-5

Printed at Replika Press Pvt. Ltd.

Dedicated to

My dear teacher
Professor Sir Alfred Cuschieri

Foreword

I am honored to have been asked by Professor RK Mishra to write the foreword to his *Textbook of Practical Laparoscopic Surgery*. Less than twenty years ago laparoscopy was a revolutionary technology available in a few select centers for which indications were unclear at best. Now laparoscopy is the preferred method of surgery for a wide range of pathology ranging from cholecystitis and gastroesophageal reflux to morbid obesity and colon carcinoma; virtually every gastrointestinal tract operation can be laparoscopically undertaken. In most circumstances the laparoscopic approach has been shown to have numerous advantages including less pain, less morbidity, shorter hospitalization and less cost. In addition to being the access technique of choice from the esophagus to the rectum it has also gained significant popularity for urologic,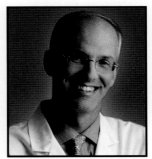
gynecologic, and other intra-abdominal procedures. Because of the overwhelming surgeon and patient preference for laparoscopy, education and training in the laparoscopic arena have been in high demand. Although many textbooks have been written to help satisfy this void, few are as easy to read and as informative about the gamut of laparoscopic themes. The 49 chapters allow the most uninformed neophyte to rapidly understand the technical considerations related to these procedures. However, the depth and breadth of the well illustrated volume also allow the experienced laparoscopic general, urologic, or gynecologic surgeon to become familiar with the new and exciting areas such as robotics and hepatopancreatic operations. The illustrations are all crystal clear, the cutaway enlargements very helpful, and the text explaining them is easy to read. The subject matter has been well researched and is written in an authoritative although not pedantic way as could only be done by a highly experienced laparoscopic surgeon with a wonderful aptitude for sharing his knowledge. Professor Mishra has beautifully detailed each area ranging from the history of sterilization techniques to the physics of energy sources to practical methods of port site closure. The constant thread throughout the book is its practical nature - this is not a book to be taken from the shelf on rare occasions to use as a reference prior to performing the occasional obscure operation. This book is instead one to read cover to cover and then to share with one's residents, fellows, theater staff, and associates to insure that each of them is fluent in the practicalities of laparoscopy. Having written a few books, I know how much work is required to produce such a well illustrated and superbly written comprehensive textbook. It was immediately apparent to me during my reading that the textbook of practical laparoscopy was a labor of love for Professor Mishra and thus will become a cherished and favorite resource for all of its readers, including me. I wish to congratulate him on his outstanding achievement and thank him for having allowed me to review it and to write this brief foreword.

Steven D Wexner MD, FACS, FRCS, FRCS Ed, FASCRS, FACG
President Society of American Gastrointestinal Endoscopic Surgeons 2006-2007.
Past President American College of Surgeons. Professor of Surgery, Ohio State University
Professor of Surgery, University of Siena, Italy, Jerusalem and Israel. Clinical Professor, Department of Surgery, Division of General Surgery, University of South Florida
College of Medicine. Chief of Staff and Chairman, Medical Executive Committee, Cleveland Clinic Hospital.
Chairman, Department of Colorectal Surgery and Chairman, Division of Research and Education,
Research Professor of Biomedical Science, Florida Atlantic University, Boca Raton, Florida

Foreword

In less than ten years so much has happened in the very young field of laparoscopic surgery. We are at a major crossroads in the approach to surgical problems that will be chronicled as the most important transition of our century: Large incision surgery to microincision surgery.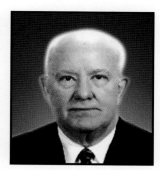

The laparoscope has literally revolutionized both general surgery and gynecology. As new procedures are developed, surgeons want to offer their patients the benefits of smaller wounds, less postoperative stress, shorter hospital stay. This rapid acceptance of laparoscopic surgery has come at a high price to some patients, however, when complications unique to this approach have lead to prolonged hospitalization or death.

In the 1970's, practicing gynecologists had taken to laparoscopy by the thousands because of the "simple" sterilization techniques and the diagnostic opportunities for chronic infertility and pelvic pain. Unique, puzzling complications of vessel injury and bowel and skin burns, as well as sterilization failures, rapidly made "simple" laparoscopic surgery problems the leading cause of gynecologic law suits. In the 1990's, general surgeons are embracing the laparoscope as enthusiastically and innocently as gynecologists did in the 1970's and are seeing unique and disastrous complications: Who had ever heard of a common iliac artery injury during a cholecystectomy? The World Association of Laparoscopic Surgeons responded to these problems with the same high purpose as the AAGL had by organizing teaching courses reviewing complications so as to prevent them.

Textbook of Practical Laparoscopic Surgery represents an historical landmark and is a must for all surgeons and gynecologist. The chapters are comprehensive, well written and up-to-date. The layout and general presentation is superb with several color illustrations throughout. The detail covered in each chapter is all encompassing and spans areas such as ergonomics of minimal access surgery, laparoscopic anatomy and the basic principles of laparoscopy. In addition to surgical techniques, this book provides a broader focus on issues pertaining to laparoendoscopic surgery, such as telerobotic surgery, use of simulators in training, and a comprehensive look at credentialing past, present, and future.

I congratulate Professor Mishra for completing this voluminous work and hope that his effort will be fruitful to the medical fraternity.

Dr Ray L Green MD, FACOG
President World Association of Laparoscopic Surgeon (USA)
Diplomate of American Board of Obstetrics and Gynecology
Fellow American College of Obstetrician and Gynecologist

Preface to the Second Edition

When the first edition of *Textbook of Practical Laparoscopic Surgery* was published, evidence-based medicine principle were starting to be embraced by the surgery community. Our second edition comes at a critical time in minimal access surgical care when laparoscopic surgeons are expected to use the best available evidence to support their every day decision in patient care, citing critical scientific evidence to support their decisions. The 2nd edition of this book has made some major improvements on the 1st edition. In particular, the book is now much more accessible.

In new edition of *Textbook of Practical Laparoscopic Surgery* the reader will quickly see the added depth and scope of coverage a marked improvement over previous edition. We have thoroughly revised every chapter and sharpened the focus of our evidence based approach. Many new chapters we have included on Colorectal Surgery, Gynecological Surgery, Sling Operations, Obesity Surgery and Complications of Minimal Access Surgery. We have also identified and given attention to cover minimal access surgical procedure for patient populations that require specialized care, including Pediatric, Urological and Obesity surgery. Even though many new chapters are added the book has kept the same basic format as its predecessor. In particular, it is written in a clear note form which emphasizes key points and makes the text very accessible. A quick flick through the book demonstrates that there are a great many more illustrations than the 1st edition, but they are all line drawings and schematics.

We believe the chapters on new emerging topic of minimal access surgery like NOTES and Robotics, strike a balance describing both the current status of practice and possibilities on the horizon. The chapters and designing of the book have been carefully edited to provide a smooth, readable text. Minimal access surgery is a challenging yet wonderfully rewarding endeavor. As this new field of minimal access surgery grows with the advances in technology and new surgical techniques, there should always be that unfatigable desire that pushes one to continually strive for the best results possible. My desire is that the readers will be the beneficiaries of this attempt of second edition of this book to harvest the collective wisdom from those who have risen to the challenge of minimal access surgery. The ultimate reward to us is enhanced results and improved outcomes for our patients, and an opportunity to advance the art and science of Minimal Access Surgery.

In summary, the second edition of *Textbook of Practical Laparoscopic Surgery* has been thoroughly updated with recent advances in both scientific evidence and clinical practice. It is hoped that the information contained within this book will prompt the reader to pay closer attention to their own outcomes with laparoscopic surgery and provide insight into the techniques that have proven effective. We hope you will agree that this book, with its consistent and long established reputation, is different from other textbooks of laparoscopic surgery. I believe that this book would be a good choice for a student, practicing surgeons or a recent graduate who wishes to either review laparoscopic surgery as a whole, or needs a reference text for those unusual cases.

I hope that this new edition of text will be an opportunity for the readers to solidify fundamental principles across the great field of laparoscopic surgery. In the spirit of community of minimal access surgeon, we welcome any suggestions you may have to improve this book for future editions.

RK Mishra

Preface to the First Edition

When I was to finish my Master's in Minimal Access Surgery from Ninewells Hospital and Medical School, UK. I was one among the few fortunate students who was called by Chancellor Sir James W Black (Nobel Prize Winner in Medicine 1988) for special meeting. Sir Black advised us to start training of minimal access surgery after completing our degree. He realized the great lack of university trained well qualified personnel who could propagate art and science of minimal access surgery to the medical fraternity. Sir Black emphasized that training of minimal access surgery is going into the profit making hands of the industry and as a qualified minimal access surgeon this is our duty to disseminate the knowledge of our skill to the entire speciality who wants to use this surgical proficiency. Keeping in mind this instruction of my Chancellor I started teaching laparoscopy to surgeon gynecologist, urologist and pediatric surgeon all over the world. This book is based on seven years of my teaching experience in minimal access surgery. Within seven years I have trained more than 1500 surgeons and gynecologists from every corner of the world.

In recent years progress in medical care has been rapid especially in areas of laparoscopic robotic and NOTES. The major reason of this progress has been the interdisciplinary approach of merging technology with medicine. However, there are limited good books available which are self sufficient and yet easy to understand. This book has been written to fill this gap. It has grown out of numerous discussions during various educational training programs. The participants have included gynecologists, urologists, and general surgeons from fresh doctors to senior surgeons.

The book is primarily intended for the reader who has some background of conventional operative surgical and gynecological procedures. It is broad in its scope and depth wherever needed is provided without being unnecessarily sophisticated. There are plenty of illustrations and diagrams to facilitate faster learning.

The essential section of the book includes the concept of ergonomics, task analysis and practical problems encountered in attempting to venture into laparoscopic operative surgery. An overall view of the latest instruments is presented and detailed explanations in appropriate sections are penned down. The medical terminology is deliberately introductory to facilitate easy understanding. Enough fundamentals are presented within the context of this book to make it reasonably self sufficient. In fewer than 200 pages, this book guides you through the process of developing a foundation of laparoscopic surgery like developing skill of dissection, suturing, knotting and tissue approximation.

The second section of book describes comprehensive laparoscopic operative procedure demonstrating a method that is tested, proven, and based upon sound instructional theory. The procedures are written according to systemic task analysis and students are advised to see the DVDs provided with this book. The latter chapters are devoted to special topics of recent advances in minimal access surgery to give the reader a true overall view of the field.

Although I have taken every care to make this book error free, nonetheless mistakes may have been overlooked. I will be grateful for any constructive criticism.

RK Mishra

Acknowledgments

I would like to express my gratitude to all those who gave me the inspiration to write this book. I want to thank my colleagues at Surgical Skill Unit, Ninewells Hospital and Medical School. I express my gratitude to all my fellow doctors and students whose constructive criticism and words of encouragement motivated me to accomplish this work.

I am very grateful to Mr AM Sinha, Department of Biotechnology (AIIMS) whose infectious enthusiasm, innovative ideas, valuable suggestions, and proofreading are largely responsible for the high quality of this publication.

I take this opportunity to thank M/s Jaypee Brothers Medical Publishers (P) Ltd. I am truly impressed by the outstanding publication team, especially Shri Jitendar P Vij (Chairman and Managing director), Mr Tarun Duneja (Director–Publishing), Mr KK Raman (Production Manager). I am grateful to them for their patience and continuous support.

I would especially like to thank Mr Sunil Dutt for excellent formatting, Mr Kshirod Sahoo for careful proofreading, and Mr Anil Sharma for working out the figures and illustrations in the book.

This work would not have been possible without the unconditional love and support from my family members. I thank my parents Dr RP Mishra and Mrs Shanti Mishra, my brothers Dr Rakesh Kumar Mishra and Dr Rajeev Kumar for their encouragement. I would like to give my special thanks to my wife Sadhana and children Nidhi, Rishi, and Ashish whose patience and love enabled me to complete this work.

Contents

Section 4: Laparoscopic Urology

Section 5: Pediatric Laparoscopy

Section 6: Miscellaneous

Essentials of Laparoscopy

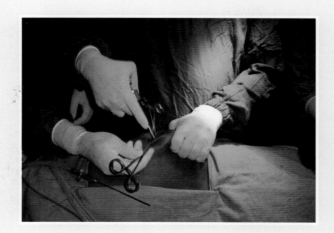

1 Chronological Advances in Minimal Access Surgery

The earliest recorded references to endoscopy date to ancient times with Hippocrates. In his description there is explanation of rectum examination with a speculum. Hippocrates advised injecting a large quantity of air into the intestines through the anus in intestinal obstruction. He advocated the insertion of suppository that was 10 digits long. These descriptions suggest that Hippocrates was well aware of ileus with intestinal obstruction and thought that there were several possible etiologies, including fecal impaction, intussusceptions, and sigmoid volvulus. Moreover, Hippocrates treated these life-threatening conditions with minimally invasive approaches.

1585 Aranzi was the first to use a light source for an endoscopic procedure, focusing sunlight through a flask of water and projecting the light into the nasal cavity.

1706 The term "trocar," was coined in 1706, and is thought to be derived from "trochartor" troise-quarts, a three-faced instrument consisting of a perforator enclosed in a metal cannula.

1806 Philip Bozzini, built an instrument that could be introduced in the human body to visualize the internal organs. He called this instrument "LICHTLEITER". Bozzini used an aluminum tube to visualize the genitourinary tract. The tube, illuminated by a wax candle, had fitted mirrors to reflect images (Fig. 1.1).

1853 Antoine Jean Desormeaux, a French surgeon first introduced the "Lichtleiter" of Bozzini to a patient. For many surgeons, he is considered as the "Father of Endoscopy".

1867 Desormeaux, used an open tube to examine the genitourinary tract, combining alcohol and turpentine with a flame in order to generate a brighter, more condensable beam of light.

1868 Kussmaul performed the first esophago-gastroscopy on a professional sword swallower, initiating efforts at instrumentation of the gastrointestinal tract. Mikulicz and Schindler, however, are credited with the advancement of gastroscopy.

1869 Commander Pantaleoni used a modified cystoscope to cauterize a hemorrhagic uterine growth. Pantaleoni thus performed the first diagnostic and therapeutic hysteroscopy.

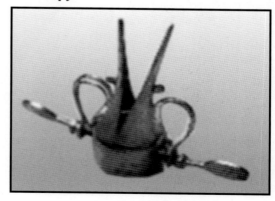

Fig. 1.1: Lichtleiter's endoscope

1901   Dimitri Ott, a Petrograd gynecologist used head mirrors to reflect light and augment visualization and used access technique in which a speculum was introduced through an incision in the prior vaginal fornix in a pregnant woman.

1901   The first experimental laparoscopy was performed in Berlin in 1901 by the German surgeon Georg Kelling, who used a cystoscope to peer into the abdomen of a dog after first insufflating it with air. Kelling also used filtered atmospheric air to create a pneumoperitoneum, with the goal of stopping intra-abdominal bleeding (Ectopic pregnancy, bleeding ulcers, and pancreatitis) but these studies did not find any response or supporters (Fig. 1.2).

Kelling proposed a high-pressure insufflation of the abdominal cavity, a technique he called the "Luft-tamponade" or "air-tamponade".

1910   HC Jacobaeus of Stockholm published a paper on discussion of the inspection of the peritoneal, pleural and pericardial cavity.

1911   Bertram M Bernheim of Johns Hopkins Hospital introduced first laparoscopic surgery to the United States. He named it the procedure of minimal access surgery as "organoscopy". The instrument used was a proctoscope of a half inch diameter and ordinary light for illumination was used.

1911   HC Jacobaeus coined the term "laparo-thorakoskopie" after using this procedure on the thorax and abdomen. He used to introduce the trocar inside the body cavity directly without employing a pneumoperitoneum.

1918   O Goetze developed an automatic pneumoperitoneum needle characterized for its safe introduction to the peritoneal cavity.

The next decade and a half witnessed a decline in technological advancement in endoscopy due to World War I.

1920   Zollikofer of Switzerland discovered the benefit of CO_2 gas to use for insufflation, rather than filtered atmospheric air or nitrogen.

1929   Kalk, a German physician, introduced the forward oblique (135°) view lens systems. He advocated the use of a separate puncture site for pneumoperitoneum. Goetze of Germany first developed a needle for insufflation.

1929   Heinz Kalk, a German gastroenterologist developed a 135° lens system and a dual trocar approach. He used laparoscopy as a diagnostic method for liver and gallbladder diseases (Fig. 1.3).

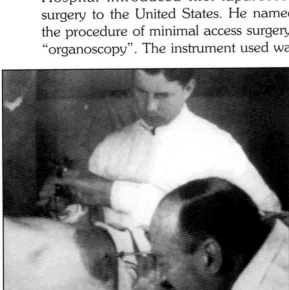

Fig. 1.2: Kelling performing laparoscopy in dog

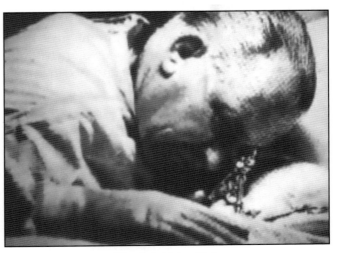

Fig. 1.3: Heinz Kalk

1934 John C Ruddock, an American surgeon described laparoscopy as a good diagnostic method, many times, superior than laparotomy. He used the instrument for diagnostic laparoscopy which consisted of built-in forceps with electrocoagulation capacity (Fig. 1.4).

1936 Boesch of Switzerland is credited with the first laparoscopic tubal sterilization.

1938 Janos Veress of Hungary developed a especially designed spring-loaded needle. Interestingly, he did not promote the use of his Veress needle for laparoscopy purposes.

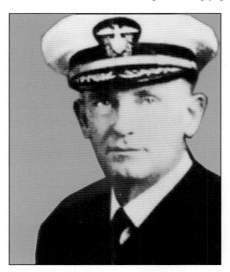

Fig. 1.4: John Ruddock

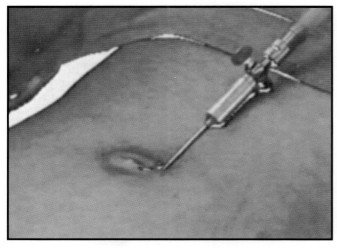

Fig. 1.5: Veress needle

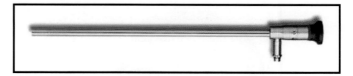

Fig. 1.6: Laparoscope

He used Veress needle for the induction of pneumothorax. Veress needle is widely used instrument today to create pneumoperitoneum (Fig. 1.5).

1939 Richard W Telinde, tried to perform an endoscopic procedure by a culdoscopic approach, in the lithotomy position. This method was rapidly abandoned because of the presence of small intestine.

1939 Heinz Kalk published his experience of over 2000 liver biopsies, performed using local anesthesia without mortality.

1944 Raoul Palmer, of Paris performed gynecological examinations using laparoscopy, (Fig. 1.6) and placing the patients in the Trendelenburg's position, so air could fill the pelvis. He also stressed the importance of continuous intra-abdominal pressure monitoring during a laparoscopic procedure.

1953 The rigid rod lens system was discovered by Professor Hopkins. The credit of videoscopic surgery goes to this surgeon who had revolutionized the concept by making this instrument.

1960 Kurt Semm was a German gynecologist, who invented the automatic insufflator (Fig. 1.7). His experience with this new device was published in 1966. Though not recognized in his own country, but on the other side of the Atlantic, both American physicians and instrument makers valued the Semm's insufflator for its simple application, clinical value, and safety (Fig. 1.8).

1960 Patrick Steptoe, a British gynecologist adapted the techniques of sterilization by two puncture technique.

1972 H Coutnay Clarke showed laparoscopic suturing technique for hemostasis.

Section One

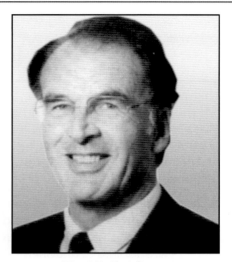

Fig. 1.7: Kurt Semm

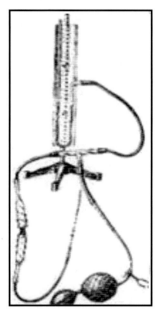

Fig. 1.8: First insufflator made by Prof Semm

1973 Gaylord D Alexander, developed techniques of safe local and general anesthesia suitable for laparoscopy.

1977 First laparoscopic assisted appendicectomy was performed by Dekok. Appendix was exteriorized and ligated outside the abdominal cavity.

1977 Kurt Semm demonstrated endoloop suturing technique in laparoscopic surgery.

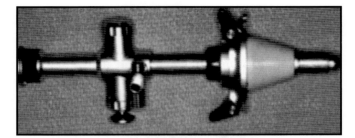

Fig. 1.9: Hasson's cannula

1978 Hasson introduced an alternative method of blunt trocar placement. He proposed a blunt mini-laparotomy which permits direct visualization of trocar entrance into the peritoneal cavity.

Hasson's cannula was a reusable device of similar design to a standard cannula but attached to an olive-shaped sleeve was developed. This sleeve would slide up and down over the shaft of the cannula and form an airtight seal at the fascial opening. In addition, the sharp trocar was replaced by a blunt obturator. This cannula is held in place by the use of stay sutures passed through the fascial edges and attached to the body of the cannula (Fig. 1.9).

1980 Patrick Steptoe started to perform laparoscopic procedures first time in UK.

1983 Semm, German gynecologist, performed the first laparoscopic appendicectomy.

1985 The first documented laparoscopic cholecystectomy was performed by Erich Mühe in Germany in 1985.

1987 Phillipe Mouret has got the credit to perform the first laparoscopic cholecystectomy in Lyons, France using video technique (Fig. 1.10). Cholecystectomy is the laparoscopic procedure which revolutionized the general surgery.

1987 Ger reported first laparoscopic repair of inguinal hernia using prototype stapler.

1987 Complete removal of gallbladder was performed by Mouret in Lyon, France.

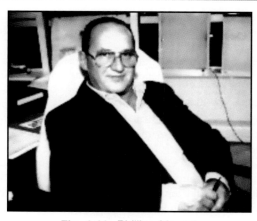

Fig. 1.10: Phillipe Mouret

1988 Harry Reich performed laparoscopic lymphadenectomy for treatment of ovarian cancer.

1988 McKernan and Sye performed first cholecystectomy in the USA (Fig. 1.11).

1989 Harry Reich described first laparoscopic hysterectomy using bipolar desiccation; later he demonstrated staples and finally sutures for laparoscopic hysterectomy.

1989 Reddick and Olsen reported that CBD injury after laparoscopic cholecystectomy is 5 times than with conventional cholecystectomy. As a result of this report, USA government announced, that surgeons should perform at least 15 laparoscopic cholecystectomy under supervision, before being allowed to do this procedure on their own.

1990 Bailey and Zucker in USA popularized laparoscopic anterior highly selective vagotomy combined with posterior truncal vagotomy.

1994 First robotic arm was designed to hold the telescope with the goal of improving safety and reducing the need of skilled camera operator (Fig. 1.12).

1996 First live telecast of laparoscopic surgery performed remotely via the Internet (Robotic Telesurgery).

2000 The US Food and Drug Administration (FDA) first time approved the da Vinci Surgical System, making it the first robotic system allowed to be used in American operating rooms.

2001 The Lindbergh operation, named in honor of American aviator Charles Lindbergh, was the first ever transatlantic surgery. Doctors Michel Gagner and Jacques Marescaux removed the gall bladder of a 68-year-old woman in Strasbourg, France from New York. The surgeons used a ZEUS robotic surgical system from Computermotion Inc. and an ATM fiberoptic connection provided by France Télécom.

2004 Robotic prostatectomy became the first most commonly performed robotic surgery. According to Intuitive Surgical Inc., the California-based manufacturers of the da

Section One

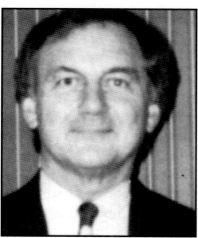

Fig. 1.11: William Sye

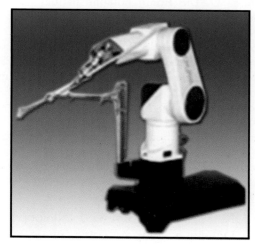

Fig. 1.12: Robotic arm

Vinci robot, the number of robotic prost-atectomies rose from 36 in 2000 to 8000 in 2004.

2005   Combining robotically assisted coronary artery bypass surgery (CABG) with stented angioplasty shows promise for treating extensive coronary artery disease, researchers reported at the American Heart Association Scientific Sessions 2005, Dallas.

The evolution of minimal access therapy aims to minimize the traumatic insult to the patient without compromising the safety and efficacy of the treatment compared with traditional open surgery. If this is achieved, patients recover more quickly, which reduces hospital stay and allows more rapid return to full activity and work within minimum time.

BIBLIOGRAPHY

1. Bernheim BM. Organoscopy: cystoscopy of the abdominal cavity. Ann Surg 1911;53:764–7.
2. Bozzini P. Lichtleiter, eine Erfi ndung zur Anschauung innerer Theile und Krankheiten. J Prakt Arzneikunde 1806;24:107–13.
3. Desormeaux AJ. Endoscope and its application to the diagnosis and treatment of affections of the genitourinary passage. Chicago Med J 1867.
4. Fervers C. Die Laparoskopie mit dem Cystoskop. Mediz Klinik 1933;31:1042–5.
5. Fourestier M, Gladu A, Vulmiere J. Perfectionnements a l'endoscopie medicale. Realisation bronchoscopique. La Presse Medicale 1952;60:1292–3.
6. Goetze O. Die Röntgendiagnostik bei gasgefüllter Bauchhöhle. Eine neue Methode. Münch Med Wochenschr 1918;65:1275–80.
7. Gordon AG, Magos AL. The development of laparoscopic surgery. Baillieres Clin Obstet Gynaecol 1989;3:429–49.
8. Gow JG, Hopkins HH, Wallace DM, et al. The modern urological endoscope. In: Hopkins HH, ed. Handbook of Urological Endoscopy. Edinburgh: Churchill Livingstone; 1978.
9. Gunning JE. The history of laparoscopy. J Reprod Med 1974;12:222–5.
10. Jacobeus HC. Ueber die Möglichkeit die Zystoskopie bei Untersuchung seröser Höhlungen anzuwenden. Münch Med Wochenschr 1910;57: 2090–2.
11. Jacobs M, Verdeja JC, Goldstein HS. Minimally invasive colon resection (laparoscopic colectomy). Surg Laparosc Endosc 1991;1:133–50.
12. Kalk H. Erfahrungen mit der Laparoskopie (Zugleich mit Beschreibung eines neuen Instrumentes). Zeitschr Klin Med 1929;111:303–48.
13. Kelling G. Ueber Oesophagoskopie, Gastroskopie und Kölioskopie. Münch Med Wochenschr 1902;49:21–4.
14. Kurze Uebersicht über meine Erfahrungen mit der Laparo-thoraskopie. Münch Med Wochenschr 1911;58:2017–9.
15. Lau WY, Leow CK, Li AK. History of endoscopic and laparoscopic surgery. World J Surg 1997;21:444–53.
16. Mühe B. The first laparoscopic cholecystectomy. Langenbecks Arch Chir 1986;369:804.
17. Nadeau OE, Kampmeier OF. Endoscopy of the abdomen: abdominoscopy. Surg Gynecol Obstet 1925;41:259–71.
18. Nitze M. Beobachtungs- und Untersuchungsmethode für Harnröhre, Harnblase and Rektum. Wiener Mediz Wochenschr. 1879;29:651–2.
19. Orndorff BH. The peritoneoscope in diagnosis of diseases of the abdomen. J Radiol 1920;1:307–25.
20. Roccavilla A. L'endoscopia delle grandi cavita sierose mediante un nuovo apparecchio ad illuminazione dirtta (laparo-toracoscopia diretta). La Riforma Medica 1914;30:991–5.
21. Rosin D. History. In: Rosin D, ed. Minimal Access Medicine and Surgery. Oxford: Radcliffe Medical Press; 1993.
22. Ruddock JC. Peritoneoscopy. Surg Gynecol Obstet 1937;65:623–39.
23. Semm K. Endoscopic appendectomy. Endoscopy 1983;15:59–64.
24. Semm K. Operative Manual for Endoscopic Abdominal Surgery. Chicago: Thieme; 1987.
25. Semm K. The history of endoscopy. In: Vitale GC, Sanfi lippo JS, Perissat J, eds. Laparoscopic Surgery: An Atlas for General Surgeons. Philadelphia: JB Lippincott; 1995.
26. Short AR. The uses of coelioscopy. Br Med J 1925;3: 254–5.
27. Steiner OP. Abdominoscopy. Surg Gynecol Obstet 1924;38:266–9.
28. Stone WE. Intra-abdominal examination by the aid of the peritoneoscope. J Kan Med Soc. 1924;24:63–6.
29. Veress J. Neues Instrument zur Ausführung von Brust- oder Bauchpunktionen and Pneumothoraxbehandlung. Deutsch Med Wochenschr 1938;40:1480–1.
30. Vitale GC, Cuschieri A, Perissat J. Guidelines for the future. In: Vitale GC, Sanfi lippo JS, Perissat J, eds. Laparoscopic Surgery: An Atlas for General Surgeons. Philadelphia: JB Lippincott; 1995.
31. Zollikofer R. Zur Laparoskopie. Schweiz Med Wochenschr 1924;5: 264–5.

2   Laparoscopic Equipments

It is well known that laparoscopy is the consequence of advances made in the field of medical engineering. Each surgical specialty has different requirement of instruments. Laparoscopy was initially criticized owing to the cost of specialized instruments and possible complications due to these sharp long instruments. Also, it necessitated difficult hand eye coordination. Gradually, the technique gained recognition and respect from the medical fraternity since it drastically reduced many of the complications of the open procedure. Minimal access surgery has developed rapidly only after grand success of laparoscopic cholecystectomy. Computer aided designing of laparoscopic instruments is an important branch of medical engineering. It is now possible to control the access through microprocessor controlled laparoscopic instruments. New procedures and instruments are innovated regularly which makes it important for the surgeon to be familiar with the developments. Laparoscopy is a technologically dependent surgery and it is expected every surgeon should have reasonably good knowledge of these instruments.

LAPAROSCOPIC TROLLEY

The mobile laparoscopic video cart is equipped with locking brakes and has four anti-static rollers. The trolley has a drawer and three shelves (Fig. 2.1). The upper shelves have a tilt adjustment and used for supporting the video monitor unit. Included on the trolley is an electrical supply terminal strip, mounted on the rear of the second shelf (from the top). Recently, ceiling mounted trolleys are launched by many

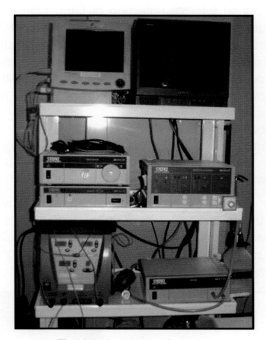

Fig. 2.1: Laparoscopic trolley

companies which are ergonomically better and consume less space in operation theater.

LIGHT CABLE

Minimal access surgery depends on the artificial light available in closed body cavity, and before the discovery of light source and light cable; mirrors were used to reflect the light onto the subject where direct light access was not possible.

In 1954, a major breakthrough in technology occurred in the development of fiberoptic cables

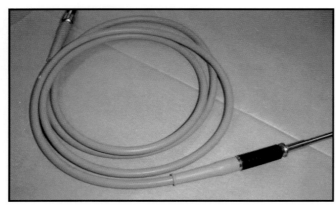

Fig. 2.2: Fibre optic light cable

(Fig. 2.2). The principle of fiberoptic cable was based on the total internal reflection of light. Light can be conducted along a curved glass rod due to multiple total internal reflections. Light would enter at one end of the fiber and emerge at the other end after numerous internal reflections with virtually all of its intensity.

Nowadays, there are two types of light cable available:
1. Fiberoptic cable
2. Liquid crystal gel cable.

Fiberoptic Cable

These cables are made up of a bundle of optical fiber glass thread swaged at both ends. The fiber size used is usually 20 to 150 micron in diameter (Fig. 2.3). They have a very high quality of optical transmission, but are fragile.

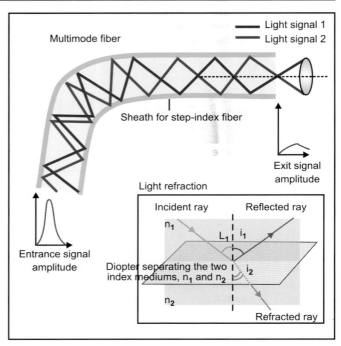

Fig. 2.4: Multimode fiber

The light inside these fibers travels on the principle of total internal reflection without losing much of its intensity (Fig. 2.4). The multimode fiber maintains the intensity of light and the light can be passed in a curved path of light cable.

As the light cables are used progressively, some optical fibers break (Fig. 2.5). The loss of optical fibers

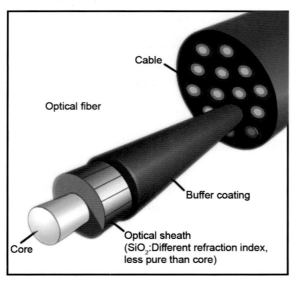

Fig. 2.3: Internal structure of fiberoptic cable

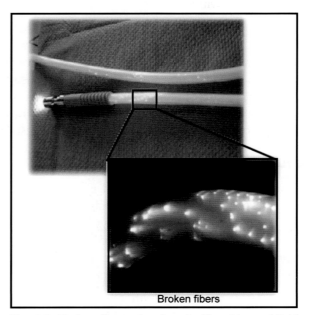

Fig. 2.5: Broken fibers showing significant loss of light

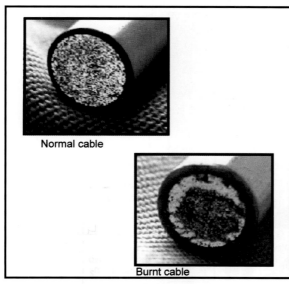

Fig. 2.6: Burnt fiber causes significant reduction in intensity of light

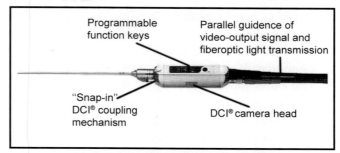

Fig. 2.7: DCI attachment of light cable

may be seen when one end of the cable is viewed in daylight. The broken fibers are seen as black spots. To avoid the breakage of these fibers the curvature radius of light cable should be respected and in any circumstances it should not be less than 15 cm in radius.

If the heat filter or cooling system of light source does not work properly, the fibers of these light cable is burnt and it will decrease the intensity of light dramatically (Fig. 2.6). If poor quality fibers are used it might burn just within few month of use.

Liquid Crystal Gel Cable

These cables are made up of a sheath that is filled with a clear optical gel (Liquid crystal). They are capable of transmitting up to 30 percent more light than optic fibers. Due to more light and better color temperature transmission, this cable is recommended in those circumstances, where documentation (movie, photography or TV) is performed.

The quartz swaging at the ends is extremely fragile, especially when the cable is hot. The slightest shock, on a bench for example, can cause the quartz end to crack and thus cause a loss in the transmission of the light.

Gel cables transmit more heat than optical fiber cables. These cables are made more rigid by a metal sheath, which makes them more difficult to maintain and to store. In conclusion, even though the choice is a difficult one, we use optical fiber cables, which are

as fragile as the gel cables but their flexibility makes them much easier to maintain.

Attachment of Light Source

Conventional attachment has at right angle connection for light source and camera. Recently, new attachment for light cable is available known as DCI interface (Fig. 2.7). The benefit of this is that it maintains upright orientation regardless of angle of viewing, using auto rotation system. It also provides single handed control of the entire endoscope camera system.

Maintenance of Light Cable

The following points should be followed for the maintenance of light cable:

1. Handle them carefully.
2. Avoid twisting them.
3. After the operation has been completed, the cable should preferably be disconnected from the endoscope and then connected to the light source (Fig. 2.8). In fact, most of the sources currently

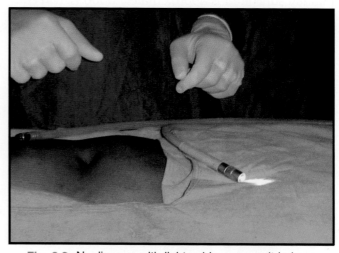

Fig. 2.8: Negligence with light cable can result in burn

Section One

available have a plug for holding the cable until it cools down.

4. The end of the crystal of cable should be periodically cleaned with a cotton swab moistened with alcohol.

5. The outer plastic covering of the cable should be cleaned with a mild cleaning agent or disinfectant.

6. Distal end of fiberoptic cable should never be placed on or under drapes, or next to the patient, when connected to an illuminated light source. The heat generated from the intensity of light may cause burns to the patient or ignite the drapes (Fig. 2.8).

7. The intensity of light source is so high that there is chance of retinal damage if the light will fall directly on eye. Never try to look directly on light source when it is lighted.

THE LIGHT SOURCE

A good laparoscopic light source should emit light as much as possible near the natural sun light. Two types of light source are in use:
- Xenon
- Halogen

Xenon has a more natural color spectrum and a smaller spot size than halogen. In practice, the yellow light of the halogen bulb is compensated for in the video camera system by white balancing. The output from the light sources is conducted to the telescope by light cables that contain either glass fiber bundles or special fluid. The halogen light source is used in the medical field since last 20 years but the spectral temperature of these lights is 3200 Kelvin which makes it too different and too low from natural sunlight. The midday sunlight has approximately 5600 Kelvin color temperature.

A more suitable light source for laparoscopic cameras involves the creation of an electrical arc in a metal halide system or in Xenon. This electrical arc is produced in same way as in flash of photographic camera. One of the main advantages of the laparoscopy is that of obtaining a virtually micro-surgical view compared to that obtained by laparotomy. Quality of the image obtained very much depends on the quantity of light available at each step of optical and electronic system. The Xenon light source emits a spectral temperature of color of approximately 6000 Kelvin on average for a power of 300 W (Fig. 2.9). Arc generated lamps have a spectral

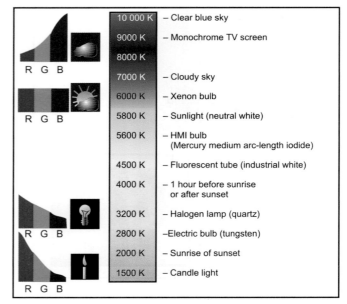

Fig. 2.9: Spectrum of light

temperature that gradually decreases with use and white balance is required before each use. The bulb needs replacing after 250 to 500 hours of usage, depending on the type of lamp.

A typical light source consists of:
- A lamp
- A heat filter
- A condensing lens
- Manual or automatic intensity control circuit.

Lamp

Lamp or bulb is the most important part of the light source. The quality of light depends on the lamp used. Several modern types of light sources are currently available (Fig. 2.10). These light sources mainly differ

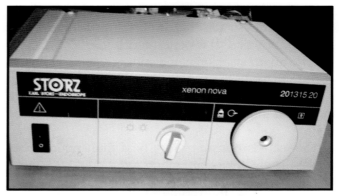

Fig. 2.10: Light source

on the type of bulb used. Four types of lamp are used more recently:

1. Quartz halogen
2. Incandescent bulbs
3. Xenon
4. Metal halide vapor arc lamp.

Halogen Bulbs

Halogen bulbs provide highly efficient crisp white light source with excellent color rendering. Electrodes in halogen lamps are made of tungsten. This is the only metal with a sufficiently high melting temperature and sufficient vapor pressure at elevated temperatures. They use a halogen gas that allows bulbs to burn more intensely. Halogen bulbs use low voltages and have an average life of 2,000 hours. The color temperature of halogen lamp is around (5000-5600 K). These lamps are economical and can be used for laparoscopic surgery if low budget setup is required.

Xenon Lamps

Xenon lamps consist of a spherical or ellipsoidal envelope made of quartz glass, which can withstand high thermal loads and high internal pressure. For ultimate image quality, only the highest-grade clear fused silica quartz is used. It is typically doped, although not visible to the human eye, to absorb harmful UV radiation generated during operation. The color temperature of xenon lamp is about 6000-6400 K. The operating pressures are tens of atmospheres at times, with surface temperatures exceeding 600°C.

The smaller, pointed electrode is called the cathode, which supplies the current to the lamp and facilitates the emission of electrons. To supply a sufficient amount of electrons, the cathode material is doped with thorium. The optimum operating temperature of the cathode tip is approximately 2000°C. To obtain this precise operating temperature, the cathode tip is pointed and in many cases has a groove on the pointed tip to act as a heat choke. This heat choke causes the tip to run at a higher temperature. This configuration of the cathode tip allows for a very high concentration of light from the cathode tip and a very stable arc.

The anode, the larger electrode, receives electrons emitted by the cathode. Once the electrons penetrate the anode face, the resulting energy is converted to

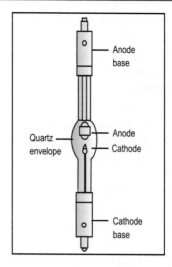

Fig. 2.11: Metal halide bulb

heat, most of which radiates away. The large, cylindrical shape of the anode helps to keep the temperature low by radiating the heat from the anode surface.

Metal Halide Vapor Arc Lamp

In metal halide lamp, a mixture of compounds (comprising mostly salts of rare earths and halides as well as the mercury which provides the conduction path) is carefully chosen to produce an output which approximates to 'white' light as perceived by the human eye (Fig. 2.11). There are two type of metal halide lamp generally used. They are iron iodide lamp and gallium iodide lamp. Iron iodide is a broad emitter and enhances the spectral output of the lamp in the 380 nm. Gallium iodide has the effect of introducing spectral lines at 403 nm and 417 nm of the electromagnetic spectrum (Fig. 2.12).

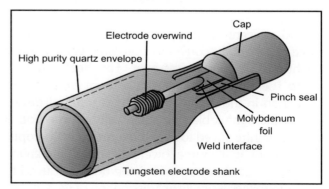

Fig. 2.12: Internal structure of metal halide tube

The intensity of the light delivered by any lamp also depends on the power supply of the source. However, increasing the power poses a real problem as it generates more heat. At present, the improvements made to the cameras means that it is possible to return to reasonable power levels of 250 W. However, 400 W units are preferable in order to obtain sufficient illumination of the abdomen even when bleeding causes strong light absorption. It is important to remember that a three chip camera require more light than single chip camera so a 400 W light source is recommended for 3 chips camera.

The two most frequently used types of lamps are halogen and xenon. The main difference between them is in the colors obtained. The xenon lamp has a slightly bluish tint. The light emitted by xenon lamp is more natural compared to halogen lamp. However, most of the cameras at present, analyze and compensate these variations by means of automatic "equalization of whites" (2100 K to 10,000 K), which allows the same image to be obtained with both light sources.

A proper white balancing before start of the operation is essential for obtaining a natural color. The white light is composed of equal proportion of red, blue and green color. At the time of white balancing, the camera sets its digital coding for these primary colors to equal proportion, assuming that the target is white. If at the time of white balancing, the telescope is not seeing a perfectly white object, the setup of the camera will be incorrect and the color perception will be poor.

The newer light source of xenon is defined as a cool light but practically it is not completely heat free and it should be cared for ignition hazard.

Heat Filter

For 100 percent of energy consumed, a normal light source (a light bulb) converts approximately 2 percent to light and 98 percent as heat. This heat is mainly due to the infrared spectrum of light and due to obstruction in the pathway of light. If infrared travels through the light cable, the cable will become hot. A heat filter is introduced to filter this infrared in fiberoptic cable. A cool light source lowers this ratio by creating more light, but does not reduce the heat produced to zero. This implies a significant dissipation of heat, which increases as the power rating increases. The sources

are protected against transmitting too much heat at present. The heat is essentially dissipated in transport, along the cable, in the connection with the endoscope and along the endoscope.

Some accidents have been reported due to burning caused by the heat of the optics system. It is therefore important to test the equipment, particularly if assemblies of different brands are used.

Condensing Lens

The purpose of condensing lens is to converge the light emitted by lamp to the area of light cable input. In most of the light source it is used for increasing the light intensity per square cm of area.

The Interface of a Standard Light Source

It is essential to know about all the switch and function of the light source. All essential details of the equipment and all the action required on the part can be found on the operating manual of the product.

Manual or Automatic Intensity Control Circuit

Manual adjustment allows the light source to be adjusted to a power level defined by the surgeon. In video cameras, close-up viewing is hampered in too much light, whereas more distant view is too dark. To address this, the luminosity of most of the current light sources is adjustable.

The advanced light source system is based on the automatic intensity adjustment technology. The video camera transforms the signal into an electronic signal. This electronic signal is coded in order to be transported. The coding dissociates the luminance and chrominance of the image. The luminance is the quantity of light of the signal (black and white) that dictates the quality of the final image. When there is too much light for the image (when the endoscope is near to the tissue), the luminance signal of the oscilloscope increases. On the other hand, when the luminosity is low (distant view or red surroundings), the luminance is low and the electronic signal is much weaker. A good quality luminance signal is calibrated to 1 millivolt. Overexposed images make the electronic signal pass above one millivolt, whereas underexposed images make the signal drop below one millivolt. Light sources equipped with adjustment analyze the luminance. If the signal is significantly higher than 1 millivolt, they lower the power and bring the signal back within the standards. Conversely, if the signal is too weak, they increase their intensity.

These systems are extremely valuable, permitting work to be performed at different distances from the target in good viewing conditions. However, the cameras currently available are often equipped with a regulation system, which is capable of automatic gain control in poor light condition and the purchase of a light source with adjustment associated with a camera equipped with an adjustment system, is a double purchase that is unnecessary.

Troubleshooting of Laparoscopic Light Source

Troubleshooting for inadequate lighting is shown in Table 2.1.

A laparoscopic surgeon should be technically well acknowledged of the principle of the instrument they are using. The purchase of a costly instrument is not an answer for achieving a good task, ability to handle them is equally important.

TELESCOPE

There are two type of telescope, rigid and flexible. The rigid scopes are based on the Hopkins rod lens system. Rigid rod lens system provides good resolution and better depth perception (Fig. 2.13). There are three important structural differences in telescope available in the market.

Table 2.1: Troubleshooting of light source	
Probable cause	*Remedy*
Loose connection at source or scope	Adjust connector
Light is on "manual-minimum"	Go to "automatic"
Bulb is burned out	Replace bulb
Fiberoptics are damaged	Replace light cable
Automatic iris adjusting to bright	Dim room lights
Reflection from instrument	Re-position instruments, or switch to "manual"

1. 6 to 18 rod lens system telescopes
2. 0 to 120° telescopes
3. 1.5 to 15 mm of telescopes.

Normally used telescope is the Hopkins Forward Oblique Telescope (30°) (Fig. 2.14). Its diameter is 10 mm length 33 cm and is autoclavable. Hopkins lens system uses more glass than air so it has improved light transmission. At the distal end, is a front lens complex (inverting real-image lens system, IRILS) which creates an inverted and real image of the subject. A number of IRILS transport the image to the eyepiece containing a magnifying lens. In the Hopkins rod-lens

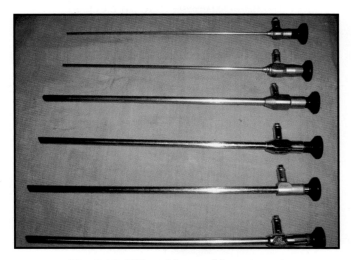

Fig. 2.13: Different types of laparoscope

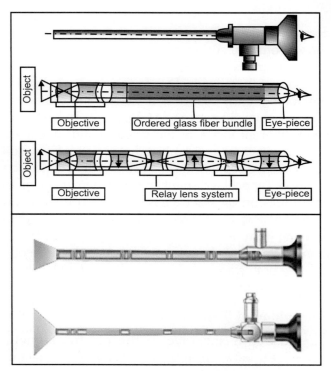

Fig. 2.14: Inside view of laparoscope

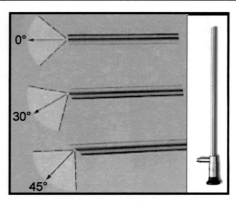

Fig. 2.15: Angle of laparoscope

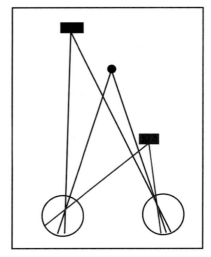

Fig. 2.16: Difference in angle of light on different retinas

system light is transmitted through glass columns and refracted through intervening air lenses.

The 30° forward oblique angle permits far greater latitude for viewing underlying areas under difficult anatomical conditions (Fig. 2.15).

One of the major limitations of minimal access surgery is the loss of depth perception. The surgeon works with an artificial two-dimensional video picture available on the monitor. There is a need to develop some mechanism to improve depth perception or stereoscopic vision.

Stereopsis

Stereopsis refers to perception of three-dimensional shape from any source of depth information. Unlike horses, humans have two eyes located side-by-side in the front of their heads. Due to the close side-by-side positioning, each eye takes a view of the same area from a slightly different angle (Fig. 2.16). The two eyes have different views of the visual world and these different views setup disparities that give us information about relative depth of the image that is third dimension of vision. Binocular disparity results when image of an object falls on different areas of the two retinas and binocular vision or Stereopsis is impression of depth resulting from differences in the images on these two retinas. We lose stereoscopic vision in laparoscopy because both eyes see same two-dimensional pictures available on the monitor.

Physiology of Three-dimensional Vision

Human eye is sensitive to the electromagnetic wavelength between 400 to 700 nm. The "electromagnetic energy" in the range of approximately "400 to 700 nm", which the human eye can transduce, is called "light". The eyes transduce light energy in the electromagnetic spectrum into nerve impulses.

In 1838, Charles Wheatstone published the first paper on stereopsis entitled "On some remarkable and hitherto unobserved, phenomena of binocular vision". In this he pointed out that the positional differences in the two eye's images due to their horizontal separation yielded depth information. Prior to this time, the principal problem in the study of binocular vision was "how the world seen as single when we have two different views of it?" People thought that only objects with the same visual directions, falling on corresponding points would be seen as single, all other points would be double. By means of the stereoscope that he invented. Wheatstone demonstrated that the stimulation of non-corresponding points yield singleness of vision, and results in the perception of depth.

Cells in visual cortex are sensitive for binocular vision. Some cells are sensitive for corresponding areas of the left and right retinas and some have sensation for non-corresponding areas of the two retinas. The difference in image on the two retinas of eye is perceived by cortex as a depth (Fig. 2.17). Binocular disparity provides the visual system with information concerning the three-dimensional layout of the environment. Recent physiological studies in the primary visual cortex provide a successful account of the mechanisms by which single neurons are able to signal disparity.

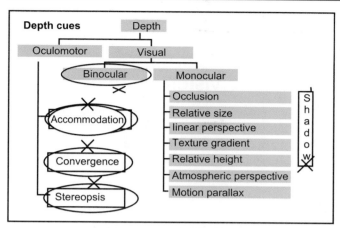

Fig. 2.17: Different depth cues: The depth cues which are crossed are lost in minimal access surgery

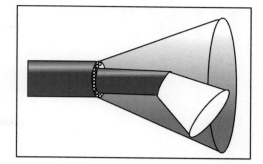

Fig. 2.18: Shadow telescope by Schurr

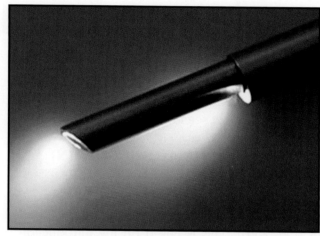

Fig. 2.19: Shadow telescope of Tübingen University

Recent studies of visual perception have begun to reveal the connection between neuronal activity in the brain and conscious visual experience. Transcranial magnetic stimulation of the human occipital lobe disrupts the normal perception of objects in ways suggesting that important aspects of visual perception are based on activity in early visual cortical areas. Recordings made with microelectrodes in animals suggest that the perception of the lightness and depth of visual surfaces develops through computations performed across multiple brain areas.

Even though the picture on the monitor is two-dimensional, the operator can assume some depth due to different cues for monocular vision. This is known as "depth cue".

Among the entire depth cue mentioned above, only few monocular are available on the monitor screen. Oculomotor binocular depth cue like convergence, accommodation and stereopsis is lost in two-dimensional monitor screen.

Even though the picture is two-dimensional, these depth cue helps our brain to interpret a two-dimensional image into virtual three-dimensional feeling. Today, the picture on the screen is 2D but our brain is continuously converting this 2D image in 3D by the help of different monocular depth cues. This conversion of two-dimensional pictures into three-dimensional pictures by brain helps the surgeon to perform a task in laparoscopic surgery.

A telescope with light delivering through a separate illumination cannula was developed by Schurr in 1996 (Fig. 2.18).

With slight modification, the section for minimally invasive surgery, University of Tübingen, and MGB Endoskopische Geräte GmbH Berlin Company have introduced a new shadow telescope in 1999 (Fig. 2.19). Shadow telescope is a rigid 10 mm endoscope with 30° view direction and uses additional illumination fibers ending in an optimized distance behind the front lens. This arrangement of illumination fibers creates a more natural and more plastic appearance, a better balanced contrast and a well-dosed visible shadow. The shadow gives additional secondary space clues and therefore improves orientation and judgment of the three-dimensional properties.

In shadow telescope, angle between the first and second source of illumination is fixed and due to this shadow is also fixed. The second problem with this telescope is that the light which is creating shadow comes from below but we do not usually experience getting illuminated from the floor. All the light in our day to day life is coming from above, and most of the

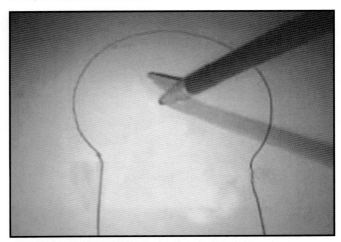

Fig. 2.20: Shadow in laparoscopy

time, the shadow we are seeing lies below the object. But in this telescope the shadow is above the object and so the shadow seems to be unnatural.

INVENTION OF IDEAL SHADOW IN LAPAROSCOPIC SURGERY

The first ideal shadow was introduced in laparoscopic surgery by Dr RK Mishra in the University of Dundee, UK (Fig. 2.20). This is based on the introduction of one additional light source through a separate port for the generation of natural shadow in minimal access surgery.

Due to the limitations of currently present shadows producing techniques, necessity was felt for development of some newer methods of shadow production. Shadow can play a very powerful role in defining form by giving the object a three-dimensional feel and it is easy to generate. Although shadow is an important depth cue, but too much shadow may cause blurred working field for surgeons and shadow in wrong direction may have adverse effect on the performance of surgeon.

To increase the task performance in minimal access surgery we recommend certain general rules about shadows. First, light which will cast shadow ideally should come from above. Second, to enhance the task performance with shadow, the contrast of shadow should be mild (22 to 42%). This useful percentage of contrast can be achieved by equal intensity setting and equal distance of both the light sources from the operating field. Third, too much shadow (more than

60%) should be avoided because very dark shadow can increase the error rate by interfering with the view of plane of dissection.

ENDOSCOPIC VISION TECHNOLOGY

In the past endoscopic procedures were done without the aid of monitors. The operator visualized the interiors of the patient directly through the eyepiece of the scope. This method was associated with many difficulties. He was the only person who could observe the procedure leading to poor coordination with other members of the team. As a result extensive and difficult procedures could not be performed. The magnification was very poor. Surgeons had to face problems with posture leading to discomfort and strain as his eye was always glued to the eyepiece. He had difficulties in orientation due to visualizing with only one eye.

As better methods of communication developed the introduction of television brought about a significant impact. A good magnification of the image was reproduced. All members of the team could visualize the procedure. Surgeons could operate more comfortably. Complex procedures began to be undertaken and were even recorded.

Soulas in France first used television for endoscopic procedures in 1956. He demonstrated the first televised bronchoscopy. A rigid bronchoscope was attached to a black and white camera that weighed about 100 lbs.

In 1959, a laparoscopic procedure was demonstrated using a closed circuit television program using the "Fourestier method". This method was developed by transmitting an intense beam of light along a quartz rod from the proximal to distal ends of the laparoscope.

The first miniature endoscopic black and white television camera was developed in Australia in 1960 (Fig. 2.21). It weighed 350 grams, was 45 mm wide and 120 mm long. Because of its small dimensions it could be attached to the eyepiece.

LAPAROSCOPIC VIDEO MONITOR

Surgical monitors are slightly different from the TV which we watch at home (Fig. 2.22). Monitor lasts long so a surgeon gets high end product with at least 600 lines resolution. The size of the screen varies from 8 to 21 inches. The closure the surgeon is to the monitor, the smaller the monitor should be to get better picture. The basic principle of image reproduction is horizontal

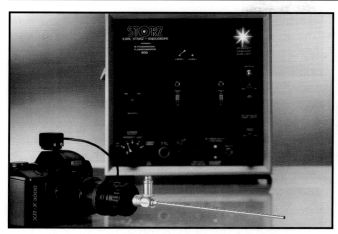

Fig. 2.21: Endoscopic camera

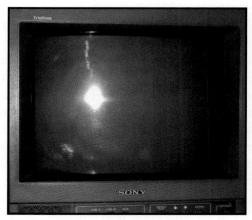

Fig. 2.22: Laparoscopic monitor

beam scanning on the face of the picture tube. This plate is coated internally with a fluorescent substance containing phosphor. This generates electrons when struck by beams from the electron gun. As the beam sweeps horizontally and back, it covers all the picture elements before reaching its original position. This occurs repetitively and rapidly. This method is called 'horizontal linear scanning'. Each picture frame consists of several such lines depending on the type of system used.

The existing television systems in use differ according to the country. The USA uses the NTSC (National Television System Committee) system. In European countries the PAL (Phase Alternation by Line) system is in use. There is also a French system called SECAM (SEquential Color And Memory). The broadcasting standards for each are summarized in Table 2.2.

The final image depends upon the number of lines of resolution, scanning lines, pixels and dot pitch. The number of black and white lines a system can differentiate gives the lines of resolution. These can be horizontal and vertical. Horizontal resolution is the number of vertical lines that can be seen and *vice versa*. Pixels denote the picture elements and they are responsible for picture resolution. The more number of pixels is, the better the resolution. They are represented on the camera chip by an individual photodiode. The restricting factor of information on a scan line is the 'dot pitch' that represents phosphor element size.

The NTSC system has certain drawbacks. Not all the lines of resolution are used. The maximum number of lines visible is reduced by 40. Improving the resolution of the camera will not improve monitor resolution. This is due to a fixed vertical resolution. In addition to these problems, if the phase angle is disturbed even a little, it produces unwanted hues.

The PAL system is superior in certain aspects. It can overcome this problem by producing alternations over the axis of modulation of the color signed by line. This system also deals with problems of flickering. It involves a process called 'inter-lacing' where odd and even lines in a field are scanned alternatively. Sequential color and memory systems are similar to PAL in these aspects except that the signals are transmitted in sequence.

Another important aspect one has to keep in mind is the formation of the color image. This is done by super-imposing the data for color on the existing black and white picture. The black and white signal is monochromatic and combines with the composite color signal. This gives the final color signal. Luminance (brightness) is delivered by the black and white signal. Chrominance (color) is delivered by the color signal. It is called composite as it contains the three primary color

Table 2.2: Different types of monitor systems

System	PAL	SECAM	NTSC
Number of lines	625	625	525
Visible lines (max)	575	575	486
Field frequency cycles (cps) per second	50	50	60
Frames per second	25	25	30

information (red, green and blue). A system that combines luminance and chrominance into one signal is called a "compound system".

Color values can be problematic as they can go out of phase. This is due to their high sensitivity. Applying a reference mark for the signal on the scanning line called as "color burst" can prevent this. The color on a monitor can be calibrated. This can be done manually by using the standard color bars of NTSC or by using other methods like "blue gun". New monitors do not require this, as calibration can be done automatically.

Images cannot be visualized on the monitor unless they are wired. Monitor cables are of three types. The RGB cable has 3 wires, one for each primary color. The Y/C cable has two wires, one for the luminance (Y) and one for the chrominance (C) component. The composite cable consists of one pair of wires. An important factor to realize is that no matter what type of cable is used, whether it has better bandwidth or other advantages, the final resolution depends upon the monitor used.

We face many problems with monitors in regard to minimal access surgery. But before dealing with them, a mention of the frames of reference in vision would be apt. NJ Wade's paper on 'Frames of reference in vision' mentions various frames namely retinocentric, egocentric, geocentric and pattern centric. He applies these to minimal access surgery and finds a dissociation of pattern centric motion (seen on the monitor) and the area of manipulation. Any visual motor task requires a match between the coordinate systems operating in both vision and motor control. Knowledge of these frames can alter our perspective of the way things happen in minimal access surgery with respect to vision.

After routine use we encounter many drawbacks with the monitor. Only a 2D image can be seen on present day monitors. The operative field is represented only by monocular depth cues. Monitor positioning is such that the visual motor axis is disrupted. The monitor distance from the surgeon is also quite far. As a result, the efficiency of the surgeon decreases. Apart from pictorial depth cues the picture can be further disturbed by anti-cues. These may originate from the monitor. Glaring effect due to reflection is one of these important anti-cues.

The endoscopes transmit resolution and contrast to the monitor. The efficacy by which this occurs determines the more delicate aspects of the image. Resolution and contrast can be measured on a especially designed optical bench and expressed as modulation transfer function (MTF). If there is excessive glare in the picture then contrast and resolution decrease. Distortions of the image can occur and if these lines seem to curve outwards they are called "barrel distortion". Field curvature occurs when there is improper focus of the center from other parts. Astigmatism can occur when some lines of different orientation are present in focus and others are not.

When a moving object is shown on a monitor, unless the speed with which it is moving is similar to the refresh rate, then jerky movements will occur. This is called "temporal aliasing". This can be prevented by the use of filters, or by performing slow movements. Fatigue and headache can occur due to disturbance of saccadic eye movements. These are rapid eye movements used to visualize the borders of a field.

When a surgeon has to constantly look in a different direction and operate in another his efficiency to perform declines. The job becomes even more difficult if the monitor is positioned at a further distance, giving rise to spatial disorientation. A surgeon can perform optimally if he can look and operate in the same direction as in open surgery. This can also be called the "gaze-down position".

THREE-DIMENSIONAL VIDEO SYSTEMS

Stereoscopic vision is needed for precise and fast complex manipulations because perception of space and depth are necessary in surgery. The most commonly used systems depend on rapid time sequential imaging with two cameras and one monitor and are based on the physiological phenomenon of retinal persistence. Both channels alternate (open/close) with sufficient speed (50-60 Hz) to avoid detection of flicker by the human eye. The monitors must therefore have double the frequency (100-120 Hz). Sequential switching between the two eyes is necessary to ensure that the correct image (left and right) falls on the corresponding retina otherwise picture will overlap. This is achieved by wearing special optical glasses that act as alternating shutters to each eye. The current problem with these optical shutters, especially the active battery operated liquid crystal display type shutter is loss of brightness and color degradation. There is no clinically proved evidence that current three-dimensional systems improve performance of laparoscopic surgery.

The current 3D technology is harmful to the surgeon on prolonged use as it gives incorrect depth perception and results in headache and eyestrain. Another way in which 3D images can be obtained is a mechanism by which the surgeon wears a polarized glass. The shutter mechanism is present in the monitor. The final image, however, occurs by the fusion of the two images in the brain. The current 3D systems can only be operated from a very close distance and if placed further will not produce the desired 3D effect.

With the increasing demands for technological development many new techniques are currently under trial. These seem to eliminate some of the problems encountered, but only time and repeated use will tell.

Head mounted display (HMD) is an interesting technique that aims at normalizing the visual- motor axis. It consists of a monitor and the necessary connections mounted to the surgeon's head with the power supply pack attached to the back of the surgeon's shirt. It is not very heavy and also allows the surgeon to view peripherally. The optical characteristics are:
1. Lines of resolution- 420 × 320 lines
2. Contrast ratio- 100: 1
3. Horizontal field of vision- 22°
4. Diagonal field- 27.5°
5. Vertical field- 19°.

The surgeon using the display will have to make adjustments to the inter-pupillary distance, focus and the distance from his eyes each time. Studies have shown HMD to have certain advantages. It is light weight, comfortable to position, reduces mental stress, is cheaper than monitor systems, and decreases eye strain. It allows the surgeon to visualize the operative field directly (the abdomen and ports). The problems, however, are that the picture is granular, definition is not very good and nausea can occur.

As mentioned before, the gaze down position is said to improve the performance of the surgeon as it brings the alignment between his hands and eyes to normal. This principle has been used in a project called "view-

site". This mechanism is used to project the operative field image onto a sterile screen placed on the patient's abdomen close to the original area of surgery. However, it cannot be used for extensive procedures as the image field is small, resolution is not up to the mark and separation and identification of tissue planes becomes difficult if bleeding were to occur.

Image display systems are now available which project the image on to a sterile screen overlying the chest of the patient. This aids both cerebral processing of the image and endoscopic manipulations and improves both quality and efficiency of performance (Fig. 2.23). The limitation of the current "gaze down" image display systems are diminished resolution and encroachment of the operative field by the sterile screen. An experimental system (suspended image system) being developed at the University of Dundee and the Central Research Laboratory (EMI) projects the image in air on top of the patient, which means there is no screen to obstruct the surgeon's movement. This is called the suspended image system (SIS). It consists of two components: a high precision retro-reflector and a beam splitter. With the help of these, the system can produce images with good resolution and can suspend them on top of the patient in close vicinity to the operative site. The advantages of this method are that there is no distortion, object can be placed anywhere, focal length is not specific and the image is similar to the original in size. This system is also said to improve the sense of depth, as there are

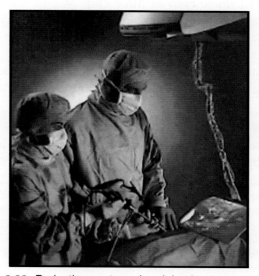

Fig. 2.23: Projection systems in minimal access surgery

no anti-cues. Also, the visual motor axis is correctly aligned for optimal performance.

VISTRAL is a system currently under trial. The advantage of this system is that it does not allow flatness cues to occur in 2D pictures. This improves the sense of depth and it does not require binocular depth cues. It is also said to reduce fatigue and eye strain. However, this system does not bring about any changes to resolution, brightness and color.

Another remarkable advancement in technology is the High Definition Television (HDTV). It uses component signals, the resolution of the picture is much better, and there are no distortions. They use about 1,100 lines of resolution.

Some systems are currently under evaluation and their requirements are given in Table 2.3.

These systems, however, require large amounts of space and can cause problems during transmission. Due to the increased definition, small unwanted movements can be magnified and visual stress can be increased. The alternatives to HDTV are the PALPLUS which is an advanced modification of PAL and D2-MAC, HD-MAC which are used for satellite transmissions.

LAPAROSCOPIC CAMERA

First medical camera was introduced by Circon Corporation in 1972. Laparoscopic camera is one of the very important instruments and should be of good quality (Fig. 2.24). Laparoscopic camera available is either of single chip or three chip. We all know that there are three primary colors (Red, Blue and Green). All the colors are mixture of these three primary colors in different proportion.

Within the head of camera is a CCD that "sees" an image taken by telescope. All modern miniature

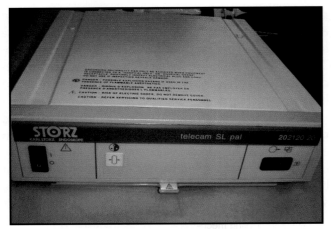

Fig. 2.24: Laparoscopic camera

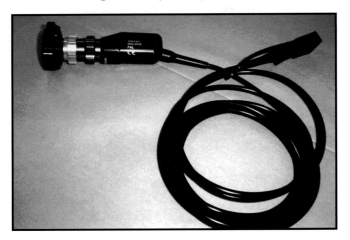

Fig. 2.25: Head of camera (CCD)

cameras used in minimal access surgery are based on the charged couple device (chip). The camera system has two components: the head of the camera (Fig. 2.25), which is attached to the ocular of the telescope, and the controller, which is usually located on the trolley along with the monitor. The camera head consists of an objective zoom lens that focuses the image of the object on the chip (Figs 2.26A and B). The CCD then converts optical image into an electrical signal that is sent through the camera cable to CCU (camera control unit). The chip has light sensitive photoreceptors that generate pixels by transforming the incoming photons into electronic charges. The electronic charges are then transferred from the pixels into a storage element on the chip. A subsequent scanning at defined time intervals results in a black and white image with grey tones.

Table 2.3: Different types of TV system

System	Japan (NHK/Sony)	Europe (EUREKA 95)	USA
Number of lines	1125	1250	1050
Visible lines (92%)	1035	1150	966
Pixels per line	1831	2035	1709
Total number of pixels	1895085	2340250	1650894
Field frequency (cps)	60	50	59, 94
Luminance	20	20	20
Chrominance	7	7	7

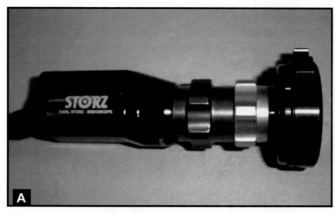

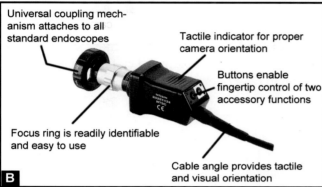

Figs 2.26A and B: CCD camera

The number of pixels determines the resolution. The average chip contains 250000-380000 pixels. Cameras are classified according to the number of chips. These differ, among other things, in the way they relay color information to the monitor. Color separation is used to create a colored video image from the original black and white. In single chip cameras, color separation is achieved by adding a stripe filter that covers the whole chip. Each stripe accepts one of the complementary colors (magenta, green, cyan, or yellow) and each pixel is assigned to one stripe.

In single chip camera, these 3 primary colors are sensed by single chip. In three chip camera there are 3 CCD chips for separate capture and processing of 3 primary colors. In three chip cameras color separation is achieved with a prism system that overlies the chips. Each chip receives only one of the three primary colors (red, green, or blue). This system gives a higher resolution and better image quality because the pixel number is three times greater.

The video information, color and light are scanned at a rate of 525 lines per frame and 30 frames per second. Picture resolution determines the clarity and detail of the video image. Higher the resolution the better will be quality of image. The resolution of picture is ascertained by the number of distinct vertical line that can be seen in the picture. The higher the resolution numbers, the sharper and cleaner image will form. The CCU of camera is connected with monitor and monitor converts the electrical image back to the original optical image.

These 3 chip camera has unprecedented color reproduction and highest degree of fidelity. Three chip cameras have high horizontal image resolution of more than 750 lines.

Chip on Stick Technology

Currently chip on stick technology has been introduced in which CCD will be at the tip inside the abdominal cavity. It is proved that the resolution of picture will be more than 250 k pixels (Fig. 2.27).

Focusing of Laparoscopic Camera

Laparoscopic camera need to be focused before inserting inside the abdominal cavity. At the time of focusing it should be placed at a distance of approximately 5 cm away from the target. This distance is optimum for focusing because at the time of laparoscopic surgery, most of the time we keep the telescope at this distance.

White Balancing of Camera

White balancing should be performed before inserting camera inside the abdominal cavity. White balancing is necessary every time before start of surgery because every time there is some added impurities of color due to following variables:
• Difference in voltage
• Different cleaning material used to clean the tip of telescope which can stain the tip

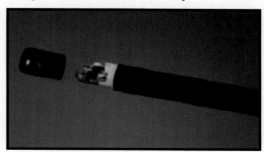

Fig. 2.27: Chip on stick technology

Section One

- Scratches, wear and tear of the telescopes eye-piece, object piece and CCD of camera.

White balancing is done by keeping any white object in front of telescope attached with camera that senses white object as reference. It adjusts its primary color (red, blue and green) to make a pure natural white color.

LAPROFLATTOR

The electronic CO_2 Laproflattor is a general purpose insufflation unit for use in laparoscopic examinations and operations (Fig. 2.28). Controlled pressure insufflation of the peritoneal cavity is used to achieve the necessary work space for laparoscopic surgery by distending the anterolateral abdominal wall and depressing the hollow organs and soft tissues. Carbon dioxide is the preferred gas because it does not support combustion. It is very soluble which reduces the risk of gas embolism, and is cheap. Automatic insufflators allow the surgeon to preset the insufflating pressure, and the device supplies gas until the required intra-abdominal pressure is reached. The insufflator activates and delivers gas automatically when the intra-abdominal pressure falls because of gas escape or leakage from the ports. The required values for pressure and flow can be set exactly using jog keys and digital displays. Insufflation pressure can be continuously varied from 0 to 30 mm Hg; total gas flow volumes can be set to any value in the range 0-9.9 liters/mm.

Patient safety is ensured by optical and acoustic alarms as well as several mutually independent safety circuits. The detail function and quadro-manometric indicators of insufflator is important to understand safety point of view. The important indicators of insufflators are preset pressure, actual pressure, flow rate and total gas used.

Suction Irrigation Machine or Pelvis Cleaner

It is used for flushing the abdominal cavity and cleaning during endoscopic operative intrusions (Fig. 2.29). It has been designed for use with the 26173 AR suction /instillation tube. Its electrically driven pressure/suction pump is protected against entry of bodily secretions. The suction irrigation machine is used frequently at the time of laparoscopy to make the field of vision clear. Most of the surgeons use normal saline or Ringer Lactate for irrigation purposes. Sometime heparinized saline is used to dissolve blood clot to facilitate proper suction in case of excessive intra-abdominal bleeding.

Disposable or Reusable Instrument

Several factors should be considered at the time of choosing laparoscopic instrument, including cost, availability and reliability. Reusable instruments are expensive initially but in long run they are cost effective. The cost of disposable instruments is less compared to reusable but patient cost is increased. In developing countries, disposable instruments are very rarely used because labor cost is low compare to the cost of disposable instrument. In Europe and USA, surgeons often choose to use disposable instrument in order to save high labor cost. The main advantage of disposable instrument is high performance due to its sharpness

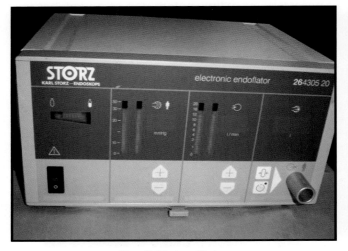

Fig. 2.28: Insufflator

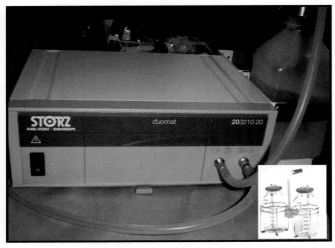

Fig. 2.29: Laparoscopic suction irrigation machine

and reduced chance of disease transmission due to certified high-end factory sterilization. However, once discarded, environment concerns are raised about disposal and biodegradability of disposable instruments. Ideally disposable instrument should not be used repeatedly because handling, sorting, storing and sterilization make these instrument questionable. The disposable instruments are not sterilized properly by dipping in glutaraldehyde because they are not dismountable. Insulation of disposable instrument also can be torn easily which can lead to electrosurgical injuries.

VERESS NEEDLE

Veress needle was invented by a chest physician for aspiration of pleural effusion keeping in mind that its spring mechanism and blunt tip will prevent the injury of lung tissue (Fig. 2.30). Veress needle consists of an outer cannula with a beveled needle point for cutting through tissues. Inside the cannula is an inner stylet, which is loaded with a spring that "springs forward" in response to the sudden decrease in pressure encountered upon crossing the abdominal wall and entering the peritoneal cavity. The lateral hole on this stylet enables CO_2 gas to be delivered intra-abdominally.

Veress needle is used for creating initial pneumoperitoneum so that the trocar can enter safely and the distance of abdominal wall from the abdominal viscera should increase. Veress needle technique is the most widely practiced way of access. Before using Veress needle every time it should be checked for its potency and spring action. Veress needle is available in three length 80 mm, 100 mm, 120 mm. In obese

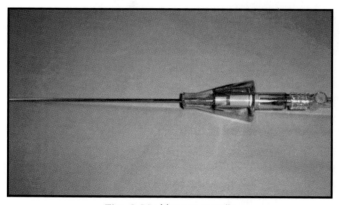

Fig. 2.30: Veress needle

patient 120 mm and in very thin patient with scaphoid abdomen 80 mm veress needle should be used. Veress needle should be held like a dart at the time of insertion. The proper technique of veress needle insertion, different safety measures and indicators are discussed later in access technique.

TROCAR AND CANNULA

The word "trocar" is usually used to refer to the entire assembly but actual trocar is a stylet which is introduced through the cannula. The trocars are available with different type of tips. The cutting tips of these trocars are either in the shape of a three edged pyramid or a flat two edged blade.

Conical tipped trocars are supposed to be less traumatic to the tissue. The tip can be penetrated through the parietal wall without cutting and decreased risk of herniation or hemorrhage is reported.

Cannulas are in general made from plastic or metal. Plastic devices whether they are transparent or opaque, need to be designed in such a way as to minimize the reflection of light from the telescope. Reusable and disposable trocars are constructed by a combination of metal and plastic. The tip of disposable trocar has a two edged blade. These are very effective at penetrating the abdominal wall by cutting the tissue as they pass through. Most of the disposable plastic trocar have a spring loaded mechanism that withdraws the sharp tip immediately after it passes through the abdominal wall to reduce the incidence of injury of viscera. Trocar and cannula are of different sizes and diameter depending upon the instrument for which it is used. The diameter of cannula ranges from 3 to 30 mm; the most common size is 5 mm and 10 mm. The metal trocar has different type of tips, i.e. pyramidal tip, Eccentric tip, conical tip or blunt tip depending on the surgeon's experience (Fig. 2.31).

All the cannula have valve mechanism at the top (Figs 2.33 and 2.34). Valves of cannula provide internal air seals, which allow instruments to move in and out within cannula without the loss of pneumoperitoneum. These valves can be oblique, transverse, or in piston configuration.

These valves can be manually or automatically retractable during instrument passage. Trumpet type valves are also present which provide excellent seals,

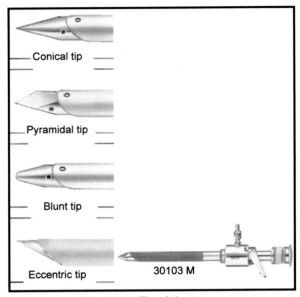

Fig. 2.31: Tip of the trocar

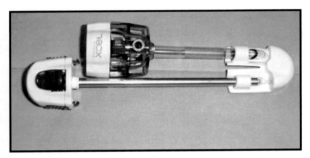

Fig. 2.32: Disposable trocar and cannula

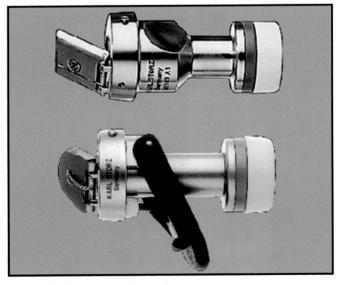

Fig. 2.33: Different valve mechanism of cannula

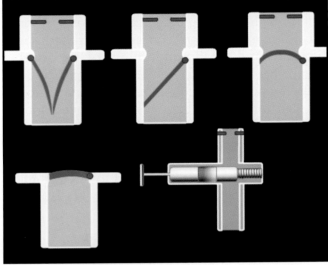

Fig. 2.34: Different valve mechanism of cannula (internal view)

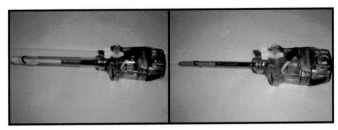

Fig. 2.35: Disposable trocar and cannula

but they are not as practical as some of the other systems. They require both hands during instrument insertion, which may explain why they are less often used in advanced laparoscopic cases. The flexible valves, limits the leakage of carbon dioxide during work whatever the diameter of the instrument used.

It should be remembered that sharp trocars although looking dangerous are actually better than blunt one because they need less force to introduce inside the abdominal cavity and chances of inadvertent forceful entry of full length of trocar is less. There is always a difference in the marked exterior diameter of the cannula and the interior usable diameter. The end of the cannula is either straight or oblique. An oblique tip is felt to facilitate the easy passage of the trocar through the abdominal wall.

Trocar and cannula should be held in proper way in hand so that head of the trocar should rest on the thenar eminence, the middle finger should rest over the gas inlet and index finger is pointed towards the sharp end of the trocar.

Laparoscopic Hand Instruments

Laparoscopic hand instruments vary in diameter from 1.8 to 12 mm but majority of instruments are designed to pass through 5 to 10 mm of cannula. The hand instrument used in laparoscopic surgery are of different length (varies company to company and length of laparoscopic instrument varies from 18 to 45 cm) but they are ergonomically convenient to work if they have same length of approximately 36 cm in adult and 28 cm in pediatric practice. Shorter instruments 18 to 25 cm are adapted for cervical and pediatric surgery. Certain procedures for adult can also be performed with shorter instruments where the space is constricted. 45 cm instruments are used in obese or very tall patients. For better ergonomics half of the instruments should be inside the abdomen and half outside. If half of the instrument is in and half out, it behaves like class 1 lever and it stabilizes the port nicely so the surgery will be convenient.

Most of the laparoscopic procedures require a mixture of sharp and blunt dissection techniques, often using the same instrument in a number of different ways. Many laparoscopic instruments are available in both reusable and disposable version (Figs 2.32 and 2.35). Most reusable instruments are partially dismountable so that it can be cleaned and washed properly. Some manufacturer have produced modular system where part of the instrument can be changed to suit the surgeons favorite attachment like handle or working tip.

Most laparoscopic instruments like graspers (Figs 2.37 and 2.38) and scissors have basic opening and closing function. Many instrument manufacturers

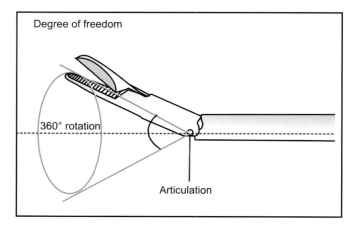

Fig. 2.36: Articulation of hand instrument

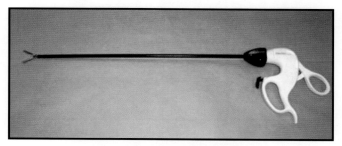

Fig. 2.37: Disposable grasper

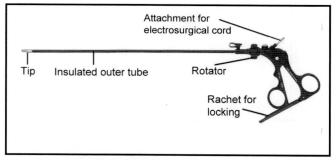

Fig. 2.38: Reusable graspers

during past few years are able to rotate at 360° angle which increases the degree of freedom of these instruments (Fig. 2.36).

Certain types of instrument offer angulations at their tip in addition to usual 4° of freedom. These instruments are used to avoid obstacles and for the lateral grasping when the instrument is placed outside of the visual field. This feature is available for both reusable as well as disposable instrument. The complex mechanism of such instrument makes their sterilization very difficult.

A variety of instruments, especially retractors have been developed with multiple articulations along the shaft. When these are fixed with the tightened cable the instrument assumes a rigid shape which could not have been introduced through the cannula.

Most of the hand instrument has three detachable parts:
- Handle
- Insulated outer tube
- Insert which makes the tip of the instrument.

Different Handles of Hand Instrument

Certain instruments handle are designed to allow locking of the jaw (Fig. 2.39). This can be very useful when the tissue needs to be grasped firmly for long period of time preventing the surgeons hand from

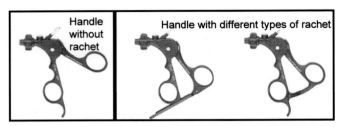

Fig. 2.39: Different type of handle of hand instruments

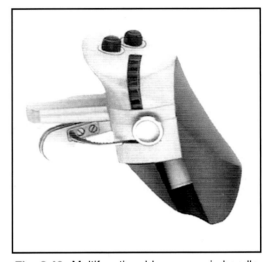

Fig. 2.40: Multifunctional laparoscopic handle

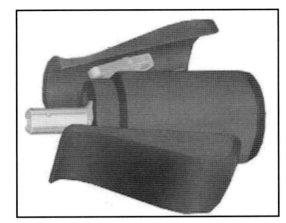

Fig. 2.41: Cuschieri ball handle

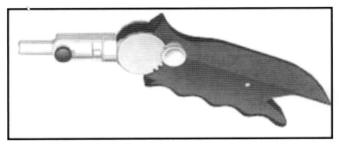

Fig. 2.42: Cuschieri pencil handle

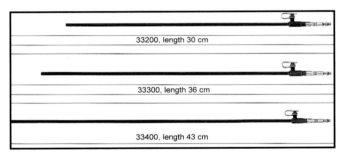

Fig. 2.43: Outer sheath of hand instrument

getting fatigue. The locking mechanism is usually incorporated into the handle so that surgeon can easily lock or release the jaws. These systems usually have a ratchet so that the jaws can be closed in different position and to different pressure. Most of the laparoscopic instruments handle has attachments for unipolar electrosurgical lead and many have rotator mechanism to rotate the tip of the instrument.

Some multifunctional laparoscopic handle has attachment for suction and irrigation and some time hand switch for cutting and coagulation switch of electrosurgery.

Cuschieri Ball Handle, invented by Prof. Sir Alfred Cuschieri, lies comfortably in surgeon's palm (Fig. 2.41). This design reduces the fatigue of surgeon and eases rotation of the instrument by allowing rotation within the palm rather than using wrist rotation. Squeezing the front of the handle between the thumb and the first fingers increases the jaw closing force; squeezing the rear of the handle between the thenar eminence of the thumb and last fingers opens the jaws.

Cuschieri pencil handle also has great ergonomic value especially when used with needle holder (Fig. 2.42). This handle allows the angle between the handle and the instrument to be altered to suit the surgeon's wrist angle. The conveniently placed lever of this pencil handle when pressed can change the angle. Just like ball handle, pressure at the front increases the jaw closing force while pressure at the rear opens the jaw (Fig. 2.40).

Outer Sheath of Hand Instrument

The insulation covering of outer sheath of hand instrument should be of good quality in hand instrument to prevent accidental electric burn to bowel or other viscera (Fig. 2.43).

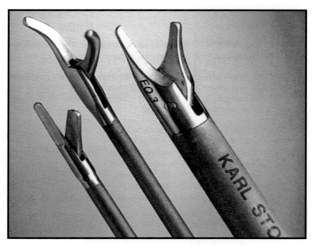

Fig. 2.44: Insert of hand instrument

Insulation covering may be of silicon or plastic. At the time of cleaning the hand instrument, utmost care should be taken so that insulation should not be scratched with any sharp contact. A pin hole breach in insulation is not easily seen by naked eye but may be dangerous at the time of electrosurgery.

Insert of Hand Instrument

Insert of hand instrument varies only at tip (Fig. 2.44). It may be grasper, scissors, or forceps. This grasper may have single action jaw or double action jaw. Single action jaw opens less than double action jaw but close with greater force. Thus, most of the needle holders are single action jaw. The necessary wider opening in double action jaw is present in grasper and dissecting forceps. Single action graspers and dissectors are used where more force is required (Fig. 2.45).

Single Action Jaw Graspers

These graspers are good when you don't have control over depth and surgeon wants to work in single plane in controlled manner particularly during adhesiolysis.

Double Action Jaw Graspers

These are shown in Figures 2.46 and 2.47.

INSTRUMENTS FOR SHARP DISSECTION

1. Scissors
2. Electrosurgery hook
3. HF electrosurgery spatula (Berci)

4. HF electrosurgery knife
5. Knife.

Scissors

Jean-Claude Margueron of Emar in 14th century BC invented scissors. Scissors are one of the oldest surgical instruments used by surgeons. Scissors are used to perform many tasks in open surgical procedure but its use in minimal access surgery is restricted. In minimal access surgery scissors require greater skill because in inexperienced hand it may cause unnecessary bleeding and damage to important structures.

Mechanism of cutting:

The scissors has three parts (Fig. 2.48):
1. Blade
2. Fulcrum
3. Handle.

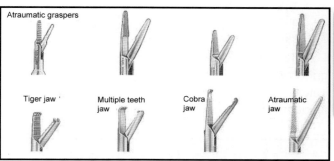

Fig. 2.45: Different jaw of graspers

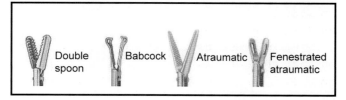

Fig. 2.46: Double action jaw graspers

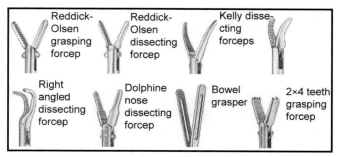

Fig. 2.47: Serrated jaw graspers

Section One

The cutting force of the scissors works on the law of lever. The force applied on the blade can be calculated by length of the handle and force applied on the grip of handle. A pair of scissors is an example of first class levers connected together at the joint known as fulcrum.

There are three type of lever:

Scissors works on the principle of class 1 lever (Fig. 2.49). In class 1 lever, the Pivot (fulcrum) is between the effort and the load. The more the length of the handle or the fulcrum of the scissors, the less force of cutting will be required. The laparoscopic scissors do not apply the exact law of lever because of the cylinder action of the long shaft, but the design of handle helps in the amplification of force by lever action.

Scissors function by the combination of:
1. Gripping
2. Squeezing
3. Tearing.

When the blades of scissors close, its sharp edges grind against each other and any tissue which comes between the blades of scissors will get cut. The scissors-tissue interaction can be described in five stages:

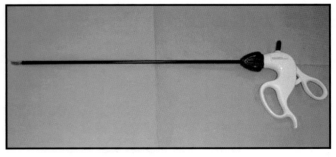

Fig. 2.48: Disposable scissors

A. Engagement

In the process of engagement, the two blades of the scissors engage a piece of tissue to cut. The amount of tissue engaged should not be more than the space between the jaw of blades otherwise the chance of slipping of tissue is more. After engagement, the force applied on the handle of the scissors initiate cutting.

B. Elastic Deformation

This stage starts just after the engagement of tissue between the blades of the scissors. In this process, the tissues between the two blades of scissor start deforming. This stage is called elastic deformation, because if the force on the handle of scissors is removed then the tissue deformity will return to its normal state.

C. Plastic Deformation

Further force on the handle of scissors will cause the tissue between the blades to go into a plastic deformed state, which is irreversible. After undergoing this state of tissue deformation, even if further process of cutting is stopped the impression on the tissue remains.

D. Fracture

Further increased force on the fulcrum of scissors will result in the fracture of intercellular plane of the tissue. This stage of cutting is peculiar to scissors because unlike the scalpel, the site of tissue fracture is intercellular.

E. Separation

After the fracture the tissue separates along line of the blade of scissors, and then this whole process of cutting will continue on the engaged tissue.

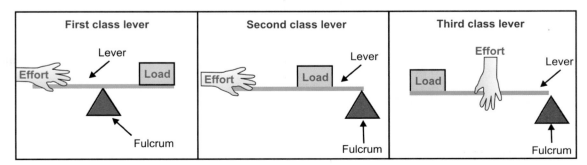

Fig. 2.49: Types of lever

Histology of the Tissue After Cutting

Histological examination of the tissue after cutting with scissors shows that there is separation of tissue through intracellular plane. Microscopic examination shows serrated cut margin along the line of tissue separation.

TYPES OF LAPAROSCOPIC SCISSORS

The blade of this scissor is straight and it is widely used as an instrument for mechanical dissection in laparoscopic surgery. Straight scissor can give controlled depth of cutting because it has only one moving jaw (Fig. 2.50). At the time of cutting the fixed jaw should be down and moving jaw should be up.

The blade of this scissors is slightly curved and this is the most widely used scissor in laparoscopic surgery (Fig. 2.51). These scissors are mounted on a curved handle which is either fixed or retractable. The type with a fixed curvature proximal to the scissor blades require introduction through flexible valveless ports. The surgeon prefers this scissor because the curvature of the blade of the scissors abolishes the angle of laparoscopic instruments manipulation and better view through telescope is achieved.

The main advantage of this scissors is that the serrated edges prevent the tissue to slip out of the blades. It is a useful instrument in cutting a slippery tissue or ligature. Serrated scissors may be straight or curved (Fig. 2.52).

The sharp edge of both blades is in the shape of a flattened C. The blades can be partially closed, trapping tissue in the hollow of the blades without dividing it and allowing it to be slightly retracted. This allows the surgeon to double check before he closes the blades completely.

The main advantage of this scissors is that, it encircles the structure before cutting: Tissue is held between its jaws and there is no chance of slipping. The hook scissor is especially useful for cutting secured duct or artery in laparoscopic surgery. The cutting of nerve bundle in neurectomy becomes very easy with the help of this scissor. Hook scissors is also helpful in partial cutting of cystic duct for intraoperative cholangiography. All the other scissors cut from proximal to distal whereas the hook scissors cut distal to proximal (Fig. 2.53).

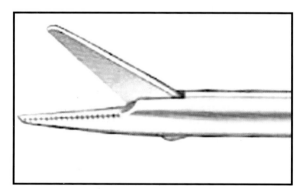

Fig. 2.50: Straight scissors

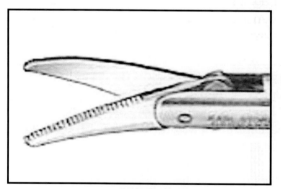

Fig. 2.52: Serrated scissors

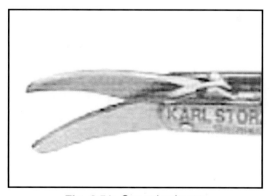

Fig. 2.51: Curved scissors

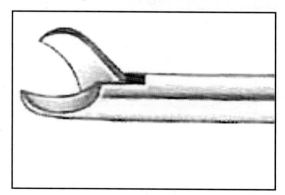

Fig. 2.53: Hook scissors

Section One

These very fine scissors, are either straight or angled, and are used to partially transect the cystic duct. The main advantage of this scissor is to cut the ducts partially for facilitating cannulation. It may be used for cutting the cystic duct for performing intraoperative cholangiogram. Exploration of small ducts like common bile duct is very helpful with micro scissors due to its fine small blades. Fine micro scissors are also available in its curved form (Fig. 2.54).

The use of scissors endoscopically requires little modification of open techniques. The basic instrument is a miniaturized, long handled version of conventional scissors and can be single or double action. There are some special types of scissors used in endoscopic surgery.

INSULATED SCISSORS

These allow the use of electrocautery through the scissors. However, when using non-disposable instruments, electrocoagulation using the open blades leads to blunting of the edges. Electrocoagulation using the scissors is thus limited, and when carried out is applied only with the blades closed. Scissor dissection is usually carried out with a grasper in the other hand. If this instrument is insulated then any vessels encountered can be easily coagulated by the grasper. A further disadvantage associated with electro-coagulation with the scissors results from the long non-insulated segment required to accommodate the blades and hinge mechanism. For safe practice this requires to be kept in view, and this limits the magnification available to the surgeon.

Scissors have following advantages:

1. Inexpensive
2. Safe in safe hand

3. Operator determined precise action
4. Closed blades can work for blunt dissection and electrocautery
5. Piercing tissue with closed blades and then opening helps in obtaining a good plane of dissection.

Scissors have following disadvantages:

1. Non-hemostatic
2. Accidental chances of cutting small ducts and vessels
3. If overlooked, due to its pointed end, there is chance of injury to viscera
4. If used for electric coagulation, its blades get blunt easily.

Endoknife (Scalpel)

The knife is not used frequently in endoscopic surgery due to the problems associated with the safety of a blade, which cannot be closed or deactivated. However, it does have some important uses.

In our practice, a disposable blade (Beaver) is mounted on a metal rod, which has a socket at the distal end into which it can be screwed (Fig. 2.55).

The most common use of the knife is for opening the hepatic duct or common bile duct during exploration for stones. A small, clean cut, linear stab wound is created in the anterior wall. Great care is required during incision and removal of the knife. However, a sharp curved scissor is better and safer than the endoknife for the choledochotomy.

BIOPSY FORCEPS

Punch, cutting and dissecting biopsy forceps are used to take biopsies at the time of laparoscopic surgery

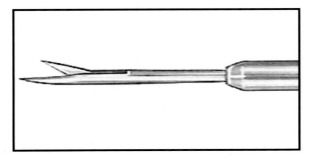

Fig. 2.54: Micro-tip scissors

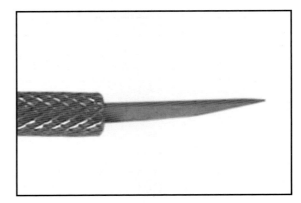

Fig. 2.55: Endoknife

(Fig. 2.56). The toothed punch biopsy forceps has special teeth which prevent accidental drop of tissue inside the abdominal cavity.

Coagulating and Dissecting Electrodes

Spatula and hook is the main electrode used for monopolar cutting and coagulation (Fig. 2.57). Spatula is either "W" shaped or blunt. Hooks are also of various shapes, e.g. "L" shaped, "J" shaped or "U" shaped (Fig. 2.58).

Hooks are simple instrument whose distal tip can vary slightly. They must be insulated along the entire length because they are used with the monopolar current. The hook with ceramic cone protecting the distal end is available which protects efficiently against current diffusion (Fig. 2.59).

Some ball shaped, Barrel shaped or straight coagulation electrodes are also available to achieve proper hemostasis. These blunt electrodes are particularly useful when there is generalized oozing of blood and surgeon cannot see specific bleeder point, e.g. bleeding from the gallbladder bed at the time of laparoscopic cholecystectomy. These blunt electrosurgical instruments are also used for fulguration at the time of ablation of endometriosis.

BIPOLAR FORCEPS

Bipolar forceps are one of the very important electrosurgical instruments in minimal access surgery (Fig. 2.60). It is safer than monopolar instruments because electron travels only through the tissue held between the jaw and patients body is not a part of circuit. Both the jaw of bipolar is insulated and the patients return plate is not necessary to be attached (Fig. 2.61). The detailed principle of electrosurgery is discussed later in laparoscopic dissection techniques.

ASPIRATION NEEDLE

These long needles are used in laparoscopy to aspirate fluid from distended ovarian cysts, gallbladder, or any localized pocket of pus in liver (Fig. 2.62). It may be

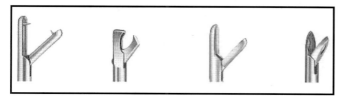
Fig. 2.56: Biopsy forceps

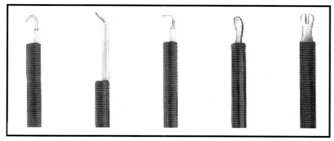
Fig. 2.57: Spatula

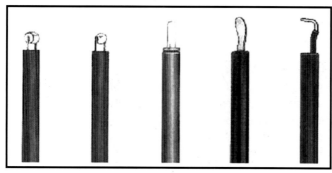
Fig. 2.58: Various types of hooks

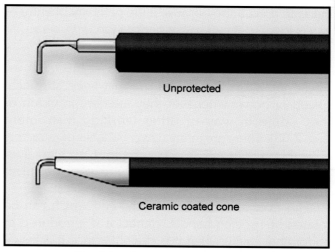
Unprotected

Ceramic coated cone

Fig. 2.59: Ceramic coating of hook

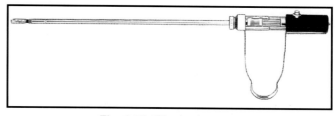
Fig. 2.60: Bipolar forceps

Section One

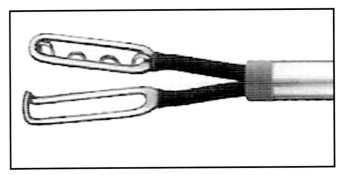

Fig. 2.61: Jaw of bipolar forceps

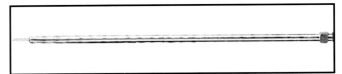

Fig. 2.62: Aspiration needle

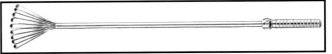

Fig. 2.63: Fan retractor

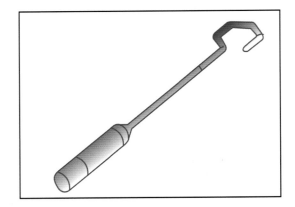

Fig. 2.64: Cuschieri liver retractor

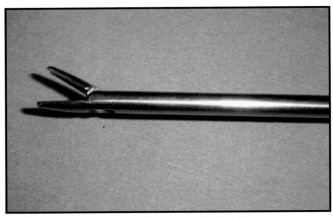

Fig. 2.65: Jaw of needle holder

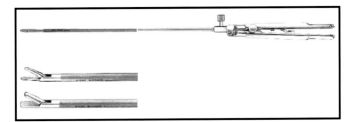

Fig. 2.66: Laparoscopic straight handle needle holder

used for drilling of polycystic ovary. Aspiration needle should be inserted inside the abdominal cavity with extreme precaution because if the pathway of entry or exit is ignored it can cause perforation of viscera.

Fan Retractor

These retractors are used to retract liver, stomach, spleen or bowel whenever they interfere in vision or they come in way of other working instrument (Fig. 2.63). There are many newer varieties of retractors available which are less traumatic. Cuschieri liver retractor is one of them which are very useful in fundoplication (Fig. 2.64).

This liver retractor has a distal end which can be rotated by moving handle. Retractor is introduced in abdominal cavity when it is straight. Once it is inside the abdomen, the distal end can take various shapes just like serpent. This retractor can also be used for simple, atraumatic manipulation of bowel.

Needle Holders

Needle holders should grasp the needle rock solid hard to prevent rotation (Figs 2.65 and 2.66). Hence, until now, reusable needle holders are not available. Needle

holders have different type of jaws (Fig. 2.67). Flat grasping surface makes it possible to turn needle in all direction as in conventional surgery. Dome shaped indentation at the tip automatically orients the needle in a particular direction although this function is not always useful, it can sometime make it easier to grasp the needle. Laparoscopic knotting and suturing should be learnt on a good quality endotrainer. The art and science of laparoscopic suturing and knotting is explained later in tissue approximation technique. Surgeons should slowly learn these techniques.

Section One

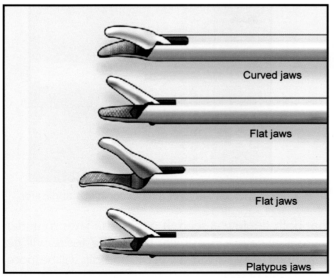

Fig. 2.67: Different types of jaw of needle holder

Curved jaws

Flat jaws

Flat jaws

Platypus jaws

They will develop their confidence once capable of suturing inside abdominal cavity and as a result conversion rate will also decrease.

Many automatic laparoscopic suturing devices are invented for intracorporeal suturing but none of them are substitutes of manual laparoscopic suturing because these devices can work only under appropriate tissue plane suitable for their application (Figs 2.68 to 2.70).

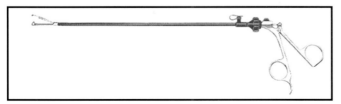

Fig. 2.68: Laparoscopic autosuturing instrument

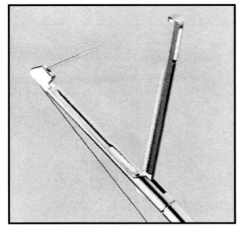

Fig. 2.69: Autosuturing device

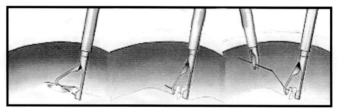

Fig. 2.70: Autosuturing device (Mechanism)

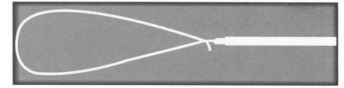

Fig. 2.71: Pretied loop

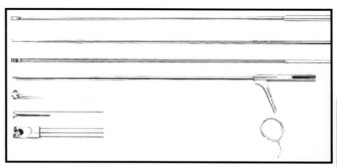

Fig. 2.72: Laparoscopic knot pusher

Knot Pusher

Although pre-tied loops are available in the market but surgeon should learn how to tie these extracorporeal knot.

Pre-tied loop can be used for any free structure like appendix but for continuous structure like cystic duct surgeon has to perform extracorporeal knotting intra-operatively (Fig. 2.71). For extracorporeal knotting, knot pushers are used. These knot pushers are of either closed jaw or of open jaw type (Fig. 2.72).

Laparoscopic Clip Applicator

Disposable preloaded clip applicators are available in 5 mm and 10 mm diameter (Figs 2.73 and 2.74). These are expensive, but nice to use because the loading time of clip can be minimized. Disposable clip applier comes with 20 preloaded clips (Fig. 2.75). In case of emergency, when bleeding has to be stopped immediately one after another, clip can be applied rapidly with the help of these clip applicators.

Section One

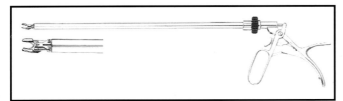

Fig. 2.73: Laparoscopic clip applicator

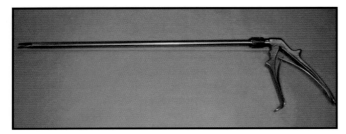

Fig. 2.74: Laparoscopic reusable clip applicator

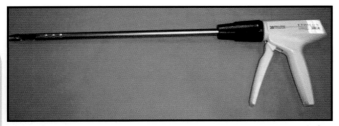

Fig. 2.75: Laparoscopic disposable clip applicator

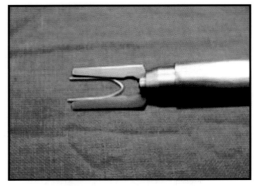

Fig. 2.76: Clip loaded over laparoscopic clip applicator

Titanium is most widely used metal in minimal access surgery for tissue approximation. It rarely reacts with human body and this is why it is popular. It is easy to apply and can be left inside abdominal cavity. After few weeks it is covered by fibrous tissue. Titanium clip is used by 99 percent of surgeons for clipping cystic duct and cystic artery at the time of laparoscopic cholecystectomy. Recently, silicon clips has been launched. Absorbable clips (Absolok, Ethicon) are preferred to clip cystic ducts nowadays. It adds to safety by working at the tip and it does not have chance to form cystic duct clip stone. The absorbable soft clips can also be used in running stitches at the beginning and at the termination of knotting.

Medium large size clip is of 9 mm and used most frequently for cystic duct and cystic artery (Fig. 2.76). The medium size clip is 7 mm in length and can be used to clip cystic artery or thin cystic duct. The large size clip is 11 mm in length and it is used to control thick wide cystic ducts or large mesenteric vessels. The jaw of clip applicator should be at right angle to the structure and before clipping surgeon should take care

that both the jaw is seen. If one of the jaws is hidden there is always a possibility that some tissue will get entrapped between the jaw of clip and clip will be loose. At the time of securing any duct or artery with titanium clip, three clips are generally applied. Two clips are left towards the structure which is secured and one clip is towards the tissue which surgeon wants to remove to prevent spillage of fluid (Fig. 2.77). The distance between first and second clip should be 3 mm and distance between second and third clip should be 6 mm so that after cutting in between second and third clip there will be 3 mm stump both the side. The clip should not be applied very near to each other, because clips are held in position by dumbbell formation and if they are very near to each other, they will nullify the dumbbell formation of each other and both the clip will be loose.

Cystic Duct Clip Stone

Recently, many cases have been reported of cystic duct clip stone and this is the reason why in many institutions

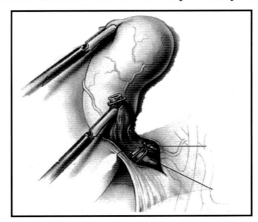

Fig. 2.77: Clip on cystic duct and artery

clipping of cystic duct is replaced by extracorporeal knotting. If titanium clip is applied on the cystic duct sometime it may crush one of the walls of cystic duct and it may get internalized inside the lumen of cystic duct. Inside the lumen of cystic duct it acts as a niddus for the deposition of bile pigment and the formation of stone. The cross-section of these stone the clip inside is seen glistening like pupil of a cat and so it is also known as "Cat eye stone". These stone can slip inside the CBD and may cause CBD obstruction. Although the reported case of CBD obstruction is very less, the surgeon should try to ligate cystic duct to avoid this complication.

Irrigation and Suction Tube

A suction-irrigation probe can be a versatile instrument. Laparoscopic suction and irrigation tube is one of the very important instruments which surgeon should practice frequently (Fig. 2.78). Vision is one of the limitations of laparoscopic surgery. The blood is the darkest color inside abdominal cavity and excess of blood inside absorbs most of the light. Whenever there is bleeding, one should first try to suck it out. Controlled suction and irrigation enhance the observation and improve operative technique. Suction irrigation tube also can be used for blunt dissection. At the time of using suction and irrigation, the tip of the suction irrigation cannula should be dipped inside blood, otherwise the gas will be sucked and surgeon will lose his vision due to loss of pneumoperitoneum. 10 mm suction tube should be used if there is more than 1,500 ml of hemoperitoneum or if there is blood clots inside the abdominal cavity. Sometime small spilled stones can also be sucked with the help of laparoscopic irrigation suction tube at the time of laparoscopic cholecystectomy. It is very useful instrument for doing peritoneal toilet in case of appendicular or duodenal perforation.

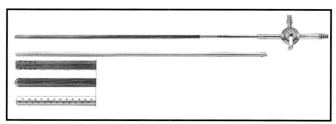

Fig. 2.78: Laparoscopic irrigation and suction tubes

Fallop Ring Applicator

Fallop ring applicator is used for application of silastic ring to perform tube ligation. These may be fitted with one or two silastic rings (Figs 2.79 to 2.81).

Myoma Fixation Screw

When performing a laparoscopic myomectomy, it is difficult to stabilize a smooth, hard fibroid. This is used to fix the subserous or intramural myoma at the time of laparoscopic myomectomy. Myoma screw can also be used to fix and retract big size uterus at the time of laparoscopic hysterectomy (Fig. 2.82).

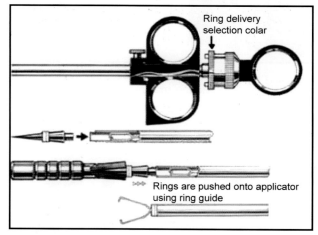

Fig. 2.79: Fallop ring

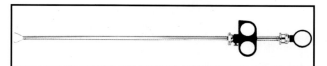

Fig. 2.80: Fallop ring applicator

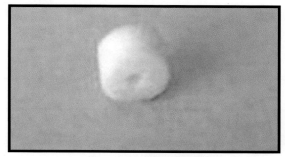

Ring delivery selection colar

Rings are pushed onto applicator using ring guide

Fig. 2.81: Handle of fallop ring applicator (Mechanism)

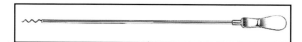

Fig. 2.82: Myoma screw

Section One

Uterine Manipulator

Uterine manipulator is one of the very essential instruments for mobilization of the uterus, identification of the vaginal fornices and sealing of the vagina during hysterectomy (Fig. 2.83). Uterine manipulator is used in most of the advanced gynecological procedures (Figs 2.84 to 2.86).

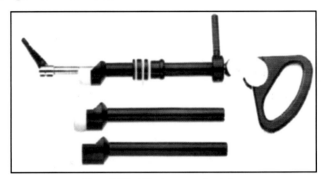

Fig. 2.83: Uterine manipulator

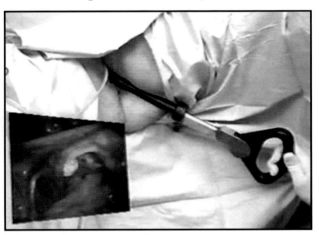

Fig. 2.84: Lateral traction over uterus by uterine manipulator

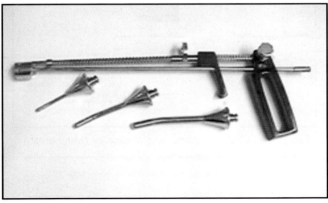

Fig. 2.85: Different attachments of uterine manipulator

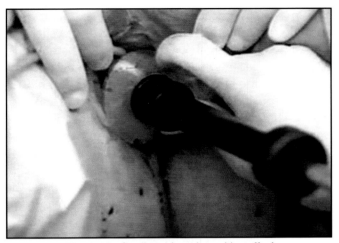

Fig. 2.86: Sealing of vagina with cuff of uterine manipulator for TLH

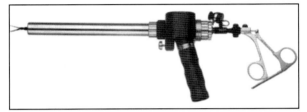

Fig. 2.87: Tissue morcellator

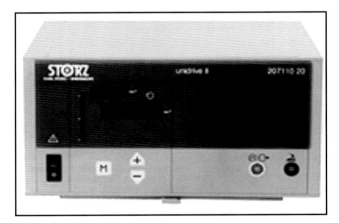

Fig. 2.88: Base unit of tissue morcellator

Tissue Morcellator

The morcellator is used to grasp the tissue to be removed and cuts it into small bits, which are forced into the hollow part of the instrument (Figs 2.87 to 2.89). It can be designed to remove a myoma or an ovary. It can be introduced through a 10 mm port or through the colopotomy wound (Figs 2.90A and B).

Hernia Stapler, Endoanchor and Tacker

For fixing mesh in hernia surgery many preloaded devices are available (Fig. 2.91). Currently, three popular brands of implants to fix the mesh are available. These are Tacker, Protack or Anchor. The comparative chart of these implants is shown in Table 2.4.

There are many varieties of laparoscopic stapler (Fig. 2.92). The LONG45A Endocutter manufactured by Ethicon has a shaft that is 10 cm and it allows easier access during laparoscopic weight loss surgery, such as gastric bypass, where longer instruments are needed for morbidly obese patients. The ETS45 and ETS-FLEX45 Endoscopic Linear cutters provide a 45 mm

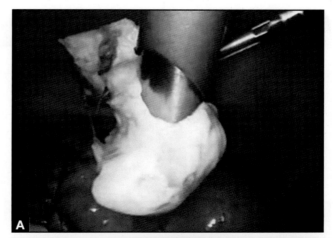

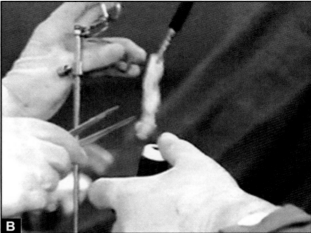

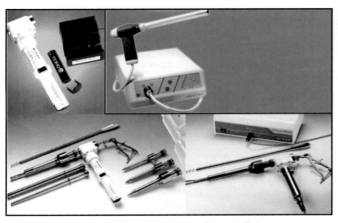

Fig. 2.89: Different type of morcellator

Figs 2.90A and B: Morcellation of myoma in myomectomy

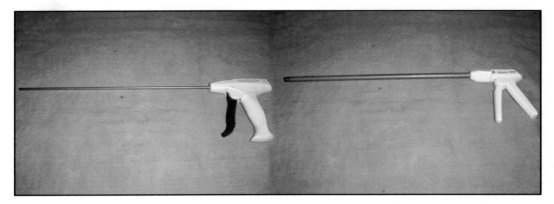

Fig. 2.91: Endoanchor and tacker

staple and cut line (Fig. 2.93). The 34 cm shaft length makes the device suitable for many minimally invasive surgical procedures. The cutters are intended for transaction, resection, and/or creation of anastomosis in minimally access surgical procedures.

Complications related to the use of laparoscopic instruments are numerous and varied, surgeon must understand and look for two types of complications.
- *Electrical insulation:* Use of monopolar current through the hooks, graspers and scissors requires

Section One

Feature	ESS endoanchor	Tyco protack	Tyco tacker
Number of implants	20	30	20
Geometry of implant	Anchor	Helical Fastener	Helical Fastener
Implant material	Nitinol	Titanium	Titanium
Implant length	5.9 mm	3.8 mm	3.6 mm
Implant width	6.7 mm	4 mm	3.4 mm
Port size required	5 mm	5 mm	5 mm
Shaft length	360 mm	356 mm	356 mm
Trigger fire orientation	Release to deploy	Depress to deploy	Depress to deploy

Table 2.4: Different types of implant for fixing mesh

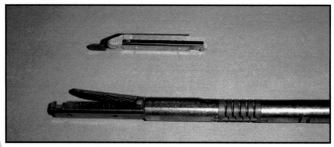

Fig. 2.92: Jaw of stapler

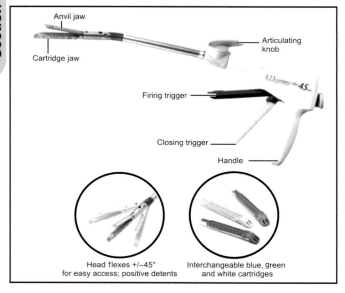

Fig. 2.93: Endopath ETS compact-flex45 articulating endoscopic linear cutters

that instrument have perfectly insulated sheath. Repeated cleaning and sterilization can lead to insulation failure and leakage of current.
- *Instrument breakage:* Repeated exposure to high pressure and high temperature sterilization can degrade the mechanism of instrument. Consi-

derable mechanical strain applied on the instrument articulation can cause these to break. If mechanical part gets lost in the abdominal cavity then they must be retrieved. If laparoscopic retrieval of lost part of instrument is not possible conversion to open surgery may be necessary.

Laparoscopic surgical instruments are extremely variable and increasing number of instruments is being designed for specific application. Instruments are getting complex with greater functionality and freedom of movement. Such instruments reflect the trend towards the automation of procedure. In the future, such developments ultimately will lead to full robotization.

BIBLIOGRAPHY

1. Bhayani SB, Andriole GL. Three-dimensional (3D) vision: does it improve laparoscopic skills? An assessment of 3D headmounted visualization system. Rev Urol 2005;7: 211–4.
2. Byrn JC, Schluender S, Divino CM, et al. Three dimensional imaging improves surgical performance for both novice and experienced operators using the da Vinci Robot System. Am J Surg 2007;193:519–22.
3. Chan AC, Chung SC, Yim AP, et al. Comparison of two dimensional vs. three dimensional camera systems in laparoscopic surgery. Surg Endosc 1997;11:438–40.
4. Ericsson KA. Deliberate practice and the acquisition and maintenance of expert performance in medicine and related domains. Acad Med 2004;79: S70–S81.
5. Everbusch A, Grantcharov TP. Learning curves and impact of psychomotor training on performance in simulated colonoscopy: a randomized trial using a virtual reality endoscopy trainer. Surg Endosc 2004;18:1514–8.
6. Fraser SA, Freldman LS, Stanbridge D, et al. Characterizing the learning curve for a basic laparoscopic drill. Surg Endosc 2005;19:1572–8.
7. Ganai S, Seymour NE. VR to OR for Camera Navigation. In: Westwood JD, et al. (eds), Medicine Meets Virtual Reality IOC press, Amsterdam, 2005;111(13):45–8.

8. Grantcharov TP, Bardram L, Funch-Jensen P, et al. Impact of hand dominance, gender and experience with computer games on performance in virtual reality laparoscopy. Surg Endosc 2003;17:1082–5.

9. Grantcharov TP, Bardram L, Funch-Jensen P, et al. Learning curves and impact of previous operative experience on performance on virtual reality simulator to test laparoscopic surgical skills. Am J Surg 2003;185:146–9.

10. Haluck RS, Gallagher AG, Satava RM, Webster R, Bass TL, Miller CA. Reliability and validity of Endotower, a virtual reality trainer for angled endoscope navigation. Stud Health Technol Inform 2002;85:179–84.

11. Haluck RS, Webster RW, Snyder AJ, Melkonian MG, Mohler BJ, Dise ML, Lefever A. A virtual reality surgical trainer for navigation in laparoscopic surgery. Stud Health Technol Inform 2001;81:171–6.

12. Hanna GB, Cuschieri A. Influence of two-dimensional and three-dimensional imaging on endoscopic bowel suturing. World J Surg 2000;24:444–9.

13. Hanna GB, Shimi SM, Cuschieri A. Randomized study of the influence of two dimensional versus three dimensional imaging on performance of laparoscopic cholecystectomy. Lancet 1998;351:248–51.

14. Hart SG, Staveland LE. Development of a multi-dimensional workload rating scale: Results of empirical and theoretical research. In: Hancock PA, Meshkati N (eds), Human Mental Workload. Elsevier, Amsterdam, 1988;139–83.

15. Jones DB, Brewer JD, Soper NJ. The influence of threedimensional video systems on laparoscopic task performance. Surg Laparosc Endosc 1996;6:191–7.

16. Korndorffer JR Jr, Hayes DJ, Dunne JB, Sierra R, Touchard CL, Markert RJ, Scott DJ. Development and transferability of a cost-effective laparoscopic camera navigation simulator. Surg Endosc 2005;19:161–7.

17. Korndorffer JR Jr, Stefanidis D, Sierra R, Clayton JL, et al. Validity and reliability of a videotrainer laparoscopic camera navigation simulator. Surg Endosc 2005;19: S246.

18. Maithel S, Sierra R, Korndorffer J, Neumann P, Dawson S, Callery M, Jones D, Scott D. Construct and face validity of MIST-VR, Endotower, and CELTS: are we ready for skills assessment using simulators? Surg Endosc 2006;20:104–12.

19. McDougall EM, Soble JJ, Wolf JS Jr, et al. Comparison of three-dimensional and two-dimensional laparoscopic video systems. J Endourol 1996;10:371–74.

20. O_Donnell RD, Eggemeier FT. Workload assessment methodology. In: Boff KR, Kaufman L, Thomas JP (eds). Handbook of perception and performance, Cognitive processes and performance Wiley, New York, 1986;42;1(2): 42-9.

21. Peitgen K, Walz MV, Walz MV, et al. A prospective randomized experimental evaluation of three dimensional imaging in laparoscopy. Gastrointest Endosc 1996;44:262–7.

22. Perkins N, Starkes JL, Lee TD, et al. Learning to use minimal access surgical instruments and 2-dimensional remote visual feedback: how difficult is the task for novices? Adv Health Sci Educ 2002;7:117–31.

23. Perkins N, Starkes JL, Lee TD, Hutchison C. Learning to use minimal access surgical instruments and 2-dimensional remote visual feedback: how difficult is the task for novices? Adv Health Sci Educ Theory Pract 2002;7: 117–31.

24. Peters JH, Fried GM, Swanstrom LL, Soper NJ, Sillin LF, Schirmer B, Foffman K, SAGES FLS Committee Development and validation of a comprehensive program of education and assessment of the basic fundamentals of laparoscopic surgery. Surgery 2004;135:21–27.

25. Powers TW, Bentrem DJ, Nagle AP, et al. Hand dominance and performance in a laparoscopic skills curriculum. Surg Endosc 2005;19:673–77 World J Surg 2008;32:110–118 17.

26. Reed JF. Analysis of two treatment, two period cross trials in emergency medicine. Ann Emerg Med 2004;43:54–8.

27. Risucci D, Geiss A, Gellman L, et al. Surgeon-specific factors in the acquisition of laparoscopic surgical skills. Am J Surg 2001;181:289–93.

28. Scott DJ, Jones DB. Virtual reality training and teaching tools. In: Soper NJ, Swanstrom LL, Eubanks WS (eds). Mastery of Endoscopic and Laparoscopic Surgery. Lippincott Williams and Wilkins, Philadelphia, 2005;2:146–60.

29. Stefanidis D, Korndorffer JR Jr, Sierra R, Touchard C, Dunne JB, Scott DJ. Skill retention following proficiency-based laparoscopic simulator training. Surgery 2005;138:165–70.

30. Stefanidis D, Korndorffer JR, Scott DJ. Robotic laparoscopic fundoplication. Curr Treat Options Gastroenterol 2005;8: 71–83.

31. Sun CC, Chiu AW, Chen KK, et al. Assessment of a three dimensional operating system with skill tests in a pelvic trainer. Urol Int 2000;64:154–8.

32. Taffinder N, Smith SG, Huber J, et al. The effect of a second-generation 3D endoscope on the laparoscopic precision of novices and experienced surgeons. Surg Endosc 1999;13:1087–92.

33. Thomsen MN, Lang RD. An experimental comparison of 3-dimensional and 2-dimensional endoscopic systems in a model. Arthroscopy 2004;20:419–23.

34. Torkington J, Smith SG, Rees B, et al. The role of the basic surgical skills course in the acquisition and retention of laparoscopic skills. Surg Endosc 1001;15:1071–5.

35. Wickens CD, Hollands J. Engineering psychology and human performance. Prentice Hall, Upper Saddle River, NJ 2000;1164.

36. Windsor JA, Zoha F. The laparoscopic performance of novice surgical trainees: testing for acquisition, loss, and reacquisition of psychomotor skills. Surg Endosc 2005;19:1058–63.

Section One

3

Sterilization of
Laparoscopic Instruments

Sterilization is the process by which surgical items are rendered free of viable microorganisms, including spores. The purpose of effective laparoscopic instruments sterilization is to provide the surgeon with a sterile product.

HISTORY OF STERILIZATION

According to ancient writings, most primitive people regarded disease as the work of evil spirits or as coming from supernatural powers. Hippocrates (460 - 370 BC) began the shift of the healing process from mystical rites to a practical approach. Marcus Terentius Varro (117-26 BC), proposed a germ theory by stating, "Small creatures, invisible to the eye, fill the atmosphere, and breathed through the nose cause dangerous diseases." Seventeenth century advancements in anatomy, physiology and medical instrumentation included the development of the microscope in 1683 by Anton van Leeuwenhoek which allowed bacteria to be studied. Research into surgery and anatomy continued during the eighteenth century. In the 1850s, Pasteur proved that fermentation, putrefaction, infection and souring are caused by the growth of microbes. Lord Joseph Lister was the one who successfully identified the implications for surgical infections. Lister believed that infection could be prevented if he could prevent the airborne microbes from entering the wound. Further advances in aseptic techniques from 1881 to 1882 were possible when a German bacteriologist, Robert Koch, introduced methods of steam sterilization and developed the first non-pressure flowing steam sterilizer.

LEGISLATION IN STERILIZATION

The sterilization of laparoscopic instruments must comply with safety standards. These vary depending upon legislation of the individual countries.

In Germany legislation requires steam autoclaving at 134°C for 5 minutes. However, in France sterilization is practiced at this temperature for 18 minutes. In USA, Food and Drug Administration (FDA) has established different sterilization criteria regarding sterilization of re-usable instruments. General requirement for characterization of sterilizing agent and the development, validation and routine control of a sterilization process for laparoscopic instrument is provided by the manufacturer and sterilization should be performed strictly according to the manufacturer's guidelines.

Cleaning

All used instruments, regardless of size, should be completely immersed in distilled water before leaving the operating room. The first step of the high level disinfection process is thorough cleaning (Fig. 3.1). Cleaning removes debris, mucous, blood and tissue (bioburden) which would interfere with the action of the disinfectant. Current recommendations specify disassembly of most laparoscopic equipment prior to sterilization. If the surgical assistants are unfamiliar with the proper assembly of laparoscopic instruments, it may cause patient injury from equipment malfunction. Because of the intricate internal parts of laparoscopic instruments, questions have been raised about the efficacy of cleaning and sterilization techniques.

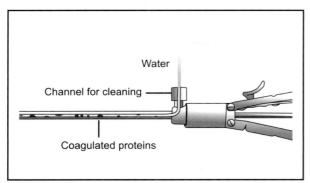

Fig. 3.1: Incomplete cleaning can result in accumulation of coagulated protein inside channel of the instrument

In the instruments which can not be dismantled there is separate channel to irrigate water under pressure to clean it properly. At least 300 ml of water should be flushed through these instruments to clean it properly.

Approximately 99.8 percent of the bioburden can be removed by meticulous cleaning. Cleaning may be accomplished via manual or mechanical washing.

ULTRASONIC TECHNOLOGY FOR CLEANING

- Energy from high-frequency sound waves
- Vigorous microscopic implosions of tiny vapor bubbles
- Millions of scrubbing bubbles do the job of cleaning
- Ultrasonic cleaners facilitate removal of organic material, decreasing the risk of contaminants (Fig. 3.2).

The cleaning agent selected should be:

- Able to remove organic and inorganic soil
- Able to prevent water-borne deposits
- Low foaming
- Able to be rinsed completely
- Compatible with the materials being cleaned.

Following cleaning, items to be disinfected must be rinsed thoroughly to remove any residual detergent. After cleaning, instruments are subjected to sterilization.

Sterilization

The two methods of sterilization most commonly used for laparoscopic instruments.

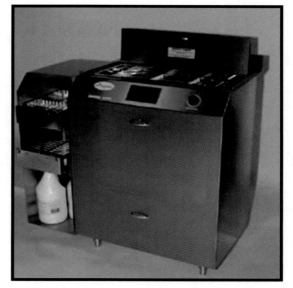

Fig. 3.2: Ultrasonic laparoscopic instrument cleaner

- Steam sterilization
- Chemical sterilization.

Autoclaving by means of steam was the oldest, safest and most cost-effective method of sterilization. When steam is placed under pressure and the temperature is raised, the moist heat produces changes within the cell protein, thereby rendering it harmless over a prescribed period of time. The relationship between temperature, pressure and time of exposure is the critical factor in the destruction of microbes. Although steam sterilization in effective an inexpensive it is not suitable for all laparoscopic instruments.

The growth and expansion of minimal access surgical procedures require specialized surgical instrumentation. Most of the laparoscopic instrument can be safely autoclaved but some of the laparoscopic instruments cannot withstand the prolonged heat and moisture of the steam sterilization process. Laparoscopic cameras, laparoscopes, light cables and flexible endoscopes are damaged by heat. Therefore, alternative methods of sterilization were needed to effectively sterilize moisture-stable, moisture-sensitive and heat-sensitive items that require rapid, frequent processing in the clinical setting.

One of the most common types of alternative of steam sterilization is chemical sterilization. Many chemicals are proven to have sterilizing property. Laparoscopic camera (CCD) is damaged by chemical sterilization with repeated exposure. In these expensive devices, a sterile plastic sleeve or sterile thick cloth sleeve should be used to avoid contamination.

Ethylene Oxide (EtO)

One of the most common types of chemical sterilization uses ethylene oxide (EtO) gas, which is in use since the 1950s. EtO is colorless at ordinary temperatures, has an odor similar to that of ether and is extremely toxic and flammable. Mixture of EtO with an inert gas such as carbon dioxide or a chlorofluorocarbon (CFC) was used to make it non-inflammable. The most common combination was 12 percent EtO and 88 percent freon. A newer formulation uses EtO plus a hydrochlorofluorocarbon (HCFC).

EtO sterilization depends on four parameters:

- Time
- Temperature
- Gas concentration
- Relative humidity.

All EtO sterilizers operate at low temperature, typically between 49 - 60° C (130 - 140° F) and relative humidity of 40 to 60 percent. The humidity must be not less than 30 percent in order to hydrate the items during the sterilization process. These characteristics make EtO sterilization suitable for complex medical equipment.

Both temperature and humidity have a profound influence on the destruction of microorganisms because they affect penetration of the gas through bacterial cell walls, as well as through the wrapping and packaging materials. It typically takes between 3 and 6 hours for the sterilization portion of the cycle to be completed.

Additionally, items sterilized by EtO must be aerated to make them safe for personnel handling and patient use. Therefore, the EtO sterilization and aeration processes can take up to 20 hours and should be used only when time is not a factor.

Hydrogen Peroxide Gas Plasma

Hydrogen peroxide is an oxidizing agent that affects sterilization by oxidation of key cellular components. Plasma is a state of matter distinguishable from a solid, liquid, or gas. The cloud of plasma is composed of ions, electrons and neutral atomic particles that produce a visible glow. Hydrogen peroxide is bactericidal, virucidal, sporicidal and fungicidal, even at low concentration and temperature.

A solution of hydrogen peroxide and water (59% nominal peroxide by weight) is vaporized and allowed to surround and interact with the devices to be sterilized. Applying a strong electrical field then creates plasma. The plasma breaks down the peroxide into a "cloud" of highly energized species that recombine, turning the hydrogen peroxide into water and oxygen. No aeration time is required and the instruments may either be used immediately or placed on a shelf for later use. A load of surgical instruments may be sterilized in less than 1 hour.

Peracetic Acid

Liquid paroxyacetic, or peracetic acid, is a biocidal oxidizer that maintains its efficacy in the presence of high levels of organic debris. Peracetic acid is acetic acid plus an extra oxygen atom and reacts with most cellular components to cause cell death. The peracetic acid solution is heated to 50 - 56° C (122 - 131° F) during the 20 to 30 minutes cycle. Peracetic acid must be used in combination with anticorrosive additives.

Parameters for peracetic acid sterilizers include:

- Relatively short cycle times
- Availability of the items for immediate use
- Sterilant can be discharged into the drainage system since it is not hazardos
- No aeration time is required for the sterilized items
- Items must be rinsed with copious amounts of sterile water after the sterilization process.

Items processed by this method should be used immediately after processing, since the containers are wet and are not protected from the environment. This system must also be monitored for sterility with live spores.

Glutaraldehyde

An activated 2 percent aqueous glutaraldehyde solution is recognized as an effective liquid chemical sterilant. Glutaraldehyde is most frequently used as a high-level disinfectant for lensed instruments because it is non-corrosive and has minimal harmful effect on the instrument (Fig. 3.3).

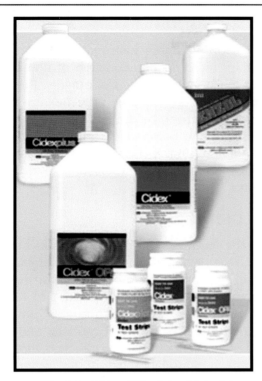

Fig. 3.3: Cidex (2% glutaraldehyde)

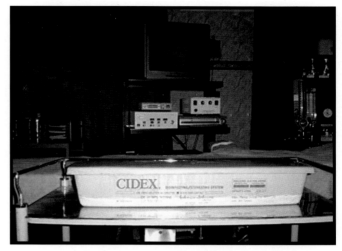

Fig. 3.4: Cidex tray used for laparoscopic instrument sterilization

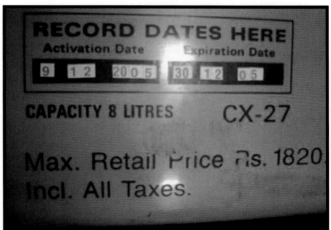

Fig. 3.5: Labeling of cidex tray (Activation date and expiration date)

Sterilization can be achieved with an activated 2 percent glutaraldehyde solution after the item is completely immersed for 10 hours at 25° C in especially designed tray. Before immersion, the item must be thoroughly cleaned and dried. During immersion, all surfaces of the item must be in contact with the solution. After immersion, the item must be rinsed thoroughly with sterile water prior to use (Fig. 3.4).

Cidex should be used maximum 15 times or 21 days after activation, whichever may be earlier. Once activated, the solution should be discarded after 21 days, so it is important to write the date of activation and date of expiry in the space provided on the Cidex tray (Fig. 3.5). If the instrument is not cleaned properly, the activated glutaraldehyde becomes dirty just after few use and turns into blackish solution. In this case it should be rejected before specified period of time. It is important that surgeon should read carefully the literature provided by the manufacturer.

Ortho-phthalaldehyde

For laparoscopic instruments, 0.55 percent ortho-phthalaldehyde is good option, it is non-glutaraldehyde solution for disinfection of delicate instruments. In fact, ortho-phthalaldehyde solution is one of the gentlest reprocessing options available, which means it can substantially reduce instrument damage and repair costs. It is good not only because of its speed and efficiency but also because of its environmental safety. It comes with the trade name of Cidex OPA. It has following advantage:

- No activation or mixing required
- It can be used in both automated and manual reprocessing
- 2-years shelf life and 75 days open-bottle shelf life

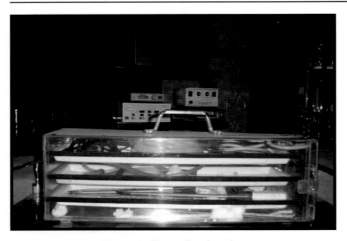

Fig. 3.6: Formalin chamber

- Rapid 5 minutes immersion time at a minimum of 25°C in an automatic endoscope reprocessor
- Efficient 12 minutes soak time at room temperature (20 °C) for manual reprocessing
- Effective against glutaraldehyde-resistant mycobacterium.

Formaldehyde

Bactericidal properties and use of formaldehyde include: 37 percent aqueous solution (formalin) or 8 percent formaldehyde in 70 percent isopropyl alcohol kills microorganisms by coagulating intracellular protein. Solution is effective at room temperature.

Specially designed airtight formalin chambers are available (Fig. 3.6). Eight to ten formalin tablets wrapped with moist gauge piece should be placed in the chamber and the door should be closed. The vapor of formalin acts for one week, after one week tablets should be changed. Although known to destroy spores, it is rarely used because it takes from 12 to 24 hours to be effective. Formalin chamber is used by many surgeons to carry their sterilized instrument from one hospital to another. Pungent odor of formalin is quite objectionable and irritating to the eyes and nasal passages. The vapors can be toxic and ongoing controversy exists regarding its carcinogenic effects. However, low-temperature steam with formaldehyde has been widely used in health care facilities in Northern Europe for the sterilization of reusable medical devices that cannot withstand steam sterilization.

Other Chemical Disinfectant

Recently, non-aldehyde instrument disinfectant is available for rapid decontamination of non-invasive and heat labile laparoscopic instruments. It contains halogenated tertiary amines, poly hexamethylene biguanide hydrochloride, Ethyl alcohol B, Dodecylamine and Sulphamic acid. Contact time for bactericidal and fungicidal and virucidal protection is 10 minutes. For sporicidal protection, contact time is 30 minutes.

CONCLUSION

Most of the laparoscopic instrument can be easily sterilized if the person knows how to dissemble, clean and use specific chemical for sterilization. Manufactures instruction is important to follow if desired effect has to be achieved. Expensive instruments should be handled carefully and all the insulated instruments should be checked thoroughly for any breach in insulation before sterilization. Apart from newer generation chemical disinfectant, low-temperature steam with formaldehyde has been widely used in health care facilities in Northern Europe for the sterilization of reusable medical devices that cannot withstand steam sterilization.

Other key considerations in the sterilization process which should be taken care are:
- Packaging of the items after sterilization
- Monitoring the sterilization process
- Shelf life of the sterilized items
- Cost implications.

BIBLIOGRAPHY

1. Barthram C, McClymont W. The use of a checklist for anaesthetic machines. Anaesthesia 1992;47:1066–69.
2. Berge JA, Gramstad L, Grimnes S. An evaluation of a time-saving anaesthetic machine checkout procedure. Eur J Anaesthesiol 1994;11:493–498.
3. Berge JA, Gramstad L, Jensen O. A training simulator for detecting equipment failure in the anaesthetic machine. Eur J Anaesthesiol 1993;10:19–24.
4. Blike G, Biddle C. Preanesthesia detection of equipment faults by anesthesia providers at an academic hospital: comparison of standard practice and a new electronic checklist. Aana J 2000;68:497–505.
5. Burner ST, Waldo DR, McKusich DR. National health expenditures projections through 2030. Health Care Finance Rev 1992;14(1):1-29.

6. Calland JF, Guerlain S, Adams RB, Tribble CG, Foley E, Chekan EG A systems approach to surgical safety. Surg Endosc 2002;16:1005–1014-5.

7. Cival Aviation Authority (CAA) 2000 Guidance on the design, presentation, and use of electronic checklists. CAP 708. Safety Regulation Group. Retrieved July 2008 at http://www.caa.co.uk/ docs/33/CAP708.PDF.

8. Cival Aviation Authority (CAA). 2006 Guidance on the design presentation and use of emergency and abnormal checklists. CAP 676. Safety Regulation Group. Retrieved July 2008 at http://www.caa.co.uk/docs/33/CAP676.PDF.

9. Dankelman J, Grimbergen CA. Systems approach to reduce errors in surgery. Surg Endosc 2005;19:1017–21.

10. Degani A, Wiener EL. Human factors of flight deck checklists: the normal checklist. NASA Contractor Report 1990;177-49.

11. Diamond T, Mole DJ. Anatomical orientation and crosschecking, the key to safer laparoscopic cholecystectomy. Br J Surg 2005;92:663–4.

12. Eiseman B, Borlase BC. Measurement of cost effectiveness. In: Eiseman B, Stahlgren L (eds) Cost effective surgical practice. WB Saunders Co, Philadelphia, 1978;1-5.

13. Ginzberg E. High-tech medicine and rising health care costs. JAMA 1990;263(13):1820-22.

14. Gwinnutt CL, Driscoll PA. Advanced trauma life support. Eur J Anaesthesiol 1996;13:95–101.

15. Hart EM, Owen H. Errors and omissions in anesthesia: a pilot study using a pilot's checklist. Anesth Analg 2005;101:246–250. table of contents Surg Endosc 2009 23:715–726.725.

16. Helmreich RL . On error management: lessons from aviation. BMJ 2000;320:781–5.

17. Jordan AM. Hospital charges for laparoscopic and open cholecystectomies. 1991;266(24): 3425.

18. Kendell J, Barthram C. Revised checklist for anaesthetic machines. Anaesthesia 1998;53:887–90.

19. Kohn LT, Corrigan JM, Donaldsen MS. To err is human. Institute of Medicine, Washington DC, 1999;1–14.

20. Kwaan MR, Studdert DM, Zinner MJ, Gawande AA. Incidence, patterns, and prevention of wrong-site surgery. Arch Surg 2006;141:353–7 discussion 357–8.

21. Leape L. The preventability of medical injury. In: Bogner MS (ed) Human error in medicine. Lawrence Erlbaum Associates, Hillsdale, NJ. 1994.

22. Leonard M, Graham S, Bonacum D. The human factor: the critical importance of effective teamwork and communication in providing safe care. Qual Saf Health Care 2004;13(1):i85–i90 19. DeFontes J, Surbida S. Preoperative safety briefing project. Permanente J 2004;8:21–27.

23. Lingard L, Espin S, Rubin B, Whyte S, Colmenares M, Baker GR, Doran D, Grober E, Orser B, Bohnen J, Reznick R. Getting teams to talk: development and pilot implementation of a checklist to promote interprofessional communication in the OR. Qual Saf Health Care 2005;14(5):340–6.

24. Makary MA, Holzmueller CG, Thompson D, Rowen L, Heitmiller ES, Maley WR, Black JH, Stegner K, Freischlag JA, Ulatowski JA, Pronovost PJ. Operating room briefings: working on the same page. Jt Comm J Qual Patient Saf 2006;32(6):351–5.

25. Makary MA, Mukherjee A, Sexton JB, Syin D, Goodrich E, Hartmann E, Rowen L, Behrens DC, Marohn M, Pronovost PJ. Operating room briefings and wrong-site surgery. J Am Coll Surg 2007;204:236–43.

26. Manley R, Cuddeford JD. An assessment of the effectiveness of the revised FDA checklist. Aana J 1996;64:277–82.

27. March MG, Crowley JJ. An evaluation of anesthesiologists' present checkout methods and the validity of the FDA checklist. Anesthesiology 1991;75:724–9.

28. McIntyre RC, Foster MA, Weil KC, Cohen MM. A comparison of outcome and cost of open vs. laparoscopic cholecystectomy. J Laparoendosc Surg 1992;2:143-8.

29. Meijer DW. Safety of the laparoscopy setup. Minim Invasive Ther Allied Technol 2003;12:125–8.

30. Michaels RK, Makary MA, Dahab Y, Frassica FJ, Heitmiller E, Rowen LC, Crotreau R, Brem H, Pronovost PJ. Achieving the National Quality Forum's "Never Events": prevention of wrong-site, wrong-procedure, and wrong-patient operations. Ann Surg 2007;245:526–32.

31. Palmer E, Degani A. Electronic checklists: evaluation of two levels of automation. In: Proceedings of the Sixth International Aviation Psychology Symposium. Ohio State Univeristy, Columbus, OH. 1994.

32. Peters JH, Ellison L, Innes JT, Liss JL, Nichols KE, Lomano JM, Roby SR, Front ME, Carey LL. Safety and efficacy of laparoscopic cholecystectomy. A prospective analysis of 100 initial patients. Ann Surg 1991;213:3-12.

33. Punt MM, Stefels CN, Grimbergen CA, Dankelman J. Evaluation of voice control, touch panel control, and assistant control during steering of an endoscope. Minim Invasive Ther Allied Technol 2005;14:181–7.

34. Reason J. Human error. Cambridge University Press 33. Degani A, Wiener EL. Cockpit checklists: concepts, design, and use. Hum Factors 1990;1993;35(2):28–43.

35. Reason J. Human error: models and management. BMJ 2000;320:768–70.

36. Reichert M. Laparoscopic instruments. AORN J 1993;57(3): 637-55.

37. Rouse SH, Rouse WB. Computer-based manuals for procedural information. IEEE Trans Syst Man Cybern 1980;10(8):506–510.

38. Saufl NM. Universal protocol for preventing wrong-site, wrong-procedure, wrong-person surgery. J Perianesth Nurs 2004;19:348–51.

39. Schieber GJ, Poulhir JP, Greenwald LM. US. health expenditure performance: an international comparison and data update. Health Care Finance Rev 1992;13(4):1-15.

40. Stufflebeam DL. Guidelines for developing evaluation checklists: the checklists development checklist (CDC). Retrieved May 2007 at http://www.wmich.edu/evalctr/checklists/ guidelines_cdc.pdf] 2000.

41. Technology Assessment Committee of the American Society for Gastrointestinal Endoscopy Position statement report on transmission of microorganisms. Gastrointestinal Endosc 1993;36(6): 885-8.

Section One

42. Undre S, Healey AN, Darzi A, Vincent CA. Observational assessment of surgical teamwork: a feasibility study. World J Surg 2006;30:1774–83.

43. Universal protocol for preventing wrong-site, wrong-procedure, wrong-person surgery. Retrieved June 2007 at www.joint commission.org/PatientSafety/UniversalProtocol]

44. Verdaasdonk EG, Stassen LP, van der Elst M, Karsten TM, Dankelman J. Problems with technical equipment during laparoscopic surgery: an observational study. Surg Endosc 2007;21:275–9.

45. Vincent C, Moorthy K, Sarker SK, Chang A, Darzi AW. Systems approaches to surgical quality and safety: from concept to measurement. Ann Surg 2004;239:475–82.

46. Wagner C, de Bruijne M. Onbedoelde schade in Nederlandse ziekenhuizen. Nederlands Instituut voor onderzoek van de gezondheidszorg (NIVEL) 2007;20.

Anesthesia in Laparoscopic Surgery

The anesthetic problems during minimal access surgery are related to the cardiopulmonary effects of pneumoperitoneum, carbon dioxide absorption, extraperitoneal gas insufflation, venous embolism and inadvertent injuries to intra-abdominal organs. Optimal anesthetic care of patients undergoing laparoscopic surgery is very much important. Good anesthetic techniques facilitate risk free surgery and allows early detection and reduction of complications.

In young patients, fit for diagnostic laparoscopy, general anesthesia is the preferred method and does not impose any increased risk. Adequate anesthesia and analgesia are essential and endotracheal intubation and controlled ventilation should be considered. The pneumoperitoneum can be created safely under local anesthesia provided that the patient is adequately sedated throughout the procedure. For successful laparoscopy under local anesthesia intravenous medication for sedation should be given.

EVALUATION AND PREPARATION OF PATIENT FOR LAPAROSCOPIC SURGERY

There are laparoscopic operations that are emergencies. Therefore, all patients should receive the same evaluation and preparation that they would receive for an open, elective abdominal operation. There are several unique concerns with laparoscopy and the type of patients who undergo these procedures.

Many of the patients scheduled to undergo laparoscopic surgery are young women undergoing gynecological laparoscopy. Young women are at high-risk for postoperative nausea and vomiting following general anesthesia, and gynecological procedures may provoke nausea and vomiting as well. Laparoscopy itself is also associated with postoperative nausea and vomiting, probably due to stretching of the abdominal cavity or residual irritant effects of retained carbon dioxide. Anesthesiologists should plan their anesthetic to prevent and treat postoperative nausea and vomiting in these patients.

A second group of patients that cause concern are those with significant cardiac disease. Most of these patients tolerate abdominal insufflation at low pressures currently used (<18 mm Hg) surprisingly well. If the operation is to be of short duration, few patients with cardiac disease, other than those with severe congestive heart failure, require invasive monitoring. However, insufflation can be associated with a moderately reduced cardiac index, increased cardiac filling pressures, systemic blood pressure, and systemic vascular resistance. In addition, hypercarbia from insufflated carbon dioxide may be detrimental to patients with cardiac disease by stimulating the sympathetic nervous system and vasopressin release. Therefore, for extensive laparoscopic procedures direct arterial and pulmonary artery catheterization and/or transesophageal echocardiography may be necessary for monitoring.

A third group of patients of concern are those with severe emphysema, asthma, cystic fibrosis or other pulmonary disease. Often these are patients who would benefit from a laparoscopic operation as opposed to an open procedure because of improved postoperative pulmonary function following procedures performed laparoscopically. However, some of these patients may not be able to be adequately ventilated to eliminate the carbon dioxide absorbed during laparoscopy. It is important for patients with severe lung disease to be in optimum medical condition prior to having surgery.

The anesthesiologist must be certain that the patient does not have an upper respiratory tract infection or other conditions that may impair pulmonary function at the time of surgery. Prior preparation with a course of bronchodilators, steroids and/or antibiotics may be necessary. In these patients, an intra-arterial catheter for arterial blood sampling for gas analysis as well as direct arterial pressure monitoring is essential, since the end-tidal carbon dioxide tension often does not accurately reflect the arterial carbon dioxide tension and may be significantly lower.

A laparoscopic surgeon should develop communication and understanding with his anesthetist. Adequate preoperative assessment of the patient and the disease minimizes the risk of general anesthesia. Necessary measures should be undertaken to correct any metabolic or hematological abnormalities. These include hypokalemia, hyponatremia, hyperglycemia, azotemia, anemia and coagulation defects. All the required pre-anesthetic laboratory data should be available, including blood grouping and testing for the hepatitis B antigen and HIV. Patients should have an electrocardiogram and chest X-ray.

Physiological Changes During Laparoscopy

The introduction of gas into the peritoneal cavity under pressure may cause pain, respiratory distress, and possibly cardiac embarrassment. Further, Trendelenburg's position is necessary for access but extreme Trendelenburg's position enhances respiratory and cardiac embarrassment.

Pneumoperitoneum at the time of laparoscopic surgery causes upward displacement of the diaphragm, resulting in the reduction in lung volumes including functional residual capacity. Pulmonary compliance is reduced and airway resistance is increased due to high intra-abdominal pressure· The anesthetist often uses high airway pressure to overcome the intra-abdominal pressure for a given tidal volume, which increases the risk of hemodynamic changes and barotraumas.

The impaired diaphragmatic mobility gives rise to uneven distribution of ventilation to the nondependent part of the lung, resulting in ventilation-perfusion mismatch with hypercarbia and hypoxemia. The ventilatory impairment is even more severe if there is associated airway and alveolar collapse. Increased intra-abdominal pressure also predisposes to regurgitation of gastric contents and pulmonary aspiration.

Insufflation of CO_2 is usually accompanied by hypercapnia. The reason initially proposed to explain this hypercapnia was that CO_2 was reabsorbed from the peritoneal cavity. This explanation was all the more plausible in that it was based on the capacity of CO_2 to diffuse, and the exchange capacities of the peritoneal serosa. Recent studies reveal a two phase phenomenon, with absorption proportional to intraperitoneal pressure for low insufflation pressures, then a drop in the rate of this re-absorption probably due to the peritoneal circulation being crushed under the effect of the pressure. The variations in $PaCO_2$ observed during the second phase with high intra-abdominal pressures which act against re-absorption essentially depend on a change in the ventilation/perfusion ratio with an increase in the dead space.

The hypercapnia mechanism is different with extra-peritoneal insufflation. In this case, the pressure effect limiting re-absorption from the peritoneum no longer applies. The increase in pressure increases the diffusion space by dilacerations of the tissues, and thus the CO_2 re-absorption surface. Re-absorption is thus directly proportional to the pressure and volume of CO_2 insufflated in extraperitoneal insufflation. Severe hypercapnia is thus possible, if not to say frequent, in these situations. On the other hand, provided the hypercapnia is controlled, the circulatory effect of extra-peritoneal insufflation is lower than those of intraperitoneal insufflation.

The increase in intrathoracic pressures induced by the increase in intra-abdominal pressure can be limiting factors for laparoscopic surgery in certain patients. Insufflation of the pneumoperitoneum in laparoscopic surgery is accompanied by a decrease of some 30 percent in pulmonary compliance. The resistance of the air passages increases in the same proportions. The resulting increase in pressure in the air passages can have adverse consequences for patients with bubbles of emphysema. These patients and all those who suffer from dystrophy of the pulmonary parenchyma will find it difficult to cope with the often considerable hyperventilation required by hypercapnia, with volumes per minute sometimes reaching 2 or 3 times than normal.

Venous gas embolism is a fatal complication of pneumoperitoneum. Veress needle or the trocar may directly puncture the arteries or blood flow across an opening in an injured vessel, may sometimes draw gas into the vessel and lead to gas embolism.

A slow infusion of air less than 1 liter/minute is absorbed across the pulmonary capillary-alveolar membranes without causing any damage. At higher infusion rates, the gas bubbles lodging in the peripheral pulmonary arterioles provoke neutrophil clumping, activation of the coagulation cascade and platelet aggregation. This may lead to pulmonary vaso-constriction, bronchospasm, pulmonary edema and pulmonary hemorrhage. Gas bubbles attached to fibrin deposits and platelet aggregates mechanically obstruct the pulmonary vasculature and increases the pulmonary vascular resistance.

The increased right heart after load leads to acute right heart failure with arrhythmia, ischemia, hypotension and elevated central venous pressure. Sometimes, paradoxical embolism is seen through a patent foramen ovale.

Elevated intra-abdominal pressure produces physiological changes in the hemodynamic by its effects on systemic vascular resistance, venous return and myocardial performance. Systemic venous return increases when intra-abdominal pressure is elevated. Effects on venous return and cardiac output depend on the magnitude of the intra-abdominal pressure. Venous return initially increases with intra-abdominal pressure below 10 mm Hg. This paradox is due to reduction in the blood volume sequestrated in the splanchnic vasculature which increases cardiac output and arterial pressure. When intra-abdominal pressure exceeds 20 mm Hg, the inferior vena cava is compressed. Venous return from the lower half of the body is impeded resulting in a fall in cardiac output.

A number of animal studies have been devoted to variations in cardiac output induced by the increase in intraperitoneal pressure. The results are consistent with a fall in cardiac output proportional to the intraperitoneal pressure. In low abdominal pressure (5 mm Hg), cardiac output remains unchanged. The drop in right transmural auricular pressure indicates a reduction in the venous return which is demonstrated by a reduction in flow, through the vena cava, the degree of which is proportional to the intra-abdominal pressure.

The cardiac output is governed by the myocardial function, the post-loading and by the venous return, the latter in turn depending on venous resistance and mean systemic pressure. With an intra-abdominal pressure of 5 mm Hg, the venous return improves. Under these conditions the intraperitoneal pressure remains lower than the pressure in the vena cava which results in a flushing effect, with no obstructive phenomena in the lower vena cava. When the intraperitoneal pressure rises above the intravascular pressure, a sub-diaphragmatic narrowing of the lower vena cava slows the flow of blood. The abdominal blood volume is reduced due to the pressure and a reflux into the venous system of the lower members occurs.

The increase in vascular resistance can be explained by the splanchnic vascular compression, but the persistence of high resistance after exsufflation, means a humoral factor could be suggested. During the increase in intraperitoneal pressure a considerable rise in antidiuretic hormone is found, and its vasopressive effects are well-known. This secretion would seem to be dependent on the drop in cardiac flow rate. A simultaneous rise in the level of plasma norepinephrine, whose vasoconstrictor effects are equivalent to those of vasopressin, has also been reported. The increase in vascular resistance is correlated with a rise in arterial pressure insofar as inotropism is sufficient.

The circulation of kidney becomes much compromised with increased intra-abdominal pressure. Renal blood flow and glomerular filtration rate decreases because of increase in renal vascular resistance, reduction in glomerular filtration gradient and decrease in cardiac output. The increase in systemic vascular resistance impairs left ventricular function and cardiac output. Arterial pressure however remains relatively unchanged, which conceal the fall in cardiac output. High intrathoracic pressure during intermittent positive pressure ventilation add in impairment of venous return and cardiac output, particularly if positive end expiratory pressure (PEEP) is also applied. The elevation in intra-abdominal pressure produces lactic acidosis, probably by severely lowering cardiac output and by impairing hepatic clearance of blood lactate.

Stretching of the peritoneum sometimes leads to stimulation of vagus nerve and can provoke arrhythmias such as AV dissociation, nodal rhythm, sinus bradycardia and asystole. This shock is more commonly seen with rapid stretching of the peritoneum at the beginning of peritoneal insufflation.

Faulty pneumoperitoneum may give rise to subcutaneous emphysema, pneumomediastinum, pneumopericardium and pneumothorax. However, gas can also dissect through existing defects in the diaphragm or along surgically traumatized tissue planes in the retroperitoneum, the diaphragm or the falciform ligament. Gas can leak into the subcutaneous tissues connected with poor positioning of a trocar sleeve (2.7% of cases of severe hypercapnia in a series of cholecystectomies published by Wieden, CO_2 is seen to spread outside the abdominal cavity during laparoscopic assisted hysterectomy, with or without lymphadenectomy, and during bladder neck suspensions. In laparoscopic gynecological surgery, because this effusion originates in the pelvis, it mostly affects the sides and loins and generally remains hidden by the drapes until the end of the operation. Only the very abundant, rare forms can be diagnosed by the anesthetist during the operation, when they shift towards to the upper part of the thorax. In this case, the capnographic signs (slow and regular increase in CO_2 expired) will provide an alert during the anesthesia.

REGIONAL ANESTHESIA

Spinal anesthesia is reported enthusiastically for diagnostic laparoscopy without significant complications. Regional anesthesia may be useful for pelvic procedures but if high block is used it interferes with the respiratory status of patient. Bilateral lower intercostal nerve block has also been used, but it is time-consuming and it can cause pneumothorax (Figs 4.1A and B).

GENERAL ANESTHESIA

Many centers use general anesthesia as a routine in all laparoscopic cases. General anesthesia is advisable in pediatric patients also. Endotracheal anesthesia with muscle relaxants and controlled ventilation is generally preferred especially in elderly or high-risk cases.

Anesthesia for laparoscopy can be achieved with a variety of agents and techniques. General anesthesia using balanced anesthesia technique including intravenous induction agents like: Thiopentone, propofol, etomidate, and inhalational agents like nitrous oxide, isoflurane can be used.

A variety of muscle relaxants including succinyl choline, mivacurium, atracurium, vecuronium is available for rapid recovery and cardiovascular stability. Total intravenous anesthesia using agents like propofol, midazolam and ketamine, alfentanil and vecuronium has been reported for outpatient laparoscopy.

Few anesthetist advocates open anesthesia, which avoids the post-intubation sore throat and laryngeal sequelae, but this is associated with a risk of inhalation of gastric content and gastric distension. The chances of latter is not by the passage of a nasogastric tube.

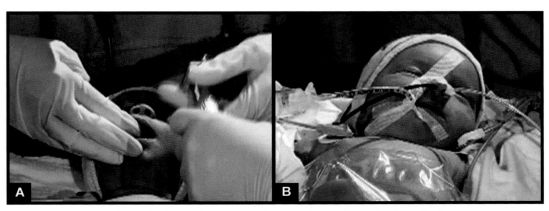

Figs 4.1A and B: Endotracheal intubation in pediatric patient

Halothane should be avoided or used sparingly in patients with several previous operations and in the presence of liver disease.

LOCAL ANESTHESIA

Many surgeons have done sufficient number of laparoscopic procedures under local anesthesia with intravenous sedation and results are encouraging with minimal morbidity and negligible mortality. Laparoscopy under local anesthesia should be performed with an anesthetist being present to monitor the patient's cardiac and respiratory functions. Intravenous sedation should be administered with IV. diazepam and pethidine. Preferred local anesthetic agent is 1 percent lignocaine without adrenaline or lidocaine without epinephrine. The anesthetic agent should be administered at the sites of insertion of the needle, and all trocars.

If local anesthesia is used, anesthetist should perform valuable service by providing "vocal local technique". Anesthetist should talk constantly to the patient that everything is going well. One of the most difficult situations of local anesthesia is that, the patient, rather than the surgeon, becomes the center of attraction for all noises and comments made in the room during surgery.

It is important to understand that under local anesthesia adequate sedation and analgesia are administered to keep the patient somnolent but responsive. Continuous monitoring of all the vitals is essential throughout the procedure. Secondly, it is essential that a pneumoperitoneum of approximately 1.5 to 3 liters be present under pressure.

Anesthetist's Role in Laparoscopy

The role of anesthetist in laparoscopic surgery is vital. The laparoscopic surgery should never be performed if anesthetist has no experience in minimal access surgical anesthesia. It is up to anesthetist to identify whether he is capable of performing realistically without compromising the safety of the patients. It is only on these clearly established bases that safe laparoscopy can be contemplated.

The following monitoring device should routinely used at the time of minimal access surgical general anesthesia:

- Electrocardiogram
- Sphygmomanometer
- Airway pressure monitor
- Pulse oximeter
- End tidal CO_2 concentration ($PETCO_2$) monitor
- Peripheral nerve stimulator
- Body temperature probe.

A balanced anesthesia using appropriate amount of muscle relaxant, intravenous and epidural narcotics and artificial ventilation is essential to combat the insult and the effects of pneumoperitoneum, namely the resorption of carbon dioxide, diaphragmatic movement impairment and the reduction in lung volumes. The direct arterial pressure monitoring and records of blood pressure and the blood gases estimation is needed. The CVP monitoring helps in assessing the preload status. The ECG monitoring demonstrates the rhythm status continuously.

The prophylactic heparin should be used in accordance with prevention of deep venous thrombosis and subsequent pulmonary embolism. The use of intermittent inflated pneumatic cast compression helps in maintaining circulation in the legs during the operation. Now, epidural anesthesia is also considered as a safe alternative to general anesthesia for outpatient laparoscopy without associated respiratory depression.

INTRAOPERATIVE COMPLICATIONS

If anesthetic consideration is not taken properly arrhythmias have been associated with laparoscopy. The most common are junctional rhythms, bigemini and asystole. Bradycardia has been reported due to rapid insufflation especially in older patients. The increasing pressure on the peritoneum increases vagal tone and bradycardia may develop. This bradycardia may be increased secondary to absorption of CO_2. Atropine has proven effective in restoring vagal tone.

The development of a CO_2 gas embolus is a rarely encountered emergency. It develops due to intravasations of CO_2 used in laparoscopic surgery. Some apparent sign of air embolism include a sudden drop in end tidal CO_2, a drop in blood pressure and development of an arrhythmia. A classic "water wheel" or "mill wheel" murmur will be heard in cardiac auscultatory area. Should such an event be suspected further insufflation should be immediately stopped and abdomen should be deflated. The patient should be turned towards left and head down to deviate the bubbles of CO_2 away from heart. The patient should be hyperventilated with 100 percent O_2. If a central line is present, aspiration of the embolus should be attempted.

Pulmonary edema can result from aggressive fluid replacement or irrigating fluid absorption. Fluid management is even more difficult in gynecological procedure where hysteroscopy is combined. Pulmonary edema is prevented by monitoring fluid input and output. Intraoperative diuretics should be administered if a large discrepancy between fluid input and output is found. If a patient develops respiratory distress, pulmonary edema should always be considered. Rales couples with classic chest radiographic findings will confirm the diagnosis.

Patient Selection

- Patients with cardiac pathology must be subjected to a thorough preoperative assessment taking the particular hemodynamic conditions imposed by laparoscopic surgery into account.
- Patients presenting with decompensated congestive cardiopathy are at highest risk of laparoscopic surgery because the hemodynamic repercussions would be too difficult to manage, even with the help of invasive monitoring techniques.
- The increase in systemic vascular resistance and the oxygen requirements of the myocardium could be the risk factor in cardiac patients. For these patients, the postoperative benefits of laparoscopic surgery must be weighed against the intraoperative risks. Preoperative investigation in these patients enables this risk to be evaluated more closely. The cardiac reserve must be assessed carefully; in particular myocardial contractility and the ejection fraction should be estimated.
- The drop in venous return during peritoneal insufflation is one of the important factors which are responsible for drop in cardiac output during laparoscopic surgery. This drop in venous return is more important when the hypovolemia develops due to excessive bleeding, indicating that hypovolemia is a contraindication, at least for as long as their circulating volume has not been

restored to normal. This point is particularly important for ruptured ectopic pregnancy or during laparoscopic surgical exploration of abdominal injuries.

Monitoring

Careful monitoring of a patient undergoing laparoscopic surgical procedure is very important. Monitoring has certain elements in common for all patients. Others are more specific to patients with cardiopathy. A multi parameter monitor (Fig. 4.2) is essential and minimum parameters are important to look for:
1. ECG
2. Rate of respiration
3. SpO_2
4. NIBP
5. Temperature
6. Pulse rate
7. Cardiac output
8. $EtCO_2$

Routine Monitoring

The stethoscope remains an important instrument enabling anesthetist to auscultate both the lungs after any change in position and after insufflation of the pneumoperitoneum, because it pushes back the tracheal carina, can displace intubation to the right. The use of a stethoscope in the precordial position is a good practice in order to detect gas embolism, but requires permanent auscultation.

Electrocardioscopic monitoring during laparoscopy enables arrhythmia, which may occur due to

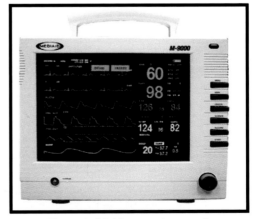

Fig. 4.2: Multiparameter monitor

hypercapnia, to be rapidly detected. At the time of laparoscopic surgery, sudden appearance of a microvoltage can be the sign of subcutaneous emphysema or pneumomediastinum.

Oximetry monitoring (SpO_2) is essential part of any surgery but it is especially important in laparoscopic surgery because the dim lighting in the laparoscopic surgery theatre and the wearing of protective glasses, if a laser is being used make it difficult to recognize cyanosis. In any case, the latter is a late clinical sign of hypoxia. Variations in saturation are not specific during laparoscopic surgery. Desaturation is a late sign of complications such as gas embolism, pneumothorax, selective intubation or a shunt effect due to excessively high intraperitoneal pressure.

During laparoscopic surgery, control of intraperitoneal pressure is an integral part of the anesthesia monitoring. The insufflator must be microprocessor controlled; it must be reliable and subjected to regular checks. Excessive intraperitoneal pressure must trigger an alert and an immediate halt in insufflation. As the majority of older insufflators do not have safety valve for a reduction in intraperitoneal pressure, this must be carried out by manual exsufflation via opening the valve of cannula.

Monitoring of the neuromuscular block is also important. Proper relaxation is good for laparoscopic surgery. Stable and deep myoresolution improves the laparoscopic surgeon's view and limits the peritoneal insufflation pressures. In addition, the wide range of operating times and the rapidity with which an operation is terminated means it is essential to know exactly what the neuromuscular block situation is at any point in time. When equipment for reading the muscular activity in the thumb is not available, the simplest stimulation is a train of four on a temporal branch of the facial nerve and observation of the contraction of the orbicular eye muscle.

Intraperitoneal insufflation of dry and unheated gas, possibly accompanied by irrigation with cold liquids results in heat loss during laparoscopic surgery which is at least equal to that with laparotomy. Temperature monitoring associated with measures to combat heat loss is also essential when procedures take several hours. It is important to remember that excessive leakage of gas through the cannula causes rapid hypothermia to the patient.

Cardiovascular Monitoring

Measurement via the bloodstream enables arterial pressure to be monitored in real time. In addition the appearance of cyclic variations in time with ventilation is an excellent indication of drops in pre-loading which prompt the intraperitoneal insufflation pressure to be limited, to increase filling or even to accentuate the Trendelenburg's position when possible. Installation of an arterial entry point, also helps with blood gas measurements.

Measurement of central venous pressure is traditionally used to supervise the filling pressures in the right heart. This becomes difficult during laparoscopic surgery because of the changes in position which require continual changes at cell level, and particularly because of the increase in intrathoracic pressure transmitted from the peritoneal area via the diaphragm. It is important to perform simultaneous measurement of intrathoracic pressure which is obtained by esophageal pressure, and to deduct this from the measured central venous pressure.

Catheterization of the right heart using a Swan Ganz probe has been used for monitoring during laparoscopic surgery (Fig. 4.3). As for central venous pressure, the values measured need to be corrected according to the intrathoracic pressure. An increase in pulmonary arterial pressure is an early sign of gas embolism. Aspiration of the gas bubbles by the proximal orifice placed in the right atrium theoretically

Section One

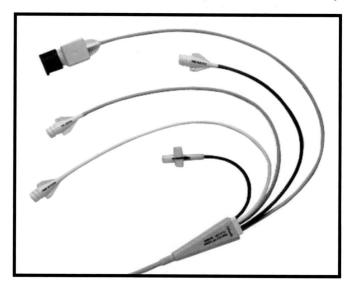

Fig. 4.3: Swan Ganz catheter

helps to minimize the consequences of air embolism. The use of a Swan Ganz probe during laparoscopy for patients with coronary disease helps adapt the anesthesia protocol and therapy, for simple measurement of arterial pressure is insufficient in 80 percent of these cases. Nevertheless in the course of general anesthesia with controlled ventilation when SaO_2, hemoglobin and oxygen consumption are stable, a change in SvO_2 is often the sign of a change in cardiac flow rate.

Because right heart catheterization is an invasive procedure, several studies have reported the use of cardiac flow rate monitoring by electrical bio-impedance during laparoscopic surgery. The principle is founded on continuous measurement of the blood flow rate in the thorax by analysis of the variations in conductivity relative to an electrical field. Transthoracic electrical bio-impedance brings a certain number of advantages:

- Low-risk (non-invasive monitoring)
- Easy and simple to use
- Continuous measurement in real time
- Not limited in time
- Inexpensive
- Reliability seems to be satisfactory compared to other methods.

It is important that the skin be carefully prepared and the electrodes are of good quality and correctly positioned. However, its use in standard monitoring is still limited due in large part to the frequent difficulties encountered in interpreting the variations.

Some studies have been made of hemodynamic monitoring during laparoscopic surgery using trans-esophageal ultrasound cardiography. Whereas the advantages of this technique for monitoring and diagnosis are considerable, the cost remains an important barrier. Interpretation can also be difficult because of the variations in the viewing axis of the heart according to peritoneal pressure and the variable patient's position.

Measurement of the cardiac flow rate by pulsed Doppler velocimetry can be carried out by either the transesophageal or the supra-sternum route at the time of laparoscopic surgery. The basic principle is the same as with any Doppler device with a piezoelectric transducer transmitter and a transducer receiver which receives the return echoes modified by the Doppler

effect when they bounce off mobile structures like wall of the heart, vessels or red blood cells. Based on the effective diameter of the aorta which can either be calculated from the cardiac flow rate measured by another method, or estimated from the patients biometric factors, the ejection volume can be deduced and thus the continuous cardiac flow rate.

Respiratory Monitoring

The CO_2 end tidal pressure ($PetCO_2$) provides evidence of production of carbon dioxide by the cellular metabolism, absorbed through the peritoneal cavity and pulmonary exchanges (Fig. 4.4). A rapid increase in $PetCO_2$ is a complication:

- A rapid rise of a few millimeters of mercury returning a few minutes later to the base figures may be the sign of minimal CO_2 gas embolism.
- A more gradual and persistent rise is often the sign of extraperitoneal diffusion of CO_2 (preperitoneal, subcutaneous, retroperitoneal, mediastinal, etc.). This increase in expired CO_2 continues after exsufflation of the pneumoperitoneum, indeed often several hours after the laparoscopic procedure, justifying a follow-up of hypercapnia in the recovery room.
- The CO_2 is transported by the circulatory system from the peripheral areas towards the lungs. Any disturbance in the circulation will reduce the CO_2 expired. A rapid drop in $PetCO_2$ may be the sign of a drop in cardiac flow rate or a decreased venous return, but also pulmonary arterial obliteration. This is what happens in massive gas embolism which shows up as a drop in $PetCO_2$ proportional in size and duration to the volume of the CO_2 embolus.

Classically the $PetCO_2$ values are 2 to 6 mm Hg lower than $PaCO_2$. During anesthesia with artificial ventilation, the ventilation/perfusion ratio of often greater than 1, so a $PaCO_2$-$PetCO_2$ gradient of 10 to 15 mm Hg must be expected. However, during laparoscopic surgery, the change in the arterial CO_2-$ETCO_2$ gradient is very variable.

Changes in position such as the Trendelenburg's or the lateral reclined position can modify the value of the $PetCO_2$. Furthermore, it is shown that in cases of cardiovascular disease, the correlation between $PetCO_2$ and $PaCO_2$ was less good when compared

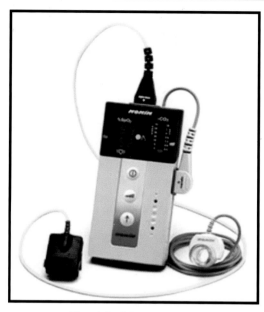

Fig. 4.4: CO_2 monitor

with patients with no such pathology, and the same is true with obese patients. A recent study confirms that in patients with respiratory impairment; the increases in $PaCO_2$ are underestimated by $PetCO_2$. So for these patients with respiratory or heart pathology, it is particularly useful to duplicate the $PetCO_2$ measurement by arterial gasometry at the beginning of the operation and every time there is an important variation in $PetCO_2$.

In view of this uncertainty, transcutaneous CO_2 monitoring would give a better idea of $PaCO_2$, but this also raises a certain number of technical problems (heating of electrodes, difficulties with measurements in adults, etc.).

Anesthetist should keep following points in mind at the time of laparoscopic surgery:

1. The patient voids urine just prior to entering the operating room.
2. No shaving is necessary.
3. All patients undergoing laparoscopy should have an empty bowel. In the unlikely event of bowel damage, there is much less risk of contamination if the bowel is empty.
4. The position of leg is important considering different laparoscopic procedure. Pressure stocking prevents DVT.

5. Good muscle relaxation reduces the intra-abdominal pressure required for adequate working room in abdominal cavity.
6. The inflation of stomach should be avoided during artificial ventilation using mask as this increases the risk of gastric injury during trocar insertion or instrumentation.
7. The distended stomach also hampers the visibility of Calot's triangle at the time of laparoscopic cholecystectomy or laparoscopic bile duct surgery.
8. Tracheal intubation and intermittent positive pressure ventilation should be routinely used. This ensures airway protection and controls pulmonary ventilation to avoid hypocarbia.
9. The ventilatory pattern should be adjusted according to respiratory and hemodynamic performance of the individual patient.
10. Ventilation with large tidal volumes (12-15 ml/kg) prevents alveolar atelectasis and hypoxemia and allows adequate alveolar ventilation and CO_2 elimination.
11. Halothane increases the incidence of arrhythmia during laparoscopic surgery especially in the presence of hypercarbia.
12. Isoflurane is the preferred volatile anesthetic agent in minimal access surgery as it has less arrhythmogenic and myocardial depressant effects.
13. Patients should receive adequate airway humidification and protection against unintentional hypothermia because generally the duration of operation is more in laparoscopic surgery.
14. Excessive intravenous sedation should be avoided because it diminishes airway reflexes against pulmonary aspiration in the event of regurgitation.
15. Monitoring of $PetCO_2$ is mandatory during laparoscopic surgery. The continuous monitoring of $PetCO_2$ allows adjustment of the minute ventilation to maintain normal concentration of carbon dioxide and oxygen.
16. Airway pressure monitor is mandatory for anesthetized patients receiving intermittent positive pressure ventilation.

Section One

Postoperative Considerations

At the end of the procedure, antagonism of the residual muscle relaxation should be reversed by appropriate dose of neostigmine. When patient is awake he or she should be extubated and transferred to the recovery room in a semi-recumbent position. Before extubation, the patient's stomach may be emptied with an orogastric tube. During the next five hours in the postoperative period, analgesia should be achieved. Patients spend a minimum of an hour in the recovery room. Vital signs and O_2 saturation are monitored and supplemental O_2 is administered by mask or nasal prongs.

Nausea is frequent after general anesthesia. Intravenous droperidol, ondensetrone or metoclopramide can be administered if nausea persists. Vomiting is also common after recovery from anesthesia. Ondem or vomiset, given half an hour before reversal agent is very helpful in preventing postoperative nausea and vomiting.

The urine output should be at rate of 100 ml/h and that should continue for 18 hours postoperatively. The nursing management included oxygen therapy, early mobilization, incentive spirometry and chest physiotherapy. These should repeat at 2 hour interval. On the morning of the second post operative day the patient should be mobile, pain free, and should start soft diet. She or he should be transferred to the surgical ward and may be discharged home next day if everything is alright.

It is very common to expect some pain after the procedure. Shoulder pain may occur as a result of distension of the abdomen with gas. As the gas absorbs into the bloodstream and is exhaled through the lungs the pain will gradually disappear, usually over 24 or 48 hours. Depending on the surgery carried out, there may be some interference in bowel function leading to abdominal distension and colicky discomfort. Tramadol hydrochloride is effective for these types of pain. Initial loading dose of these analgesics if administered can give smooth painless recovery.

All procedures under anesthesia carry small but inherent risks and patient should understand these before agreeing to undergo the procedure. However, the risks of anesthesia for elective surgery under modern conditions are very small indeed.

BIBLIOGRAPHY

1. Cunningham AJ, Turner J, Rosenbaum S, Rafferty T. Transoesophegeal echocardiographic assessment of haemodynamic function during laparoscopic cholecystectomy. Br J Anaesth 1993;70: 621–5.
2. Dorsay DA, Greene FL, Baysinger CL. Hemodynamic changes during laparoscopic cholecystectomy monitored with transesophegeal echocardiography. Surg Endosc 1995;9: 128–34.
3. Gannedahl P, Odeberg S, Brodin LA, Sollevi A. Effects of posture and pneumoperitoneum during anaesthesia on the indices of left ventricular filling. Acta Anaesthesiol Scand 1996;40:160–66.
4. Girardis M, Broi UD, Antonutto G, Pasetto A. The effect of laparoscopic cholecystectomy on cardiovascular function and pulmonary gas exchange. Anesth Analg 1996;83:134–40.
5. Hachenberg T, Ebel C, Czorny M, Thomas H, Wendt M. Intrathoracic and pulmonary blood volume during CO2-pneumoperitoneum in humans. Acta Anaesthesiol Scand 1998;42:794–8.
6. Ho HS, Saunders CJ, Gunther RA, Wolfe BM. Effector of hemodynamics during laparoscopy: CO2 absorption or intraabdominal pressure? J Surg Res 1995;59:497–503.
7. Ido K, Suzuki T, Taniguchi Y, Kawamoto C, Isoda N, Nagamine N, Ioka T, Kimura K, Kumagai M, Hirayama Y. Femoral vein stasis during laparoscopic cholecystectomy: effects of graded elastic compression leg bandages in preventing thrombus formation. Gastrointest Endosc 1995;42:151–55.
8. Ishizaki Y, Bandai Y, Shimomura K, Abe H, Ohtomo Y, Idezuki Y. Safe intraabdominal pressure of carbon dioxide pneumoperitoneum during laparoscopic surgery. Surgery 1993;114: 549–54.
9. Joris JL, Noirot DP, Legrand MJ, Jacquet NJ, Lamy ML. Hemodynamic changes during laparoscopic cholecystectomy. Anesth, Analg 1993;76: 1067–71.
10. Koivusalo AM, Kellokumpu I, Scheinin M, Tikkanen I, Makisalo H, Lindgren L. A comparison of gasless mechanical and conventional carbon dioxide pneumoperitoneum methods for laparoscopic cholecystectomy. Anesth Analg 1998;86:153–158.
11. Matzen S, Perko G, Groth S, Friedman DB, Secher NH. Blood volume distribution during head-up tilt induced central hypovolaemia in man. Clin Physiol 1991;11: 411–22.
12. Myre K, Rostrup M, Buanes T, Stokland O. Plasma catecholamines and haemodynamic changes during pneumoperitoneum. Acta. Anaesthesiol Scand 1998;42: 343–47.
13. O'Leary E, Hubbart K, Tormey W, Cunningham AJ. Laparoscopic cholecystectomy: haemodynamic and neuroendocrine responses after pneumoperitoneum and changes in position. Br J Anaesth 1996;76: 640–4.
14. Schwenk W, Bohm B, Fugener A, Muller JM. Intermittent pneumatic sequential compression (ISC) of the lower extremities prevents venous stasis during laparoscopic cholecystectomy: a prospective randomized study. Surg Endosc 1998;12:7–11.

15. Shuto K, Kitano S, Yoshida T, Bandoh T, Mitarai Y, Kobayashi M. Hemodynamic and arterial blood gas changes during carbon dioxide and helium pneumoperitoneum in pigs. Surg Endosc 1995;9: 1173–8.

16. Walder AD, Aitkenhead AR. Role of vasopressin in the haemodynamic response to laparoscopic cholecystectomy. Br J Anaesth, 1997;78:264–266-77.

17. Mariano ER, Furukawa L, Woo RK et al. Anesthetic concerns for robot-assisted laparoscopy in an infant. Anesth Analg 2004;99:1665–7.

18. Wilcox S, Vandam LD. Alas, poor Trendelenburg and his position! A critique of its uses and effectiveness. Anesth Analg, 1998;67:574–8.

19. Sprung J, Whalley DG, Falcone T et al. The impact of morbid obesity, pneumoperitoneum and posture on respiratory system mechanics and oxygenation during laparoscopy. Anesth Analg 2002;94:1345–50.

20. Oliver SB, Cucchiara RF, Warner MA et al. Unexpected focal neurologic deficit on emergence from anesthesia: a report of three cases. Anesthesiology 1987;67:823–6.

21. Winter R, Munro M. Lingual and buccal nerve neuropathy in a patient in the prone position: a case report. Anesthesiology, 1989;71:452–4.

22. Case EH, Stiles JA. The effects of various surgical positions on vital capacity. Anesthesiology 1946;7:29–31.

23. Collins VJ. Principles of anesthesiology, 2nd edn. Lea and Febiger, Philadelphia. 1976.

24. Henderson Y, Haggard HW. The circulation in man in head down position and a method for measuring the venous return to the heart. J Pharm Exp Therap 1918;11:189–201.

25. Donald JS, Gamble CJ, Shaw R. The cardiac output in man. Am J Physiol 1934;109:666.

26. Kubal K, Komatsu T, Sanchala V et al. Trendelenburg position used during venous cannulation increases myocardial oxygen demands. Anesth Analg 1984;63:239.

27. Hirvonen EA, Nuutinen LS, Kauko M. Hemodynamic changes due to Trendelenburg positioning and pneumoperitoneum during laparoscopic hysterectomy. Acta Anaesthesiol Scand 1995;39:949–955.

28. Irwin MG, Ng JKF. Transoesophageal acoustic quantification for evaluation of cardiac function during laparoscopic, surgery. Anaesthesia 2001;56:623–9.

29. Taura P, Lopez A, Lacy AM et al Prolonged pneumo-peritoneum at 15 mmHg causes lactic acidosis. Surg Endosc 1998;12:198–201.

30. Andrei VE, Schein M, Margolis M et al. Liver enzymes are commonly elevated following laparoscopic cholecys-tectomy—is elevated intra-abdominal pressure the cause? Dig Surg 1998;15:256–9.

31. Glantzounis GK, Tselepis AD, Tambaki AP et al. Laparoscopic surgery-induced changes in oxidative stress markers in human plasma. Surg Endosc 2001;15:1315–19.

32. Bandyopadhyay D, Kapadia CR. Large bowel ischemia following laparoscopic inguinal hernioplasty. Surg Endosc, 2003;17:520–1.

33. Andrei VE, Schein M, Wise L. Small bowel ischemia following laparoscopic cholecystectomy. Dig Surg 1999;16: 522–4.

34. Hasson HM, Galanopoulos C, Langerman A. Ischemic necrosis of small bowel following laparoscopic surgery. JSLS 2004;8:159–63.

35. Razvi HA, Fields D, Vargas JC et al. Oliguria during laparoscopic surgery—evidence for direct renal parenchymal compression as an etiologic factor. J Endourol 1996;10: 1–4.

36. Nguyen NT, Perez RV, Fleming N et al. Effect of prolonged pneumoperitoneum on intraoperative urine output during laparoscopic gastric bypass. J Am Coll Surg 2002;195: 476–83.

37. McDougall EM, Monk TG, Wolf JS et al. The effect of prolonged pneumoperitoneum on renal function in an animal, model. J Am Coll Surg 1996;182:317–28.

38. Ben-Haim M, Rosenthal RJ. Causes of arterial hypertension and splanchnic ischemia during acute elevations in intra-abdominal pressure with CO_2 pneumoperitoneum: a complex central nervous system mediated response. Int J Colorectal Dis 1999;14:227–36.

39. Walder AD, Aitkenhead AR. Role of vasopressin in the haemodynamic response to laparoscopic cholecystectomy. Br, J Anaesth 1997;78:264–66.

40. Dorsay DA, Green FL, Baysinger CL. Hemodynamic changes during laparoscopic cholecystectomy monitored with transesophageal echocardiography. Surg Endosc 1995;9:128–34.

41. Cunningham AJ, Turner J, Rosenbaum set al. Trans-esophageal echocardiographic assessment of haemodynamic function during laparoscopic cholecystectomy. Br J Anaesth 1993;70:621–5.

42. Odeberg S, Ljungqvist O, Svenberg T et al. Haemodynamic effects of pneumoperitoneum and the influence of posture during anesthesia for laparoscopic surgery. Acta Anaesthesiol Scand 1994;38:276–83.

43. Miller R. Miller's Anesthesia, 6th edn. Elsevier, Philadelphia 28. Joris JL, Noirot DP, Legrand MJ et al (1993) Hemodynamic changes during laparoscopic cholecystectomy. Anesth Analg 2005;76:1067–1071.

44. Joris JL, Hamoir EE, Hartstein GM et al. Hemodynamic changes and catecholamine release during laparoscopic adrenalectomy for pheochromocytoma. Anesth Analg 1999;88:16–21.

45. Feig BW, Berger DH, Dougherty TB et al. Pharmacologic intervention can reestablish baseline hemodynamic parameters during laparoscopy. Surgery 1994;116:733–71.

46. Root B, Levy MN, Pollack S et al. Gas embolism death after laparoscopy delayed by "trapping" in portal circulation. Anesth Analg 1978;37:232–7.

47. Brunner F, Frick P, Bu¨hlmann A. Post decompression shock due to extravasation of plasma. Lancet 1964;1:1071–3.

48. Boussuges A, Blanc P, Molenat F et al. Haemoconcentration in neurological decompression illness. Int J Sports Med 1996;17:351–5.

49. Diakun TA. Carbon dioxide embolism: Successful resuscitation with cardiopulmonary bypass. Anesthesiology 1991;74:1151–3.

50. Makinen MT. Comparison of body temperature changes during laparoscopic and open cholecystectomy. Acta Anaesthesiol Scand 1997;41:736–40.

51. Stewart BT, Stitz RW, Tuch MM et al. Hypothermia in open and laparoscopic colorectal surgery. Dis Colon Rectum 1999;42:1292–1295, 66 J Robotic Surg 2008;2:59–66.

5 Abdominal Access Techniques

Minimal access surgery, a new surgical and interventional approach was called by different name and one of the popular is minimally invasive surgery. However, this terminology is considered inappropriate by Prof. Cuschieri for two reasons. Firstly, it carries connotations of increased safety, which is not the case. Secondly, it is semantically incorrect since to invade is absolute, and indeed such interventions are as invasive as open surgery in terms of reach of the various organs and tissues. The hallmark of the new approaches is the reduction in the trauma of access. Hence, a more appropriate generic term is minimal access therapy.

In minimal access surgery, the technique of first entry inside the human body with telescope and instruments is called access technique. Technique of access is different for different minimal access surgical procedures. Thoracoscopy, retroperitoneoscopy, axilloscopy have different ways of access.

It is important to know that approximately 20 percent of laparoscopic complications are caused at the time of initial access. Developing access skill is one of the important achievements for the surgeon practicing minimal access surgery. First entry or access in laparoscopy is of two types, closed and open access.

CLOSED ACCESS

In closed access technique, pneumoperitoneum is created by Veress needle. This is a blind technique and most commonly practiced way of access by surgeons and gynecologists worldwide. Closed technique of access merely by Veress needle insertion and creation of pneumoperitoneum is an easy way of access but it is not possible in some of the minimal

access surgical procedures like axilloscopy, retroperitoneoscopy and totally extraperitoneal approach of hernia repair. In general, closed technique by Veress needle is possible only if there is a preformed cavity like abdomen.

OPEN ACCESS

In this, there is direct entry by open technique, without creating pneumoperitoneum and insufflator is connected once blunt trocar is inside the abdominal cavity under direct vision. There are various ways of open access like Hasson's technique, Scandinavian technique and Fielding technique.

Some surgeons and gynecologists practice blind trocar insertion without pneumoperitoneum. The incidence of injury due to this type of access is much higher. This type of direct trocar entry is practiced by gynecologists for sterilization. Sterilization may be performed because in multipara patients the lower abdominal wall is lax; making the fascia thinner and easy elevation by hand is possible.

Bleeding due to accidental damage to a major vessel during this initial stage is one of the most dangerous complications of laparoscopic surgery.

Anatomy of Anterior Abdominal Wall

There are three large, flat muscles (External oblique, internal oblique, and transverses abdominis) and one long vertically oriented segmental muscle (rectus abdominis) on each side. Four major arteries on each side are also present which form an anastomotic arcade that supplies the abdominal wall. The superior and inferior epigastric artery and the branches provide the major blood supply to the rectus abdominis muscle and other medial structures (Fig. 5.1).

Among all these arteries, the most important for laparoscopic surgeon is the inferior epigastric artery and vein. The inferior epigastric vessels landmark is less variable compared to superior epigastric. Bleeding from inferior epigastric is a big problem because it is larger in diameter than superior epigastric.

Umbilicus is the site of choice for access. It is the scar remaining after the umbilical cord obliterates. At the level of umbilicus, skin fascia and peritoneum are fused together, with the minimum fat. The midline is free of muscle fibers, nerves and vessels except at its inferior edge where pyramidalis muscle is sometimes found. Trocar site in these locations rarely cause much bleeding. The colon is attached to the lateral abdominal wall along both gutters and puncture laterally should be under video control to avoid visceral injury.

When left subcostal site is chosen for access it should be 2 cm below the costal margin. The costal margin provides good resistance as the needle is introduced. When puncture site lateral to the midline is used, it is prudent to choose location lateral to the linea semilunaris to avoid injury of superior and inferior epigastric vessels. In obese patients, the linea semilunaris may not be visible. In these, location of inferior artery can be localized by careful trans-illumination.

Access to preperitoneal space is gained by penetrating almost all the layer of abdominal wall except peritoneum. The open technique of access is preferable in this situation. After incising the fascia with the scalpel, fingered dissection is advisable to avoid puncture of peritoneum.

CLOSED ACCESS TECHNIQUE

Creation of pneumoperitoneum is one of the most important steps in laparoscopy. The aim is to build up a good protective cushion to ensure the safe entry of trocar and cannula.

Veress Needle Insertion

The standard method of insufflations of the abdominal cavity is via a Veress needle inserted through a small skin incision in the infraumbilical region. The Veress needle consists of a sharp needle with an internal spring loaded trocar. The trocar is blunt ended with a lumen and side hole. Disposable and non-disposable metal Veress needles are available commercially in different lengths, i.e. long for obese patients, short for thin or pediatric patients.

Before using Veress needle, it should be checked for its patency and spring action (Fig. 5.2). Spring action of Veress needle can be checked by pulling the head out. The disposable Veress needle spring action can be checked by pressing the sharp end against any sterilized draping (Fig. 5.3).

Insufflation via the Veress needle creates a cushion of gas over the bowel for insertion of the first trocar. Insufflation then retracts the anterior abdominal wall, exposing the operative field.

Preparation of Patient

The patient should be nil orally since the morning of surgery. In some of the procedure like LAVH or

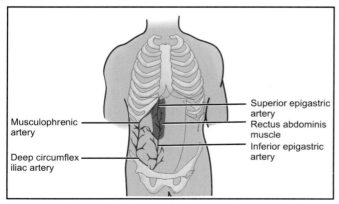

Fig. 5.1: Anterior abdominal wall anatomy

Musculophrenic artery

Deep circumflex iliac artery

Superior epigastric artery

Rectus abdominis muscle

Inferior epigastric artery

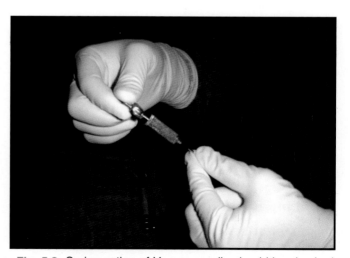

Fig. 5.2: Spring action of Veress needle should be checked

Section One

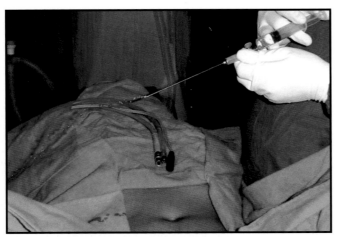

Fig. 5.3: Patency of Veress needle should be checked

colorectal surgery where distended bowel may interfere, it is good to prepare bowel prior to the night of surgery by giving some mild purgative. Bowel preparation can minimize the need of accessory port to retract the bowel.

Before coming to operation theater patient should always void urine. The full urinary bladder may get perforation at the time of insertion of Veress needle or trocar. If the laparoscopic procedure is going to be performed of upper abdomen then Foley's catheterization is not necessary. If gynecological operative surgery or any general surgical lower abdominal procedure has to be performed (like hernia or adhesiolysis) it is wise to insert Foley's catheter.

If surgeon is going to perform any upper abdominal procedure like cholecystectomy, fundoplication, Duodenal perforation, hiatus hernia, etc it is good practice to have nasogastric tube in place. A distended stomach will not allow proper visualization of Calot's triangle and then surgeon has to apply more traction over fundus or Hartman pouch and this may cause tenting of CBD followed by accidental injury. In gynecological or lower abdominal laparoscopic procedure, it is not necessary to put nasogastric tube.

In minimal access surgery, shaving of skin is not must and if necessary it should be done on operation table itself by surgeon.

Operating Room Set-up

An organized well equipped operation theater is essential for successful laparoscopy. The entire surgical team should be familiar with the instruments and their function. Each instrument should be inspected periodically for loose or broken tips even if the same instrument was used during a previous procedure. It is necessary to confirm proper sterilization of instruments because the surgeon ultimately is responsible for the proper functioning of all instrument and equipment.

The entire instrument should be placed according to wish of the surgeon so that it should be ergonomically perfect for that surgery. The co-axial alignment should be maintained. Co-axial alignment means the eye of the surgeon, target of dissection and monitor should be placed in same axis.

Patient Position

Initially at the time of pneumoperitoneum by Veress needle, patient should be placed supine with 10-20 degrees head-down. The benefit of this steep Trendelenburg's position is that bowel will be pulled up and there will be more room in pelvic cavity for safe entry of veress needle. It is important to remember that, patient should be placed in head down position only if surgeon is planning to insert veress needle pointing towards pelvis cavity. If surgeon is planning to insert Veress needle perpendicular to abdominal wall as in case of very obese patient or diagnostic laparoscopy in local anesthesia, the patient should be placed in supine position otherwise all the bowel will come just below the umbilicus and there is increased risk of bowel injury.

In gynecological laparoscopic procedures or if laparoscopy is planned to be performed together with hysteroscopy, patient should be positioned in lithotomy position and one assistant should be positioned between the leg of patient. Patient's leg should be comfortably supported by padded obstetric leg holders or Allen stirrups which minimizes the risk of venous thrombosis. In these procedure, surgeon need to use uterine manipulator for proper visualization of female reproductive organs. The assistant seating between the legs of patient will keep on watching the hand movement of surgeon on monitor and he should give traction with the handle of uterine monitor in appropriate direction.

If thoracoscopy or retroperitoneoscopy is planned then patient is placed in lateral position (Fig. 5.4).

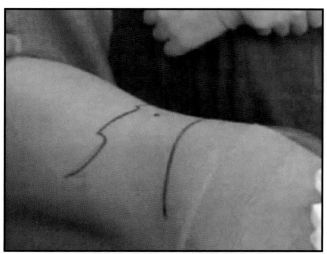

Fig. 5.4: Patient position in retroperitoneoscopy

Position of Surgical Team

The laparoscopic surgeon is very much dependent and helpless with eye fixed on monitor. At the time of laparoscopic surgery, surgeon is largely depending on the skill of his assistant. If the surgery is of upper abdomen, French surgeons like to stand between the legs of patient, popularly known as "French position" (Fig. 5.5).

The American surgeons like to operate from left in cases of upper abdominal surgery like fundoplication and hiatus hernia called as "American position".

It is not wise to remain standing in any one position and surgeon can walk to the other side of operation table to achieve proper ergonomics. In most of the cases at the time of access, surgeon should stand on left side of the patient. If surgeon is left handed, he should stand right to the patient at the time of access. This helps in inserting Veress needle and trocar towards pelvis by dominant hand. Once all the ports are in position, the surgeon should come opposite to the side of pathology to start surgery. In cholecystectomy, appendectomy, right sided hernia or right ovarian cyst, surgeon should stand left to the patient. In left sided pathology like left ovarian cyst and left sided hernia it is ergonomically better for surgeon to stand right to the patient (Fig. 5.6).

In most of the upper abdominal surgery, camera assistant should stand left to the surgeon and in lower abdominal surgery he or she should stand right to the surgeon. Camera assistant while holding telescope can pass his or her hand between body and arm of surgeon so that some time surgeon can help him to focus his camera correctly. Camera assistant can be placed opposite to the surgeon to stand but in this case it is better to have two monitor on both the side of patient, one for surgeon and one for camera stand and other members of surgical team.

The surgeon should work in the most comfortable and less tiring position possible with shoulder relaxed, arms alongside of the body, elbows at 90° angle and forearm horizontal.

Preparation for Access

Before starting access, abdomen should be examined for any palpable lump. It is wise to tell the patient to void urine before coming to operating room but if the bladder is found full at the time of palpation. Foley's should be applied. Remember that full bladder may be injured very easily by veress needle or trocar (Figs 5.7A to D).

Section One

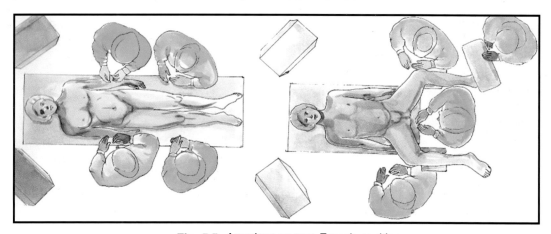

Fig. 5.5: American versus French position

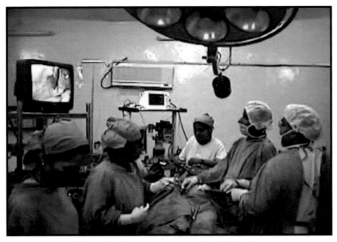

Fig. 5.6: Surgeons stands left to the patient in most of the right sided pathology

Once the patient is cleaned painted and draped, all the connection should be attached, followed by focusing and white balancing of camera. At the time of focusing, the distance between the gauge piece and tip of the telescope should be 6 to 8 cm.

Choice of Gas for Pneumoperitoneum

At first, pneumoperitoneum was created by filtered room air. Carbon dioxide and nitrous oxide are now preferred gas because of increased risk of air embolism with room air. CO_2 is used for insufflation as it is 200 times more diffusible than oxygen. It is rapidly cleared from the body by the lungs and will not support combustion. N_2O is only 68 percent as rapidly absorbed in blood as CO_2. N_2O has one advantage over CO_2 that it has mild analgesic effect, and hence no pain if diagnostic laparoscopy is performed under local anesthesia. CO_2 has the advantage of being non-combustible and allows the concomitant use of electro-coagulation and laser irradiation. For short operative procedures like sterilization or drilling, under local anesthetic N_2O may also be used. During prolonged laparoscopic procedure, N_2O should not be a preferred gas for pneumoperitoneum because it supports combustion better than air. CO_2 when comes in contact with peritoneal fluid converts into carbonic acid. Carbonic acid irritates diaphragm causing shoulder tip pain and discomfort in abdomen. Carbonic acid has one advantage also that it alters pH of peritoneal fluid (acidotic changes) and it is mild antiseptic so the chances of infection may be slightly less compared to

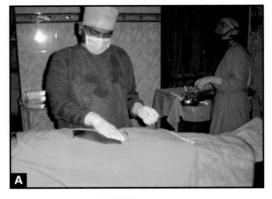

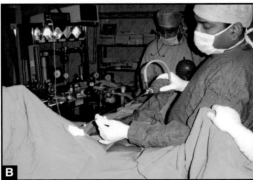

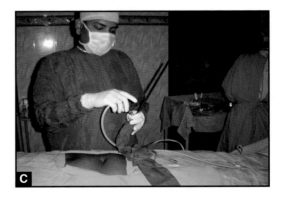

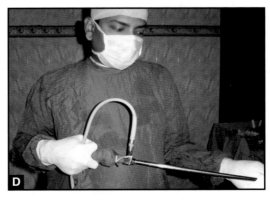

Figs 5.7A to D: Preparation before access; palpation of abdomen, attachment of cables, focusing and white balancing

any other gas. Helium gas being inert in nature is also tried in many centers but it does not have any added benefit over CO_2.

Site of Veress Needle Entry

There are many sites of Veress needle entry tried for Veress needle insertion but central location of umbilicus and ability of umbilicus to hide scar makes it most attractive site for primary port.

Umbilical is good site for access because it is:
- Thinnest abdominal wall (easy access)
- Cosmetically better
- No significant blood vessels
- Ergonomically better (center point of abdomen).

Initially there was controversy regarding use of umbilicus for first port access. First concern was regarding infection. Umbilicus is a naturally dirty area and many surgeons were having this impression that it may cause infection of port site. The umbilical skin cannot be cleaned of all bacteria even with modern iodophor solution. Carson and associates (1997) demonstrated that the bacteria introduced inside the abdominal cavity through this dirty skin but these bacteria do not have many dead cells to act as culture medium to grow and the normal defense mechanism of body destroys these bacteria rapidly. Second fear of using umbilicus was ventral hernia. Umbilicus is the weakest abdominal wall so the chances are more that ventral hernia may develop if umbilicus is used for access. A survey of American Association of Gynecological Laparoscopists members reported in 1994 a study of 3127 surgeons and there were 840

hernia reported. 86 percent of cases of incisional hernia after laparoscopy were due to unrepaired 10 mm or larger port wound.

Due to these two possible complications of using umbilicus for access, many surgeons started using supraumbilical or infraumbilical region of abdominal wall for access. Even the port wound of 10 mm away from the umbilical site has reported higher incidence of incisional hernia. Recent study has proved that umbilicus does not have increased incidence of infection or ventral hernia compared to other site if few precautions are taken.

1. Umbilicus should be cleaned meticulously before incision (Fig. 5.8).
2. Rectus sheath of all the 10 mm port should be repaired.
3. If umbilical route is used for tissue retrieval, infected tissue should be removed after putting in endobag. It should not contaminate the port wound.
4. Any hematoma formation at the port wound site should be discouraged by maintaining proper hemostasis.

Where in Umbilicus?

- Superior or inferior crease of umbilicus, in non-obese patients (for abdominal procedure).
- Transumbilical in obese patients or if diagnostic laparoscopy is going to be performed under local anesthesia.

In most of the patients, inferior crease of umbilicus is best site of incision. This is called as smiling incision (Fig. 5.9). In obese patient, transumbilical incision is

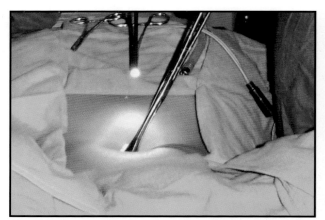

Fig. 5.8: Proper cleaning of umbilicus is necessary before inserting port

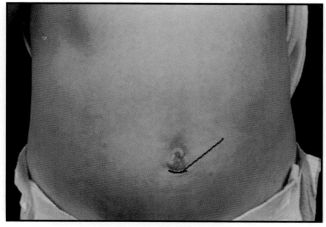

Fig. 5.9: Smiling incision

preferred because this area has minimum thickness of fat. In obese patient veress needle should be inserted perpendicular to the abdominal wall because if oblique entry is tried, the full length of Veress needle will be some where within the fat pad and there is chance of creation of pre-peritoneal space.

Stabilization of Umbilicus and Incision

Before incision along the inferior crease of umbilicus it should be stabilized with the help of two Ellis forceps. Once Ellis forceps will hold the umbilicus, the crease of umbilicus will be everted and it is easy to give smiling incision. Initial 1 mm incision with blade no. 11 should be given (Figs 5.10A and B).

Some surgeon give 11 mm incision in beginning itself, but this is not good because gas may leak from the side of puncture of veress needle due to tear in rectus and this will interfere with the quadro-manometric indicator of insufflator.

Stab wound should be given just skin deep and any puncture of rectus or peritoneum should be avoided. After this initial incision tip, mosquito forceps is introduced to clear the subcutaneous fat and any remaining septa of skin (Fig. 5.11).

INTRODUCTION OF VERESS NEEDLE

Veress needle should be held like a dart (Fig. 5.12). At the time of insertion there should be 45° of elevation angle. Elevation angle is angle between instrument and body of patient. To get an elevation angle of 45° the distal end of the Veress needle should be pointed toward anus.

To prevent creation of pre-peritoneal slip of tip of Veress needle, it is necessary that Veress needle should be perpendicular to the abdominal wall. However, there is a fear of injury of great Vessels or bowel if Veress needle is inserted perpendicular to the abdominal wall. To avoid both the difficulty (creation of pre-peritoneal space and injury to bowel or great vessels), the lower abdominal wall should be lifted in such a way that it should lie at 90° angle in relation to the Veress needle but in relation to the body of patient Veress needle will be at an angle of 45° pointed towards anus. Lifting of abdominal wall should be adequate so that the distance of abdominal wall from viscera should increase. If less than required dose of muscle relaxant is given in muscular patient, lifting of abdominal wall may be difficult. In multipara patient, lifting lower abdominal wall is very easy.

For many years surgeons have been using towel clip to elevate the abdominal wall. This towel clip technique of lifting abdominal was advocated by Johns Hopkins University but after some time it was realized that towel clip technique increases the distance of skin from rest of the abdominal wall more than distance of abdominal wall from viscera. Abdominal wall should be held full thickness with the help of thenar, hypothenar and all the four fingers (Fig. 5.13). It is lifted in such a way that angle between Veress needles to abdominal wall should be 90° and angle between Veress needle and patient should be 45°. At the time of entry of Veress needle surgeon can hear and feel two click sounds. The first click sound is due to rectus sheath and second click sound

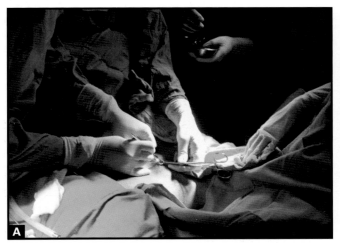
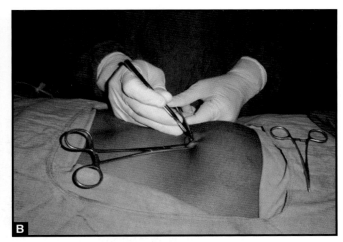

Figs 5.10A and B: Two mm Stab wound with 11 number of knife

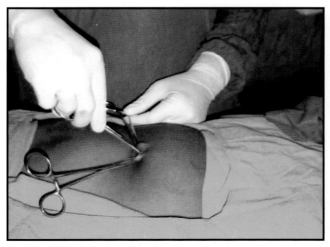

Fig. 5.11: Mosquito forceps tip introduced through stab wound

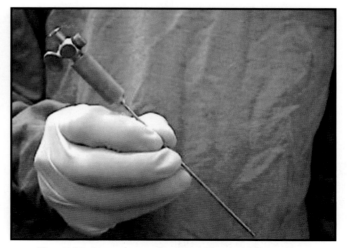

Fig. 5.12: Veress needle should be held like a dart

is due to puncture of peritoneum. Anterior and posterior rectus forms one sheath at the level of umbilicus so there will be only one click for rectus.

If any other area of abdominal wall is selected for access surgeon will get three click sounds. Once these two click sound is felt, surgeon should stop pushing Veress needle further inside and he should use various indicators to know how far he has accessed.

Indicators of Safe Veress Needle Insertion

Needle Movement Test

Once the Veress needle is inside the abdominal cavity the tip of Veress needle should be free and if surgeon will gently move the tip of needle there should not be feel of any resistance. It is very important to remember that Veress needle should not be moved inside the abdominal cavity much, otherwise there is a risk of laceration of bowel to be punctured (Fig. 5.14).

Irrigation Test

A 10 ml syringe should be taken in one hand and surgeon should try to inject at least 5 ml of normal saline through Veress needle. If tip of veress needle is inside the abdominal cavity, there will be free flow of saline otherwise some resistance is felt in injecting saline (Fig. 5.15).

Aspiration Test

After injecting saline, surgeon should try to aspirate that saline back through Veress needle (Fig. 5.16). If the tip of Veress needle is in abdominal cavity, the

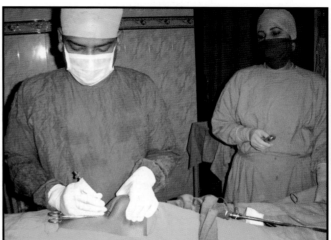

Fig. 5.13: Lifting lower abdominal wall

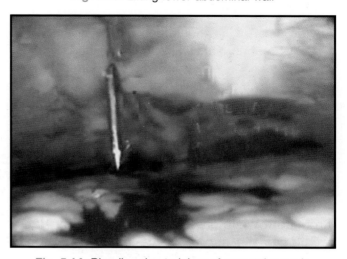

Fig. 5.14: Bleeding due to injury of omental vessels

Section One

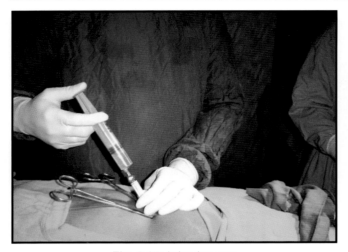

Fig. 5.15: Irrigation test

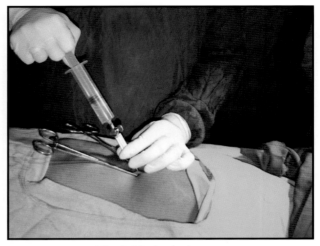

Fig. 5.16: Aspiration test

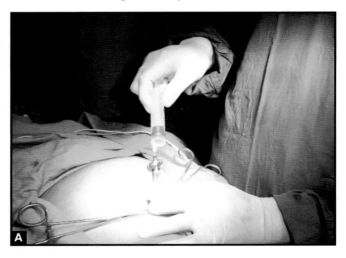

irrigated water cannot be sucked. But if it is in pre-peritoneal space on in muscle fiber of above; the rectus the injected water can be aspirated back. In aspiration test, if more irrigated fluid is coming, then surgeon should suspect ascites, some cyst or perforation of urinary bladder. If fecal mater is seen then perforation of bladder may be the reason and if blood is coming then the Vessel injury is the cause. If any fresh blood or fecal fluid is aspirated in the syringe surgeon should not remove the Veress needle and urgent laparotomy is required. Leaving veress needle in position is helpful in two ways. First it is easy to find the punctured area after laparotomy and secondly the further bleeding will be less.

Hanging Drop Test

Few drops of saline should be pored over the Veress needle and abdominal wall should be lifted slightly, if tip of the Veress needle is inside the abdominal cavity. The hanging drop should be sucked inside because inside the abdomen there is negative pressure. If tip of the Veress needle is any where else the hanging drop test will be negative (Figs 5.17A and B).

Once it is confirmed that Veress needle is inside the abdominal cavity the tubing of insufflator is attached and flow is started.

It is important to keep nice hold on Veress needle throughout while gas is flowing; otherwise Veress needle can slip out and may create preperitoneal insufflation (Figs 5.18 and 5.19).

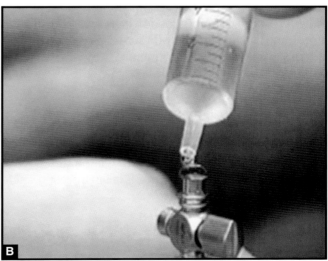

Figs 5.17A and B: Hanging drop test

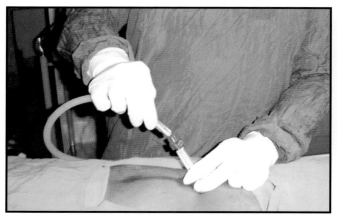

Fig. 5.18: Attaching gas tubing with careful hold of Veress needle and counter twist over leur lock of insufflator tubing

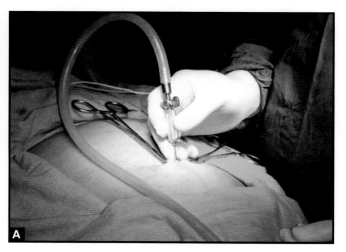

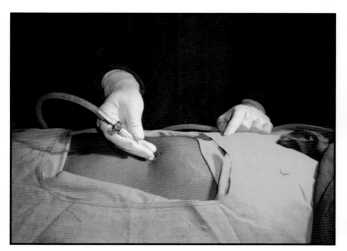

Fig. 5.19: Beginning of insufflation with careful hold over Veress needle

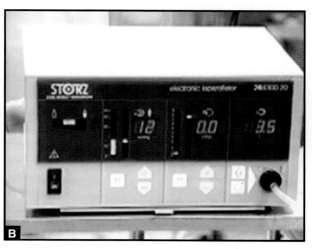

Figs 5.20A and B: Quadro-manometric indicators

Insufflation of Gas Test, Quadro-manometric Test

For safe access, surgeon should always see carefully all the four indicators of insufflator at the time of creation of pneumoperitoneum. If the gas is flowing inside the abdominal cavity there should be proportionate rise in actual pressure with total gas used. Suppose only with the entry of 400 to 500 ml of gas, if actual pressure is equal to preset pressure of 12 mm Hg, that means gas is not going in free abdominal cavity, it may be in pre-peritoneal space or inside omentum or may be in bowel. If gas is flown more than 5 liter without any distension of abdomen that may be due to leakage or gas may be going inside the vessel.

Quadro-manometric indicators of insufflator (Figs 5.20A and B)

Quadro-manometric indicators are the four important readings of insufflator.
The insufflator is used to monitor:
- Preset insufflation pressure
- Actual pressure
- Gas flow rate
- Volume of gas consumed.

Preset Pressure

This is the pressure adjusted by surgeon before starting insufflation. This is the command given by surgeon to insufflator to keep intra-abdominal pressure at this level.

The preset pressure ideally should be 12 mm of Hg. In any circumstance, it should not be more than 18 mm of mercury. Good quality insufflator always keeps intraabdominal pressure at preset pressure. Whenever intra-abdominal pressure decreases due to leak of gas outside, insufflator eject some gas inside to maintain the pressure, equal to preset pressure. If intra-abdominal pressure increases due to external pressure; insufflator sucks some gas from abdominal cavity, to maintain the pressure to preset pressure.

When surgeon or gynecologist wants to perform diagnostic laparoscopy under local anesthesia, the preset pressure should be set to 8 mm Hg. In some special situation of axilloscopy or arthroscopy, we need to have pressure more than 19 mm Hg.

Actual Pressure

This is the actual intra-abdominal pressure sensed by insufflator. When veress needle is attached there is some error in actual pressure reading because of resistance of flow of gas through small caliber of Veress needle. Since continuous flow of insufflating gas through Veress needle usually gives extra 4 to 8 mm Hg of measured pressure by insufflator, the true intra-abdominal pressure can actually be determined, by switching the flow from insufflator off for a moment. Many microprocessor controlled good quality insufflator deliver pulsatile flow of gas when Veress needle is connected, in which the low reading of actual pressure measures the true intra-abdominal pressure.

If there is any major gas leak, actual pressure will be less and insufflator will try to maintain the pressure by ejecting gas through its full capacity.

Actual pressures of more than 20 to 25 mm Hg has following disadvantage over hemodynamic status of patient.
- Decrease venous return due to vena caval compression leading to:
  a. Increased chance of DVT (Deep vein thrombosis of calf).
  b. Hidden cardiac ischemia can precipitate due to decrease cardiac output.
- Decrease tidal volume due to diaphragmatic excursion.
- Increase risk of air embolism due to venous intravasation.
- Increased risk of surgical emphysema.

Flow Rate

This reflects the rate of flow of CO_2 through the tubing of insufflator. When veress needle is attached the flow rate should be adjusted to 1 liter per minute. Studies were performed over animal in which direct IV CO_2 were administered and it was found that risk of air embolism is less if rate is within 1 liter/minute. At the time of access using Veress needle technique sometime Veress needle may inadvertently enter inside a vessel but if the flow rate is 1 liter/minute there is less chance of serious complication. When initial pneumo-peritoneum is achieved and cannula is inside abdominal cavity, the insufflators flow rate may be set at maximum, to compensate loss of CO_2 due to use of suction irrigation instrument. This should be remembered that if insufflator is set to its maximum flow rate then also it will allow flow only if the actual pressure is less than preset pressure otherwise it will not pump any gas. Some surgeons keep initial flow rate with veress needle to 1 liter/minute and as soon as they confirm that gas is going satisfactorily inside the abdominal cavity (Percussion examination and seeing obliteration of liver dullness), then they increase flow rate. No matter how much flow rate you set for Veress needle, the eye of normal caliber Veress needle can give away CO_2 flow at maximum 2.5 liter/minute. When the flow of CO_2 is more than 7 liter/minute inside the abdominal cavity through cannula, there is always a risk of hypothermia to patient. To avoid hypothermia in all modern microprocessor controlled laproflattor, there is electronic heating system which maintains the temperature of CO_2.

Total Gas Used

As soon as 100 to 200 ml of gas is inside the abdominal cavity surgeon should do percussion of the right hypochondrium and liver dullness should obliterate with tympanic sound (Fig. 5.21). This is the fourth indicator of insufflator. Normal size human abdominal cavity need 1.5 liter CO_2 to achieve intra-abdominal actual pressure of 12 mm Hg. In some big size abdominal cavity and in multipara patients sometime we need 3 liter of CO_2 (rarely 5 to 6 liters) to get desired pressure of 12 mm Hg. Whenever there is less or more amount of gas used to inflate a normal abdominal cavity, surgeon should suspect some error in pneumo-

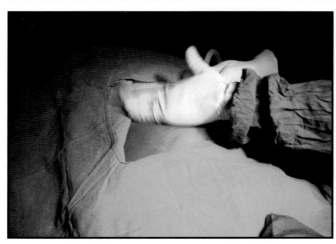
Fig. 5.21: Tapping over right hypochondrium will demonstrate obliteration of liver dullness

peritoneum technique. These errors may be leakage or may be pre-peritoneal space creation or extravasation of gas.

PRIMARY TROCAR INSERTION

Technical errors in the insertion of trocars after creation of pneumoperitoneum are the most common causes of injury, resulting from inadequate stabilization of the abdominal wall, excessive resistance to trocar insertion, and excessive, misdirected or uncontrolled force applied by the surgeon along the axis of the trocar.

It is important to stabilize the abdominal wall by full insufflation, complete muscle relaxation, to increase the distance between the anterior abdominal wall and the retroperitoneal vessels and the abdominal organs. It is important to ensure that the skin incision is of sufficient length and that the reusable trocar tip is sharp so that no resistance is offered.

Trocar and cannula designs currently available have a number of basic features in common. They come in a variety of sizes and the central trocar may have a pyramidal, conical or rounded tip. They have a valve system and a gas input with a tap (Fig. 5.26).

The disposable cannula has flap valves and care should be taken when passing instruments through the port. Some disposable cannula have a safety system. A cylinder jumps forward after penetration of abdominal wall and forms a shield over the sharp trocar tip. This is not foolproof due to shield lag. In the most recent disposable cannula the trocar itself is spring loaded. New designs of cannula, some quite minimalist are currently under investigation.

The first trocar and cannula inserted is a 11 mm disposable trocar. This will accommodate a 10 mm telescope and leave sufficient space in the cannula for rapid gas insufflation if required. Following insufflation, the Veress needle is removed and the trocar inserted with care at the same point, using a blind technique.

Steps of Primary Trocar Insertion

Patient Position

As for Veress needle insertion, patient should be placed supine with 10-20 degrees head-down. The cephalocaudal relationship between the aortic bifurcation and the umbilicus has been studied radiologically. The umbilicus is often located directly above or cephaled to the aortic bifurcation, and is consistently located cephaled to where the left common iliac vein crosses the midline. The aortic bifurcation is located more caudal to the umbilicus in the Trendelenburg's position than in the supine position.

Site

The same site of Veress needle entry should be used for primary trocar insertion. Inferior or superior crease of umbilicus can be used in average built patient and transumbilical incision can be used in obese patient. Before introduction of trocar, surgeon should confirm pneumoperitoneum. After adequate distention of abdominal cavity, the actual pressure should be equal to the preset pressure and gas flow should be stopped.

Before introduction of trocar, the initial 1 mm stab puncture wound of skin for veress needle should be extended to 11 mm. It should be remembered that most common cause of forceful entry inside the abdominal cavity with primary trocar is small skin incision. To avoid inadvertent injury of bowel due to forceful uncontrolled entry the incision of skin should not be less than 11 mm in size. The skin incision for trocar should be smiling in shape (U shaped) along the crease of umbilicus to get a better cosmetic value (Fig. 5.22).

After giving 11 mm incision with 11 number blades, surgeon should spread fatty tissues with Kelly clamp (Fig. 5.23).

Section One

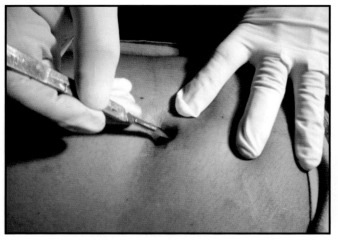

Fig. 5.22: Smiling incision along inferior crease of umbilicus

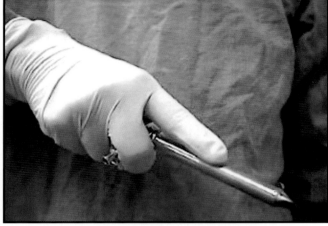

Fig. 5.24: The trocar and cannula should be held like a pistol

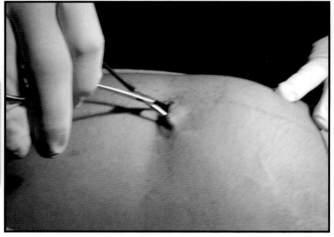

Fig. 5.23: Clearing fat and uncut subcutaneous tissue after initial skin incision

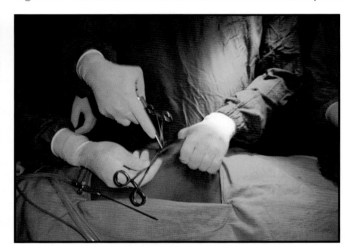

Fig. 5.25: Direction of trocar insertion

Section One

Introduction of Primary Trocar

Surgeon should hold the trocar in proper way. Head of trocar should rest on thenar eminence, middle finger should encircle air inlet and index finger should point toward sharp end (Fig. 5.24).

After holding the trocar properly in hand, full thickness of abdominal wall should be lifted by fingers thenar and hypothenar muscles. After creation of pneumoperitoneum lifting of abdominal wall is difficult because it slips. To overcome this, it should be grasped to counter the pressure exerted by the tip of trocar.

Angle of Insertion

Initially angle of insertion for primary trocar should be perpendicular to abdominal wall, but once surgeon feels giving way sensation, the trocar should be tilted to 60-70° angle.

Confirmation of Entry of Primary Trocar

- Audible click if disposable trocar or safety trocar is used.
- Whooshing sound if reusable trocar is used (gas passes from the small hole at the tip of pyramidal shaped trocar to the head of trocar).
- Loss of resistance felt both in disposable as well as reusable trocar.

Once the trocar entry in abdominal cavity is conformed, cannula is stabilized with left hand and trocar is removed by right hand. After removing trocar, cannula is pushed slightly further inside the abdominal

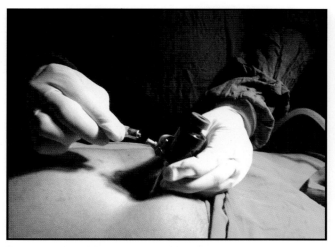

Fig. 5.26: Attaching leur lock of insufflator in primary cannula

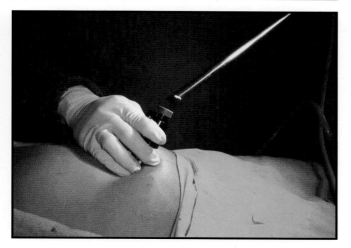

Fig. 5.27: Introduction of telescope

cavity to prevent coming cannula in pre-peritoneal space with movement of abdominal wall with respiration.

Once cannula is in place tubing of insufflator is attached again and flow is restarted to refill the CO_2 at preset pressure.

Telescope is introduced slowly keeping the oblique cut edge down in case of 30 degree telescope (Fig. 5.27).

Once the telescope is inside, the elevation angle of the telescope should be 90° with panoramic vision. The site just below the entry of primary port is examined for any vessel or bowel injury. Sometime there may be few drop of blood found just below the site of entry but these few drops of blood is trickled blood through umbilical wound. If surgeon has any doubt about perforation of bowel or injury to vessel he should evaluate this area again after putting other ports.

Working Ports

To select the site for secondary port, transillumination with illuminated telescope tip should be done first to locate avascular area to avoid injury of subcutaneous vessels.

With the help of mosquito forceps any remaining skin fiber is breached and the subcutaneous fat should be cleared.

Initially the direction of entry of trocar is perpendicular but as soon as the tip of trocar is seen the direction of trocar should be changed towards the anterior abdominal wall to prevent any injury of underlying viscera (Figs 5.25 and 5.30 to 5.32).

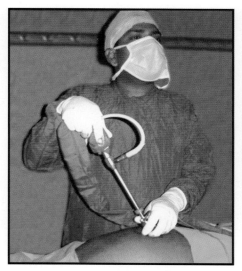

Fig. 5.28: Inspection just below entry for any possible injury

Subsequent Ports

Subsequent trocars are inserted under direct vision at locations appropriate for the procedure and to the anatomy of the individual (Fig. 5.29). If the port is on the opposite side of the patient, it can be introduced same way but if surgeon is not able to bend enough to opposite side, his right index finger can be placed over the head of the trocar and left hand should guard the shaft of cannula. With slow rotatory movement of right hand, first the tip of trocar should be perpendicular to the skin but as soon as tip of trocar is seen direction of trocar should changed towards the anterior abdominal wall. Alternatively surgeon can go to another side of the patient and he can introduce the trocar in conventional way (Figs 5.28 and 5.34A and B).

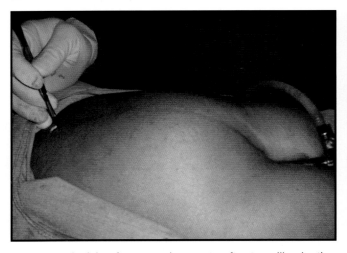

Fig. 5.29: Incision for secondary ports after transillumination

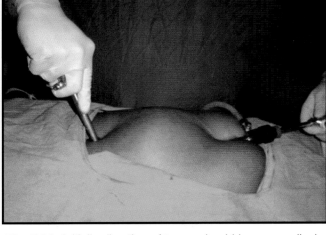

Fig. 5.31: Initially direction of trocar should be perpendicular

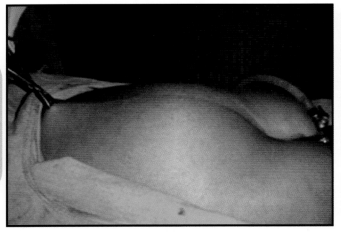

Fig. 5.30: Clearing subcutaneous tissue under
transillumination

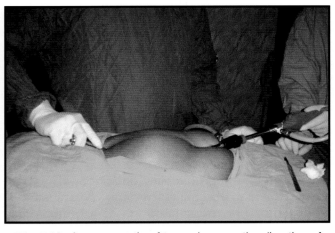

Fig. 5.32: As soon as tip of trocar is seen, the direction of
trocar should be turned towards the anterior abdominal wall

In same manner, all the working port should be
introduced and instruments are inserted to start the
surgery (Fig. 5.35). It should be remembered that
distance between two ports should never be less than
5 cm. The "Baseball Diamond Concept" discussed in
next chapter is the most appropriate method to decide
the site of introduction of working port (Fig. 5.33). The
positioning of operative ports is an important factor in
determining the ease with which a procedure is carried
out. It is a skill which must be learnt.

Slipping of Port

Sometimes the port wound becomes bigger than the
diameter of cannula and it tends to slip out frequently.
In these situation, a simple stitch over skin and fixing
of the cannula with the help of sterile adhesive helps

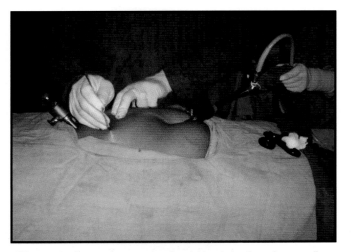

Fig. 5.33: Secondary ports should be introduced according
to baseball diamond concept

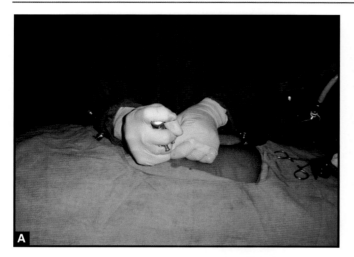

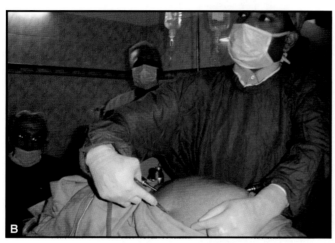

Figs 5.34A and B: Method of introduction of trocar on opposite side of the patient

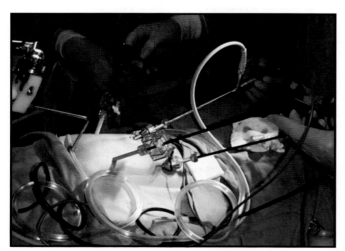

Fig. 5.35: All the ports and instruments should be positioned properly without entangling each other

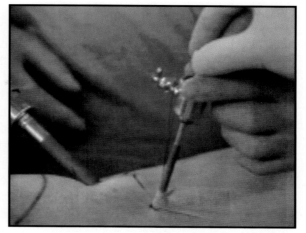

Fig. 5.36: The port can be stabilized with the help of stay suture and sterile adhesive plaster

(Fig. 5.36). In pediatric laparoscopic surgery, stabilizing the port is necessary.

Non-disposable metal cannula have trumpet or flap valves. The flap valves can be manually opened when introducing or removing an instrument. This avoids damaging delicate instruments like tip of telescope or blunting sharp instruments like aspiration needle and scissors. A reducer tube is used with large cannula to maintain the gas seal and this automatically opens the valve.

A number of cannula modeled on the Hasson cannula is available for use during open laparoscopic procedures. Different sized converters (gaskets) are available for disposable cannula to maintain the gas seal.

Open access technique was developed by Hasson in 1974. Open access technique is similar to mini-laparotomy and the cannula is introduced inside.

Hasson's technique involves direct open visualization of the tissues at every layer until the peritoneum is opened, followed by placement of anchoring sutures in the fascia to secure a conical collar (Fig. 5.37). The trocar is then placed through the collar to establish pneumoperitoneum and access. Disadvantages include persistent uncontrolled carbon dioxide leakage in many cases, increased incision size and increased time for placement.

Advantages of Open Technique

1. Definite, small risk of injury with blind Veress needle technique irrespective of experience.

2. Particularly useful in previous abdominal surgery or underlying adhesions.
3. The incidence of injury to adhesion although not eliminated is significantly reduced by entry into the peritoneal cavity under direct vision.
4. There is a decreased risk of injury to the retroperitoneal vessels. The trocar is blunt and the angle of entry allows the surgeon to maneuver the cannula at an angle, which avoids viscera, while still assuring peritoneal placement.
5. The risk of extraperitoneal insufflation is eliminated. Placement under direct vision ensures that insufflation of gas is actually into the peritoneal cavity.
6. The likelihood of hernia formation is decreased because the fascia is closed as part of the technique.
7. Increasing number of surgeons performing laparoscopy without experience and in these group open technique may be easy.
8. Useful in muscular man and children with strong abdominal wall.
9. Useful for gynecologists or surgeon lacking sufficient upper arm strength to elevate the abdominal wall of patient.

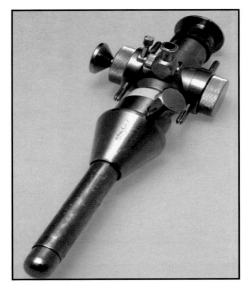

Fig. 5.37: Hasson's trocar and cannula

An open technique, which involves creating a mini-laparotomy into which a special cannula is inserted, may be adopted. This procedure has its own complications and requires skilled execution.

The Hasson trocar system was initially developed for laparoscopy in patients who have had a previous laparotomy. After seeing benefit of open access technique, many surgeons started using open access technique routinely in all their patients. An access wound was made using traditional open techniques and the Hasson trocar and cannula was designed to both fix the port and seal this larger wound round the port. It requires the use of sutures to prevent slippage of port. This involved making a small entry wound directly through the scar tissue of the umbilicus and then dilating this up by passage of a blunt, preferable conically tipped trocar and cannula (Fig. 5.41).

Steps of Open Access Technique

A transverse incision is made in the sub-umbilical region and the upper skin flap is retracted with a 4 inch Allis forceps. The lower flap is retracted using a small right angled retractor. Subcutaneous tissue is dissected till

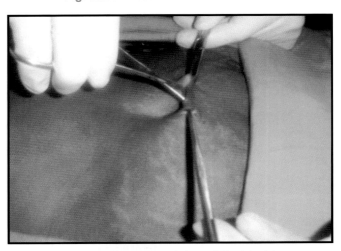

Fig. 5.38: Transverse infraumbilical incision

the linea alba and the rectus sheath is visualized. Stay sutures are taken on either side of the midline.

Transverse incision for Open Access

- Stay suture is given both the end of transverse incision (Fig. 5.38).
- Both the stays are pulled up to make a bridge like elevation of rectus.
- Rectus sheath is incised in the midline along the line of linea alba pointing upwards. Incision should not penetrate the peritoneum; otherwise any adhesion with the peritoneum may be punctured (Fig. 5.39).

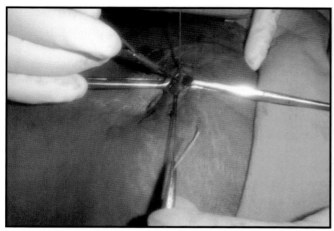

Fig. 5.39: Rectus is pulled up by two stay sutures on both the side and rectus is cut in midline longitudinally

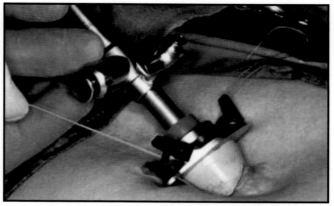

Fig. 5.41: Hasson's Cannula in proper position

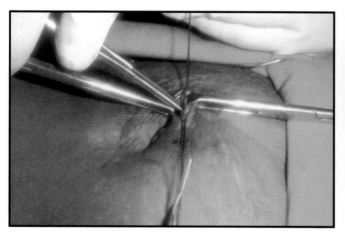

Fig. 5.40: Digging of hemostat to puncture peritoneum

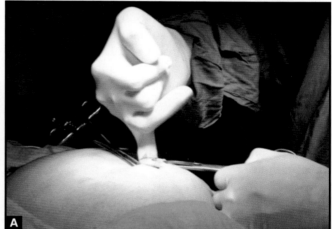

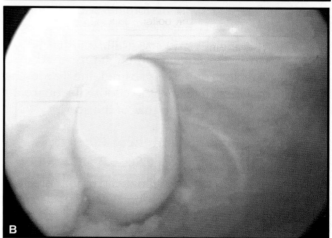

Figs 5.42A and B: Finger insertion after open access will confirm adhesion

- A hemostat is stabbed into the peritoneum, holding the stays up (Fig. 5.40).
- The give-way of the peritoneum can be felt as peritoneum is perforated and then the hemostat is opened to widen the opening.
- Surgeon should insert his finger to feel all around inside the abdominal cavity to feel any possible adhesion (Figs 5.42A and B).
- Small tiny adhesion felt can be broken with gentle sweeping movement of finger. Blunt trocar-cannula should be inserted for the first port after visualizing the intraperitoneal viscera.
- Care is taken not to make a big incision; cannula dilates the smaller incision to give an airtight fit.
- If incision is big, a purse string suture should be applied to hold the port in proper position.

Open Fielding Technique

This technique developed by Fielding in 1992 involves a small incision over the everted umbilicus at a point where the skin and peritoneum are adjacent. Fielding technique is useful in patients with abdominal incisions from previous surgery provided there is no midline incision, portal hypertension and reanalyzed umbilical vein, and umbilical abnormalities, such as urachal cyst, sinus or umbilical hernia. Thorough skin preparation of the umbilicus is carried out and the everted umbilicus is incised from the apex in a caudal direction. Two small retractors are inserted to expose the cylindrical umbilical tube running from the undersurface of the umbilical skin down to the linea alba. This tube is then cut from its apex downwards towards its junction with the linea alba. Further, blunt dissection through this plane permits direct entry into the peritoneum. Once the peritoneal cavity is breached, the primary port can be inserted directly and insufflation started. A blunt internal trocar facilitates insertion of this port and an external grip that can be attached to the port assist to secure it in position. Suture is usually not required to prevent gas leakage because the umbilicus has been everted so the angle of insertion of the laparoscopic port becomes oblique and the incision required is relatively small. However, one may be needed to stabilize the port.

The Scarred Abdomen

Additional precautions are necessary during the access procedure in patients with abdominal scars. It may be inadvisable to insert the Veress needle below the umbilicus in a patient with a scar in this area (or an umbilical hernia). Insufflation through unscarred such as subcostal region, or if this is scarred, the iliac fossae is better. A general guideline is to choose the quadrant of the abdomen opposite to that of the scar.

Contraindications of Umbilical Entry

- Previous midline incision
- Portal hypertension with reanalyzed umbilical artery with advanced cirrhosis of the liver
- Umbilical abnormalities viz. urachal cyst, sinus, hernia.

PNEUMOPERITONEUM IN SPECIAL CONDITIONS

Palmer's Technique

A small incision is made to allow the insertion of the Veress needle through left subcostal margin. This

access was advocated by Palmer in the 1940s because visceral parietal adhesions are rarely encountered in this area (Fig. 5.43).

In addition, some authors feel that because the abdominal wall in the area is supported by the rigid thoracic wall, insertion of the needle is more controlled than in the periumbilical area.

In cases where umbilical entry is contraindicated, it is preferred to use left upper quadrate for entry of Veress needle.

The Veress needle is introduced through left hypochondria, i.e. Palmer's point. Special care should be taken that there should not be hepatosplenomegaly (Figs 5.44 and 5.45).

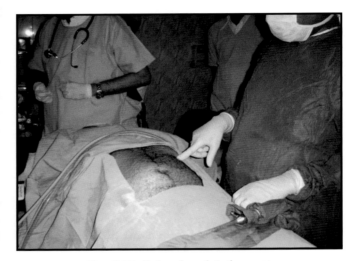

Fig. 5.43: Palmer's point of access

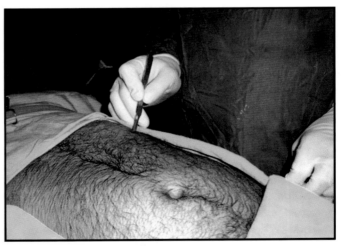

Fig. 5.44: A stab wound of 2 mm is given over Palmer's point

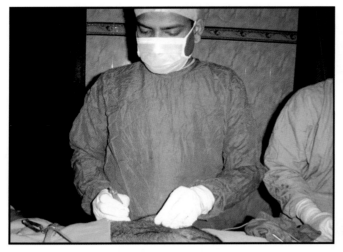

Fig. 5.45: Veress needle introduction in right hypochondrium

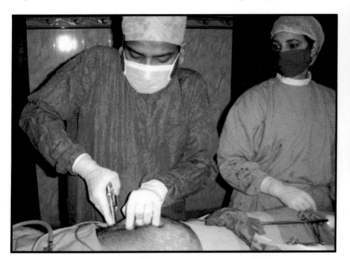

Fig. 5.46: After achieving proper pneumoperitoneum the trocar and cannula is introduced perpendicular to abdominal wall

After access, umbilicus site is re-checked for any adhesion or other abnormalities. If necessary, umbilicus port may be introduced under vision (Fig. 5.47).

Diagnostic Laparoscopy may be Performed Under Local Anesthesia

Intravenous sedation should be given, Veress needle and trocar should be inserted perpendicular to skin and slow insufflation 0.5 L/minute should be administered to prevent pain (Fig. 5.46). Pressure should not exceed 8 mm Hg otherwise the patient will feel pain. N$_2$O can be used if diagnostic laparoscopy is planned under local anesthesia because it has an analgesic effect.

Obese Patients

In obese patient incision site should be transumbilical (base of umbilicus) for the insertion of Veress needle, because it is the thinnest abdominal wall and even in obese patient, the amount of fat in transumbilical region is less compared to other areas of the abdominal wall. Direction of Veress needle entry in obese patient should be perpendicular to abdominal wall and patient should be in supine position not in Trendelenburg's position (Fig. 5.48). Once the Veress needle is inside pneumoperitoneum should be created up to

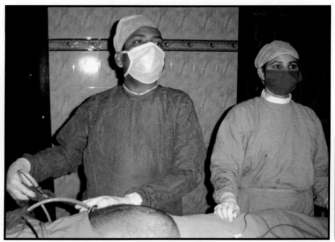

Fig. 5.47: After access through Palmer's point umbilicus should be inspected for any possible adhesion

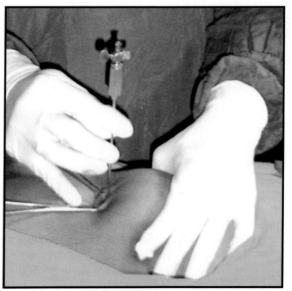

Fig. 5.48: Veress needle should be introduced perpendicular in obese patient

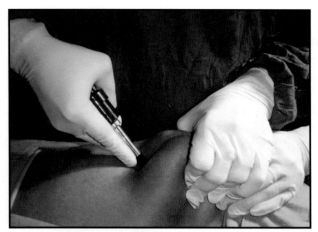

Fig. 5.49: Assistant hand should be asked for help, to lift the abdominal wall in obese patients

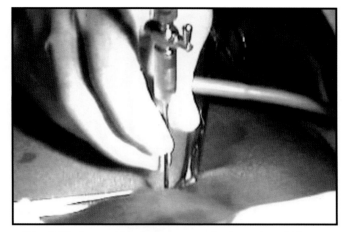

Fig. 5.50: In morbid obese perpendicular entry of Veress needle should be without lifting the abdominal wall

18 mm Hg. Once the actual pressure is equal to preset pressure and at least 1.5 to 3 liter of gas is introduced, Veress needle is removed. After removing Veress needle the initial incision is enlarged up to 11 mm.

After enlarging the initial incision, fat should be cleared up to anterior rectus sheath with the help of hemostat and little finger.

In obese patients, it is difficult to lift the abdominal wall alone, assistant's hand should be asked for help to have a better grip (Fig. 5.49).

ENTRY IN CASES OF MORBID OBESITY

In morbid obese patient, the umbilicus is well below the aortic bifurcation in supine position. Perpendicular entry of Veress needle is necessary. In morbid obese patient, it is virtually impossible to lift the abdominal wall and veress needle need to be introduced perpendicular to the abdominal wall transumbilically without lifting. At least 18 mm Hg pressure is necessary to leave the heavy abdominal wall in case of morbid obese patient (Fig. 5.50).

Ultrasound Visceral Slide

There is a simple preoperative test that can help to identify a safe region for Veress needle insertion in the scarred abdomen. The preoperative detection of anterior abdominal wall adhesions by ultrasonic scanning is a simple and reliable technique of ultrasonic detection and mapping of abdominal wall adhesions.

Once the Veress needle has been inserted, there should still be concern about the risk of causing damage with the trocar. The following techniques have been described for this situation.

Sounding Test

A fine spinal needle, attached to a saline filled syringe, is passed into the inflated abdomen. As the needle is slowly advanced, while aspirating, a stream of bubbles is seen in the saline until the needle tip contacts tissue. The needle is then withdrawn towards the surface and the process repeated several times, in different directions, thereby "mapping" the gas filled cavity and any solid structures.

Visually Guided Entry

Optical trocars are used for visual guided entry (Figs 5.51 and 5.52). These permit smaller skin incisions and better visualization of tissues as they are penetrated, and have been shown in large series to be safe and fast way to access the peritoneal space. Injuries can be recognized immediately, thereby reducing their potential morbidity. Disadvantages include the inability to remove the trocar during its initial advancement, which may change the original tract and confuse orientation, in addition to making it difficult to recognize the peritoneal layer. FDA reports also confirm deaths from major vascular injuries associated with the use of optical trocars.

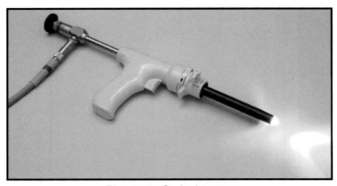

Fig. 5.51: Optical trocar

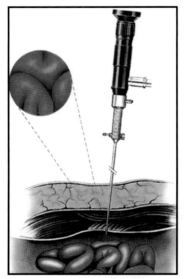

Fig. 5.52: Optical needle

Some Veress needle with in-built fiberoptic telescope is also used for direct visualization at the time of its introduction but quality of picture is not optimum for very safe access.

Postoperative Chest and
Shoulder Pain After Laparoscopy

Residual CO_2 left inside the abdominal cavity sometime cause considerable discomfort like chest pain and shoulder tip pain. The cause of this discomfort is that residual CO_2 gets trapped in the subdiaphragmatic recesses and then irritate diaphragm. Irritation of diaphragm causes referred pain in chest and over shoulder tip. This pain is more when patient sits upright. To avoid this entrapment of CO_2 it is good practice to put the patient in the Trendelenburg's position at the time of removing gas at the end of surgery. Only after removing the last telescopic cannula the Trendelenburg's position of the patient is discontinued.

Some surgeon leave some fluid like ringer lactate inside the abdominal cavity to divert gas away from sub diaphragmatic space but effect of this is controversial.

Subdiaphragmatic gas which remains inside is absorbed completely within 24 to 48 hours after surgery.

Complications of Access Technique

Improper trocar insertion causes most of the operative complications of laparoscopic surgery. Examples are injury to the bowel, major Vessels, bladder, inferior epigastric vessels and subcutaneous emphysema. Other complications include thermal injury to the bowel, abdominal wall contusions, trocar-site herniation with possible bowel obstruction, and trocar-site tumor implants. However, the overall incidence of complications is relatively low (about 2%).

Visceral Injuries

Incidence of Injury of Hollow Viscus

- Small bowel (2.7%)
- Large bowel (0.15%)
- Bladder (0.5%)
- Stomach (0.02%).

Solid organs

- Liver
- Spleen.

Vessel injury

- Inferior epigastric
- Omental
- Mesenteric vessels
- Aorta
- Inferior vena cava.

Other Complications

- Gas embolism (1:10 000 to 1:60 000, but lethal)
- Pneumo-omentum
- Surgical emphysema

Section One

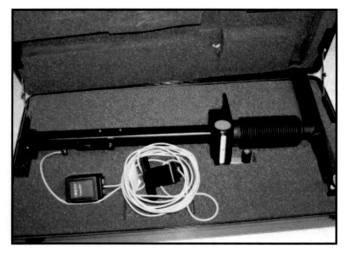

Fig. 5.53: Laparolift

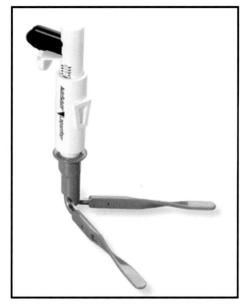

Fig. 5.54: Laparofan attached with laparolift after introduction inside abdominal cavity

- Pneumomediastinum
- Sudden collapse.

The anesthetist should check for conditions such as drug reactions pneumothorax, gas embolism which may give rise to myocardial arrhythmias.

If Cardiac Arrhythmia is found:
- Stop insufflation
- Withdraw instrument and remove CO_2 by opening the valve but leave port in position.
- Turn the patient to left
- Correct hypoxia and resuscitate
- Postpone surgery.

If case of severe hypotension, proceed to immediate laparotomy with all instruments left *in situ*. Assume retroperitoneal bleeding to be the cause.

Mild to Moderate Hypotension

In cases of moderate hypotension the surgeon should consider discontinuing gas insufflation immediately and reducing intra-abdominal pressure to 8.0 mm Hg. 360° scan of the abdominal cavity should be performed immediately to rule out retroperitoneal bleeding.

If bleeding or expanding hematoma is seen, one should proceed immediately to long midline laparotomy and compression of the bleeding vessel. Blood should be aspirated, bleeder is exposed and bleeding should be controlled with vascular clamps. When necessary, operator should obtain assistance of a vascular surgeon.

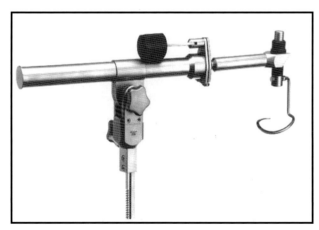

Fig. 5.55: Abdolift (another variety of abdominal lifting device)

Withdrawal of Instrument and Ports

Once the surgery is finished all the instrument should be removed carefully under vision. All the accessory port should be removed and the gas is removed by releasing the valve of 10 mm cannulas. The primary port should be taken out in the end (Fig. 5.57).

If last port is suddenly withdrawn sudden suction effect of cannula can pull the omentum or bowel inside the port wound, the chances of port site hernia and adhesion is much higher in this case. It is a good practice to insert some blunt instrument or telescope

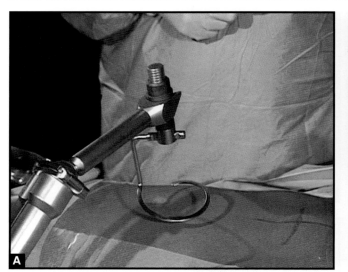
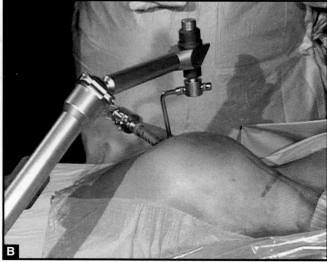

Figs 5.56A and B: Abdolift lifting the abdominal cavity

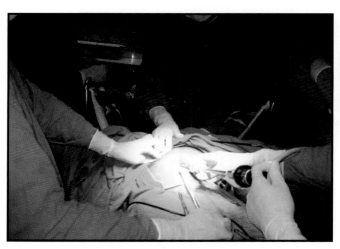

Fig. 5.57: The tip of telescope should be introduced in and cannula is pulled over telescope to prevent suction of omentum or bowel

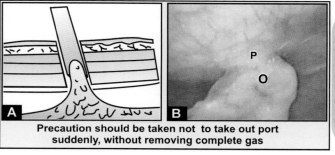

Precaution should be taken not to take out port suddenly, without removing complete gas

Figs 5.58A and B: Adhesion may form if cannula is pulled rapidly at the end of surgery
P: Peritonium, O: Omentum

inside the abdomen while removing the last cannula out over that instrument, to prevent inadvertent entrapment of omentum or bowel (Figs 5.58A and B).

PORT CLOSURE TECHNIQUES

The access technique will result in breach in continuity of abdominal wall which need to be repaired at the end of surgery. All the 10 mm or greater than 10 mm port should be repaired properly to prevent any future possibility of hernia. The rectus sheath is only necessary to suture with Vicryl. Only one stitch is required in middle which will convert 10 mm wound into 5 mm. The 5 mm port wounds are not necessary to repair (Figs 5.59A to D).

Various types of port closure instruments are available. The suture passer is a convenient instrument for port closure it is used to pass the thread on the side of cannula and then it is tied externally (Figs 5.60A and B).

For port closure specially designed port closure instruments are also available commercially, like port closure needle and aneurism needle.

After closing the rectus sheath the skin can be closed by intradermal, skin stapler or by any of the surgical skin glues available (Fig. 5.61).

Section One

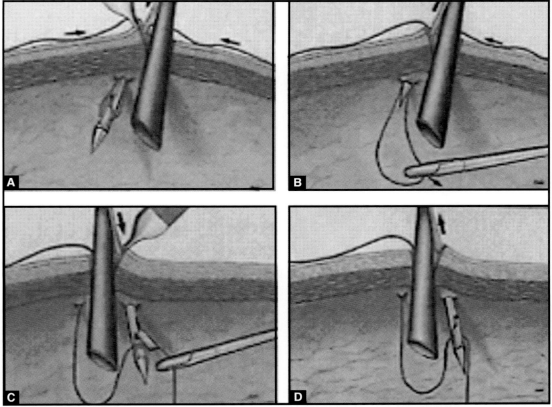

Figs 5.59A to D: Port closure with the help of suture passer

Gasless Laparoscopic Surgery

Conventional laparoscopic surgery requires pneumoperitoneum to elevate the abdominal wall for proper exposure. A continuous insufflation of a non-combustible gas in a sealed environment is essential part of minimal access surgery. Many undesirable physiological side effects have been observed with CO_2 pneumoperitoneum. Furthermore, it has been necessary to retrain surgeons to use specialized instruments in order to operate on video images. Abdominal lifting mechanical devices can provide working space without pneumoperitoneum. With gasless technique, conventional instruments can be used, direct visualization of abdominal viscera is possible, and digital examination of abdominal contents can be performed without the fear of losing exposure. Since these procedures are being performed in an isobaric abdominal cavity, the risk of body fluid contamination to operating team is diminished when compared to open or traditional laparoscopic surgery. Gasless laparoscopic surgery is primarily advocated for the patients who are at high risk of pneumoperitoneum.

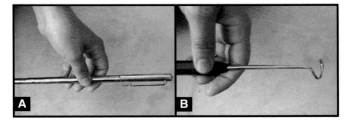

Figs 5.60A and B: Port closure needle and aneurysm needle

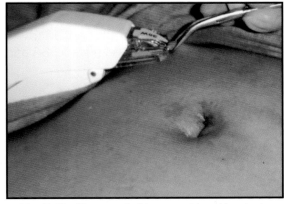

Fig. 5.61: Closure of skin wound by skin stapler

A variety of abdominal lift devices have been developed recently to provide working space. Although gasless laparoscopic surgery is good for patient with high risk of pneumoperitoneum, due to intraoperative problems and complications and because of suboptimal exposure, gasless laparoscopic surgery is still not considered as the prime modality for every patient.

All the gasless systems can be used on their own or with low pressure insufflation (4-6 mm Hg).

Three Basic Types

1. Rubber tube sling abdominal wall lifts.
2. Planar intraperitoneal abdominal wall retraction lift devices.
3. Subcutaneous abdominal wall lift devices.

None of these techniques gives as good a laparoscopic exposure as the pressurized pneumoperitoneum because they produce a tent-like elevation of the abdominal wall rather than an elevated expansion and they do not depress the hollow organs and omentum. Exposure is improved when low pressure insufflation is added (Table 5.1).

Several devices for gasless laparoscopy have been developed recently. The Laparolift (Origin Med systems) is commercially available device routinely used by many surgeons and gynecologist worldwide (Figs 5.53 to 5.55).

It consists of an adjustable arm that is attached to the side of the operating table and sterilely draped (Fig. 5.56A and B). The surgeon can raise and lower it electronically. The arm is connected to the Laparofan, a disposable sterile device with two metal blades (available in 10 and 15 cm lengths) that are inserted through the umbilical incision in an overlapped position. After entering the peritoneal space, the

Table 5.1: Problems due to pneumoperitoneum

Hypothermia
Cardiac arrhythmia
Cardiovascular collapse
Pulmonary insufficiency
Gas embolism
Venous thrombosis
Cerebral edema/ischemia
Ocular hypertension
Extraperitoneal insufflation (subcutaneous emphysema, pneumomediastinum)

Laparofan paddles are spread. Using the dovetail connector, the Laparofan retractor is attached to the Laparolift arm and raised, creating a working cavity for laparoscopic surgery. It is intended to be used as a substitute for, or in conjunction with, pneumoperitoneum for abdominal wall retraction. The blades are then splayed out and locked into a V by tabs on the plastic handle, which is fixed to the end of the adjustable arm. The maximum lifting force of 13.6 kg is equivalent to a pneumoperitoneum pressure of 15 mm Hg. The laparoscope is inserted through the same incision, cephalad to the Laparofan.

The physiologic changes associated with CO_2 pneumoperitoneum are well tolerated in healthy patients but may result in life-threatening cardiac arrhythmia, myocardial infarction, cardiac failure, or pulmonary insufficiency in compromised patients who cannot compensate for these alterations in

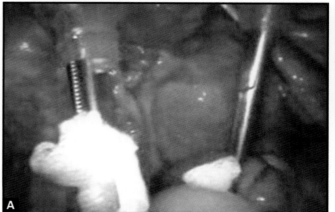

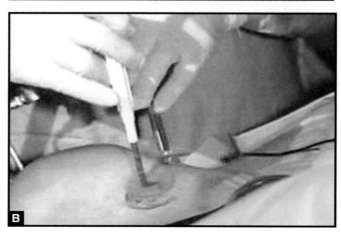

Figs 5.62A and B: Use of open surgical instrument in gasless laparoscopic surgery

Section One

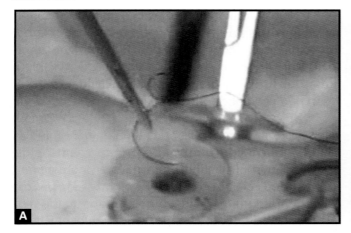

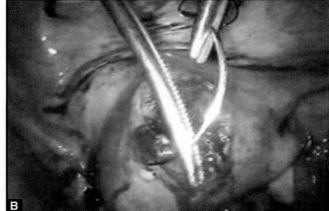

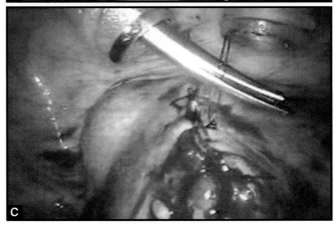

Figs 5.63A to C: Use of open needle holder and suturing technique in gasless laparoscopic

hemodynamic. A gasless laparoscopic approach could provide an added margin of safety for these patients. Patients undergoing laparoscopic surgery for malignancy or laparoscopically assisted vaginal hysterectomy may also benefit from gasless laparoscopy. Another potential advantage of gasless laparoscopy is the ability to use continuous suction and conventional laparotomy instruments (Figs 5.62A to 5.63C).

Disadvantages of Gasless Laparoscopic Surgery

• Marked guttering effect of lateral abdominal wall result after lifting anterior abdominal wall.
• Anterior abdominal adhesion can make insertion of these mechanical devise difficult and visualization almost impossible.
• It is a space occupying as instrument takes all the ergonomically good space of port position.
• It only elevates anterior abdominal wall whereas gas creates workable space in whole abdominal cavity.
• Sometime causes pressure necrosis of superior or inferior epigastric vessels.
• Bigger incision is required in the umbilicus.
• Difficult to perform in presence of ileus.
• Difficult peritoneal toileting at remote places.

Studies to date have demonstrated that surgical procedures with gasless laparoscopy are technically more difficult than those performed with adequate pneumoperitoneum owing to impaired visualization from bowel in the pelvis. As with any new laparoscopic device, the initial enthusiasm over gasless laparoscopy has been tempered by actual clinical experience.

However, because gasless laparoscopy still promises significant advantages over CO_2 pneumoperitoneum in high-risk patient, it is anticipated that interest in this technique will continue with improvements that will eliminate the current limitations to its use.

BIBLIOGRAPHY

1. Approach matter? J Urol 2004; 172:2218–23.
2. Bemelman WA, Dunker MS, Busch ORC, Den Boer KT, De Wit LTH, Gouma DJ. Efficacy of establishment of pneumoperitoneum with the Veress needle, Hasson trocar, and modified blunt trocar (TrocDoc): a randomized study. J Laparoendosc Adv Surg Tech 2000;10:325–9.
3. Bernik TR, Trocciola SM, Mayer DA, Patane J, Czura CJ, Wallack MK. Balloon blunt-tip for laparoscopic cholecystectomy: improvement over the traditional Hasson and Veress needle methods. J Laparoendosc Adv Surg Tech 2001;11:73–8.
4. Bhoyrul S, Payne J, Steffes B, Swansrtom L, Way LW. A randomized prospective study of radially expanding trocars in laparoscopic surgery. J Gastrointestinal Surg 2000;4: 392–7.

5. Bhoyrul S, Vierra MA, Nezhat CR, Krummel TM, Way LW) Trocar injuries in laparoscopic surgery. Am Coll Surg 2001;6: 677–83.

6. Bonjer HJ, Hazebroek EJ, Kazemier G, Giuffrida MC, Meijer WS, Lange JF. Open vs closed establishment of pneumoperitoneum in laparoscopic surgery. Br J Surg 1997;84:599–602.

7. Champault G, Cazacu F, Taffinder N. Serious trocar accidents in laparoscopic surgery: a French survey of 103, 852 operations. Surg Laparosc Endosc 1996;6: 376–70.

8. Cogliandolo A, Manganaro T, Saitta FP, Micali B. Blind vs open approach to laparoscopic cholecystectomy. Surg Laparosc Endosc 1998;8:353–55.

9. Eden CG, King D, Kooiman GG, et al. Transperitoneal or extraperitoneal laparoscopic radical prostatectomy: does the

10. Endogru T, Teber D, Frede T, et al. Comparison of transperitoneal and extraperitoneal laparoscopic radical prostatectomy using match-pair analysis. Eur Urol 2004; 46:312–20.

11. Gill IS, Clayman RV, Albala DM, et al. Retroperitoneal and pelvic extraperitoneal laparoscopy: an international perspective. Urology 1998; 52:566–71.

12. Guillonneau B, Vallancien G. Laparoscopic radical prostatectomy: the Montsouris experience. J Urol 2000; 163:1643–9.

13. Gutt CN, Oniu T, Schemmer P, Kraus T, Buchler MW. Circulatory and respiratory complications of carbon dioxide insufflation. Dig Surg 2004;21:95–105.

14. Hanney RM, Carmalt HL, Merret N, Tait N. Use of the Hasson cannula producing major vascular injury at laparoscopy. Surg Endosc 1999;13:1238–40 .

15. Hashizume M, Sugimachi K . Needle and trocar injury during laparoscopic surgery in Japan. Surg Endosc 1997;11: 1198–1201.

16. Hasson HM. Open laparoscopy as a method of access in laparoscopic surgery. Gynaecol Endosc 1999;8:353–62.

17. Hoznek A, Antiphon P, Borkowski T, et al. Assessment of surgical technique and perioperative morbidity associated with extraperitoneal versus transperitoneal laparoscopic radical prostatectomy. Urology 2003;61:617–22.

18. Khoury N. A comparative study of laparoscopic extraperitoneal and transabdominal preperitoneal hernioplasty. J Laparoendosc Surg 1995;5:349–55.

19. Liao CH, Chueh SC, Lai MK, et al. Laparoscopic adrenalectomy for potentially malignant adrenal tumors greater than 5 centimeters. J Clin Endocrinol Metab 2006; 91:3080–3.

20. Magrina JF. Complications of laparoscopic surgery. Clin Obstet Gynecol 2002;45:469–80.

21. McCormack K, Wake BL, Fraser C, et al. Transabdominal pre-peritoneal (TAPP) versus totally extraperitoneal (TEP) laparoscopic techniques for inguinal hernia repair: a systematic review. Hernia 2005;9:109–14.

22. Merlin TL, Hiller JE, Maddern GJ, Jamieson GG, Brown AR, Kolbe A. Systematic review of the safety and effectiveness of methods used to establish pneumoperitoneum in laparoscopic surgery. Br J Surg 2003;90:668–79.

23. Neudecker J, Sauerland S, Neugebauer E, Bergamaschi R, Bonjer J, Cuschieri A, Fuchs KH, Jacobi Ch , Jansen FW, Kovusalo AM, Lacy A, McMahon MJ, Millat B, Schwenk W. The European Association for Endoscopic Surgery clinical practice guideline on the pneumoperitoneum for laparoscopic surgery. Surg Endosc 2002;16:1121–43.

24. Peitgen K, Nimtz K, Hellinger A, Walz MK. Offener zugang oder Veress-nadel bei laparoskopischen eingriffen? Ergebnisse einer prospektiv randomisierten studie. Chirurg 1997;68:910–13.

25. Porpiglia F, Terrone C, Tarabuzzi R, et al. Transperitoneal versus extraperitoneal laparoscopic radical prostatectomy: experience of a single center. Urology 2006;68:376–80.

26. Raboy A, Ferzli G, Albert P. Initial experience with extraperitoneal endoscopic radical retropubic prostatectomy. Urology 1997; 50:849–53.

27. Remzi M, Klingler HC, Tinzl MV, et al. Morbidity of laparoscopic extraperitoneal versus transperitoneal radical prostatectomy versus open retropubic radical prostatectomy. Eur Urol 2005; 48:83–9.

28. Rodriguez AR, Kapoor R, Pow-Sang JM. Laparoscopic extraperitoneal radical prostatectomy in complex surgical cases. J Urol 2007;177:1765–70.

29. Rozet F, Galiano M, Cathelineau X, et al. Extraperitoneal laparoscopic radical prostatectomy: a prospective evaluation of 600 cases. J Urol 2005; 174:908–11.

30. Ruiz L, Salomon L, Hoznek A, et al. Comparison of early oncologic results of laparoscopic radical prostatectomy by extraperitoneal versus transperitoneal approach. Eur Urol 2004; 46:50–6.

31. Semm K, Semm I Safe insertion of trocars and the Veress needle using standard equipment and the 11 security steps. Gynaecol Endosc 1999;8: 339–347.

32. Stolzenburg JU, Do M, Rabenalt R, et al. Endoscopic extraperitoneal radical prostatectomy: initial experience after 70 procedures. J Urol 2003;169:2066–71.

33. Tamme C, Scheidbach H, Hampe C, et al. Total extraperitoneal endoscopic inguinal hernia repair (TEP). Surg Endosc 2003;17:190–5.

Section One

6 Principle of Laparoscopic Port Position

The relative position of the instrument ports is very important in the performance of surgical procedures endoscopically. The angle the instruments make with the operative site and to each other should mimic, as far as possible to the natural relationship of the hands and eyes during conventional surgery. It is proved that the most common cause of stressful minimal access surgery is wrong port position. Ninty five percent of surgeon and gynecologists use umbilicus as primary port but at the time of inserting secondary port there is controversy among operator and they lack the principles behind secondary port position.

PRIMARY PORT POSITION

The central location and ability of the umbilicus to camouflage scars makes it an attractive primary port site for laparoscopic surgery. There are many drawbacks with umbilicus as well. Umbilicus is a naturally weak area due to absence of all the layers. Weakness is also due its location at the midpoint of the abdomen's greatest diameter.

It is easy to believe that there is a difference between the umbilicus and other trocar sites in both susceptibility to infection and postoperative incisional herniation.

The study showed that the increased infection rate at the umbilicus seems to be related to retrieval of infected organs through the umbilicus and not to the umbilicus itself. When umbilicus was used to retrieve gallbladder after cholecystectomy the rate of infection was high due to port contamination with infected gallbladder. Excluding cholecystectomy, the umbilical infection rate was two percent, similar to that of any

alternative site. The postoperative ventral hernia rate was at 0.8 percent, the same at the umbilicus as elsewhere if the port more than 10 mm size is not repaired. It is now proved that the wound infection at the umbilicus is similar to that at other sites; postoperative ventral hernia at the umbilicus is similar to that at other sites and most of the infection after laparoscopic cholecystectomy is due to the contamination of wound due to infected gallbladder.

SECONDARY PORT POSITION

The obligatory passage of the laparoscopic instruments through the abdominal wall generates a fixed point after which all movements are reversed. For instance, when the hand moves to the left, the end of the instruments moves right, and when the hand moves downwards, the end of the instrument moves upwards. For some surgeon's the fulcrum effect is not a problem, but for others it is an insurmountable obstacle to the performance of advanced laparoscopy.

Because the handling of laparoscopic instruments is through the fixed point at abdominal wall, the force feedback felt by the surgeon will depend on the length of the instrument inferior to this fixed point.

Base Ball Diamond Concept of Port Position

A satisfactory relationship includes (Fig. 6.1):
- An angle of 60° between the two instrument tips
- Tangential approach to the site
- Appropriate working distance

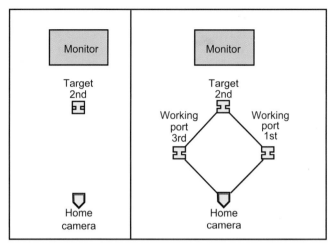

Fig. 6.1: Base ball diamond concept of port position

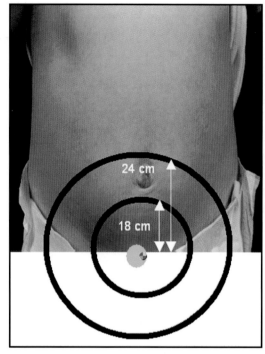

Fig. 6.3: Draw two arcs on the abdominal wall at 18 and 24 cm from that point and note area in between

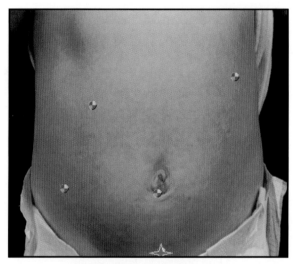

Fig. 6.2: First, decide the target

FIRST DECIDE THE TARGET

Target may be in suprapubic region for LAVH, right iliac fossa for appendicectomy, right upper quadrant for laparoscopic cholecystectomy or left upper quadrant for fundoplication (Fig. 6.2).

Draw the Line of Optimum Area

For optimum task performance, half to two-third instrument should be inside the abdomen. The size of adult laparoscopic instrument is 36 cm and pediatrics instrument is 28 cm (Figs 6.3 and 6.4).

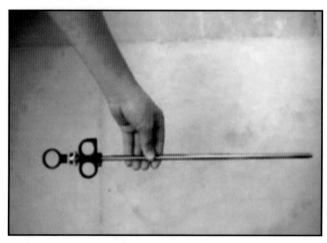

Fig. 6.4: Measure the length of instrument

Telescope and Instruments

- Telescope should be in the middle of working instrument (Figs 6.5)
- Manipulation angle of instruments should be 60 degree (Fig. 6.7).

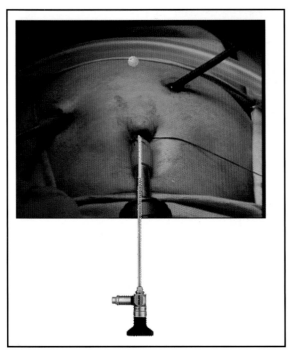

Fig. 6.5: Telescope should in the center of working instrument

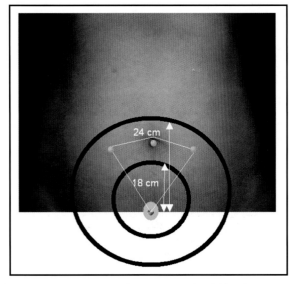

Fig. 6.6: 18 cm and 24 cm arc should be drawn

Rule of Diamond for LAVH

These factors combined with the specific anatomy will determine individual port sites. For standard operations like cholecystectomy, standard port sites related to surface marking may suffice but as more advanced or varied situations are tackled we recommend that you master the skill of individual port placement using the

internal view. In general, the optic and the two main operating ports usually lie at the points of a flattened triangle, the optic being centrally and more distally placed. Try to keep ports at least 5 cm apart (Figs 6.6 and 6.8).

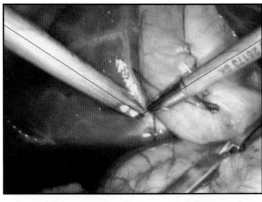

Fig. 6.7: Manipulation angle 60° is angle between tips of instrument

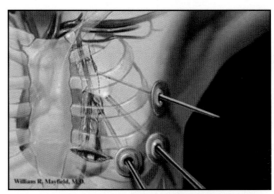

Fig. 6.8: Port position in thoracoscopic surgery

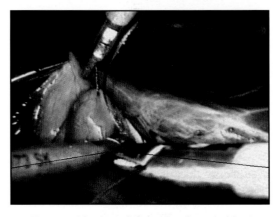

Fig. 6.9: Manipulation angle of 60° is ideal

Manipulation angle 60° is essential for optimum task performance in laparoscopic surgery (Figs 6.7 and 6.9).

PORT POSITION IN VARIOUS SURGERIES (FIGS 6.10 TO 6.14)

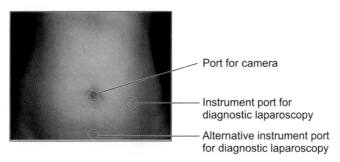

Port for camera

Instrument port for diagnostic laparoscopy

Alternative instrument port for diagnostic laparoscopy

Fig. 6.10: Port position for diagnostic laparoscopy

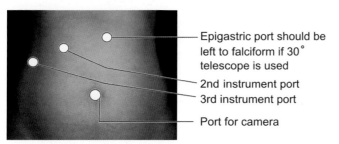

Epigastric port should be left to falciform if 30° telescope is used

2nd instrument port
3rd instrument port

Port for camera

Fig. 6.11: Port position for cholecystectomy

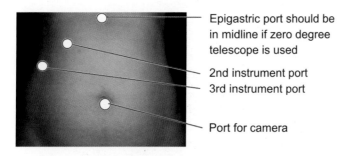

Epigastric port should be in midline if zero degree telescope is used

2nd instrument port
3rd instrument port

Port for camera

Fig. 6.12: Alternative port position for cholecystectomy

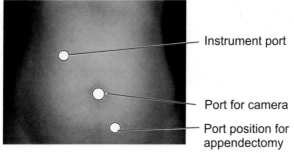

Instrument port

Port for camera

Port position for appendectomy

Fig. 6.13: Port position for appendectomy

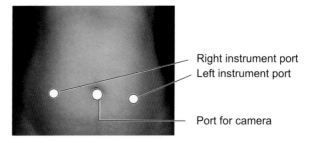

Right instrument port
Left instrument port

Port for camera

Fig. 6.14: Position for bilateral hernia, LAVH and most of the gynecological procedures

DRAWBACKS OF INCORRECT PORT POSITION

Swording

Swording occurs when the telescope or the shaft of the assistant's instrument obstruct the operator's instruments. If this occurs you may need to consider:

- Repositioning retracting instruments
- Rotation of an angled telescope allowing alteration of the position of the end of the telescope
- Withdrawal of the telescope
- Transposition of the operator's instruments
- Additional port placement
- Changing the instruments to a different port.

BIBLIOGRAPHY

1. Abu-Rafea B, Vilos GA, Vilos AG, Ahmad R, Hollett-Caines J, Al Omran M. High-pressure laparoscopic entry does not adversely affect cardiopulmonary function in healthy women. J Minim Invasive Gynecol 2005;12(6):475–9.
2. Abu-Rafea B, Vilos GA, Vilos AG, Hollett-Caines J, Al Omran M. Effect of body habitus and parity on insufflated CO2 volume at various intraabdominal pressures during laparoscopic access in women. J Minim Invasive Gynecol 2006;13(3):205–210.
3. Agresta F, De Simone P, Ciardo LF, Bedin N. Direct trocar insertion vs Veress needle in nonobese patients undergoing laparoscopic procedures: a randomized prospective single-center study. Surg Endosc 2004;18(12):1778–81.
4. Ahmad G, Duffy JMN, Watson AJS. Laparoscopic entry echniques and complications. International Journal of Gynecology and Obstetrics 2007;99(1):52–5.
5. Angelini L, Lirici MM, Papaspyropoulos V, Sossi FL. Combination of subcutaneous abdominal wall retraction and optical trocar to minimize pneumoperitoneum-related effects and needle and trocar injuries in laparoscopic surgery. Surg Endosc 1997;11(10):1006–1009.
6. Azevedo OC, Azevedo JL, Sorbello AA, Miguel GP, Wilson Junior JL, Godoy AC. Evaluation of tests performed to

confirm the position of the Veress needle for creation of pneumoperitoneum in selected patients: a prospective clinical trial. Acta Cir Bras 2006;21(6):385–91.

7. Baggish MS. Analysis of 31 cases of major-vessel injury associated with gynecologic laparoscopy operations. J Gynecol Surg 2003;19(2):63–73.

8. Bateman BG, Kolp LA, Hoeger K. Complications of laparoscopy–operative and diagnostic. Fertil Steril 1996;66(1):30–35.

9. Bemelman WA, Dunker MS, Busch OR, Den Boer KT, de Wit LT, Gouma DJ. Efficacy of establishment of pneumoperitoneum with the Veress needle, Hasson trocar, and modified blunt trocar (TrocDoc): a randomized study. J Laparoendosc Adv Surg Tech A 2000;10(6):325–30.

10. Bhoyrul S, Payne J, Steffes B, Swanstrom L, Way LW. Arandomized prospective study of radially expanding trocars in laparoscopic surgery. J Gastrointest Surg 2000;4(4):392–397.

11. Bhoyrul S, Vierra MA, Nezhat CR, Krummel TM, Way LW. Trocar injuries in laparoscopic surgery. J Am Coll Surg 2001;192(6):677–83.

12. Bishoff JT, Allaf ME, Kirkels W, Moore RG, Kavoussi LR, Schroder F. Laparoscopic bowel injury: incidence and clinical presentation. J Urol 1999;161(3):887–890.

13. Bonjer HJ, Hazebroek EJ, Kazemier G, Giuffrida MC, Meijer WS, Lange JF. Open versus closed establishment of pneumoperitoneum in laparoscopic surgery. Br J Surg 1997;84(5):599–602.

14. Briel JW, Plaisier PW, Meijer WS, Lange JF. Is it necessary to lift the abdominal wall when preparing a pneumoperitoneum? A randomized study. Surg Endosc 2000;14(9):862–864.

15. Brosens I, Gordon A, Campo R, Gordts S. Bowel injury in gynecologic laparoscopy. J Am Assoc Gynecol Laparosc 2003;10(1):9–13.

16. Byron JW, Markenson G, Miyazawa K. A randomized comparison of Verres needle and direct trocar insertion for laparoscopy. Surg Gynecol Obstet 1993;177(3):259–62.

17. Catarci M, Carlini M, Gentileschi P, Santoro E. Major and minor injuries during the creation of pneumoperitoneum. A multicenter study on 12,919 cases. Surg Endosc 2001;15(6):566–569 34. Schafer M, Lauper M, Krahenbuhl L. Trocar and Veress needle injuries during laparoscopy. Surg Endosc 2001;15(3):275–80.

18. Champault G, Cazacu F. Laparoscopic surgery: injuries caused by trocars. (French Survey 1994) in reference to 103,852 interventions. J Chir (Paris) 1995;132(3):109–13.

19. Chandler JG, Corson SL, Way LW. Three spectra of laparoscopic entry access injuries. J Am Coll Surg 2001;192(4):478–90.

20. Chapron C, Cravello L, Chopin N, Kreiker G, Blanc B, Dubuisson JB. Complications during set-up procedures for laparoscopy in gynecology: open laparoscopy does not reduce the risk of major complications. Acta Obstet Gynecol Scand. 2003;82(12):1125–9.

21. Chapron C, Fauconnier A, Goffinet F, Breart G, Dubuisson JB. Laparoscopic surgery is not inherently dangerous for patients presenting with benign gynaecologic pathology. Results of a meta-analysis. Hum Reprod 2002;17(5):1334–42.

22. Chapron C, Pierre F, Harchaoui Y et al. Gastrointestinal injuries during gynaecological laparoscopy. Hum Reprod 1999;14(2):333–7.

23. Chapron C, Pierre F, Querleu D, Dubuisson JB. Major vascular complications from gynecologic laparoscopy. Gynecol Obstet Fertil 2000;28(12):880–7.

24. Chapron C, Pierre F, Querleu D, Dubuisson JB. Complications of gynaecological laparoscopy. Gynecol Obstet Fertil 2001;29(9):605–12.

25. Chapron C, Querleu D, Bruhat MA et al. Surgical complications of diagnostic and operative gynaecological laparoscopy: a series of 29,966 cases. Hum Reprod 1998;13(4):867–72.

26. Chapron C, Querleu D, Mage G et al. Complications of gynecologic laparoscopy. Multicentric study of 7,604 laparoscopies. J Gynecol Obstet Biol Reprod (Paris) 1992;21(2):207–13.

27. Chapron CM, Pierre F, Lacroix S, Querleu D, Lansac J, Dubuisson JB. Major vascular injuries during gynecologic laparoscopy. J Am Coll Surg 1997;185(5):461–5.

28. Chin K, Newton J. Survey of training in minimal access surgery in the West Midlands region of the UK. Gynacol Endosc 1996;5(6):329–3.

29. Corson SL, Chandler JG, Way LW. Survey of laparoscopic entry injuries provoking litigation. J Am Assoc Gynecol Laparosc 2001;8(3):341–7.

30. Cravello L, Banet J, Agostini A, Bretelle F, Roger V, Blanc B. Open laparoscopy: analysis of complications due to first trocar insertion. French. Gynecol Obstet Fertil 2002;30(4):286–90.

31. Driscoll V. Bowel injury during laparoscopic sterilization – Vanessa Palmer v Cardiff and Vale NHS Trust. The AvMA Med Legal J 2004;10(3):109–111.

32. El Banna M, Abdel-Atty M, El Meteini M, Aly S. Management of laparoscopic-related bowel injuries. Surg Endosc 2000;14(9):779–82.

33. Ellis H. Medicolegal consequences of postoperative intrabdominal adhesions. J R Soc Med 2001;94(7):331–332.

34. Epstein J, Arora A, Ellis H. Surface anatomy of the inferior epigastric artery in relation to laparoscopic injury. Clin Anat 2004;17(5):400–08.

35. Ferriman A. Laparoscopic surgery: two thirds of injuries initially missed. West J Med 2000;173(6):372.

36. Fuller J, Ashar BS, Carey-Corrado J. Trocar-associated injuries and fatalities: an analysis of 1399 reports to the FDA. J Minim Invasive Gynecol 2005;12(4):302–07.

37. Galen DI, Jacobson A, Weckstein LN, Kaplan RA, DeNevi KL. Reduction of cannula-related laparoscopic complications using a radially expanding access device. J Am Assoc Gynecol Laparosc 1999;6(1):79–84.

Section One

38. Garry R. A consensus document concerning laparoscopic entry techniques: Middlesbrough, March 19–20 1999. Gynacol Endosc 1999;(8):403–406.
39. Geers J, Holden C. Major vascular injury as a complication of laparoscopic surgery: a report of three cases and review of the literature. Am Surg 1996;62(5):377–9.
40. Gett RM, Joseph MG. A safe technique for the insertion of the Hasson cannula. ANZ J Surg 2004;74(9):797–8.
41. Gordts S, Watrelot A, Campo R, Brosens I. Risk and outcome of bowel injury during transvaginal pelvic endoscopy. Fertil Steril 2001;76(6):1238–41.
42. Gunenc MZ, Yesildaglar N, Bingol B, Onalan G, Tabak S, Gokmen B. The safety and efficacy of direct trocar insertion with elevation of the rectus sheath instead of the skin for pneumoperitoneum. Surg Laparosc Endosc Percutan Tech 2005;15(2):80–81.
43. Hanney RM, Alle KM, Cregan PC. Major vascular injury and laparoscopy. Aust N Z J Surg 1995;65(7):533–35.
44. Harkki-Siren P, Kurki T. A nationwide analysis of laparoscopic complications. Obstet Gynecol 1997;89(1):108–12.
45. Harkki-Siren P, Sjoberg J, Kurki T. Major complications of laparoscopy: a follow-up Finnish study. Obstet Gynecol 1999;94(1):94–98.
46. Hart R, Doherty DA, Karthigasu K, Garry R. The value of virtual reality-simulator training in the development of laparoscopic surgical skills. J Minim Invasive Gynecol 2006;13(2):126–33.
47. Hasson HM. Open laparoscopy as a method of access in laparoscopic surgery. Gynacol Endosc 1999;8(6):353–62.
48. Hasson HM, Rotman C, Rana N, Kumari NA. Open laparoscopy: 29-year experience. Obstet Gynecol 2000;96 (5 Pt 1):763–766.
49. Hender K. What is the safety of open (Hasson) technique versus closed (blind Veress needle) technique for laparoscopy? Centre for Clinical Effectiveness – Evidence Report. Centre for Clinical Effectiveness (CCE), Clayton, Victoria. 2001.
50. Hill DJ, Maher PJ. Direct cannula entry for laparoscopy. J Am Assoc Gynecol Laparosc 1996;4(1):77–79.
51. Hurd WW, Amesse LS, Gruber JS, Horowitz GM, Cha GM, Hurteau JA. Visualization of the epigastric vessels and bladder before laparoscopic trocar placement. Fertil Steril 2003;80(1):209–12.
52. Hurd WW, Bude RO, DeLancey JO, Newman JS. The location of abdominal wall blood vessels in relationship to abdominal landmarks apparent at laparoscopy. Am J Obstet Gynecol 1994;171(3):642–6.
53. Jacobson MT, Osias J, Bizhang R et al. The direct trocar technique: an alternative approach to abdominal entry for laparoscopy. Journal of the Society of Laparoendoscopic Surgeons 2002;6(2):169–74.
54. Jansen FW, Kapiteyn K, Trimbos-Kemper T, Hermans J, Trimbos JB. Complications of laparoscopy: a prospective multicentre observational study. Br J Obstet Gynaecol 1997;104(5):595–600.
55. Jansen FW, Kolkman W, Bakkum EA, de Kroon CD, Trimbos-Kemper TC, Trimbos JB. Complications of laparoscopy: an
inquiry about closed- versus open-entry technique. Am J Obstet Gynecol 2004;190(3):634–638 Surg Endosc 2008; 22:2686–2697. 2693.
56. Jansen FW, Wind J, Cremeres JEL, Bemelman WA. 146: Entry Related Complications in Laparoscopy and Their Medical Liability Insurance. J Minim Invasive Gynecol 2007;14(6,1):S54–S55.
57. Kaali SG, Barad DH. Incidence of bowel injury due to dense adhesions at the sight of direct trocar insertion. J Reprod Med 1992;37(7):617–8.
58. Kaloo P, Cooper M, Molloy D. A survey of entry techniques and complications of members of the Australian Gynaecological Endoscopy Society. Aust N Z J Obstet Gynaecol 2002;42(3):264–6.
59. Kaloo P, Cooper M, Reid G. A prospective multicentre study of laparoscopic complications related to the direct-entry technique. Gynaecol Endosc 2002;11(2):67–70.
60. Kolkman W, Wolterbeek R, Jansen FW. Gynecological laparoscopy in residency training program: Dutch perspectives. Surg Endosc 2005;19(11):1498–1502.
61. Lalchandani S, Philips K. Laparoscopic entry technique-a survey of practices of consultant gynaecologists. Gynecol Surg 2005;2(4):245–49.
62. Larobina M, Nottle P. Complete evidence regarding major vascular injuries during laparoscopic access. Surg Laparosc Endosc Percutan Tech 2005;15(3):119–23.
63. Leng J, Lang J, Huang R, Liu Z, Sun D. Complications in laparoscopic gynecologic surgery. Chin Med Sci J 2000;15(4):222–6.
64. Leonard F, Lecuru F, Rizk E, Chasset S, Robin F, Taurelle R. Perioperative morbidity of gynecological laparoscopy. A prospective monocenter observational study. Acta Obstet Gynecol Scand 2000;79(2):129–134.
65. Lingam K, Cole RA. Laparoscopic entry port visited: a survey of practices of consultant gynaecologists in Scotland. Gynaecol Endosc 2001;10(5):335–42.
66. Mac CC, Lecuru F, Rizk E, Robin F, Boucaya V, Taurelle R. Morbidity in laparoscopic gynecological surgery: results of a prospective single-center study. Surg Endosc 1999;13(1):57–61.
67. Marret H, Golfier F, Cassignol A, Raudrant D. Methods for laparoscopy: open laparoscopy or closed laparoscopy? Attitude of the French Central University Hospital. Gynecol Obstet Fertil 2001;29(10):673–9.
68. Marret H, Harchaoui Y, Chapron C, Lansac J, Pierre F. Trocar injuries during laparoscopic gynaecological surgery. Report from the French Society of Gynaecological Laparoscopy. Gynacological Endoscopy 1998;7(5):235–41.
69. Mayol J, Garcia-Aguilar J, Ortiz-Oshiro E, Diego Carmona JA, Fernandez-Represa JA. Risks of the minimal access approach for laparoscopic surgery: multivariate analysis of morbidity related to umbilical trocar insertion. World J Surg 1997;21(5):529–533.
70. McKernan JB, Champion JK. Access techniques: veress needle–initial blind trocar insertion versus open laparoscopy with the Hasson trocar. Endosc Surg Allied Technol 1995;3(1):35–8.
71. Merlin TL, Hiller JE, Maddern GJ, Jamieson GG, Brown AR, Kolbe A. Systematic review of the safety and effectiveness of

Section One

methods used to establish pneumoperitoneum in laparoscopic surgery. Br J Surg 2003;90(6):668–79.

72. Merlin TL, Hiller JE, Maddern GJ, Jamieson GG, Brown AR, Kolbe A (2001) A systematic review of the methods used to establish laparoscopic pneumoperitoneum. ASERNIP-S Report No. 13. Adelaide, South Australia: ASERNIP-S. http://www. surgeons.org/asernip-s. 2001.

73. Moberg AC, Montgomery A. Primary access-related complications with laparoscopy: comparison of blind and open techniques. Surg Endosc 2005;19(9):1196–99.

74. Molloy D, Kaloo PD, Cooper M, Nguyen TV. Laparoscopic entry: a literature review and analysis of techniques and complications of primary port entry. Aust N Z J Obstet Gynaecol 2002;42(3):246–254.

75. Munro MG. Laparoscopic access: complications, technologies, and techniques. Curr Opin Obstet Gynecol 2002;14(4):365–74.

76. Narendran M, Baggish MS. Mean Distance Between Primary Trocar Insertion Site and Major Retroperitoneal Vessels During Routine Laparoscopy. J Gynecol Surg 2002;18(4):121–7.

77. Nezhat C, Childers J, Nezhat F, Nezhat CH, Seidman DS. Major retroperitoneal vascular injury during laparoscopic surgery. Hum Reprod 1997;12(3):480–3.

78. Nezhat CH, Nezhat F, Brill AI, Nezhat C. Normal variations of abdominal and pelvic anatomy evaluated at laparoscopy. Obstet Gynecol 1999;94(2):238–42.

79. Nezhat FR, Silfen SL, Evans D, Nezhat C. Comparison of direct insertion of disposable and standard reusable laparoscopic trocars and previous pneumoperitoneum with Veress needle. Obstet Gynecol 1991;78(1):148–150.

80. Nordestgaard AG, Bodily KC, Osborne RW Jr., Buttorff JD. Major vascular injuries during laparoscopic procedures. Am J Surg 1995;169(5):543–5.

81. Pasic RP, Kantardzic M, Templeman C, Levine RL. Insufflation techniques in gynecologic laparoscopy. Surg Laparosc Endosc Percutan Tech 2006;16(1):18–23.

82. Philips PA, Amaral JF. Abdominal access complications in laparoscopic surgery. J Am Coll Surg 2001;192(4):525–36.

83. Rahman MM, Mamun AA. Direct trocar insertion: alternative abdominal entry technique for laparoscopic surgery. Mymensingh Med J 2003;12(1):45–7.

84. RANZCOG. Use of the Veress needle to obtain pneumoperitoneum prior to laparoscopy. Statement C-Gyn 7. Consensus statement of the Royal Australian and New Zealand College of Obstetricians and Gynaecologists (RANZCOG), the Australian Gynaecological Endoscopy Society (AGES). Royal Australian and New Zealand College of Obstetricians and Gynaecologists, Australia. 2006.

85. Reich H, Rasmussen C, Vidali A. Peritoneal hyperdistention for trocar insertion. Gynaecological Endoscopy 1999; 8(6):375–77.

86. Reich H, Ribeiro SC, Rasmussen C, Rosenberg J, Vidali A. High-pressure trocar insertion technique. JSLS 1999; 3(1):45– 48.

87. Rein H. Complications and litigation in gynecologic endoscopy. Curr Opin Obstet Gynecol 2001;13(4):425–9.

88. Rosen DM, Lam AM, Chapman M, Carlton M, Cario GM. Methods of creating pneumoperitoneum: a review of techniques and complications. Obstet Gynecol Surv 1998;53(3):167–74.

89. Roviaro GC, Varoli F, Saguatti L, Vergani C, Maciocco M, Scarduelli A. Major vascular injuries in laparoscopic surgery. Surg Endosc 2002;16(8):1192–6.

90. Roy GM, Bazzurini L, Solima E, Luciano AA. Safe technique for laparoscopic entry into the abdominal cavity. J Am Assoc Gynecol Laparosc 2001;8(4):519–28.

91. Saber AA, Meslemani AM, Davis R, Pimentel R. Safety zones for anterior abdominal wall entry during laparoscopy: a CT scan mapping of epigastric vessels. Ann Surg 2004; 239(2):182–5.

92. Saville LE, Woods MS. Laparoscopy and major retroperitoneal vascular injuries (MRVI). Surg Endosc 1995;9(10):1096–1100.

93. Schrenk P, Woisetschlager R, Rieger R, Wayand W. Mechanism, management, and prevention of laparoscopic bowel injuries. Gastrointest Endosc 1996;43(6):572–4.

94. Soderstrom RM. Bowel injury litigation after laparoscopy. J Am Assoc Gynecol Laparosc 1993;1(1):74–7.

95. Soderstrom RM. Injuries to major blood vessels during endoscopy. J Am Assoc Gynecol Laparosc 1997;4(3): 395–8.

96. Sokol AI, Chuang K, Milad MP. Risk factors for conversion to laparotomy during gynecologic laparoscopy. J Am Assoc Gynecol Laparosc 2003;10(4):469–73.

97. Sriprasad S, Yu DF, Muir GH, Poulsen J, Sidhu PS. Positional anatomy of vessels that may be damaged at laparoscopy: new access criteria based on CT and ultrasonography to avoid vascular injury. J Endourol 2006;20(7):498–503.

98. Sutton CJ. Medico-legal implications of keyhole surgery. Medico-Legal J 1996;64(Pt 3):101–13.

99. Sutton CJG, Philips K. Preventing Gynaecological Laparoscopic Injury. Guideline No. 2007;48.

100. Teoh B, Sen R, Abbott J. An evaluation of four tests used to ascertain Veres needle placement at closed laparoscopy. J Minim Invasive Gynecol 2005;12(2):153–8.

101. Ternamian AM. Laparoscopy without trocars. Surg Endosc 1997;11(8):815–18.

102. Ternamian AM, Deitel M. Endoscopic threaded imaging port (EndoTIP) for laparoscopy: experience with different body weights. Obes Surg 1999;9(1):44–7.

103. Tsaltas J, Pearce S, Lawrence A, Meads A, Mezzatesta J, Nicolson S. Safer laparoscopic trocar entry: It's all about pressure. Aust N Z J Obstet Gynaecol 2004;44(4):349–50.

104. Vilos AG, Vilos GA, Abu-Rafea B, Hollett-Caines J, Al Omran M. Effect of body habitus and parity on the initial Veres intraperitoneal CO_2 insufflation pressure during laparoscopic access in women. J Minim Invasive Gynecol 2006; 13(2):108–13.

105. Vilos GA. Litigation of laparoscopic major vessel injuries in Canada. J Am Assoc Gynecol Laparosc 2000;7(4):503–09.

106. Vilos GA (2002) Laparoscopic bowel injuries: forty litigated gynaecological cases in Canada. J Obstet Gynaecol Canada: JOGC 24(3):224–30.

Section One

107. Vilos GA, Ternamian A, Dempster J, Laberge PY. Laparoscopic entry: a review of techniques, technologies, and complications. Society of Obstetricians and Gynaecologists of Canada Clinical Practice Guideline. J Obstet Gynaecol Can 2007;29(5):433–47.

108. Wang PH, Lee WL, Yuan CC et al. Major complications of operative and diagnostic laparoscopy for gynecologic disease. J Am Assoc Gynecol Laparosc 2001;8(1):68–73.

109. Wind J, Cremers JE, Berge Henegouwen MI, Gouma DJ, Jansen FW, Bemelman WA. Medical liability insurance claims on entry-related complications in laparoscopy. Surg Endosc 2007;5.

110. Woolcot R. The efficacy and safety of different techniques for trocar insertion in laparoscopic surgery. Minim Invasive Ther Allied Technol 2001;10(1):11–14.

111. Yim SF, Yuen PM. Randomized double-masked comparison of radially expanding access device and conventional cutting tip trocar in laparoscopy. Obstet Gynecol 2001;97(3):435–38.

Section One

7 Laparoscopic Dissection Techniques

Dissection is defined as the separation of tissues with hemostasis. It consists of a sensory visual and tactile component, an access component involving tissue manipulation and instrument maneuverability. These are combined to achieve exposure, i.e. developing a suitable space for seeing and handling target structures.

Precision and meticulous hemostasis is essential requirement in minimal access surgery. Endoscopic dissection, in contrast to dissection in conventional surgery, possesses several limitations. Three-dimensional direct visions are replaced by two-dimensional indirect visions in laparoscopic surgery. Illumination and the video image quality are still limited despite recent advances in video systems such as digitization and 3-chip endocamera. Movement of the functional tip of laparoscopic instruments is restricted along with the kinematics response. The loss of tactile sensation in endoscopic surgery is yet another limiting factor.

Endoscopic dissection and manipulation of tissue within a confined space requires a two handed approach, assisting and dissecting both task is performed by surgeon himself. A passive assisting instrument (usually a grasper) provides counter traction and exposure for the active dissecting instrument. The active instrument may be non-energized (e.g. scissors and scalpel) or energized with electricity (diathermy), ultrasound or light energy.

TYPES OF LAPAROSCOPIC DISSECTION

A variety of mechanisms have been used to divide tissue and enable hemostasis. They all involve some form of physical energy being applied to the appropriate tissue. The amount of energy required for dissection depends on the type and constituency of the tissue. The properties of tissues may vary in different directions and for different disease states. This in totality influences the choice of the modality for dissection.

The ideal dissection technique requires a modality that can accomplish meticulous hemostasis and will be tissue selective without causing inadvertent tissue damage. It must be safe for both patient and surgical team when in regular use and when inactive in storage. In this respect built-in safety measures are mandatory. An ideal dissecting modality should be efficient in both power delivery and in space requirement. The modality must be cost-effective also. The initial expenditure needed to acquire and set-up the necessary equipment must be taken into account along with subsequent operational and maintenance costs.

In reality there is no single "ideal" dissecting modality for entire minimal access surgical procedures. In actual practice, a combination of energy forms is applied with selection of the most appropriate one at each particular phase or type of the operation.

The available modalities for dissection in minimal access surgery include:
1. Blunt dissection
2. Sharp scalpel and scissors dissection
3. High frequency radio wave electrosurgery
4. Radio frequency ablation
5. Ultrasonic dissection
6. High velocity and high pressure water-jet dissection
7. Laser surgery.

Blunt Dissection

Instrument Used

1. Closed scissors tips used as blunt dissector
2. Scissor points used to separate by spreading the jaw
3. Grasper, straight and curved
4. Inactive suction cannula
5. Heel of inactive electrosurgery (Hook or Spatula)
6. Pledget.

Methods

1. Distraction
2. Separation
3. Teasing
4. Wiping.

Pledget Dissection

Endoscopic pledget dissection was first introduced in University of Dundee in 1987. A special endoscopic pledget or peanut swab 5.0 mm ratcheted holder, manufactured by Storz (with strong jaws and inward facing tongs at the end of the jaws for security), is used in a manner similar to that employed in open surgery. The holder grasping the pledget is introduced inside a reducer tube through a 11.0 mm cannula. The blunt dissection is safe and is used to open planes and expose structures especially when the anatomy is obscured by adhesions. The movement consists of forward and backward wipes accompanied by clockwise/counterclockwise rotation of the pledget swab. It is also useful for controlled small bleeder by compressions before this is secured by clipping or electrocoagulation. The pledget swab is particularly useful for blunt dissection in Calot's triangle during cholecystectomy. It is economical, simple to use and maintains a dry operative field while performing dissection. This type of dissecting modality is also utilized in hemostatically separating gallbladder from its bed, bladder from the uterus or the rectum from the sacral attachment (Fig. 7.1).

Removal of pledget must be carried out under vision, to ensure that the swab is inside the reducer tube before withdrawal of the instrument, otherwise there is a real risk of losing the small pledget swab in the peritoneal cavity.

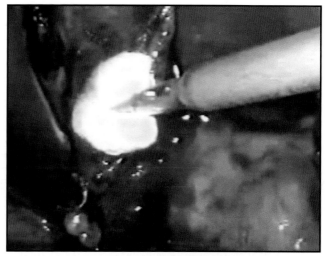

Fig. 7.1: Pledget dissection

The pledget is an invaluable tool for the rapid dissection of loose areolar planes when it is wiped or pushed against the line of cleavage to separate the tissues.

Pledget is useful in maneuvers to control minor hemorrhage. The pledget can be placed over the bleeding point to apply pressure. When used on an oozing operative field, it adsorbs some of the blood and may clarify the anatomical position.

It is important to follow routine practice, to minimize loss of the peanut swab inside the abdomen:

1. Always use a reducer tube to insert and remove the swab.
2. Employ a safe system (ratchet and elastic band) to maintain the grip of instrument used for insertion.
3. Keep the pledget in view from insertion to retraction into the introducer tube. Be sure it is retrieved into the introducer, not the cannular end.

Tissue Stripping and Tissue Distraction

These are other safe and effective forms of blunt dissection. The later is applied for seromyotomy. Insignificant hemostatic capability is the main disadvantage of blunt dissection (Fig. 7.2).

Sharp Dissection

Sharp scalpel is used mainly for division by cutting. Although inexpensive, its use is restricted in laparoscopic surgery. The lack of hemostasis, the potential of injury from the tip when inserting through

Section One

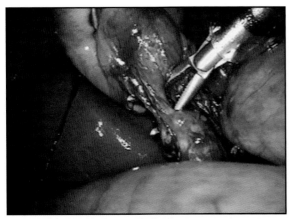

Fig. 7.2: Tissue stripping and dissection

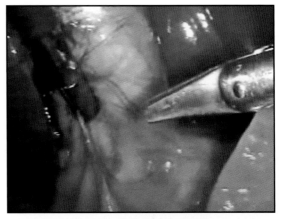

Fig. 7.3: Scissor Dissection

the port and the kinematics problems restricts its use to common bile duct division.

Scissors Dissection

It is one of the most frequent methods in laparoscopic surgery. It offers the benefits of being cheap, safe and precise operator determined action. However, being non-hemostasis renders it far from ideal as a dissecting modality (Fig. 7.3).

Electrosurgical Dissection

Electrosurgery is the most convenient way of dissection in minimal access surgery combined with most risky method of dissection. Most of the complication in laparoscopic surgery is due to use of energized instrument (1%) (Fig. 7.4).

Before understanding the principle of electrosurgery following definitions should be known.
• Current = Flow of electrons
• Circuit = Pathway for flow of electrons
• Voltage = Force that causes electron to flow
• Resistance = Obstacle to the flow of electron.

There are two basic principles of electricity:
1. Electrical current ultimately flows to ground
2. It always follows the path of least resistance.

HIGH FREQUENCY (HF) ELECTROSURGICAL DISSECTION

Our household appliances have the 50 to 60 Hz frequency. This frequency is beneficial because if faulty instrument has current and inadvertently someone touches, then he will be thrown away and the person

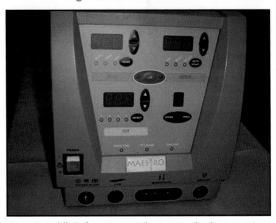

Fig. 7.4: High frequency electrosurgical generator

getting shock will be safe. If the frequency is more than 100 kHz, muscle and nerve stimulation ceases, whereas, all other property of electric current is still there. High frequency electrosurgery is the application of HF currents (in the frequency range of 300 kHz up to several MHz) to coagulate, fulgurate, spray coagulates or ablates tissue. Knowledge of how this and other physical modes interact with biological materials is becoming increasingly important to the surgeon for safe and consistent surgery (Fig. 7.5).
• Standard electrical current alternates at a frequency of 50 cycles per second (Hz).
• Nerve and muscle stimulation cease at 100,000 cycles/second (100 kHz).
• Electrosurgery can be performed safely at frequencies above 100 kHz.

HF Monopolar Electrosurgery

The monopolar circuit is composed of the generator, active electrode, patient, and patient return electrode.

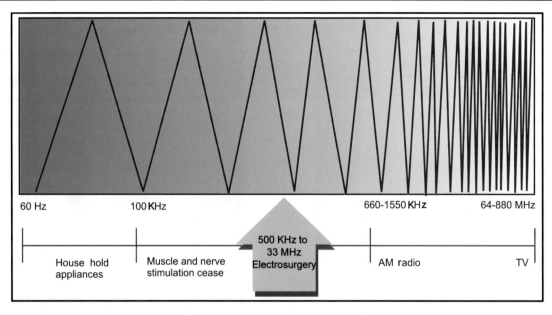

Fig. 7.5: Frequency range of electrosurgery

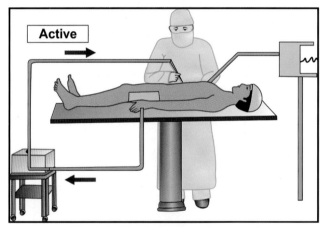

Fig. 7.6: Circuit of monopolar current

The patient's tissue provides the resistance, producing heat (Fig. 7.6).

Monopolar diathermy is used in endoscopic surgery for coagulation and for dissection (cutting). During monopolar diathermy, current is conducted from the instrument through the tissues to a skin pad (neutral electrode) connected back to the generator. Heating occurs at site of small cross section and low electrical conductivity. A high current density occurs in the tissue in immediate contact with the instrument and heat is generated.

Burn = Intensity of current × Time/area

Burn is directly proportional to the intensity of current. Intensity of current can be adjusted by the knob provided in the generator's control panel. If the intensity setting is more the burn will be more. Intensity actually denotes ampere or number of electrons that flows through the pathway.

Burn is also directly proportional to time. Time is paddle application time. Surgeon should always keep in mind that continuous activation of paddle can result in many complications. Intermittent activation is always better than continuous activation (Figs 7.7 and 7.8).

Burn is inversely proportional to area. One of the major problem in electrosurgery is patient will get burn at the site where area is narrowest. This may cause remote injury with the use of monopolar diathermy. The surgeon should hold the tissue with the point of instrument to catch the minimum amount of tissue at one time. If a bunch of tissue is caught there is always fear of remote injury.

Patient Return Electrodes

Silicon and metal patient return plates are available. The silicon is better because it does not have any sharp edge and the resistance is less (Fig. 7.9). Patient return electrode is required only in unipolar electrosurgery because the patients body is a part of circuit and the patient return plate will take the current back to the generator. If the patient return plate is not attached properly to the body of the patient, or the size of the patient return plate is very small, patient can get electric

Section One

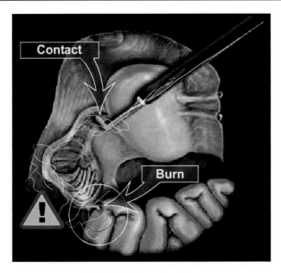

Fig. 7.7: Remote injury

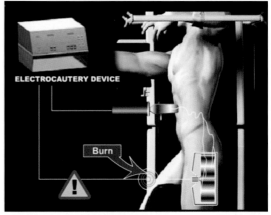

Fig. 7.8: Remote injury with electrocautery device

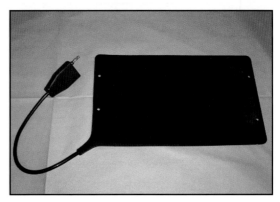

Fig. 7.9: Silicon pad

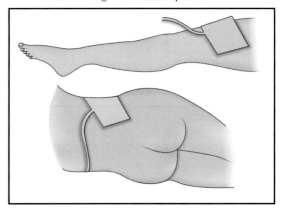

Fig. 7.10: Patient return pad

burn at the point of attachment of this patient return plate. Ideally the size of patient return plate should not be less than 100 square cm.

At the time of location of patient return plate attachment surgeon should keep in mind the following points (Fig. 7.10).

Choose

Well vascularized muscle mass to have more area of contact.

Avoid

* Vascular insufficiency should be avoided because of high resistant
* Irregular body contours can prevent plate to be in firm contact
* Bony prominences will not allow the surrounding skin to be in contact.

Consider

* Plate should be nearer to incision site
* Plate should be placed according to patients position so should not be displaced
* Plate should be away from other equipments like cardiac monitor.

The effect of HF current on the tissues depends on:
* Temperature generated.

Remote Injury

* Shape and dimensions of the contact point (broader damage with broader contact)
* Time of activation (short bursts reduce depth and charring)
* Distance from the electrode (Fig. 7.11)
* Conductivity of the tissue (bleeding results in a change in conductivity)

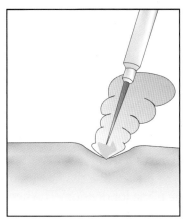

Fig. 7.11: Effect of cutting current

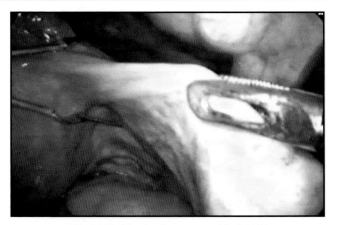

Fig. 7.13: Bipolar forcep used in LAVH

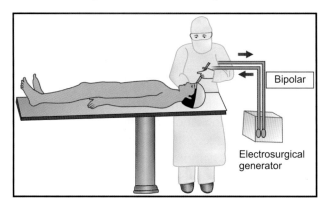

Fig. 7.12: Circuit of bipolar current

- Power output from the generator (voltage)
- Amplitude and current wave form time curve of the signal (cutting or coagulating settings).

Bipolar Diathermy

A bipolar system is inherently safer as the interaction is restricted to the immediate vicinity of contact and the current does not pass through the patient but instead returns to the generator via the receiving pole after passage through the grasped tissue (Fig. 7.12).

BIPOLAR ELECTROSURGERY

- Active output and patient return functions are both are at the site of surgery.
- Current path is confined to tissue grasped between forceps (Fig. 7.13).
- Return electrode should not be applied for bipolar procedures.

Tripolar Electrosurgery

Bipolar probes are now available for coagulation as well as for cutting. The cutting system is not strictly bipolar and is hence referred to as tripolar (Fig. 7.14).

It has four functions in one and the same instrument namely:
- Dissecting
- Grasping
- Bipolar coagulation
- Bipolar cut.

USE OF THE DIATHERMY HOOK

These are generally L or open C shaped, blunt ended rods mounted on an insulated handle. The active, non-insulated part is limited in size. The hook is a delicate

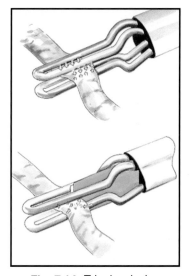

Fig. 7.14: Tripolar device

Section One

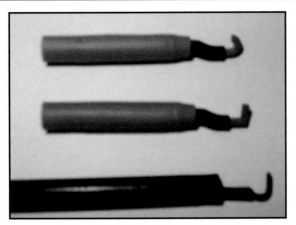

Fig. 7.15: Different types of hook

instrument and should be protected during insertion by manual opening of the cannula valve or use of a reducing tube. As electrosurgery generates smoke (which is harmful), many handles of electrosurgical hooks have a suction attachment at the other end of the handle.

Electrosurgical Hooks (Fig. 7.15)

Electrosurgical instruments like the hook are useful as blunt dissectors prior to activation. They are used to isolate the tissue to be divided by the current. The tip is passed into or under a layer of the tissue being dissected, which is then hooked and tented up (to increase its impedance and thus limit the spread of current when applied). Small portions of tissue are tackled so that an assessment of the tissue caught on the hook can be made before coagulation or cutting current is applied to the instrument. The hook can be used to clear unwanted tissue beside linear structures by passing the hook into the tissues parallel to the structure, and then rotating it to hook up strands of unwanted tissue. The tissue to be divided is held away from underlying tissue to prevent inadvertent damage. Short bursts of coagulating current can be followed by the use of cutting current, if the tissue has not already separated. The use of the hook can be summarized as "HOOK, LOOK, COOK".

The hook or the spatula may be used to mark out and coagulate a line for division. The heel of the hook is used with the HF current set to soft coagulation. Short bursts are applied and the hook moved along to create a "dotted" line of coagulated tissue. When deeper penetration is desired, the hook is appropriate instrument. This type of contact is best reserved for situation where no significant damage can be caused by current penetration (Fig. 7.16).

Monopolar electrosurgery has become the most widely used cutting and coagulating technique in minimal access surgery. It has proven to be versatile, cost effective and demonstrated superior efficacy for coagulation. By varying the voltage, current or waveform, tissue can be cut cleanly ("pure cut"); coagulated to achieve hemostasis ("coag mode") or a "blend cut" that combines these two functions can also be produced. Finally, a dispersed coagulation mode known as fulguration, allows coagulation of diffuse bleeding (Fig. 7.17).

Cutting current is low voltage high frequency current. Due to high frequency, the ions inside the cell

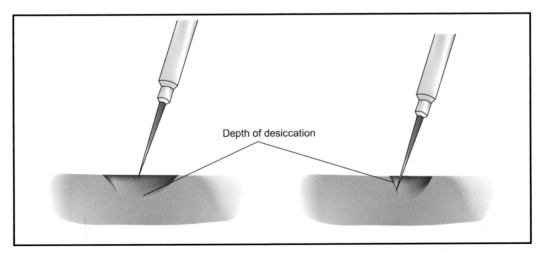

Depth of desiccation

Fig. 7.16: Depth of desiccation is proportional to paddle application time

Section One

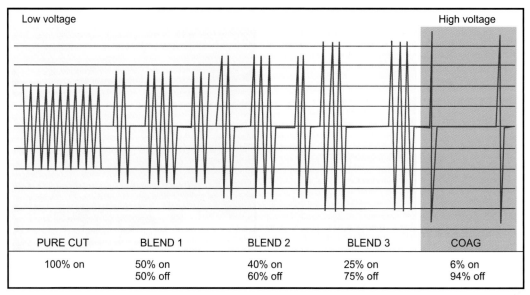

Low voltage				High voltage
PURE CUT	BLEND 1	BLEND 2	BLEND 3	COAG
100% on	50% on 50% off	40% on 60% off	25% on 75% off	6% on 94% off

Fig. 7.17: Different types of electrosurgery

get turbulence and cells brust (explode or evaporize). Cutting current can be obtained by pressing the yellow paddle of electrosurgical generator. To cut any structure it is important that surgeon should apply the sharp tip of electrosurgical instrument and the tissue should not be held firmly. At the time of cutting it is wise that tissue should be under tension. Ideally direct touch with the tissue should be avoided in case of cutting current. It should be spark wave from some distance (Fig. 7.18).

Electrosurgical coagulation is achieved by high voltage low frequency current. This low frequency is not sufficient to cause the explosion of cell but heat inside the cell is increased. Due to increased intracellular temperature, the protein inside the cell coagulates and shrinks. Shrinkage of protein will cause constriction in the lumen of bleeding vessels and the vessels are sealed. Permanency of coagulated tissue and its sealing effect depends upon melted collagen. At the time of electrosurgical monopolar coagulation the temperature of tissue cause the collagen to melt. These melted collagens solidify again once the active instrument is off from the tissue. It is important to remember that if the tissue is burnt more than required, the melted collagen burns, turns into charcoal and the sealing strength of the lumen of any vessel will decrease. Surgeons and gynecologists should always try to avoid overcooking of the tissue.

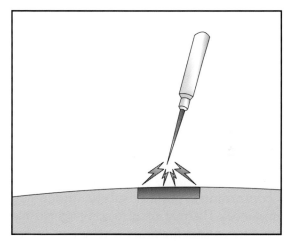

Fig. 7.18: Fulguration

Electrosurgical coagulation is of two types:

1. *Fulguration*

Fulguration is coagulation current from some distance.It is also known as spray mode. At the time of fulguration lateral spread of energy is more than depth. We want to use fulguration everywhere, where superficial burn is required and deeper injury may cause damage of underlying structure. The example of good use fulguration is ablation in cases of endometriosis, fulguration of gallbladder bed at the time of cholecystectomy, if there is generalized oozing from liver. Direct touch with tissue should be avoided

Section One

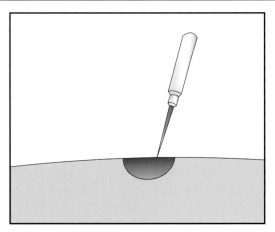

Fig. 7.19: Desiccation with more collateral damage

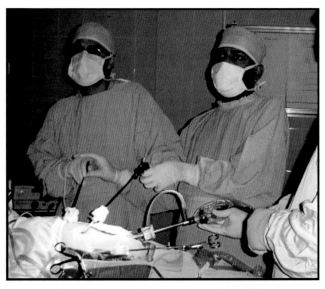

Fig. 7.21: Overshooting should be avoided

to achieve maximum effect. Fulguration is coagulation current from some distance.

2. *Desiccation*

Electrosurgical desiccation occurs when the electrode is in direct contact with the tissue. Most of the time with the unipolar or bipolar electrosurgery we do desiccation only. The tissue damage in depth and width is same in desiccation. The extent of collateral damage in desiccation is more compared to cutting current. The extent of collateral damage of desiccation can be minimized by minimizing the paddle application time (Figs 7.19 and 7.20).

However, monopolar laparoscopic electrosurgery can compromise patient safety under certain circumstances. Thermal injury to non-targeted internal organs may occur firstly as a result of imprecise mechanical operation of a laparoscopic instrument and secondly through diversion of electrical current to other

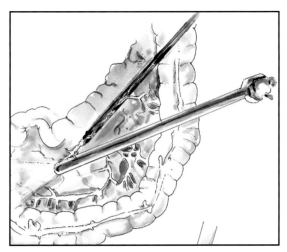

Fig. 7.22: Direct coupling

paths. These stray current may be released either through insulation failure, direct coupling or capacitive coupling. Other problems encountered include effect on pacemakers; return electrode burns, toxic smoke, charring of instruments and minimal control of energy delivery (Fig. 7.21).

Bipolar electrodes design although virtually eliminating complication from insulation failure, capacitive coupling and direct coupling (Figs 7.22 to 7.25).

The primary electrothermal tissue effect is limited to desiccation, not cutting. It requires slightly more time than monopolar coagulation because of lower power settings and bipolar generator output characteristics.

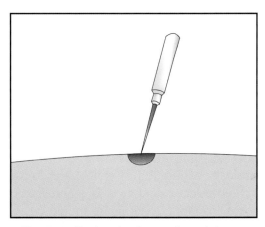

Fig. 7.20: Desiccation less collateral damage

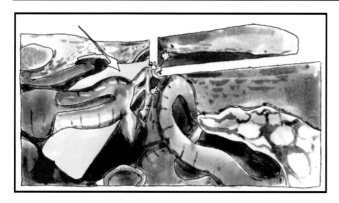

Fig. 7.23: Direct coupling

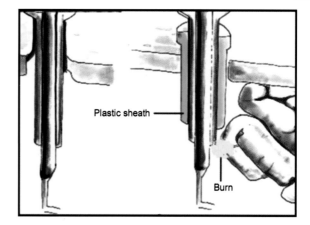

Fig. 7.25: Burn due to capacitive coupling

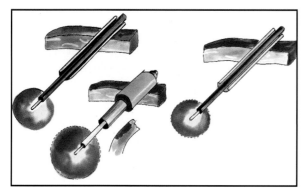

Fig. 7.24: Capacitive coupling

Safety Considerations in MAS

The potential for accidental damage with electrosurgery must always be borne in mind at the time of minimal access surgery. Following are the most commonly encountered problems specific to the minimal access surgery.

1. Overshooting
2. Overcooking
3. Direct coupling
4. Capacitive coupling
5. Insulation failure.

It is not an effective method of making a "pure cut".
• Hemostasis over a large area is not possible
• Grasping dense tissue between both the active and return electrodes is difficult.

SAFETY DURING ELECTROSURGERY

Laparoscopic dissection requires more extensive dissection and thus meticulous hemostasis becomes particularly important. Any loss of view will result in loss of control and hence decreased safety. Hemorrhage, even to a minor extent, tends to obscure their operative field and is to be avoided. This means that vessels of a size that in open surgery could be divided without particular attention need to be secured prior to division when working endoscopically. Dissection must be more meticulous to proceed smoothly to avoid any unacknowledged injury.

The magnification produced by the endoscope may initially confuse the surgeon as to the extent of electrical injury. However, an inexperienced endoscopic surgeon is well advised to convert should he have any doubt about his ability to control the situation expeditiously.

Overshooting

Overshooting means the tip of energized instrument going beyond the field of vision during electrosurgery. Over shooting is one of the common mistakes done by beginners. Surgeon should be careful that if they are cutting any structure they should apply less force otherwise their instrument will overshoot once the structure is cut and the energized instrument can heat any nearby viscera leading to perforation.

During initial learning phase of laparoscopy the trainer surgeon should keep hold on the hand of trainee at the time of electrosurgery to prevent any inadvertent injury by overshooting. At the time of laparoscopic cholecystectomy, if hook overshoots it may hit diaphragm or duodenum. If overshooting is not under the control of surgeon he should try to keep the tip of hook towards the anterior abdominal wall so that only peritoneum will be injured.

Section One

Overcooking

Proper hemostasis requires optimum application of energy over the tissue. Due to visual limitations and fear of impending bleeding, laparoscopic surgeons have a tendency of overcooking. It is important to remember that instead of more secure coagulation overcooking can create rebleeding. To understand the effect of overcooking it is important to know physiology of tissue sealing.

Coagulation current is high voltage low frequency current. At this current, the ions inside the cell will move but it cannot explode. Due to increase in intracellular heat, the protein inside the cell will be denatured, coagulated and shrink. Due to shrinkage of tissue the lumen of small bleeder obliterates and bleeding stops. At the same time due to heat, the collagen of tissue melts and once the paddle of electrosurgical generator is off the melted collagen will cool down and solidify.

Overcooking results in charring of melted collagen and the sealing strength of tissue is decreased. It could be understood just by the example of sealing of polythene over a flame of candle. If you want to seal the polythene bag but applying more temperature on polythene by putting it over direct flame, instead of getting sealed the polythene will start burning. One should know the sealing temperature of polythene so that required temperature is applied, the polythene will melt and once cooled will solidify. Similarly, the burnt collagen does not have any tissue sealing property and bleeding may start again if it is overcooked.

Most common causes of overcooking or charring of tissue are:
• High power setting of electrosurgical generator
• Prolonged activation of foot paddle
• Keeping the jaw closed permanently in contact of tissue
• Poorly engineered electrosurgical generator.

Direct Coupling

If the active electrode touches a non-insulated metal instrument within the abdomen, it will convey energy to the second instrument, which may in turn, if the current density is high enough, transfer it to surrounding tissues and cause a thermal burn. For example, the active electrode could come in contact or in close proximity (less than 2 mm) to a laparoscope, creating an arc of current between the two. The laparoscope could then brush against surrounding tissue, causing a severe burn to the bowel and other structures. The burns may not be in the visual field of the surgeon and therefore will not be recognized and dealt with in a timely fashion.

To prevent direct coupling, the active electrode should not be in close proximity to or touching another metal instrument before the generator is activated. Bowel is particularly susceptible to this kind of collateral damage from sparks and stray currents. Recognition of this complication maybe delayed until the postoperative period with serious consequences. Check that the electrode is touching the target tissue, and only that tissue, before you activate the generator. Note that when target tissue is coagulated (desiccated), the impedance increases and the current may arc to adjacent tissue, following the path of least resistance.

We should be careful that all metal instruments, such as laparoscopes pass through conductive metal trocars. This way, if the active electrode touches the instrument, the current will simply flow from the instrument to the metal trocar. As long as the trocar is in contact with a relatively large portion of the abdominal wall, the current will not concentrate. Instead, it will dissipate harmlessly from the trocar through the abdomen and back through adjacent tissue to the return electrode. If the trocar is completely or partially constructed of plastic, however, the energy may not be able to dissipate back through the body. The metal within the trocar will build up a charge, which could eventually arc to adjacent tissue and back to the return electrode, but at a harmful level of current. In doing so, it may travel through the bowel, skin, or even the operator's hands, causing burns (Fig. 7.24).

To avoid direct coupling surgeon should not activate the generator while the active electrode is touching or in close proximity to another metal object.

Capacitance Coupling

This now never arise but occurred in the early days of laparoscopic surgery with the use of plastic fixation screws to fix metal ports to the abdominal wall so as to prevent them from being accidentally pulled out or pushed when instruments were withdrawn during the course of an operation.

The physics underling this injury is fairly straight forward. Whenever current is applied through an insulated instrument inserted through a metal trocar (port) some radio frequency electric charge is transferred to the metal cannula by every activation (even if the insulation of the instrument is perfect). This effect is known as capacitance coupling.

There is absolutely no problem if the metal cannula is in contact with the full thickness of the abdominal wall, as the charge accumulated by the cannula is immediately discharged over a wide contact area (low power density, like the neutral return electrode plate) and hence no damage is done.

However, if the cannula is isolated from the abdominal wall, by a plastic screw (acting as an insulator), the cannula cannot discharge and thus accumulates a substantial charge with repeated activation of the electrosurgical instrument. Thus, in essence it becomes an electric accumulator! Should at any stage, the tip of the cannula inside the abdomen touch tissue or bowel, the accumulated charge will discharge immediately through a single point of contact, i.e. with a high power density sufficient to cause an electrical burn. Since this occurs away from the site of action of the operation, it is usually overlooked. Capacitance coupling is not a problem if plastic fixation screws are not used.

The phenomenon of "capacitance" is the ability of two conductors to transmit electrical flow even if they are separated by an intact layer of insulation. Capacitive coupling can occur even in the best-case scenario, that is, when the insulation around the active electrode is intact and the tip of the electrode isn't touching anything metal. If the active, insulated electrode is wrapped around a towel clamp, or placed inside a metal trocar sleeve, or comes in close contact with any conductive substance for an extended period of time, the current in the active electrode may induce a current in the second conductor.

As long as the induced current can dissipate easily, through a large surface of tissue, it won't present a problem. The danger occurs if the second conductor contains some insulating material, as in the case of a metal cannula held in place by a plastic anchor. The plastic anchor will prevent the energy from dissipating

and increase the likelihood of a thermal burn. Burns from capacitance current may occur when the surface area is less than 3 cm^2 or the current density is approximately 7 W/cm^2.

As with direct coupling, the best way to prevent this phenomenon is to use the active electrode monitoring system that prevents current from capacitive coupling from building to dangerous levels. Also, you should avoid all plastic-metal hybrid instruments, including cannulas, trocars, and clamps, when doing electrosurgery.

Insulation Failure

During a laparoendoscopic procedure, only about 10 percent of an insulated instrument is visible on the video monitor at any one time, which means about 90 percent of that electrode remains outside the surgeon's field of view, where it can cause the most damage. Whenever a defective instrument is introduced into the patient, electric current can escape to contiguous tissue or organs, but the surgeon is not aware that a thermal burn at a peripheral site has occurred. It is estimated that 67 percent of such injuries are not recognized at the time of surgery. Sadly, manifestations of these unsuspected injuries don't appear until several days after the actual surgery and so, when the impaired patient presents, his or her clinical symptoms are already severe. Diagnosis is difficult and often delayed, and the damage can be irreversible. Complications include perforated bowel diaphragm, urinary bladder, permanent disfigurement, fecal peritonitis cases, etc (Fig. 7.26).

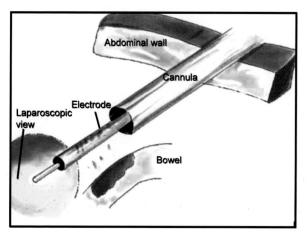

Fig. 7.26: Insulation failure

Continued regular use of cleaning and sterilization can cause the layer of insulation covering the shaft of the active electrode to break down. Tiny, visually undetectable tears are actually more dangerous than large cracks, since the current escaping from these miniscule breaks is more concentrated, and therefore capable of causing sparks (averaging 700° C). These sparks can cause severe burns and even ignite fires, especially in oxygen-rich environments. In fact, all insulated electrodes should be considered suspicious, unless adequate safety measures are introduced.

Unfortunately, many surgeons unknowingly contribute to the problem. Routine use of the high voltage "coagulation" current may actually compromise insulation integrity. The higher the voltage, the greater the risk that the current will break through weak insulation.

Surgeon should always use the lowest voltage. All electrosurgery systems will allow you to use a "coagulation" or "cutting" waveform of current.

In most cases, we should try to use the cutting current for both cutting and coagulation. The coagulation mode is necessary only when you need to fulgurate, or stop diffuse bleeding on highly vascularized tissue. Using the lowest voltage may reduce the wear on the insulation and minimize the chance that the current can escape through hairline cracks.

The surgeon should test for insulation defects in the operating room, after the set has been opened. This step can significantly reduce the number of accidental electrosurgical burns because it will prevent a surgeon from inserting a potentially lethal instrument into the patient's abdomen. Insulation that degraded during that final sterilization cycle cannot be detected until this point in time, so it is critical that inspection in the operating room itself be made an integral part of hospital protocol. It is advisable to keep a supply of single-use electrodes available to replace any found to be faulty during the preoperative scan. One can also devise a vigorous and ongoing inspection plan with a qualified technician to ensure that all reusable electrosurgical tools are scanned and reinsulated as needed.

If the instruments are re-scanned in the operating room following surgery, the surgeon can be secure in the knowledge, that no stray electrical current escaped into adjacent, but unseen sites, and so if any post-operative clinical complications were to arise, he or she could more easily isolate the cause. Conversely, if the postoperative scan revealed that insulation was damaged during the procedure, he or she may elect to take aggressive steps to investigate further. For documentation purposes, the results of both scans can be recorded in the patient record.

We should always keep in mind that using the cutting current minimizes, but does not eliminate, the risk of insulation failure. To really be sure that the insulation is not compromised, it is recommended to use an electrosurgical unit that employs active electrode monitoring technology (AEM). This technology is called "Electro-Shield" (ElectroScope Inc., Boulder, Colo.) and it virtually eliminates these types of electrical burns.

The traditional system for inspection in the sterile processing department is hardly foolproof, and its weaknesses must be addressed. Because the margin for error is so great, risk managers and physicians alike are insisting on alternatives that will ensure patient safety and reduce liability exposure. Active electrode monitoring protects against thermal burns in two ways. First, it encases the insulated electrode in a protective metal shield that is connected to the generator; the entire probe is also covered with an extra layer of insulation. The extra conductive and insulating layers ensure that stray current is contained and flows right back to the generator. Second, the system monitors the electrical circuit so if stray energy reaches dangerous levels, the unit shuts off automatically and sounds an alarm before a burn can occur. Electroscope's AEM system operates on a principle similar to ground fault interrupt (GFI) outlets in our home. It protects against insulation breaks by grounding electricity is unpredictable elements, eliminating stray burns to the patient. This is presently considered the standard of care in endoscopic electrosurgery.

SURGICAL SMOKE

Dissection with electrocautery produces a great deal of smoke. Carbon monoxide at levels as high as 1900 ppm, many times higher than the environmental Protection Agency standard of 35 ppm for a one hour exposure, are produced by electrocautery in the hypoxic environment of the carbon dioxide filled abdomen. Fortunately carbon monoxide is a very insoluble molecule and does not cross the peritoneum. Carbon monoxide absorption is therefore not a problem for patients undergoing laparoscopy. However, contamination by carbon monoxide and other toxic or infectious byproducts of electrocautery may affect the operating room personnel if the smoke is vented into the room.

When an electrosurgical probe heats tissue and vaporizes cellular fluid, one by product is surgical smoke. We know that these fumes, which can contain viral DNA, bacteria, carcinogens and irritants are malodorous and can cause upper respiratory irritation. We do not yet know whether they are capable of causing cancer or spreading infectious disease. Surgical smoke can also obscure the operative site and cause the surgeon to inadvertently touch the electrode to non-targeted tissue.

Surgical masks do not adequately filter surgical smoke, the particles are too small. A much better solution is a smoke evacuation system, a high-flow suction and filtering device that removes the particles from the air. Two kinds are available commercially. One uses a handheld nozzle, which is intended to be positioned at the surgical site.

To avoid complication of laparoscopic electro-surgery following important points are:
- Inspect insulation carefully
- Use lowest possible power setting
- Use a low voltage waveform (cut)
- Use brief intermittent activation vs. prolonged activation
- Do not activate in open circuit
- Do not activate in close proximity or direct contact with another instrument
- Use bipolar electrosurgery when appropriate
- Select an all metal cannula system as the safest choice. Do not use hybrid cannula systems that mix metal with plastic
- Utilize available technology, such as a tissue response generator to reduce capacitive coupling or an active electrode monitoring system, to eliminate concerns about insulation failure and capacitive coupling.

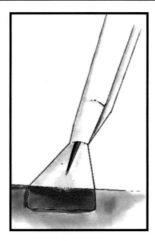
Fig. 7.27: Argon electrosurgery

ARGON BEAMER COAGULATOR

The argon beamer is used in conjunction with monopolar electrosurgery to produce fulguration or superficial coagulation (Fig. 7.27). Less smoke is produced because there is lesser depth of tissue damage. Despite these advantages, the argon beamer suffers from a very significant drawback in laparoscopic surgery, namely, increased intra-abdominal pressure to potentially dangerous levels due to high-flow infusion of argon gas.

ULTRASONIC DISSECTION

Ultrasonic dissectors are of two types: low power which cleaves water containing tissues by cavitations leaving organized structures with low water content intact, e.g. blood vessels, bile ducts, etc. and high power systems which cleave loose areolar tissues by frictional heating and thus cut and coagulate the edges at the same time. Thus, low power systems are used for liver surgery (Cusa, Selector) and do not coagulate vessels. High power systems (Autosonix, Ultracision) are used extensively especially in fundoplication and laparoscopic colon surgery. It is important to remember that high power ultrasonic dissection systems may cause collateral damage by excessive heating and this is well documented in clinical practice.

Ultrasonic surgical dissection allows coagulation and cutting with less instrument traffic (reduction in operating time), less smoke and no electrical current.
- Mechanical energy at 55,500 vibrations/sec
- Disrupts hydrogen bonds and forms a coagulum

Section One

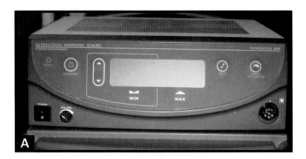

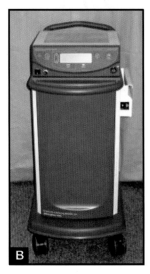

Figs 7.28A and B: Ultrasonic generator

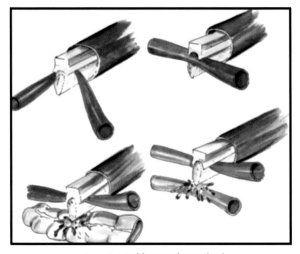

Fig. 7.29: Harmonic scalpel

- Temperature by harmonic scalpel, 80-100°C
- Temperature through electrocoagulation, 200-300°C
- Less collateral damage, less tissue necrosis.

The ultrasonic shears (harmonic scalpel) is ideal for dividing and simultaneously sealing small and medium vessels by tamponade and heat. However, larger vessels, greater than 2 mm in diameter, need additional measures (clips, tie or staple) to control bleeding. Other disadvantages of the harmonic scalpel include lack of tissue selectivity and relatively expensive. Ultrasonic dissecting applicators are also designed in hook, spatula or ball coagulator shapes (Figs 7.28A and B).

The Cavitational Ultrasonic Aspirator has the advantage of removing debris and is tissue selective, e.g. divides liver but spares bile ducts and vessels. It affords safe rapid dissection with reduction in tissue damage and blood loss compared to the harmonic scalpel. The problems associated with its use are evacuation of the pneumoperitoneum together with vibration and irrigation which cloud the telescope lens necessitating frequent cleaning (Fig. 7.29).

It is not correct that ultrasonic generators are without any risk. If bowel or blood vessels touch directly to the vibrating jaw it can be punctured.

High Velocity Water Jet Dissection

High velocity high pressure water-jet dissection involves the use of relatively simple devices to produce clean cutting of reproducible depth. Other advantages are the cleansing of the operating field by the turbulent flow zone and the small amount of water required to complete dissection.

Specific problems were identified with the use of this modality. The "hail storm" effect result in excessive misting which obscures vision. This has been solved to some extent by incorporating a hood over the nozzle. The non-hemostatic nature of this modality, difficulty in gauging distance and poor control of the depth of the cut are additional drawbacks. The spraying of tissue fragments renders it also oncologically unsound. The present use of water-jet dissection is limited to dissection of solid organs.

Hydrodissection

Hydrodissection uses the force of pulsatile irrigation with crystalloid solutions to separate tissue planes. The operating field at the same time is kept clear. Like water jet dissection no hemostasis is achievable. The use of this dissecting modality is restricted to pelvic lymphadenectomy and pleurectomy in thoracoscopic surgery.

Laser Dissection

The laser devices release photons which induce molecular vibration and create heat when they interact with the tissue and create heat. LASER is an acronym for "light amplification by stimulated radiation. Each lasing substance has a unique atomic and molecular structure and so the waveform and frequency. Laser light is monochromatic and cannot be separated into colors when passed through prism. The amount of power delivered by laser is measured in Watts. The basic components in a laser unit are a pumping system, lasing medium, optical cavity and operating system. The operating system controls delivery of laser into tissue when activated by surgeon. The surgeon controls power control knob. There are many modes of power delivery like: Continuous mode, pulse mode, super pulse mode and ultra pulse mode.

The primary difference from other source of energy is that, generally tissue is not directly touched by surgical instrument. Thus, the depth of incision is not controlled by pressure exerted on the tissue but by the power density delivered by surgeon. The unique property of laser is determined by its wavelength and tissue absorption. By changing the power setting, desired tissue effect such as ablation, fulguration, coagulation or vaporization can be achieved. These days laser are not used frequently in general laparoscopic surgery as they offer no advantages over more user friendly and safer forms of energized dissection and coagulation systems.

The previous generation of lasers (with gas vapor chambers) was large, very expensive and required special power supply (3-phase electricity) and maintenance. In addition they lacked portability. The current generation of solid state diode-array lasers has overcome all these disadvantages and may well be used for certain applications of laparoscopic general surgery in the future. Currently, laser ablation is used largely in gynecological laparoscopic surgery, e.g. ablation of endometriosis and much less commonly for the photoablation of secondary tumors of the liver. The most effective use of CO_2 laser beam is laser knife gives high precision for dissection over sensitive area like bladder, ureter, and major blood vessels.

The degree and extent of thermal damage produced by laser depends on the structure, water content, pigmentation, optical and thermal properties and perfusion of the tissue. The properties of a particular laser beam are also other determinants of heat damage. Therefore, each of the various types of laser available have a specific clinical application.

In gynecology, the argon laser coagulator is the ideal method of treating small red endometriotic deposits. Tissue absorption of light is low and hemoglobin absorption high at its operating wavelengths of 488 nm and 514 nm, i.e. selective absorption.

The carbon dioxide laser is best suited for extremely superficial ablation. It is relatively inexpensive (compared to other lasers) and has the ability to vaporize a very thin surface of tissue. On the other hand, photocoagulation of vascular lesions is ineffective using CO_2 laser. This type of laser also has the potential for injuring structures in the abdomen distant from the site under laparoscopic view.

The contact Nd: YAG laser virtually eliminates the free beam effect and is therefore suitable for laparoscopic application. The thermal injury from contact laser is superficial. No additional protection is needed for the endocamera since they are already fitted with infrared filters. However, Nd: YAG laser dissection was found to be significantly slower and produced more blood loss than monopolar electrosurgery in laparoscopic cholecystectomy.

All lasers including KPT and the more recently developed solid state have several major drawbacks in common. They are expensive, inefficient, produce toxic smoke, non tunable, require specialized theatre and achieve variable penetration. Safety issues such as heat cumulative effect, burns due to accidental exposure and retinal damage also contribute towards preventing widespread use of laser.

It is now obvious that from the range of available dissecting modalities in laparoscopic surgery none has proven to be ideal. Utility of a particular modality is dictated by how close it meets the requirements to achieve safe, effective and hemostatic tissue division under the specific circumstances. The surgeon must be able to use the appropriate combination of modalities in order to exploit the benefit each has to offer during dissection.

When properly used, laser, microelectrode, ultrasonic dissector, Tissue response generator and mechanical instruments are equally effective in any

Section One

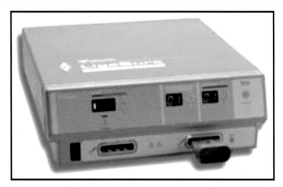

Fig. 7.30: Tissue response generator (Ligasure™)

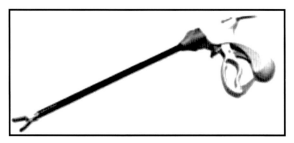

Fig. 7.31: Ligasure™

surgery. The choice of instrument should be on the instrument with surgeon is more comfortable and he has the skill and experience for that particular instrument.

CRYOTHERAPY AND RADIO FREQUENCY ABLATION

Both are used in the laparoscopic ablation of secondary tumor deposits in the liver, usually when the lesions are inoperable for whatever reason, laparoscopic cryotherapy with implantable probe destroys tumors by rapid freezing to – 40°C or lower. The lesion revascularizes for a short period (12-14 hours) on thawing but because the vasculature and the tumor parenchyma are damaged beyond repair, hemorrhagic infraction ensues. With RF thermal ablation, a radio frequency current is transmitted through the probe implanted in the tumor. The RF current causes molecular and ionic agitation which heats the tissues (much like the microwave) and hence the tumor is heated to destruction. Both modalities are operated with laparoscopic contact ultrasonographic scanning.

Tissue Response Electrosurgical Generator

The tissue response generator has unique vessel sealing ability. These vessel sealing produces significantly reduced thermal spread compared to existing bipolar instruments. These generators precisely confine its effects to the target tissue or vessel with virtually no charring and with minimal thermal spread to adjacent tissue (Fig. 7.30 and 7.31). These generator uses seal mechanism by sensing body's collagen to actually change the nature of the vessel walls by obliterating the lumen. The collagen and elastin within the tissue melt and reform to create the seal zone. These electrosurgical generator works by fusing the collagen in vessel walls to create a permanent seal. The jaw of electrosurgical forceps using this technology leaves no foreign material behind to potentially interfere with future diagnosis. The system uses the body's own collagen to reform the tissue, creating a permanent seal which resists dislodgment.

Tissue response generator has following advantages:
• It can be used with confidence on vessels up to 7 mm
• It seals all the tissue bundles without dissection and isolation
• It causes minimal thermal spread
• Its effect to the target tissue
• The unique energy output results in virtually no sticking
• Reduced sticking and charring
• Minimized need for multiple applications
• No dislodged clips
• No foreign material is left behind.

BIBLIOGRAPHY

1. Bagdasarian RW, Bolton JS, Bowen JC, Fuhrman GM, Richardson WS. Steep learning curve of laparoscopic splenectomy. J LaparoendoscAdv Surg Tech A 2000;10: 319–23.
2. Basdanis G, Papadopoulos VN, Michalopoulos A, Apostolidis S, Harlaftis N. Randomized clinical trial of stapled hemorrhoidectomy vs open with LigaSure for prolapsed piles. Surg Endosc 2005;19:235–9.
3. Berman RS, Yahanda AM, Mansfield PF, Hemmila MR, Sweeney JF, Porter GA, Kumparatana M, Leroux B, Pollock RE, Feig BW. Laparoscopic splenectomy in patients with hematologicmalignanc ies. Am J Surg 1999;178: 530–6.
4. Brunt LM, Langer JC, Quasebarth MA (1996) Comparative analysis of laparoscopic versus open splenectomy. Am J Surg 172: 596–601.

Section One

5. Carbonell AM, Joels CS, Kercher KW, Matthews BD, Sing RF, Heniford BT. A comparison of laparoscopic bipolar vessel sealing devices in the hemostasis of small-, medium, and largesized arteries. J Laparoendosc Adv Surg Tech A 2003;13: 377–80.

6. Crawford ED, Kennedy JS, Sieve V. Use of the Ligasure Vessel Sealing System in urologic cancer surgery. Grand Round Urol 1999;1: 10–17.

7. Delaitre B, Champault G, Barrat C, Gossot D, Bresler L, Meyer C, Collet D, Samama G. Laparoscopic splenectomy for hematologic disease. Study of 275 cases. French Society of Laparoscopic Surgery. Ann Chir 2000;125: 522–9.

8. Dexter SPL, Martin IG, Alao D, Norfolk DR, McMahon MJ. Laparoscopic splenectomy: the suspended pedicle technique. Surg Endosc 1996;10:393–6.

9. Diaz J, Eisenstat M, Chung R. A case-controlled study of laparoscopic splenectomy. Am J Surg 1997;173: 148–150

10. Dubay DA, Franz MG. Acute wound healing: the biology of acute wound failure. Surg Clin North Am 2003;83:463–81.

11. Franciosi C, Caprotti R, Romano F, Porta GC, Real G, Colombo G, Uggeri F. Laparoscopic versus open splenectomy: a comparative study. Surg Laparosc Endosc Percutan Tech 2000;5: 291–5.

12. Glasgow RE, Yee LF, Mulvihill SJ. Laparoscopic splenectomy. The emerging standard. Surg Endosc 1997;11: 108–12.

13. Goldstein SL, Harold KL, Lentzner A, Matthews BD, Kercher KW, Sing RF, Pratt B, Lipford EH, Heniford BT. Comparison of thermal spread after ureteral ligation with the Laparo-Sonic ultrasonic shears and the LigaSure system. J Laparoendosc Adv Surg Tech A 2002;12: 61–63.

14. Harrell AG, Kercher KW, Heniford BT. Energy sources in laparoscopy. Semin Laparosc Surg 2004;11: 201–9.

15. Heniford BT, Matthews BD, Sing RF, Backus C, Pratt B, Greene FL. Initial results with an electrothermal bipolar vessel sealer. Surg Endosc 2001;15: 799–801.

16. Horgan PG. A novel technique for parenchymal division during hepatectomy. Am J Surg 2001;181: 236–7.

17. Howard TJ, Mimms S. Use of a new sealing device to simplify jejunal resection during pancreaticoduodenectomy. Am J Surg 2005;190: 504–6.

18. Katkhouda N, Hurwitz MB, Rivera RT, Chandra M, Waldrep DJ, Gugheneim J, Mouiel J. Laparoscopic splenectomy: outcome and efficacy in 103 consecutive patients. Ann Surg 1998;228:568–78.

19. Katkhouda N, Mavor E. Laparoscopic splenectomy. Surg Clin North Am 2000;80: 1285–97.

20. Katkhouda N, Waldrep DJ, Feinstein D, Soliman H, Stain SC, Ortega AE, Mouiel J. Unsolved issues in laparoscopic splenectomy. Am J Surg 1996;172: 585–90.

21. Kennedy JS, Buysse SP, Lowes KR, Ryan TP. Recent innovation in bipolar electrosurgery. Minimally Invasive Ther Allied Technol 1999;8: 95–9.

22. Kennedy JS, Shanahan PL, Buysse SP, Ryan TP, Pearce JA, Thomsen S. Large vessel ligation using bipolar energy: a chronic animal study and histologic evaluation. 7th International meeting of the Society for Minimally Invasive Therapy 1999.

23. Kennedy JS, Shanahan PL, Taylor KD, Chandler JG. High-burst strength feed-back controlled bipolar vessel sealing. Surg Endosc 1998;12:876–8.

24. Klingler PJ, Tsiotos GG, Glaser KS, Hinder RA. Laparoscopic splenectomy: evolution and current status. Surg Laparosc Endosc 1999;9:1–8.

25. Lawes DA, Palazzo FF, Francis DL, Clifton MA. One year follow up of a randomized trial comparing LigaSure with open haemorrhoidectomy. Colorectal Dis 2004;6: 233–5.

26. Meijer DW, Gossot D, Jakimowicz JJ, De Wit LT, Bannemberg JJ, Gouma DJ. Splenectomy revised: manually assisted splenectomy with the dexterity device: a feasibility study in 22 patients. J LaparoendoscAdv Surg Tech A 1999;9: 507–10.

27. Meyer G, Wichmann MW, Rau HG, Hiller E, Schildberg FW Laparoscopic splenectomy for idiopathic thrombo-cytopenicpurpura. A 1-year follow-up study. Surg Endosc 1998;12: 1348–52.

28. Muller JM, Desambre R, Junghans T, Bohm B. Extended left emicolectomy using Ligasure Vessel Sealing System. 116th Surgical Congress, Munich, April 1999.

29. Park A, Birgisson G, Mastrangelo MJ, Marcaccio M, Witzke D. Laparoscopic splenectomy: outcomes and lessons learned from over 200 cases. Surgery 2000;128: 660–7.

30. Park A, Marcaccio M, Sternbach M, Witzke D, Fitzgerald P. Laparoscopic versus open splenectomy. Arch Surg 1999;134:1263–9.

31. Poulin EC, Mamazza J, Schlachta CM. Splenic artery embolization before laparoscopic splenectomy. An update. Surg Endosc1 1998;2: 870–5.

32. Romano F, Franciosi C, Caprotti R, Uggeri F, Uggeri F. Hepatic surgery using the LigaSure vessel sealing system. World J Surg 2005;29: 110–2.

33. Santini M, Vicidomini G, Baldi A, Gallo G, Laperuta P, Busiello L, Di Marino MP, Pastore V. Use of an electrothermal bipolar tissue sealing system in lung surgery. Eur J Cardiothorac Surg 2006;29: 226–30.

34. Schulze S, Krisitiansen VB, Fischer HB, Rosenberg J. Sealing of cystic duct with bipolar electrocoagulation. Surg Endosc 2002;16: 342–4. 2108.

35. Shields CE, Schechter DA, Tezlaf P, Baily AL, Dycus S, Cosgriff N. Method for creating ideal tissue fusion in soft-tissue structures using radio frequency energy (RF). Surg Technol Int 2004;13: 49–55.

36. Shigemura N, Akashi A, Nakagiri T, Ohta M, Matsuda H. A new tissue sealing technique using the LigaSure system for nonanatomical pulmonary resection: preliminary results of sutureless and stapleless thoracoscopic surgery. Ann Thorac Surg 2004;77: 1415–8.

37. Shimomatsuya T, Horiuchi T. Laparoscopic Splenectomy for treatment of patients with idiopathi-cthrombo cytopenicpurpura. Comparison with open splenectomy. Surg Endosc 1999;13: 563–6.

38. Steed DL. Wound-healing trajectories. Surg Clin North Am 2003;83: 547–55.

Section One

39. Stumpf M, Klinge U, Wilms A, Zabrocki R, Rosch R, Junge K, Krones C, Schumpelick V (2005) Changes of the extracellular matrix as a risk factor for anastomotic leakage after large bowel surgery. Surgery 137: 229–34.

40. Takada M, Ichihara T, Kuroda Y. Comparative study of electrothermal bipolar vessel sealer and ultrasonic coagulating shears in laparoscopic colectomy. Surg Endosc 2005;19: 226–8.

41. Targarona EM, Balague C, Marin J, Neto RB, Martinez C, Garriga J, Trias M. Energy sources for laparoscopic colectomy: a prospective randomized comparis on of conventional electrosurgery, bipolar computer-controlled electrosurgery and ultrasonic dissection. Operative outcome and costs analysis. Surg Innov 2005;12: 339–44.

42. Targarona EM, Espert JJ, Balague' C, Piulachs J, Artigas V, Trias M. Splenomegaly should not be considered a contraindication for laparoscopic splenectomy. Ann Surg 1998;228: 35– 39.

43. Trias M, Targarona EM, Espert JJ, Balague' C. Laparoscopic surgury for splenic disorders. Lessons learned from a series of 64 cases. Surg Endosc 1998;12: 66–72.

44. Walsh RM, Heniford BT, Brody F, Ponsky J. The ascendance of laparoscopic splenectomy. Am Surg 2001;67: 48–53.

45. Watson DI, Coventry BJ, Chin T, Gill PG, Malycha P. Laparoscopic versus open splenectomy for immune thrombocytopenic purpura. Surgery 1997;121: 18–22.1611.

46. Witte MB, Barbul A Repair of full-thickness bowel injury. Crit Care Med 2003;31: S538–S546.

47. Yang HR, Wang YC, Chung PK, Jeng LB, Chen RJ = Laparoscopic appendectomy using the LigaSure vessel sealing system. J Laparoendosc Adv Surg Tech A 2005;15: 353–56. 2109.

8 Laparoscopic Tissue Approximation Techniques

Knots are used since the time of primitive man for trapping animals and making weapons. Today's laparoscopic knots are basically a modification of knots used by Seamen, Fishermen, Weavers or Hangmen. In much of the literature on laparoscopic surgery, the learning curve for performing the technique is described as steep. In fact, laparoscopy is more than a new technique; it is a completely different way of operating as far as tissue approximation is concerned. The visualization is different, the instruments are different, and the tactile aspects are very different. Laparoscopic suturing and knotting is a skill that requires a great deal of practice: "As a young surgeon in training, you sit up all night, night after night, tying knots over and over and over again until you become perfect".

There are many ways of laparoscopic tissue approximation but most commonly used one are:
- Laparoscopic extracorporeal and intracorporeal knots
- Surgical glues which act as a tissue adhesive
- Laparoscopic clips
- Laparoscopic staplers
- Laser welding.

LAPAROSCOPIC SUTURING AND KNOTTING

It is important to remember that knot is either exactly right or is hopelessly wrong, and never nearly right.

There are three steps of knot tying:
- Configuration (Tying)
- Shaping (Drawing)
- Securing (Locking or snuggling).

Choice of Suture Material

Ideal Suture Characteristics

The choice of suture material influences wound healing. Ideal suture characteristics include:
- Good knot security
- Adequate tensile strength
- Flexibility and ease of handling
- Inertness and non-allergenic nature
- Resistance to infection
- Smooth passage through tissue
- Absorbability, when desirable.

Surgeons should choose sutures that they are comfortable with, and that are suited to the intended application. This choice should be based on the duration of tensile strength. For internal sutures, least number of knots should be used, to ensure knot security and avoid an excessive knot burden and consequent foreign body reaction.

Type of Suture

Sutures traditionally have been classified into natural (i.e. naturally occurring), and synthetic (man made). The use of natural sutures is declining, for a number of reasons. Examples of natural sutures include catgut and silk. Suture material is also classified into absorbable and non-absorbable.

Absorbable Sutures

The natural absorbable (catgut) tend to have unpredictable rates of absorption and tissue reaction. For the most part, these sutures have short half-lives, so they are not good for wound closure where strength is desirable. Their use is being discontinued.

The synthetic absorbable are broken down by hydrolyzation. They generally have a longer half-life, less tissue reaction, and a more consistent breakdown rate. The synthetic absorbable, polyglycolic acid (Dexon®) or polyglactin 910 (Vicryl®), have decreased tissue reaction compared to the natural absorbable. Knot security is fair and can be used for extracorporeal knotting.

Polyglactin 910 (Vicryl) keeps 75 percent of its tensile strength for about 2 weeks and 50 percent by 3 weeks. The coated sutures decrease the drag through tissue, so it is easier to use, but there are variable rates of absorption. Polyglactin is good suture material for intracorporeal suturing.

Poliglecaprone 25 (Monocryl®) is a monofilament product that has easy passage through tissue, good handling, and is inert. It keeps tensile strength for only a week, but stays in the wound for almost 4 months. It is good for anastomosis, gynecologic work, and small vessel ligation and epithelial approximation. This material can be used for both extra and intracorporeal suturing.

The delayed absorbable monofilament sutures such as polydioxanone (PDS®) and polyglyconate (Maxon®), used for abdominal wound closure have good tensile strength and low tissue reaction, but the knots are not as strong. PDS is considered as ideal material for extracorporeal knotting by many surgeons and gynecologists.

Polydioxanone (PDS) is also good for contaminated fields because it has a low affinity for bacteria. It is good for general use, tissue approximation, biliary work, anastomosis, fascial closures, heart surgery, and orthopedics.

Panacryl® is a braided synthetic absorbable suture. It has good tensile strength, low tissue reaction, and fairly good knot security. It maintains 60 percent of its tensile strength at 6 months. It may be a good substitute for a non-absorbable suture because it has complete absorption in 2½ years. It is good for fascial closures, closing tissues under tension, and it might have a role in the compromised patient where you presume there is going to be inadequate or delayed wound healing.

Non-absorbable Sutures

The natural non-absorbables, cotton and silk, should be relegated to the past. Even though they have good knot security, and are easy to tie, they provoke a lot of tissue reaction. Synthetic non-absorbable sutures in common use include nylon, polyester and stainless steel. The role of this material in laparoscopic surgery is very limited and can be used if the other materials are not available.

Suture Size

The narrower the suture, the lower is its tensile strength. Narrower sutures cause less scarring. In addition, a narrower suture will harbor fewer bacteria.

Surgeons should use the smallest suture that they are comfortable with and that will give optimal security of wound closure, with minimal wound tension.

Usually, 2/0 or 3/0 is used in most of the minimal access surgical procedure, with the exception of the fallopian tube, where 6/0 may be preferred.

Knots

The knot is the most important part of the suture closure *in vivo*, the knot is the determining factor in suture strength in 95 percent of sutures tested. Complex knots have twice the security of simple knots.

However, increasing complexity of the knot simply leads to the suture strength being the weak link. The size of the knot is also important. If you use the same suture and increase from 3 to 5 throws, the foreign body volume is increased by 50 percent.

LAPAROSCOPIC NEEDLE

In general surgery, needles are either straight or curved. With increasing proficiency, curved needle can also be used but in laparoscopic surgery most intuitive needle is endoski needle. Endoski has advantage of both straight and curved needle (Fig. 8.1).

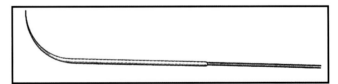

Fig. 8.1: Endoski needle

Endoski Needle

The distal end is tapered half circle and proximal shaft of the needle is straight. The shaft of the needle is 1.5 times the length of curved portion of endoski needle.

In our day to day practice we can convert half circled needle into endoski shaped by making proximal half of the needle straight.

Laparoscopic Suture Material

Although it is a personal preference and varies surgeon to surgeon but considering handicap of laparoscopic setting following is recommended.
- For extracorporeal suturing of small tubular structure like cystic duct and small blood vessels: dry chromic catgut.
- For extracorporeal suturing of thick tubular structure like appendix and large blood vessels: PDS.
- For intracorporeal continuous or interrupted suturing: Vicryl.
- For intracorporeal interrupted suturing in the repair of hernia, Fundoplication and rectopexy: Dacron (polyester) or silk.

Types of Laparoscopic Surgical Knots

- Extracorporeal (Tied outside the body and then slipped inside using a push rod)
  - Roeder's knot
  - Meltzer's knot
  - Tayside knot.
- Intracorporeal (tied with the help of needle holder within the body cavity)
  - Square knot
  - Surgeons knot
  - Tumble square knot
  - Dundee jamming knot
  - Aberdeen termination.

A long length of ligature is required (90 cm) for extracorporeal suturing. It must be long enough to have the knot pusher threaded on to it, to be passed into the abdomen, round the structure to be ligated and to be brought out again and still have sufficient length for the surgeon to tie his/her knot effectively. The type of extracorporeal knot chosen to complete the loop depends on the clinical situation and the material used.

ROEDER'S KNOT (FIGS 8.2A TO U)

Step 1:   The index finger of the assistant may be used to make extracorporeal knot. The left hand should be used to hold the short limb and the right hand long limb of thread.

Step 2:   The short limb of the thread is crossed over the long limb.

Step 3:   The intersection point of thread should be pinched by left hand index finger and thumb. At the time of making intersection, surgeon should keep sufficient length of short limb, to make it comfortably. It is important to remember that left hand is used only to hold the intersection point while the right hand will make the necessary hitches and loops.

Step 4:   The short limb is passed between the thread upward.

Step 5:   The short limb should be pulled from up by right hand to make first hitch.

Step 6:   The short limb should encircle the thread from below upward.

Step 7:   With the index finger and thumb the tail end is held.

Step 8:   The tail end of the thread is pulled to make first wind. Step 5 to 7 should be repeated two more times to make three winds.

Step 9:   After making three winds, the tail end is again passed from below up between the threads.

Step 10:   Once the tip of tail end projects up, it is pushed down by thumb inside the loop to make half knot.

Step 11:   The tail end is pulled from below to tighten the half knot.

Step 12:   Once the knot is configured properly, it should be checked by sliding over the long thread.

Step 13:   The tail end of knot should be cut short approximately to 2 cm.

Properly configured reader's knots loop diameter should be approximately 4 cm. Large size loop is difficult to manipulate inside the abdominal cavity and very short loop is difficult to reach up to the base of the structure which is to be tied.

Section One

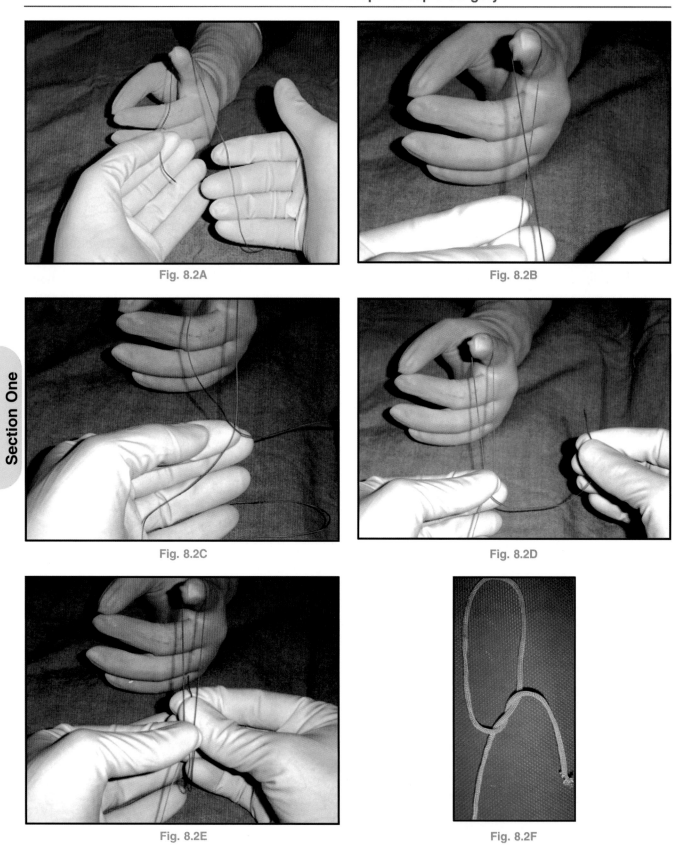

Fig. 8.2A

Fig. 8.2B

Fig. 8.2C

Fig. 8.2D

Fig. 8.2E

Fig. 8.2F

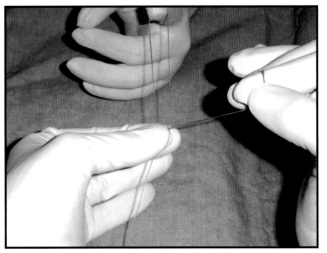

Fig. 8.2G

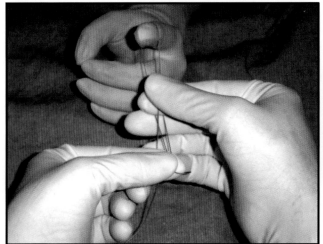

Fig. 8.2H

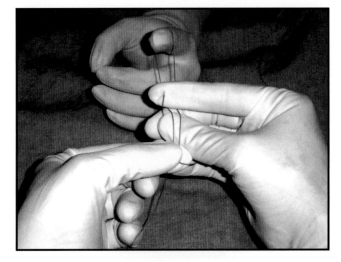

Fig. 8.2I

Figs 8.2J

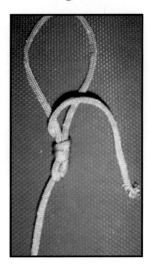

Fig. 8.2K

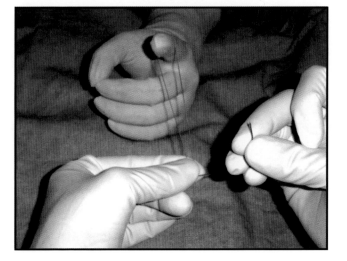

Fig. 8.2L

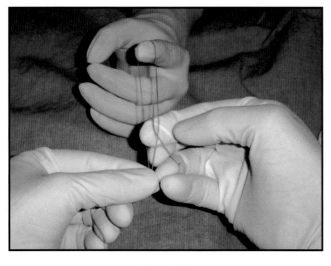

Fig. 8.2M

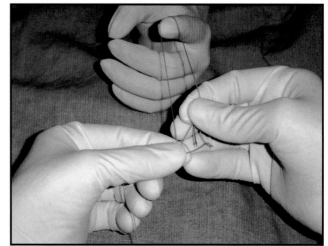

Fig. 8.2N

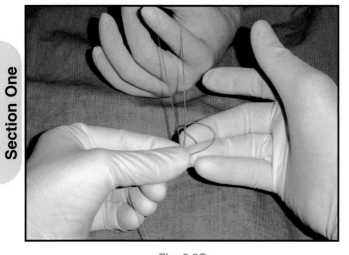

Fig. 8.2O

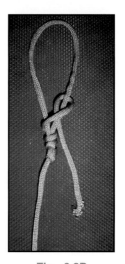

Fig. 8.2P

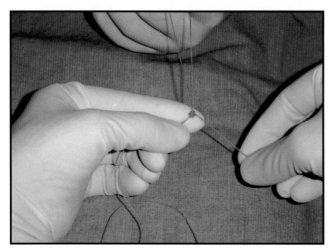

Fig. 8.2Q

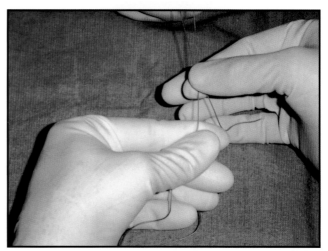

Fig. 8.2R

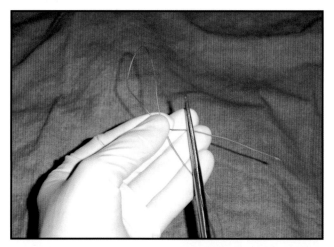

Fig. 8.2S

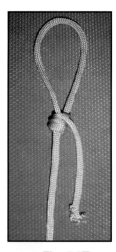

Fig. 8.2T

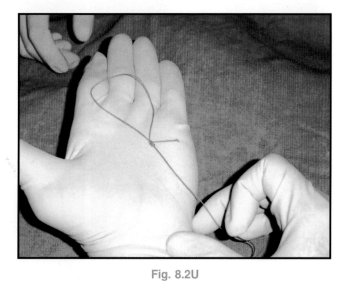

Fig. 8.2U

Figs 8.2A to U: Various steps of Roeder's knot

Roeder's knot can be remembered as 1:3:1
- One hitch
- Three winds
- One locking hitch.

The Meltzer Slip Knot

This modification of the Roeder knot was described in 1991 by Meltzer for use with PDS, and has now superseded the use of Roeder's knot. It has components:

- Two hitches
- Three winds
- Two-half locking hitches

Meltzer knot can be remembered as 2:3:2

Tying a Meltzer knot

Step 1: Two-half knot is taken first (Fig. 8.3A)

Step 2: Three rounds are taken in front of the first double half knot over both the limb of loop (Fig. 8.3B).

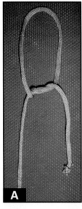

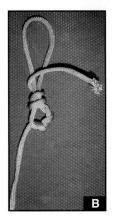

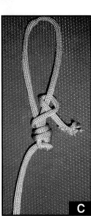

Figs 8.3A to C: Step of Meltzer slip knot

Step 3: Stack the knot and trim the short end. Slide the knot into place with knot pusher under tension (Fig. 8.3C).

APPLICATIONS

The Meltzer knot is now used by most of the surgeons instead of the Roeder knot to tie the medial end of the cystic duct during cholecystectomy and to fix the cystic duct drainage cannula after trans-cystic clearance of ductal stones, as catgut is no longer available. PDS is the suture material of choice for Meltzer knot.

The Tayside Knot (Figs 8.4A to O)

The Tayside knot is safe for use with any braided material. It supplies a degree of resistance to reverse slippage equivalent to a surgeons knot.

Step 1: A single hitch is taken first just as Roeder's knot.

Step 2: Four and a half rounds are taken approximately 1 cm below the first hitch over long limb of thread.

Step 3: A locking hitch is made by passing tail through the second and third loop.

Step 4: Finally the first hitch is brought closer to the locking hitch by spreading the first loop.

Step 5: The knot is stacked properly and the extra tail (if any) is cut. Once the knot is configured properly, it should be checked by sliding over the long thread.

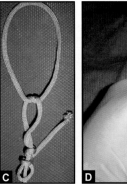
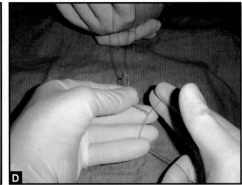

Figs 8.4A and B

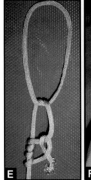
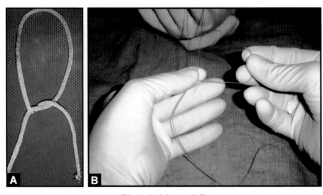

Figs 8.4C and D

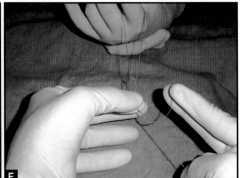

Figs 8.4E and F

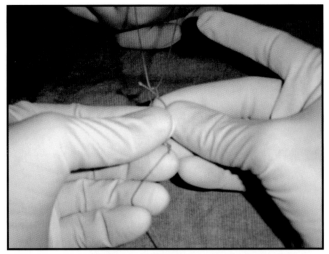

Fig. 8.4G

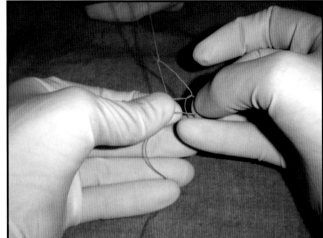

Fig. 8.4H

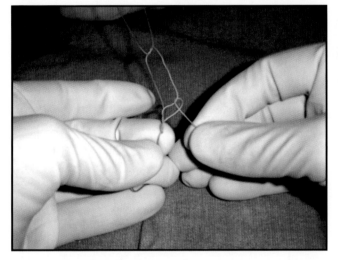

Fig. 8.4I

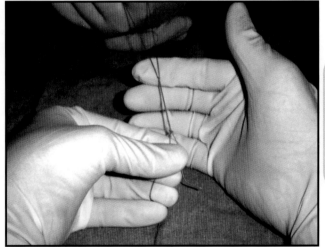

Fig. 8.4J

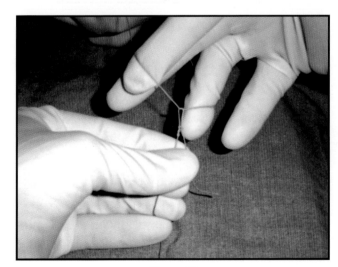

Fig. 8.4K

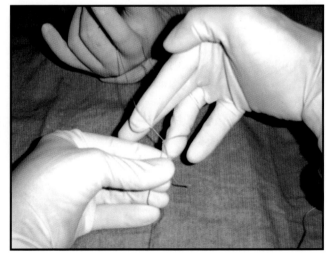

Fig. 8.4L

Section One

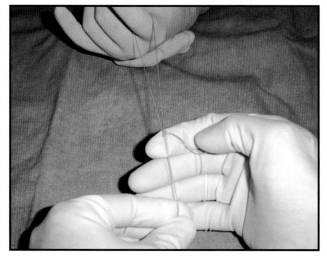
Fig. 8.4M

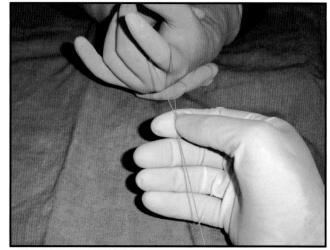
Fig. 8.4N

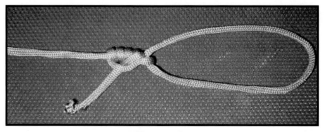
Fig. 8.4O

Figs 8.4A to O: Various step of Tayside knot

APPLICATIONS

The Tayside knot is suitable for use with all braided sutures (2/0 or stronger) as well as dacron. It is used with Dacron for ligation of vessels such as the azygous vein, splenic artery/vein or the inferior mesenteric artery/vein.

USING A PRE-TIED LOOP (FIG. 8.5)

- The loop is drawn up into the metal sleeve.
- The tube is then introduced through an abdominal port.
- Once inside the abdomen the loop is advanced using the push rod.
- A grasping forceps is placed through the loop and used to grasp the tissue to be ligated.
- The loop is delivered over the tissue and the knot and push rod positioned at the base of the tissue.
- The loop is then tightened around the tissue by tensioning the long end and applying pressure to the knot via the push rod causing it to slide.

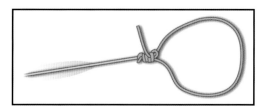

Fig. 8.5: Roeder's loop

- The knot is locked firmly in place.
- The graspers are removed and replaced by suture scissors to divide the long end prior to removal.

Pre-tied loops are available commercially. They are packaged with the following items, assembled ready for use.

- A push rod
- A pre tied loop
- A metal or silicon introducer tube.

The pre-tied loop has one long tail of suture material, which is threaded through the plastic push rod and encapsulated by the end. The region at the end of the push rod is designed to be broken so the thread may be pulled through the remainder of the rod. The push rod is passed through the metal introducer tube.

Clinical Uses

Preformed loops are used to ligate tissue, e.g. the base of the appendix, lung bullae and a hole in the gall-bladder during cholecystectomy. If multiple loops are required, the push rod and introducer can be reloaded with a length of ligature and additional loops fashioned by a surgeon with knowledge of external slip knots.

A pre-formed loop can also be used to secure a divided vessel after it has been isolated by a grasper. A slight modification of this technique allows it to be used to secure smaller identified vessels. One end is clipped and the other controlled by a grasper, which has already been passed through a loop. The vessel is divided and the loop slide into place and tightened before the grasper releases the vessel.

Endoloops are also useful for sealing a perforated organ if this is to be removed, e.g. perforation of the gallbladder during laparoscopic cholecystectomy where closure is necessary to prevent escape of gallstones into the peritoneal cavity.

On no account must endoloops be used to close a perforation in any organ that is not going to be resected and removed, as the tissue included in the closed endoloop will slough off a few days later, because of ischemia, resulting in peritonitis.

EXTRACORPOREAL KNOT FOR CONTINUOUS STRUCTURE

- A push rod is threaded onto a length of ligature material approximately 1.5 m long.
- A knot is tied at the end of the thread as it emerges from the straight end of the rod.
- The end of the ligature emerging from the tapered end is grasped by atraumatic endoscopic grasper.
- The grasper and catgut are then passed into an introducer tube.
- The introducer tube is then passed through an 11 mm cannula.
- The grasper and ligature are extended into the cavity and passed to one side and behind the structure to be ligated.
- A second grasper is introduced through a second port to grasp the ligature from the other side of the structure.

- The first grasper releases the ligature and the takes it back from the second in front of the structure.
- The first grasper and ligature are withdrawn from the abdomen through the introducer tube while the second is used to protect the structure from the suture.
- An external slip knot is tied externally. The knot tied is determined by the size of vessel to be controlled and the material in use.
- The knot is pushed into the abdomen by the push rod and positioned prior to tightening.
- The rod is withdrawn a little and scissors introduced to cut the thread leaving a reasonably long end.

Clipping

Titanium clip is most widely used tissue approximation technique used by general laparoscopic surgeon.
- Choose the correct size of clip for the structure.
- Double clip should be applied over important structures (Fig. 8.6).
- Always confirm the dumbbell effect after clipping.
- Dumbbell effect after clipping confirms the tension on tissue (Fig. 8.7).

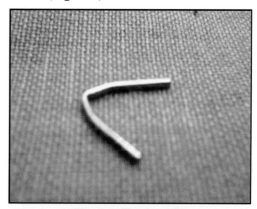

Fig. 8.6: Titanium clip

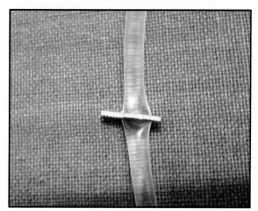

Fig. 8.7: Dumbbell formation

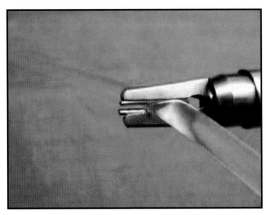

Fig. 8.8: Clip should be kept pressed for 3 seconds

- Do not clip fatty pedicles.
- Check positioning of jaws, the tips and content before clipping.
- Beware of cross clipping (Fig. 8.8).

CAT EYE STONE

Sometimes clip applied on cystic duct may internalize and it may act as foreign body. In rare cases cat eye stone has been reported with the use of Titanium clips. After many years it stimulates stone formation by deposition of bile. It is called cat eye stone because after taking a cross-section of these stone the titanium clips look like pupil of a cat seen in dark.

LAPAROSCOPIC INTERNAL SUTURING

One of the most challenging aspects of laparoscopic surgery is intracorporeal suturing and knot tying. A loss of depth perception and tactile sense and visual obstruction make placing accurate and well-tied knots a difficult and time-consuming task. The technique for suturing needs to be modified depending on the instrumentation in use. A lot of work is currently being carried out on designs for new needle holders and automatic suturing.

INSTRUMENTATION

The Needle

Endoski needle

Although conventional open surgical needles (half circle) can be used endoscopically, the endoski needle developed in Dundee is designed specifically for endoscopic use and is a hybrid of the straight and half circle needle. It carries an atraumatic suture and has a straight shaft and a terminal tapering curve (that corresponds to ¼ of a circle), giving it the shape of a miniature ski. The shaft is a modified rectangle, which becomes more and more rounded towards the tip so that the curved portion of the needle is round bodied. This combination allows for an easier grip of the shaft by the jaws of the needle holder and smooth passage of the curved portion of the needle through the tissues.

Needle Holders

The most commonly used is 5 mm Cuschieri needle holders. These have single action tapered jaws. The handles are spring loaded and the most recent versions have diamond coating for gripping the suture material without damage. A relaxed "open hand" grip is strongly recommended for these instruments. Please note that there are a wide variety of needle holders (or drivers). In practice, it is vital for each surgeon to become accustomed to a particular type and use that pair all the time. This is crucial for efficient and safe suturing.

Needle Control

Introduction into the Body Cavity

We recommend the use of the introducer tube to protect all ligatures and sutures from the cannula valve mechanisms.

The suture material on the endoski needle is trimmed to a suitable length. For a continuous suture this will be approximately 15 to 20 cm (Fig. 8.9).

The *suture length must never exceed 20 cm* as this will result in very difficult intracorporeal suturing since the length is magnified (2.5 times) by the imaging system.

The needle holder is first passed through an introducer tube. The tail of the suture is held next to the tip of the needle and the suture picked up by the needle holder at its mid point. It is then withdrawn into the introducer tube until neither the needle nor the tail is visible. The introducer tube can then be passed through a port and the needle extruded from the tube. The suture is watched into the abdomen and placed on a convenient surface, e.g. the flat, smooth anterior surface of the stomach.

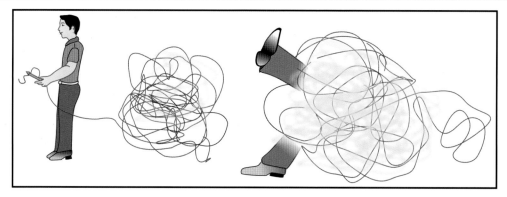

Fig. 8.9: The length of suture should not be more than 20 cm

To Insert the Needle

• Pass the needle holder through the reducing tube.
• Pick up the suture material with the needle holder at a point mid way from the tip of the needle and the tail of the thread.
• Withdraw the suture and needle inside the tube so that it is completely out of sight.
• Insert the tube through an appropriate port.
• Extrude the needle and suture from the tube by advancing the needle holder and position on a safe surface, e.g. the anterior surface of the stomach.

Manipulation

• A trailing needle is a safe needle.
• A held needle should always be in view.
• Tips of the two needle holders must always be in view.
• Two needle holders must never cross each other by moving parallel to each other from one side to the other.

The ability to maneuver the needle into the desired position in the needle holder jaw is one of the first skills you must acquire. It is well worth practicing the techniques for this as it will make all subsequent tasks much easier. This task causes much frustration until it can be achieved at will.

The first step is to arrange the needle to the required orientation on the tissues (preferably on a serosal surface and not fatty tissue). Recommended techniques to get the needle in the right attitude on the tissues include the "nudge", the "push", and the "twist" techniques. This maneuver should be better demonstrated for learning.

Position

The needle must next be positioned correctly in the jaws of the needle holder. Ideally the needle is grasped in the right orientation by the tips of the jaws. It is a mistake to grasp the needle by the back of the jaws as this impairs precision needle driving through the tissues and also reduces the grasping force so that needle swivel is more likely.

For a right handed surgeon in a straight forward situation, the needle is held in the right hand needle (RH) holder with the tip pointing to the left. The tip of the needle points upward and the shaft of the needle should make an obtuse angle with the shaft of the holder.

The key elements in achieving this are:
• The needle position on the tissues
• The angle of approach of the holder
• The pick up actions.

Adjustments to the angle can be made using:
• Other needle holder
• Surrounding tissue
• Tensioned suture material.

Passage Through the Tissues

Position the needle appropriately in the needle holder and identify the position of the first entry point. Place the tip of the needle at this position so that the sharp tip enters the tissue at right angles.

When approximately 1/2 of the curve of the needle has entered the tissue (corresponding to 2.0 mm) the wrist is supinated and lifted slightly to passage the curved section of the needle through the tissue. When the point of the needle is seen to emerge at the exit point, the grasp is maintained and the needle end (not tip) is grasped by the other (assisting) needle holder before it is released by the dominant needle holder. For the second bite (in other tissue edge) the dominant needle holder can retrieve the needle directly from the assisting needle holder provided the needle is in a favorable position for direct transfer. Otherwise it is more ergonomic to drop the needle and pick it up by the dominant holder. Once the two edges have been passaged, the needle is dropped and the suture pulled to the desired point by an instrument to instrument technique through the tissues. A trailing needle does less harm than one that is held rigid in the holder. A grasped needle must always be in view.

Tensioning

A continuous suture is initially tensioned by pulling through the suture material. Further tightening can be achieved by use of the dominant needle holder although one must be careful not to fray or damage the suture. The open jaws of needle holder are placed on the side of the suture as it exits from the tissues. They can then be used to apply counter pressure on the tissues as the suture is pulled tight by the assisting needle driver. Tension in a suture line is then maintained by occasional locking sutures and the appropriate use of an assistant. In clinical practice,

tension on the suture line is kept by the assistant using a special suture holder that does not damage the suture which has rounded jaws.

Microsurgical Tying

This is a precise choreographed set of actions. Each maneuver is designed to help make the whole process smooth and reproducible with economy of movement and structured choreography, so that suturing is efficient with minimum of wasted time. Note the following important points.

- The passive and active role of the holders
- The formation of the initial "C"
- Its relation to the tail of the suture
- The conscious assessment of position
- The use of the natural bias of the thread
- Appropriate rotations of the needle active and passive needle holder that must be manipulated in consort
- Note the importance of keeping the ends of the two needle holders in the operative field
- Note the importance of two-handedness for efficient suturing.

Steps of Surgeons Knot (Figs 8.10A to H)

- A "C" loop is made.
- The instrument of the side of "C" should be kept above the "C" and two winds are taken with the help of right instrument.
- Winds are slipped in the line of left instrument.

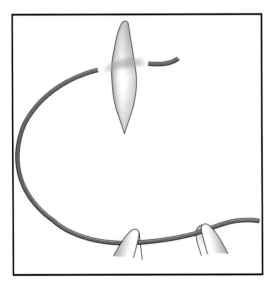

Fig. 8.10A

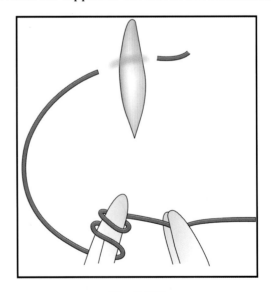

Fig. 8.10B

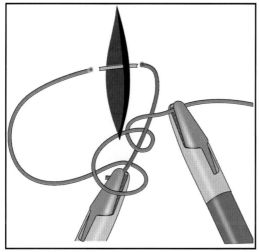

Fig. 8.10C

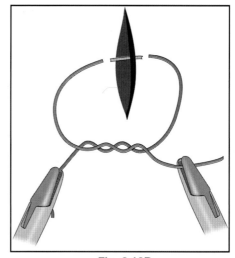

Fig. 8.10D

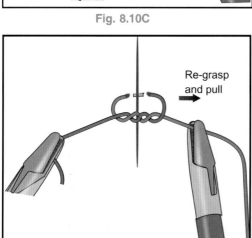

Fig. 8.10E

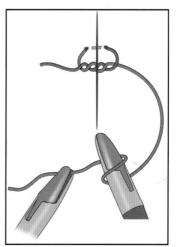

Fig. 8.10F

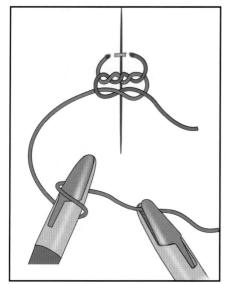

Fig. 8.10G

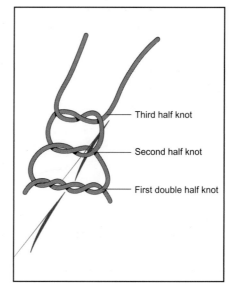

Fig. 8.10H

Figs 8.10A to H: Various steps of surgeons knot

- Knot is tightened with the help of both the instruments.
- First knot of surgeons knot is complete.
- A reverse "C" is made and single wind is taken over the right instrument with the help of left instrument.
- Again "C" loop is made and single winds are taken to complete surgeons knot.
- Surgeons knot contains double wrap on the first throw, followed by two opposing, alternating single throws.

Tumble Square Knot (Figs 8.11A to G)

This is a simple square knot which can be changed to slipping configuration by tightening of a same side of thread.
- A square knot is tied.
- Same side of thread should be straightened with the help of two Maryland or needle holders.

- After straightening of same side of thread it is ready to slide.
- Closed jaw of Maryland forceps will slide the knot.
- After tightening, the knot is locked again by pulling both the thread.
- One more knot is tied to prevent slipping of tumble square knot.

CONTINUOUS SUTURING

It is common practice to start a continuous suture with a Dundee Jamming Slip knot. An equally acceptable alternative is an internal tied knot if the surgeon is proficient.

A continuous suture can be finished in a number of ways. We recommend the Aberdeen termination, an internal tie to a convenient tail or a slipping loop tied to itself.

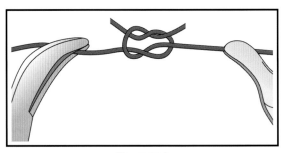

Fig. 8.11A

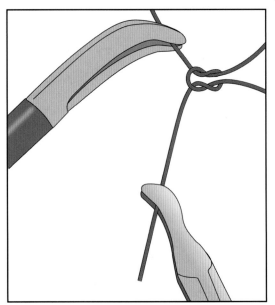

Fig. 8.11B

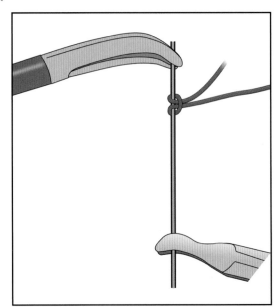

Fig. 8.11C

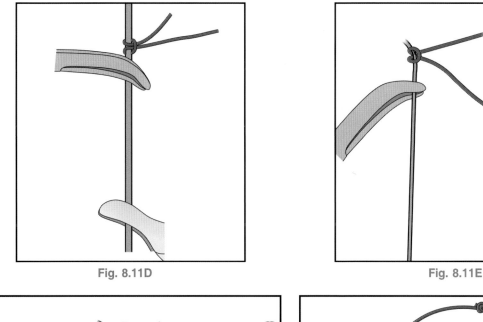

Fig. 8.11D

Fig. 8.11E

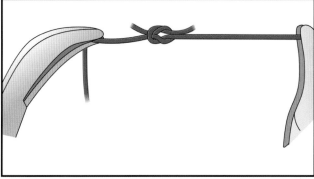

Fig. 8.11F

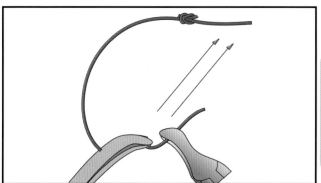

Fig. 8.11G

Figs 8.11A to G: Various steps of Tumble square knot

Dundee Jamming Slip Knot

This is a recommended way of starting a continuous suture. This knot has an external component but is completed, once inside the body cavity, after the first bite of tissue have been taken.

The external component has following steps:
- A simple slipping loop
- Passage of the tail through the first loop
- Creating a second loop
- Tensioning of the second loop.

The second loop should slip only from the tail, the knot should not be tightened at this stage and the length of both the loop and of the tail should be at least 1 cm.

Once inside, the knot is locked by passage of the standing part of the suture through the loop, which is then slipped to lock the knot.

Starting a Continuous Suture

- Tie the external component of the Dundee jamming slip knot at the end of an atraumatic suture or start with and intracorporeal surgeons knot.
- Pass an atraumatic grasper through an introducer tube.
- Pick up the suture at a point mid way from the tail of the suture to the needle tip.
- Draw suture and needle completely inside the introducer tube, being careful not to slip the Dundee jamming slip knot.
- Pass the introducer through the 11 mm cannula.
- Extrude the suture and deposit it on a safe surface (e.g. the anterior surface of the stomach).
- Pick up the needle and take the first bite of the tissue or tissues to be sutured.

Section One

- Pull the thread through until the Dundee jamming slip knot just impinges on the tissue.
- Pass the needle holder carefully through the loop of the Dundee jamming slip knot and pick up the thread attached to the needle at a point near to its exit from the tissues.
- Pull the needle holder and thread with the trailing needle back through the loop.
- Next take hold of the tail of the loop and the standing part of the thread and pull first on the tail and then on the standing part, locking the knot.
- Trim the tail. You are now ready to start your continuous suture.

APPLICATIONS

It is used in any continuous suture, e.g. closure of viscerotomies following stapled anastomosis, sutured anastomosis such as cholecystojejunostomy, gastrojejunostomy, etc. It can also be used as an interrupted suture, when additional one or two hitches are advised for security (in our practice an internally tied knot would be used in preference for an interrupted suture).

Aberdeen Termination

This is an adaptation of a termination commonly used in abdominal closure following open surgery. The continuous suture is finished by the formation of three interlocking loops. In order to simplify the maintenance of tension in the suture line, the penultimate stitch can be locked. A further bite is then taken and the suture pulled through, though not completely. A small loop of suture is left, enough that the needle holder can be passed through it to pick up the standing part of the suture. A loop of this is then drawn through the first loop, which is tightened down onto the tissues. The needle holder is then passed through the new loop to repeat the maneuver three times.

It is important that each loop be tightened as you proceed. To do this, tension must be applied to the leg of the loop, which exits, from the tissues or the preceding loop.

The standing part and needle are delivered completely through the last loop. The standing part is held up and the suture tensioned with counter pressure from the jaws of the needle holder placed on either side of the suture. The suture is cut off leaving a reasonable length (approximately 1 cm).

INTERRUPTED SUTURES

Interrupted Knots

Dundee jamming loop knot is used to create interrupted sutures. For additional safety a further hitch or two are recommended if it is to be used as an interrupted suture. More commonly interrupted intracorporeal sutures are made by the use of the surgeon's or the Tumbled square knots.

Applications of Interrupted Sutures

Interrupted sutures have a multitude of uses. Simple examples are closure of the common bile duct after exploration and fundoplication.

Stapled Anastomosis

The use of disposable stapling guns has simplified a number of endoscopic procedures such as the division of vascular pedicles and gut anastomosis.

The following important points are emphasized:
- Port positions for stapling
- Stay sutures for tensioning
- Enterotomy positioning and size
- Positioning and angulations of the instrument prior to closure
- Checking suture line
- Complete closure of residual opening
- End to end anastomosis can also be carried out by stapling closed bowel ends side by side.

Clinical Applications

An anterior or posterior, side to side anastomosis of stomach and jejunum done laparoscopically can be a satisfactory palliative procedure. Likewise, a laparoscopic cholecystojejunostomy may be performed with stapler to relieve jaundice and itching in patients with inoperable pancreatic cancer.

SUTURED ANASTOMOSIS

Sutured anastomosis can be carried out endoscopically, although the process is demanding in terms of skill and time. However, it is pertinent to note that staplers may not always be available, or appropriate, and even if a stapler is used, you require the skills to perform a sutured closure if the stapled anastomosis is not perfect.

Important points to remember are:
- Port positioning
- Use of communication with your assistant
- Positioning of sutures, especially at the corners
- Spacing the sutures (remember the magnification)
- Tensioning of sutures.

Direction of Suturing

It is important that you suture at the right height, ideally your elbows should be held adducted and at right angles. Keep you wrists loose and remember that you have two hands that must manipulate to help each other. The choreography is as follows:
- The suturing line is started with a 'starter knot' (surgeons or tumbled square knot).
- The two needle holders must be kept in view and used in concert with each other.
- Passage from right to left through the tissue edges (bites consisting of entry and exit points with dominant needle holder.
- The needle is picked up from the exit point by the passive needle holder (NH).
- It is transferred to dominant needle holder for the next bite if the orientation is correct. Otherwise it is dropped and re-orientated in the needle holder. Once the suture has passed through the two edges, the thread is pulled trough, handing the suture one needle holder to the other.
- The distance between the suture bites must be approximately equal to the depth of the bites.

TECHNIQUES TO ASSIST IN CONTROL OF BLEEDING

Methods of Securing Hemostasis

Endoscopic surgery is controlled almost entirely by vision. Any loss of view will result in loss of control and a reduction in safety. Hemorrhage, even to a minor extent, tends to obscure the operative field and consequently to be avoided. This means that vessels of a size that in open surgery could be divided without particular attention need to be secured prior to division when working endoscopically. Dissection must be more

meticulous to proceed smoothly and you must develop a disciplined approach.

Magnification of tissues by the endoscope may initially confuse an inexperienced endoscopic surgeon as to the severity of the bleeding. A moderate bleed can appear torrential but an inexperienced endoscopic surgeon is well advised to convert should he have any doubt about his ability to control the situation quickly.
- Pressure on the area applied by grasping adjacent tissue, and using this to overly and apply gentle pressure on to the area.
- Compression with pledget swab if the bleeding is not heavy until hemostasis is achieved by clipping or electrocoagulation and the sucker.
- Suction/irrigation to identify the bleeding point prior to securing it.
- Under-running by suture if the bleeding point cannot be identified.
- Argon spray coagulation for raw bleeding areas.
- Occluding the vessel with graspers before clipping it.
- Application of fibrin and other glues or hemostatic agents.

Avoid Blind Coagulation

Control the initial bleeding and then take your time to identify the bleeding point. In anatomically crowded areas containing important structures, it may be advisable to allow time for the bleeding to stop by compression for one or two minutes. If bleeding cannot be controlled inside within 5 minutes, serious consideration should be given for conversion to open surgery. This period should be shorter if bleeding is massive or arterial.

Suction and Irrigation

The availability of suction and irrigation is as important for hemostasis in endoscopic surgery as gauze swabs are in open surgery. When bleeding does occur irrigation can assist in visualization of the bleeding point and suction removes pooled blood and clears clots from the operative site. In addition, the irrigation activates Hageman factor and thus initiates spontaneous hemostasis.

Heparanized Hartmann's solution (1000 units per 500 ml bag) is ideal if clots are present. This solution is preferred to normal saline because of its lesser conductivity, an important consideration when using monopolar HF electrocautery. The heparin also reduces the stickiness of the instruments and thus improve handling especially of suture and ligature materials. It also aids removal of pooled blood. The bag of fluid is placed in a Fenwell pressure bag raised to 200 mm Hg and hung from a drip stand. As the contents of the bag are used the pressure needs to be maintained. There are several pressurized irrigation systems available, some heat the irrigating fluid to body temperature, other provide pulse irrigation which is helpful from breaking up blood clots and cleaning the peritoneal gutters.

Suction and irrigation are also essential to deal with leakage from ultra-abdominal organs, e.g. bile leakage, bowel content, perforated ulcer, appendicitis. In these acute emergency situations, laparoscopic abdominal lavage of the peritoneal quadrants is aided by shaking the patient from side to side and changing the position of the operating table (head up, head down and sideways).

BIBLIOGRAPHY

1. Ali MR, Mowery Y, Kaplan B, DeMaria EJ. Training the novice in laparoscopy. Surg Endosc 2002;16: 1732–6.
2. Champion JK, Hunter J, Trus T, Laycock W. Teaching basic video skills as an aid in laparoscopic suturing. Surg Endosc 1996;10: 23–5.
3. Croce E, Olmi S. Intracorporeal knot-tying and suturing techniques in laparoscopic surgery: technical details. JSLS 2000;4: 17–22.
4. De Beer JF, Van Rooyen K, Boezaart AP. Nicky_s knot: a new slip knot for arthroscopic surgery. Arthroscopy 1998;14: 109–10.
5. Derossis AM, Brothwell J, Sigman HH, Fried GM. The effect of practice on performance in a laparoscopic simulator. Surg Endosc 1998;12: 1117–20.
6. Dunkin BJ, Li Y, Marks JM, Ponsky JL. The "Yenni" knot: a simpler method of intracorporeal laparoscopic knot tying. J Am Coll Surg 1997;185: 492–3.
7. Faulkner H, Regehr G, Martin J, Reznick R. Validation of an objective structured assessment of technical skill for surgical residents. Acad Med 1996;71: 1363–5.
8. Figert PL, Park AE, Witzke DB, Schwartz RW. Transfer of training in acquiring laparoscopic skills. J Am Coll Surg 2001;193: 533–7.
9. Gallagher AG, McClure N, McGuigan J, Crothers I, Browning J. Virtual reality training in laparoscopic surgery: a preliminary assessment of minimally invasive surgical trainer virtual reality (MIST VR). Endoscopy 1999;31: 310–3.
10. Gaur DD. Laparoscopic suturing and knot tying: the Indian rope crick. J Endourol 1998;12: 61–6.
11. Grantcharov TP, Kristiansen VB, Bendix J, Bardram L, Rosenberg J, Funch-Jensen P. Randomized clinical trial of virtual reality simulation for laparoscopic skills training. Br J Surg 2004;91: 146–150.
12. Hamilton EC, Scott DJ, Fleming JB, Rege RV, Laycock R, Bergen PC, Tesfay ST, Jones DB. Comparison of video trainer and virtual reality training systems on acquisition of laparoscopic skills. Surg Endosc 2002;16: 406–411.
13. Harold KL, Matthews BD, Backus CL, Pratt BL, Heniford BT. Prospective randomized evaluation of surgical resident proficiency with laparoscopic suturing after course instruction. Surg Endosc 2002;16: 1729–31.
14. Hasson HM, Kumari NV, Eekhout J. Training simulator for developing laparoscopic skills. JSLS 2001;5: 255–65.
15. Hay DL, Levine RL, Von Fraunhofer JA (1990) Chromic gut pelviscopic loop ligature. Effect of the number of pulls on the tensile strength. J Reprod Med 5: 260–2.
16. Inoue H, Kumagai Y, Ami K, Nishikage T, Baba H, Yoshida T, Iwai T. A simple technique of using novel thread-holding and knot-pushing forceps for extracorporeal knot-tying. Surg Today 2000;30: 27–31.
17. Jones DB, Wu JS, Soper NJ. Laparoscopic Surgery, Principles and Procedures. Quality Medical Publishing, St. Louis, 1997;50–65.
18. Kadirkamanathan SS, Shelton JC, Hepworth CC, Laufer JG, Swain CP. A comparison of the strength of knots tied by hand and at laparoscopy. J Am Coll Surg 1996;182: 46–54.
19. Madan AK, Frantizdes CT, Shervin N, Tebbit CL. Assessment of individual hand performance in box trainers compared to virtual reality trainers. Am Surg 2003;69: 1112–14.
20. Madan AK, Frantzides CT (xxxx) Substituting virtual reality training for inanimate box trainers does not decrease laparoscopic skill acquisition. JSLS In Press.
21. Madan AK, Frantzides CT, Park WC, Tebbit CL, Kumari NVA, O_Leary PJ. Predicting baseline laparoscopic surgery skills. Surg Endosc 2005;19: 101–103.
22. Madan AK, Frantzides CT, Sasso L. Laparoscopic baseline ability assessment by virtual reality. J Laparoendosc Adv Surg Tech A 2005;15: 13–17.
23. Madan AK, Frantzides CT, Tebbit CL, Park WC, Kumari NVA, Shervin N. Evaluation of specialized laparoscopic suturing and tying devices. JSLS 2004;8: 191–3.
24. Madan AK, Frantzides CT, Tebbit CL, Quiros RM. Participant _s opinions of laparoscopic trainers during basic laparoscopic training courses. Am J Surg 2005;189: 758–61.
25. Madan AK, Frantzides CT, Tebbit CL, Shervin N, Quiros R. Self-reported versus observed scores in laparoscopic skills training. Surg Endosc 2005;19: 670–2.
26. Martin JA, Regehr G, Reznick R, MacRae H, Murnaghan J, Hutchison C, Brown M. Objective structured assessment of technical skill (OSATS) for surgical residents. Br J Surg 1997;84: 273– 8.
27. Meilahn JE. The need for improving laparoscopic suturing and knot-tying. J Laparoendosc Surg. 1992;2: 267.

28. Mori T, Hatano N, Maruyama S, Atomi Y. Significance of "hands-on training" in laparoscopic surgery. Surg Endosc 1998;12: 256–60.

29. Munz Y, Kumar BD, Moorthy K, Bann S, Darzi A. Laparoscopic virtual reality and box trainers: is one superior to the other? Surg Endosc 2004;18: 485–94.

30. Nathanson LK, Nathanson PK, Cushieri AL. Safety of vessel ligation in laparoscopic surgery. Endoscopy 1991;23: 206–209.

31. Pare A (1510–1590 A.D.). The apologies and treatise of Ambroise Pare containing the voyager made into divers places with many of his writings upon surgery. Edited by Keynes G, (ed). Galcion Educational Books, London. 1951.

32. Pearson AM, Gallagher AG, Rosser JC, Satava RM. Evaluation of structured and quantitative training methods for teaching intracorporeal knot tying. Surg Endosc 2002;16: 130–137.

33. Pennings JL, Kenyon T, Swanstrom L. The knit stitch. An improved method of laparoscopic knot tying. Surg Endosc 1995;9: 537–540.

34. Peters JH, Fried GM, Swanstrom LL, Soper NJ, Sillin LF, Schirmer B, Hoffman K. Development and validation of a comprehensive program of education and assessment of the basic fundamentals of laparoscopic surgery. Surgery 2004;135: 21–7.

35. Pietrafitta JJ. A technique of laparoscopic knot tying. J Laparoendosc Surg 1992;2: 273–5.

36. Reznick R, Regehr G, MacRae H, Martin J, McCulloch W. Testing technical skills via an innovative "bench station" examination. Am J Surg 1997;173: 226–30.

37. Roeder H. Die Technik der Mandelges-undungs bestrebungen. Artzl Rundschau Munchen 1918;57: 169–71.

38. Rosser JC, Murayama M, Gabriel NH. Minimally invasive surgical training solutions for the twenty-first century. Surg Clin North Am 2000;80: 1607–24.

39. Rosser JC, Rosser LE, Savalgi RS. Skill acquisition and assessment for laparoscopic surgery. Arch Surg 1997;132: 200–204.

40. Rosser JC, Rosser LE, Savalgi RS. Objective evaluation of a laparoscopic surgical skill program for residents and senior surgeons. Arch Surg 1998;133: 657–61.

41. Scott DJ, Bergen PC, RegeRV,LaycockR, Tesfay ST, Valentine RJ, Euhus DM, Jeyarajah DR, Thompson WM, Jones DB. Laparoscopic training on bench models: better and most cost effective than operating room experience? J Am Coll Surg 2000;191: 272–83.

42. Sedlack JD, Williams VM, DeSimone J, Page D, Ghosh BC. Laparoscopic knot security. Surg Laparosc Endosc 1996;6:144–6.

43. Semm K. Operative Manual for Endoscopic Abdominal Surgery. Year Book Medical Publishers,, Chicago. 1987.

44. Seymour NE, Gallagher AG, Roman SA, O_Brien MK, Bansal VK, Andersen DK, Satava RM. Virtual reality training improves operating room performance: results of a randomized, doubleblinded study. Ann Surg 2002;236: 458–64.

45. Sharpe LA. A new device and method for extracorporeal knot tying in laparoscopic surgery. J Gynecol Surg 1994;10: 27–31.

46. Swain CP, Kadirkamanathan SS, Gong F, Lal KC, Ratani RS, Brown GJ, Mills TN. Knot tying at flexible endoscopy. Gastrointest Endosc 1994;40: 722–9.

47. Szold A. A novel technique for simple laparoscopic extracorporeal knot tying. J Am Coll Surg 1997;184: 523–4.

48. Tarn, WW. Alexander the Great, vol II: Sources and Studies. Cambridge, 1948;262.

49. Tera H, Aberg C. Tensile strength of twelve types of knot employed in surgery, using different suture materials. Acta Chir Scand 1976;142: 1–7.

50. Youngblood PL, Srivastava S, Curet M, Heinrichs WL, Dev P, Wren SM. Comparison of training on two laparoscopic simulators and assessment of skills transfer to surgical performance. J Am Coll Surg 2005;200: 546–51. 213.

51. Zimmer CA, Thacker JG, Powell DM, Bellian KT, Decker DG, Rodeheaver GT, Edlich RF. Influence of knot configuration and tying technique on the mechanical performance of sutures. J Emerg Med 1997;9: 107–13.

Section One

Hand-assisted
Laparoscopic Surgery

In hand-assisted surgery, the surgeon can insert a hand through a small incision via a special pressurized sleeve. The surgeon makes a small incision in the abdomen and inserts his hand into the patient's body (Figs 9.1 and 9.2).

Hand-assisted laparoscopic surgery (HALS) devices allow for the introduction of the surgeon's non-dominant hand into the peritoneal cavity without loss of the pneumoperitoneum. The use of hand-assisted techniques in difficult cases facilitates the surgical procedure and offers an interesting alternative to the purely laparoscopic approach.

Hand-assisted laparoscopic surgery allows for a reduction in the number of trocars compared to the purely laparoscopic approach. The proper placement of the hand-assist device is one of the fundamental principles of HALS. The hand-assisted device should never be placed directly over the operative field. According to the principle of triangulation, the hand-assisted device is ideally placed in the same position as that of the non-dominant operating trocar in the purely laparoscopic approach (Fig. 9.3).

Hand is ideal for sensory perception and to guide the surgical instruments. Surgeon can manipulate with his other hand while observing the procedure on a monitor. With both a hand and laparoscopic instruments doing the work, the surgeon has more control over the operation and sense of depth and sensation of touch which cannot be gained through the lens of a camera. The large organ can be removed intact, making it possible to evaluate the cancer. The hand-assisted approach is also considered better for surgeons who are still learning laparoscopic techniques. Hand-assisted laparoscopic surgery is the use of the non-dominant hand intra-abdominally, together with the laparoscopic instruments in dominant hand.

The introduction of the surgeon's hand via the hand-assisted device allows for tactile feedback

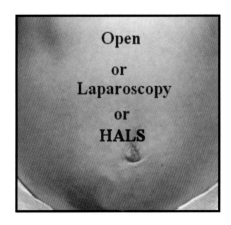
Fig. 9.1: Options before a laparoscopic surgeon

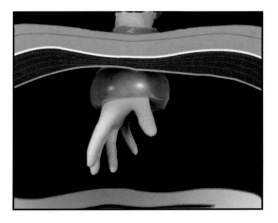
Fig. 9.2: Positioning through the abdominal wall

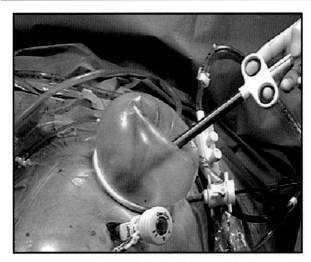

Fig. 9.3: Introduction of instruments

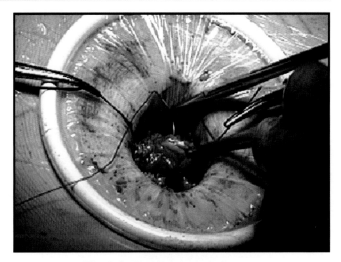

Fig. 9.4: Working through the port

and complements the information obtained visually. Hand-assisted laparoscopic surgery greatly facilitates mobilization of the organs and helps for identification of proper dissection plane, thus minimizing oozing and blood loss. HALS offers several real advantages during the procedure resulting in a significant time gain. This is especially true in obese patients as well as in cases of significant abdominal adhesions (Fig. 9.4).

The size of the incision for placement of the hand cannula is determined by the size of the surgeon's glove. A retractor-protractor which is an open ended plastic cylinder with a malleable ring at each end is then introduced into the abdominal cavity through the incision. This provides a seal for the skin wound both at the peritoneal and skin sites and keeps the incision open and also protects the wound against contamination by bacteria and malignant cells. The pneumosleeve is fitted under hand cannula and manipulated to achieve the best possible angle for the surgeon's arm during dissection. The adhesive packing is removed and the flanges are secured to the skin. A one way valve located in the sleeve's lumen prevents gas escaping from the abdomen (Fig. 9.5).

An additional cover is placed on the surgeon's arm, which is impermeable to gas. The pneumosleeve is entered and secured to the surgeon's upper arm by means of a Velcro band to prevent gas escape. The hand is then placed through the hand cannula into the abdomen. HALS, open and laparoscopic procedure is compared in Table 9.1.

Hand-assisted laparoscopic surgery (HALS) is the use of the non-dominant hand through a hand port device. It is an important adjunctive tool with other laparoscopic instruments. The hand port will be fixed via a mini-laparotomy incision, aiming for a safe maintenance of intra-abdominal gas throughout the operative procedure. The main indication for HALS is in advanced and complex laparoscopic surgical procedures.

Rationale behind HALS is that laparoscopic surgery can be used for both simple and complex procedures.

Table 9.1: Comparison of HALS, open and laparoscopic procedure

Feature	HALS	Open	Laparoscopic
Tactile feedback	Yes (+++)	Yes (++++)	No
Minimal access	Yes (+)	No	Yes (++++)
Hand-eye Coordination	Easy (+)	Easy (++++)	Difficult
Tissue retrieval	Easy (++)	Easy (++++)	Difficult
Postoperative Recovery	Fast (++)	Slow	Fast (++++)
Operative time	More (+)	Less	More (++++)
Interior mileu	Yes (++)	No	Yes (++++)
Cancer surgery	Yes (++++)	Yes (++++)	No
Cosmetic	Yes (++)	No	Yes (++++)

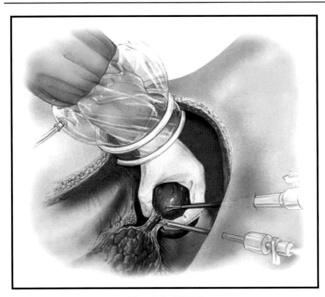

Fig. 9.5: HALS

Disadvantages of total laparoscopic surgery:
• Loss of direct tactile sensation
• Difficult hand-eye coordination
• Multiple times instrument change
• Conversion rate in complex abdominal procedures.

"Hand port" system allows surgeons the ability to insert a hand into the patient to gain a tactile sense during laparoscopic surgical procedures. This is a real improvement over previous techniques which precluded a surgeon from gaining information through touch. Commercially available to date and approved by the FDA are Dexterity Device, Intromit, Hand port and Omni port. Omni port has been extensively studied by Europe University, Dundee University as well as being clinically applied with success in the repair of abdominal aortic aneurysms in Germany and USA. Pneumo-access bubble is one of the great advances by Cuschieri and Shapiro, allowing complete visual access with the hand inside and pneumoperitoneum safely maintained.

Hand Port Devices

Devices connected to abdomen by adhesive flange:
• Dexterity (Inc., Roswell, GA, USA)
• IntroMit (Medtech Ltd., Dublin, Ireland).

Kissing Balloon Principle

Hand port device (Smith-Nephew PLC, England)

Single Piece Devices
• LapDisc (Hakko Medical, Japan)
• Omni port (Advanced Surgical Concepts Ltd., Ireland.)

The IntroMit is a single piece device that requires an adhesive to be secured to the body wall. There is no sleeve required and the device can be placed without a pneumoperitoneum.

In the HandPort system, the surgeon must wear a sleeve that attaches to the inflatable base of the device. Insertion or removal of the hand from the abdomen requires removal of the sleeve from the device, causing an immediate loss of pneumoperitoneum.

The GelPort is a three piece device that uses a wound protecting sheath (inner ring), a wound retractor (outer ring) and a gel seal cap that affixes to the wound retractor. The seal that is created maintains pneumoperitoneum, even without the insertion of the surgeon's hand. Removal of the surgeon's hand from the abdominal cavity does not cause loss of pneumoperitoneum. Moreover, the gel seal cap can be pierced by a trocar or accessory instrument while maintaining a seal at the puncture site. The large surface area of this device requires an adequate area for application on the body wall and may not be ideal for lower-quadrant hand incisions in smaller patients. However, a unique benefit of this device is that it permits the insertion instruments through the gel seal cap even while the hand is inserted in the abdomen.

The Omni port is an inflatable device through which the surgeon can rapidly remove and reinsert the hand without losing pneumoperitoneum. The device also can be insufflated to maintain pneumoperitoneum without hand insertion, allowing an accessory trocar and instrument to be inserted through this device (Figs 9.6 to 9.8).

The LapDisc consists of inner and middle rings that are connected by a silicone membrane spanning the abdominal wall. A third outermost ring rotates on the middle ring and acts as an iris, which is tightened to seal the device around the surgeon's arm. There are no pieces that require assembly with this device and insertion is quick and simple. This device has the

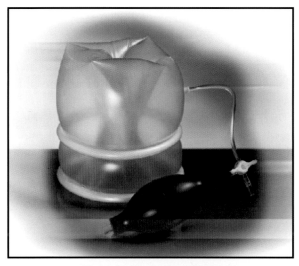

Fig. 9.6: Omni port inflated

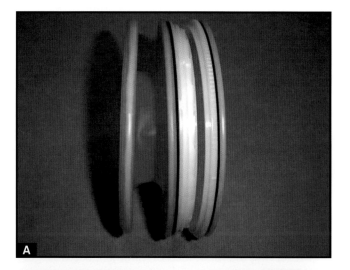

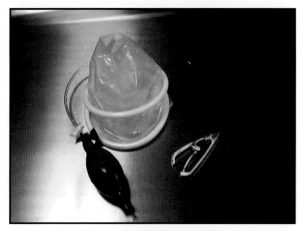

Fig. 9.7: Omni port deflated

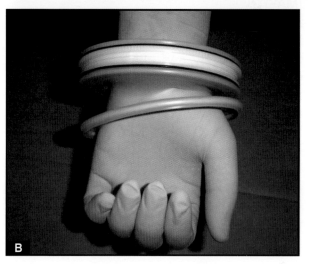

Figs 9.9A and B: LapDisc

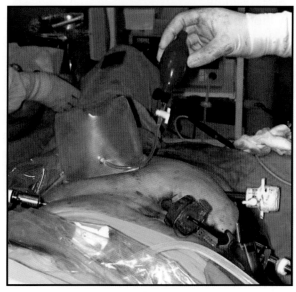

Fig. 9.8: HALS with Omni port

smallest diameter (12 cm) and can be placed on most abdominal walls without interfering with the placement of adjacent trocars (Figs 9.9A and B).

Omni Port

Omni Port is preferred device because it is:
- Single
- Simple component
- Easy to insert
- Comfortable
- Efficient pneumatic seal.

Indication of HALS

Hand-assisted laparoscopic surgery is a new addition to minimal access surgery. It has a great potential.

Many surgical operations, from the simplest to the very complicated, are greatly facilitated by the introduction of the hand into the laparoscopic arena. It is therefore purposefully designed in assisting the surgeon for complex intra-abdominal operation to be done with total laparoscopy. It stimulated many vascular surgeons throughout the world to reintroduce it into repair of complex and challenging abdominal vasculature. Nephrectomy, splenectomy, colorectal surgeries are nicely performed through hand-assisted technique.

Advantage of HALS

1. Restored tactile feedback
2. Preserving the main idea of minimal access surgery (MAS)
3. A mini-laparotomy hand port incision
4. Reduced conversion rate in total laparoscopy
5. Enhanced safety and efficiency allowing the completion of the operation with a hand inside
6. Maintenance of the intra-abdominal pressure to facilitate the better view and magnification of laparoscopic telescope
7. Improving the steep learning curve for inexperienced surgeons
8. Promising reduced cost-benefit ratio.

Limitations of HALS

Limitations can be summarized as:
1. Fatigue
2. Possible impaired tactile feedback through a lengthy complex procedure
3. Minor ergonomic restriction is due to the crowdness of the hand with the instruments
4. Not well accepted by patient and surgeons because there is already a mini-laparotomy.
5. Cosmetically inferior than total laparoscopic surgery.

LapDisc Hand Access Device

This essential product information sheet does not include all of the information necessary for selection and use of a device.

Indications

- The LapDisc hand access device is intended to provide extracorporeal extension of pneumo-peritoneum and abdominal access for the surgeon during laparoscopic surgery.
- The LapDisc is indicated for use in laparoscopic procedures, where entry of the surgeon's hand may facilitate the procedure, and for extraction of large specimens.
- The LapDisc has application in colorectal, urological and general surgical procedures. This indication for use includes the specific procedures which fall under these broad categories.

Contraindications: None known.

Warnings and Precautions

General

- Minimally invasive procedures should be performed only by persons having adequate training and familiarity with minimally invasive techniques, including laparoscopic, hand-assisted laparoscopic and open surgical procedures. Consult medical literature relative to techniques, complications, and hazards prior to performance of any minimally invasive procedure.
- Minimally invasive instruments may vary from manufacturer to manufacturer. When minimally invasive instruments and accessories from different manufacturers are employed together in a procedure, verify compatibility prior to initiation of the procedure.
- A thorough understanding of the principles and techniques involved in laser, electrosurgical, and ultrasonic procedures is essential to avoid shock and burn hazards to both patient and medical personnel and damage to the device or other medical instruments. Ensure that electrical insulation or grounding is not compromised. Do not immerse electrosurgical instruments in liquid unless they are designed and labeled to be immersed.

LD111

- This device should not be used in patients with abdominal wall thickness greater than 5 cm, or incisions less than 5 cm in length.
- Do not use the device where the incision length is greater than 9 cm as loss of pneumoperitoneum may occur.

LD112

- This device should be used in patients with abdominal wall thickness greater than 5 cm and less than or equal to 9 cm.
- Do not use the device where the incision length is greater than 9 cm as loss of pneumoperitoneum may occur.
- If pneumoperitoneum occurs:
  1. Fully close the iris valve
  2. Place damp gauze underneath the LapDisc, between the lower ring and the fascia, to stop the air flow.
- Do not allow sharp instruments such as forceps to come in contact with the silicone rubber sleeves as puncture or tearing may occur.
- Do not lay surgical instruments on the LapDisc or allow metal or sharp surgical instruments to come in contact with the LapDisc as this may weaken or damage the flexible silicone membranes.
- Sterile, water-soluble lubricant should be applied to the dorsum of the gloved hand prior to insertion through the LapDisc. Unlubricated hands may cause significant friction and tear the device.
- Do not remove the hand with the iris valve closed as it may tear the device.
- Do not overtighten the iris valve.
- Use caution when opening the iris valve when the abdomen is insufflated, as rapid loss of pneumoperitoneum may occur.
- After removing the instrument, inspect the site for hemostasis. If hemostasis is not present, appropriate techniques should be used to achieve hemostasis.
- Instruments or devices which come into contact with bodily fluids may require special disposal handling to prevent biological contamination.
- Dispose of all opened instruments whether used or unused. *Do not resterilize* the instrument. Resterilization may compromise the integrity of the device which may result in unintended injury.

Future Prospect of HALS

There are general and specific limitations, awaiting multi center prospective randomized trials in order to compare HALS in various major intra-abdominal procedures with the traditional open surgery (Fig. 9.10).

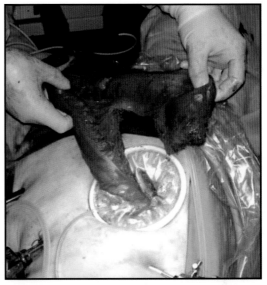
Fig. 9.10: Hemicolectomy with HALS

HALS and Colorectal Surgery

HALS can be used for all major complex abdominal surgeries like:
- Splenectomy
- Nephrectomy
- Morbid obesity surgery
- Pancreatectomy
- Nissen fundoplication
- Esophagectomy
- Rectopexy
- Repair of abdominal aortic aneurysm.

HALS is technically much easier than total laparoscopy in advanced abdominal procedures. It can help the beginning laparoscopic surgeon to practice such major operations.

BIBLIOGRAPHY

1. Antonetti MC, Killelea B, Orlando R III. Hand-assisted laparoscopic liver surgery. Arch Surg. 2002;137:407-11.
2. Ballaux KE, Himpens JM, Leman G, Van den Bossche MR. Hand-assisted laparoscopic splenectomy for hydatid cyst. Surg Endosc. 1997;11:942-3.
3. Bemelman WA, Ringers J, Meijer DW, de Wit CW, Bannenberg JJ. Laparoscopicassisted colectomy with the dexterity pneumo sleeve. Dis Colon Rectum. 1996; 39: S59-S61.
4. Bemelman WA, Witt L, Busch OR, Gouma DJ. Hand-assisted laparoscopic splenectomy. Surg Endosc. 2000;14:997-8.
5. Bleier JI, Krupnick AS, Kreisel D, Song HK, Rosato EF, Williams NN. Handassisted laparoscopic vertical banded gastroplasty: early results. Surg Endosc. 2000;14:902-7.

Section One

6. Boland JP, Kuminsky RE, Tiley EH. Laparoscopic minilaparotomy with manipulation: the middle path. Minimal Invasive Surg. 1993;2:63-67.

7. Cuschieri A, Shapiro S. Extracorporeal pneumoperitoneum access bubble for endoscopic surgery. Am J Surg. 1995;170:391-4.

8. Cuschieri A. Laparoscopic hand-assisted surgery for hepatic and pancreatic disease. Surg Endosc. 2000;14:991-996. 2001;8:104-13.

9. Cuschieri A. Whither minimal access surgery: tribulations and expectations. Am J Surg. 1995;169:9-19.

10. Darzi A. Hand-assisted laparoscopic colorectal surgery. Semin Laparosc Surg. 2001;8:153-160.

11. Darzi A. Hand-assisted laparoscopic colorectal surgery. Surg Endosc. 2000; 14:999-1004.

12. DeMaria EJ, Schweitzer MA, Kellum JM, Meador J, Wolfe L, Sugerman HJ. Handassisted laparoscopic gastric bypass does not improve outcome and increases costs when compared to open gastric bypass for the surgical treatment of obesity. Surg Endosc. 2002;16:1452-5.

13. Dunn, DC. Digitally assisted laparoscopic surgery [letter]. Br J Surg. 1994;81: 474.

14. Eijsbouts QA, de Haan J, Berends F, Sietses C, Cuesta MA. Laparoscopic elective treatment of diverticular disease: a comparison between laparoscopicassisted and resection-facilitated techniques. Surg Endosc. 000;14:726-30.

15. Fadden PT, Nakada SY. Hand-assisted laparoscopic renal surgery. Urol Clin North Am. 2001;28:167-76.

16. Fong Y, Jarnagin W, Conlon K, DeMatteo R, Dougherty E, Blumgart LH. Handassisted laparoscopic liver resection: lessons from an initial experience. Arch Surg. 2000;135: 854-9.

17. Gagner M, Gentileschi P. Hand-assisted laparoscopic pancreatic resection. Semin Laparosc Surg. 2001;8:114-25.

18. Gerhart CD. Hand-assisted laparoscopic transhiatal esophagectomy using the dexterity pneumo sleeve. J Soc Laparos Surg. 1998;2:295-8.

19. Gerhart CD. Hand-assisted laparoscopic verytical banded gastroplasty: report of a series. Arch Surg. 2000;135:795-8.

20. Gill IS. Hand-assisted laparoscopy: con. Urology. 2001;58:313-17.

21. Glasgow RE, Swanstrom LL. Hand-assisted gastroesophageal surgery. Semin Laparosc Surg. 2001;8:135-44.

22. Gorey TF, Bonadio F. Laparoscopic assisted surgery. Semin Laparosc Surg. 1997; 4:102-9.

23. Gorey TF, O'Riordain MG, Tierney S, Buckley D, Fitzpatrick JM. Laparoscopicassisted rectopexy using a novel hand-access port. J Laparoendosc Surg. 1996; 6:325-28.

24. Gorey TF, O'Riordain MG, Tierney S, et al. Laparoscopic-assisted rectopexy using a novel hand-access port. J Laproendosc Surg. 1996;6:325-28.

25. Gorey TF, Tierney S, Buckley D, et al. Video-assisted Nissen's fundoplication using a hand access port. Minimal Invasive Ther. 1996;5:364-6.

26. Gorey TF, Tierney S, O'Riordain MG, et al. Combined hand-access with laparoscopic pneumoperitoneum in intraperitoneal adhesiolysis. Ir J Med Sci. 1996; 165:297-8.

27. Gossot D, Meijer D, Bannenberg J, de Witt L, Jakimowicz J. La splenectomie laparoscopique revisite´e. Ann Chir. 1995;49:487-9.

28. HALS Study Group. Hand-assisted laparoscopic surgery vs standard laparoscopic surgery for colorectal disease. Surg Endosc. 2000;14:896-901.

29. Hanna GB, Elamass M, Cuschieri A. Ergonomics of hand-assisted laparoscopic surgery. Semin Laparosc Surg. 2001;8:92-5.

30. Hellman P, Arvidsson D, Rastad J. HandPort-assisted laparoscopic splenectomy in massive splenomegaly. Surg Endosc. 2000;14:1177-79.

31. Ichiara T, Nagahata Y, Nomura H, et al. Laparoscopic lower anterior resection is equivalent to laparotomy for lower rectal cancer at the distal line of resection. Am J Surg. 2000;179: 87-8.

32. Ichihara T, Nagahata Y, Nomura H, et al. Laparoscopic lower anterior resection is equivalent to laparotomy for lower rectal cancer at the distal line of resection. Am J Surg. 2000;179: 97-8.

33. Iwase K, Higaki J, Yoon HE, et al. Hand-assisted laparoscopic splenectomy for idiopathic thrombocytopenic purpura during pregnancy. Surg Laparosc Endosc Percutan Tech. 2001;11:53-6.

34. Jakimowicz, JJ. Will advanced laparoscopic surgery go hand-assisted? Surg Endosc. 2000;14:881-82.

35. Katkhouda N, Lord RV. Once more, with feeling: handoscopy or the rediscovery of the virtues of the surgeon's hand. Surg Endosc. 2000;14:985-6.

36. Katkhouda N, Mason RJ, Mavor E, et al. Laparoscopic finger-assisted technique (fingeroscopy) for treatment of complicated appendicitis. J Am Coll Surg. 1999;189:131-3.

37. Kawano T, Iwai T. Hand-assisted thoracoscopic esophagectomy using a new supportive approach. Surg Endosc. In press.

38. Kercher KW, Matthews BD, Walsh RM, Sing RF, Backus CL, Heniford BT. Laparoscopic splenectomy for massive splenomegaly. Am J Surg. 2002;183:192-6.

39. Kevin MS. Hand-assisted laparoscopic surgery—HALS. J Soc Laparos Surg. 2001;5:101-3.

40. Kim HB, Gregor MB, Boley SJ, Kleinhaus S. Digitally assisted laparoscopic drainage of multiple intra-abdominal abscesses. J Laparoendosc Surg. 1993;3:477- 9.

41. Klinger PJ, Smith SL, Abendstein BJ, Hinder RA. Hand-assisted laparoscopic splenectomy for isolated splenic metastasis from an ovarian carcinoma: a case report with review of the literature. Surg Laparosc Endosc. 1998;8:49-4.

42. Klingler PJ, Hinder RA, Menke DM, Smith SL. Hand-assisted laparoscopic distal pancreatectomy for pancreatic cystadenoma. Surg Laparosc Endosc. 1998; 8:180-4.

43. Kuminsky RE, Tiley EH, Lucente FC, Boland JP. Laparoscopic staging laparotomy with intra-abdominal manipulation. Surg Laparosc Endsc. 1994;4:103-5.

Section One

44. Kurian NS, Patterson R, Andrei VE, Edye MB. Hand-assisted laparoscopic surgery: an emerging technique. Surg Endosc. 2001;15:1277-81.

45. Kurokawa T, Inagaki H, Sakamoto J, Nonami T. Hand-assisted laparoscopic anatomical left lobectomy using hemihepatic vascular control technique. Surg Endosc. 2002;15:300.

46. Kurokawa T, Inagaki H, Sakamoto J, Nonami T. Hand-assisted laparoscopic anatomical right lobectomy using hemihepatic vascular control technique. Surg Endosc. In press.

47. Kusminsky RE, Boland JP, Tiley EH, Deluca JA. Hand-assisted laparoscopic splenectomy. Surg Laparosc Endosc. 1995;5:463-7.

48. Kusminsky RE, Boland JP, Tiley EH. Hand-assisted laparoscopic surgery [letter]. Dis Colon Rectum. 1996;39:111.

49. Litwin DE, Darzi A, Jakimowicz J, et al. Hand-assisted laparoscopic surgery (HALS) with the HandPort system: initial experience with 68 patients. Ann Surg. 2000; 231:715-23.

50. Lucarini L, Galleano R, Lombezzi R, Ippoliti M, Ajraldi G. Laparoscopicassisted Hartmann's reversal with the Dexterity Pneumo Sleeve. Dis Colon Rectum. 2000;43:1164-7.

51. Machi J, Oishi AJ, Mossing AJ, Furumoto NL, Oishi RH. Hand-assisted laparoscopic ultrasound-guided radiofrequency thermal ablation of liver tumors: a technical report. Surg Laparosc Endosc Percutan Tech. 2002;12: 160-4.

52. Meijer DW, Gossot D, Jakimowicz JJ, De Wit LT, Bannenberg JJ, Gouma DJ. Splenectomy revised: manually assisted splenectomy with the dexterity device— a feasibility study in 22 patients. J Laparoendosc Adv Surg Tech A. 1999; 9:507-510.

53. Meijer, DW, Bannenberg, JJG, Jakimowicz, JJ. Hand-assisted laparoscopic surgery: an overview. Surg Endosc. 2000;14:891-5.

54. Memon MA, Fitzgibbons RJ. Hand-assisted laparoscopic surgery (HALS): a useful technique for complex laparoscopic abdominal procedures. J Laparoendosc Adv Surg Tech A. 1998;8:143-50.

55. Miura Y, Mitsuta H, Yoshihara T, Ohshiro Y, Okajima M, Asahara T. Dohi Gasless hand-assisted laparoscopic surgery for colorectal cancer: an option for poor cardiopulmonary reserve. Dis Colon Rectum. 2001;44:896-8.

56. Mooney MJ, Elliott PL, Galapon DB, James LK, Lilac LJ, O'Reilly MJ. Handassisted laparoscopic sigmoidectomy for diverticulitis. Dis Colon Rectum. 1998; 41:630-5.

57. Naitoh T, Gagner M, Garcia-Ruiz A, Heniford BT, Ise H, Matsuno S. Handassisted laparoscopic digestive surgery provides safety and tactile sensation for malignancy or obesity. Surg Endosc. 1999;13:157-160.

58. Naitoh T, Gagner M. Laparoscopically assisted gastric surgery using the Dexterity Pneumo Sleeve. Surg Endosc. 1997;11:830-33.

59. Neufang T, Post S, Markus P, Becker H. Manually assisted laparoscopic surgery— realistic evolution of the minimally invasive therapy concept? Initial experiences with the "Endohand." Chirurg. 1996;67:952-8.

60. O'Reilly MJ, Saye WB, Mullins SG, Pinto SE, Falkner PT. Technique of handassisted laparoscopic surgery. J Laparoendosc Surg. 1996;6:239-44.

61. Ohki J, Nagai H, Hyodo M, Nagashima T. Hand-assisted laparoscopic distal gastrectomy with abdominal wall-lift method. Surg Endosc. 1999;13:1148- 50.

62. Ou H. Laparoscopic-assisted mini-laparotomy with colectomy. Dis Colon Rectum. 1995;38:324-6.

63. Pelosi MA, Pelosi MA III, Eim J. Hand-assisted laparoscopy for megamyomectomy: a case report. J Reprod Med. 2000;45:519-5.

64. Pelosi MA, Pelosi MA III, Eim J. Hand-assisted laparoscopy for pelvic malignancy. J Laparoendosc Adv Surg Tech A. 2000;10:143-50.

65. Pelosi MA, Pelosi MA III, Villalona E. Hand-assisted laparoscopic cholecystectomy at cesarean section. J Am Assoc Gynecol Laparosc. 1999;6:491-5.

66. Pietrabissa A, Boggi U, Moretto C, Ghilli M, Mosca F. Laparoscopic and handassisted laparoscopic live donor nephrectomy. Semin Laparosc Surg. 2001;8: 161-7.

67. Pietrabissa A, Dario P, Ferrari M, Stefanini C, Menciassi A, Moretto C, Mosca F. Grasping and dissecting instrument for hand-assisted laparoscopic surgery. Surg Endosc. 2002;16:1332-5.

68. Pietrabissa A, Moretto C, Carobbi A, Boggi U, Ghilli M, Mosca F. Hand-assisted laparoscopic low anterior resection: intial experience with a new procedure. Surg Endosc. 2002;16:431-5.

69. Posner MC, Alverdy J. Hand-assisted laparoscopic surgery for cancer. Cancer J. 2002;8:144-53.

70. Ren CJ, Salky B, Reiner M. Hand-assisted laparoscopic splenectomy for ruptured spleen. Surg Endosc. 2001;15:324.

71. Romanelli JR, Kelly JJ, Litwin DE. Hand-assisted laparoscopic surgery in the United States: an overview. Semin Laparosc Surg. 2001;8:96-103.

72. Romanelli JR, Litwin DE. Hand-assisted laparoscopic surgery: problems in general surgery. Probl Gen Surg. 2001;18:45-51.

73. Rudich SM, Marcovich R, Magee JC, et al. Hand-assisted laparoscopic donor nephrectomy: comparable donor/recipient outcomes, costs, and decreased convalescence as compared to open donor nephrectomy. Transplant Proc. 2001; 33:1106-7.

74. Ruiz-Deya G, Cheng S, Palmer E, Thomas R, Slakey D. Open donor, laparoscopic donor and hand-assisted laparoscopic donor nephrectomy: a comparison of outcomes. J Urol. 2001;166:1270-4.

75. Schweitzer MA, Broderick TJ, Demaria EJ, Sugerman HJ. Laparoscopicassisted Roux-en-Y gastric bypass. J Laparoendosc Adv Surg Tech A. 1999; 9:449-53.

76. Scoggin SD, Frazee RC, Snyder SK, et al. Laparoscopic-assisted bowel surgery. Dis Colon Rectum. 1993;36:747-50.

77. Scott HJ, Darzi A. Tactile feedback in laparoscopic colonic surgery. Br J Surg. 1997;84:1004-5.

78. Shinchi H, Takao S, Noma H, Mataki Y, Iino S, Aikou T. Hand-assisted laparoscopic distal pancreatectomy with minilaparotomy for distal pancreatic cystadenoma. Surg Laparosc Endosc Percutan Tech. 2001;11:139-43.

79. Sjoerdsma W, Meijer DW, Jansen A, den Boer KT, Grimbergen CA. Comparison of efficiencies of three techniques for colon surgery. J Laparoendosc Adv Surg Tech A. 2000;10:47-53.

80. Southern Surgeons' Club Study Group. Handoscopic surgery: a prospective multicenter trial of a minimally invasive technique for complex abdominal surgery. Arch Surg. 1999;134:477-85.

81. Stifelman M, Nieder AM. Prospective comparison of hand-assisted laparoscopic devices. Urology. 2002;59:668-72.

82. Sundbom M, Gustavsson S. Hand assisted laparoscopic bariatric surgery. Semin Laparosc Surg. 2001;8:145-52.

83. Sundbom M, Gustavsson S. Hand-assisted laparoscopic roux-en-Y gastric bypass: early results. Obes Surg. 2000;10:420-27.

84. Tanimura S, Higashino M, Fukunaga Y, Osugi H. Hand-assisted laparoscopic distal gastrectomy with regional lymph node dissection for gastric cancer. Surg Laparosc Endosc Percutan Tech. 2001;11:155-60.

85. Targarona EM, Balague´ C, Cerda´n G, et al. Hand-assisted laparoscopic splenectomy (HALS) in cases of splenomegaly: a comparative analysis with conventional laparoscopic splenectomy. Surg Endosc. 2002;16:426-30.

86. Targarona EM, Balague´ C, Trias M. Hand-assisted laparoscopic splenectomy. Semin Laparosc Surg. 2001;8:126-34.

87. Targarona EM, Gracia E, Mart1´nez- Bru C, et al. Prospective, randomized trial comparing conventional laparoscopic colectomy with hand-assisted laparoscopic colectomy: applicability, immediate clinical outcome, inflammatory response and cost. Surg Endosc. 2002;16:234-9.

88. Targarona, EM, Balague´, C. Trias, M. Laparoscopic splenectomy for splenomegaly. Probl Gen Surg. 2002;19:58-64.

89. Van de Walle P, Blomme Y, Van Outrye L. Hand-assisted staging laparoscopy for suspected malignancies of the pancreas. Acta Chir Belg. 2002;102:183-6.

90. Vassallo C, Negri L, Della Valle A, et al. Divided vertical banded gastroplasty either for correction or as a first-choice operation. Obes Surg. 1999;9:177- 9.

91. Wadstrom J, Lindstrom P. Hand-assisted retroperiton-eoscopic living-donor nephrectomy: initial 10 cases. Transplantation. 2002;73:1839-41.

92. Watson DI, Davies N, Jamieson GG. Totally endoscopic Ivor Lewis esophagectomy. Surg Endosc. 1999;13:293-7.

93. Watson DI, Game PA. Hand-assisted laparoscopic vertical banded gastroplasty: initial report. Surg Endosc. 1997;11:1218-20.

94. Wolf JS Jr, Merion RM, Leichtman AB, et al. Randomized controlled trial of handassisted laparoscopic versus open surgical live donor nephrectomy. Transplantation. 2001;27;72:284-90.

95. Woods SD, Polglase AL. Laparoscopically assisted anterior resection for villous adenoma of the rectum. Aust N Z J Surg. 1993;63:146-8.

96. Yoshida T, Inoue H, Iwai T. Hand-assisted laparoscopic surgery for the abdominal phase in endoscopic esophagectomy for esophageal cancer: an alteration on the site of minilaparotomy. Surg Laparosc Endosc Percutan Tech. 2000; 10:396-400.

Section One

Tissue Retrieval Technique

One of the limitations of minimal access surgery is difficulty in retrieval of tissue. Previously surgeons were reluctant to perform many of the advanced surgical procedure due to this difficult procedure. New techniques for removing tissue have helped increase the number and types of laparoscopic surgeries that can be done laparoscopically.

Safe removal of tissue is an important consideration in laparoscopic surgery and applies to all specimens irrespective of whether they are thought to be benign or malignant. The importance of wound protection is shown by considering laparoscopic cholecystectomy for symptomatic gallstone disease. Most of the gall-bladders at the time of retrieval can be squeezed out through an unprotected port wound. At the time of extraction exit wound must be of sufficient size, and wound protection should be used to ensure that there is no contact between the specimen and the abdominal wall during removal. We all know that the incidence of unsuspected gallbladder cancer is between 0.5% and 1% and there are reported cases of port site tumor nodules because of implantation of tumor cells after extraction of the gallbladder through an unprotected wound.

Tissue reduction enables extraction through small wounds but can be used only for benign specimens. Tissue reduction can be carried out by various techniques, including mechanical fragmentation and morcellation. It should be done inside a rip proof bag whenever possible. This is essential for laparoscopic splenectomy to prevent implantation of splenic fragments on the serosal surfaces, which leads to splenosis (Fig. 10.1).

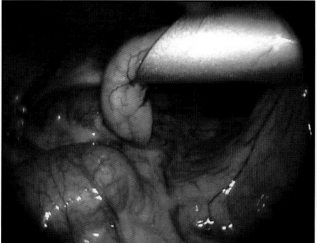

Fig. 10.1: Appendix hidden within cannula

Most commonly the resected tissue should be hidden under port and then everything should come together with port. This technique is used for most of the small size organs like appendix, gallbladder, small ovarian cyst, ectopic pregnancy, salpingectomy, small oophorectomy, etc.

Endobags

In some cases, the tissue to be removed is first encased in a specimen retrieval bag. These tissue retrieval bags are available in market and can be prepared by surgeon himself at the time of laparoscopic surgery (Fig. 10.2A).

For infected tissue and in case of suspected carcinoma, tissue retrieval bag should be used. Many sizes of disposable tissue retrieval bags are available and hard rim of these retrieval bags are easy to

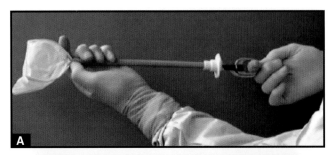

negotiate inside the abdominal cavity (Figs 10.2B to D).

One can easily make the retrieval bag by tying and cutting the fingers of sterilized gloves. If the gloves used for the retrieval of tissue, it should be used carefully. It should not puncture while removing from the abdominal cavity (Fig. 10.3).

The glove is kept stretched while one assistant will tie it in the middle (Figs 10.4A and B).

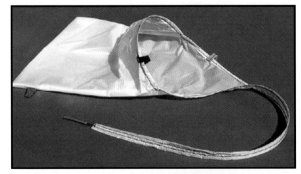

Fig. 10.3: Endobags

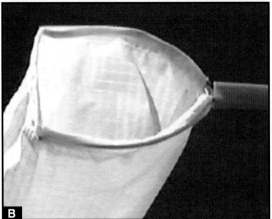

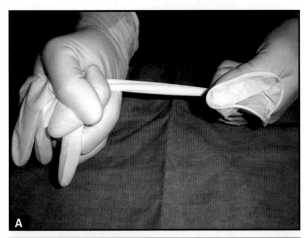

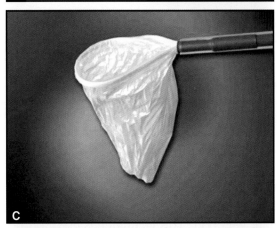

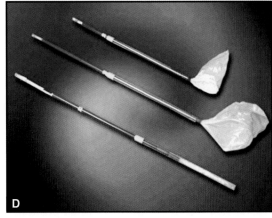

Figs 10.2A to D: Disposable endobags

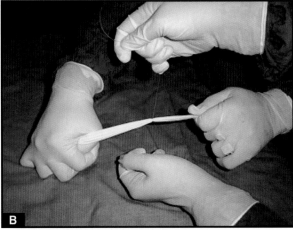

Figs 10.4A and B: Making endobag with glove

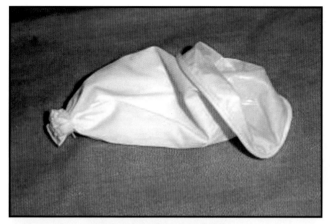

Fig. 10.5: Glove endobag

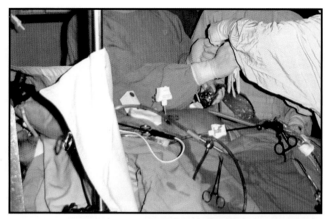

Fig. 10.7: Using glove endobag

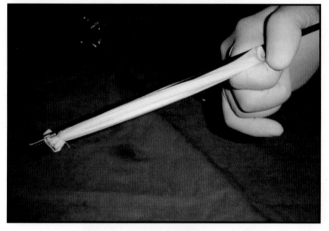

Fig. 10.6: Way of introducing endobag

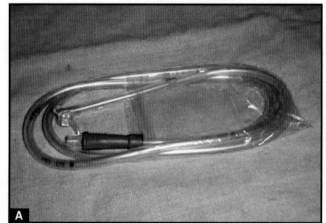

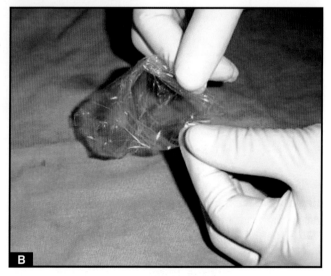

Figs 10.8A and B: Polypropylene endobag

Keeping it stretched will create a good dumbbell after knotting and so there is no chance of slipping of knot inside the abdominal cavity (Fig. 10.5).

The latex material used to manufacture gloves sometimes, react with human tissue and it can create a problem if the glove is punctured and a piece of latex is left inside human body. Most commonly this torn piece of gloves can be missed in the layers of abdominal wall (Fig. 10.6).

At the time of introduction of glove endobag, it should be held by its cut end and kept stretched over the shaft of grasper to decrease its thickness (Fig. 10.7).

The polythene covering of ryels tube can also be used as inexpensive readymade retrieval bag. This is sterilized and open at one end (Figs 10.8A and B).

These polythene bags can be used as excellent retrieval pouch if used carefully. The polythene bags has one demerit that some time the edges are difficult to find out because it is transparent and secondly because it is thin and does not have elastic property like gloves so it slips easily after once held by grasper (Figs 10.9A to E).

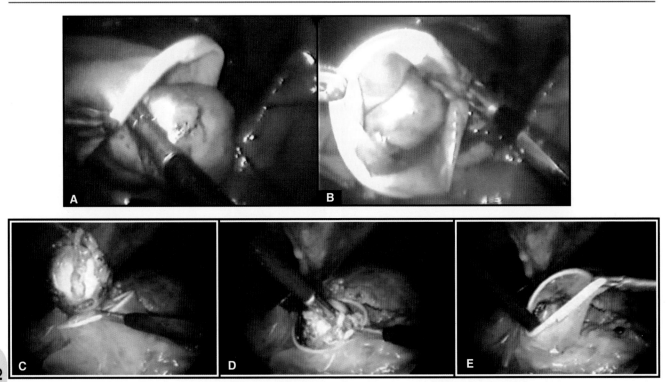

Figs 10.9A to E: Introduction of tissue in endobag

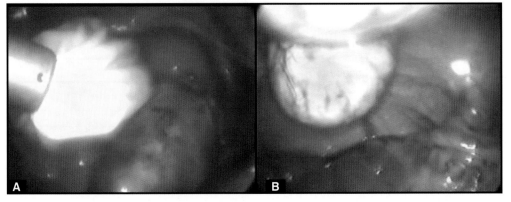

Figs 10.10A and B: Neck of endobag pulled outside the abdominal wall

Drawback of this self-made retrieval bag is that they don't have hard ream so it is difficult to manipulate inside the abdominal cavity.

These bags can be introduced inside the abdominal cavity through 10 mm ports. In special circumstances if there is difficulty is found it can be introduced directly through the port wound after withdrawing the cannula.

Once the retrieval bag is inside it should be positioned in free abdominal space and the rim of bag should be stabilized with nondominant hand and dominant hand should be used to put the specimen inside. Once the tissue is inside the abdominal cavity both the edges of the retrieval bag should be lifted to displace the specimen into the base of the bag (Figs 10.10A and B). Condom can also be used for retrieving tissue. Lubricated condom should be avoided because it can cause tissue reaction.

To take the specimen out, surgeon should hide the mouth of retrieval bag inside the cannula by pulling it and then the cannula together with the neck of bag is pulled outside the abdominal cavity.

Once the neck of the bag is out, its opening is stretched by the help of assistant. Ovum forceps can be introduced inside to morcellate the tissue manually if there is difficulty in pulling the bag out (Fig. 11.11).

Colpotomy

For large size gynecological tissue, colpotomy route is good for retrieval. Colpotomy can be done laparoscopically with the help of heal of hook. Counter pushing by other instruments is effective. Sponge over sponge holding forceps is inserted in posterior vaginal fornix by one assistant and surgeon cuts the vaginal fascia between both the uterosacral ligaments with the heel of hook (Figs 10.12A to D).

HALS

Hand-assisted technique was initially started keeping inside ease of tissue retrievals, wherein the surgeon uses his or her hand, inserted through the initial incision, to aid in the exploration, isolation, and removal of tissue.

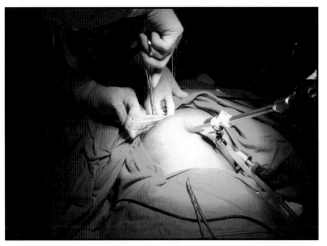

Fig. 10.11: Morcellation of tissue through endobag

Hand-assisted technique offers distinct advantages, the superior visualization afforded by the laparoscope and a tactile component that is important in many aspects of surgery and has allowed surgeons to apply a less invasive approach to surgeries that previously could not have been done laparoscopically.

Section One

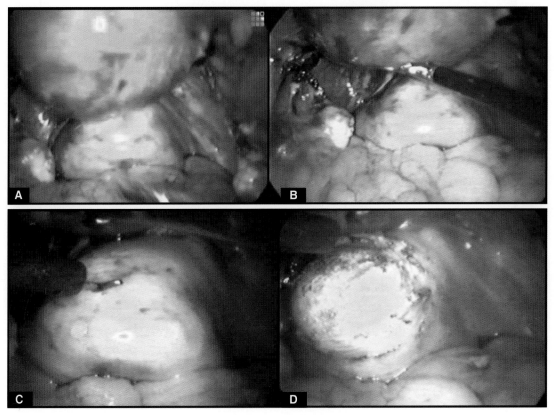

Figs 10.12A to D: Colpotomy

Hand-assisted laparoscopy can also serve as a bridge between open surgery and straight laparoscopy, making it easier for surgeons to practice and learn the skills necessary for performing laparoscopic procedures.

MORCELLATOR

Use of morcellator is another way which facilitates grinding of solid tissue and then these can be taken out without any difficulty. Recently many companies have launched battery operated morcellator. The morcellator is important instrument for tissue retrieval in myomectomy and splenectomy (Fig. 10.13).

One of the early concerns about laparoscopic procedures in cancer patient was that they caused port site metastases, i.e. the appearance of recurrent tumor tissue at the site of trocar entry (Figs 10.14A to D).

Cancer surgery, however, poses some unique challenges that make the application of laparoscopic surgery in oncology more problematic. It is critically important in cancer that whole organs should be removed intact (en bloc) so that pathologists can properly examine them and measure and document the depths and margins of tumor invasion. A second concern for surgical oncologists is cell transfer or cell spillage. Diseased tissue must be removed without contaminating adjacent tissues and structures with

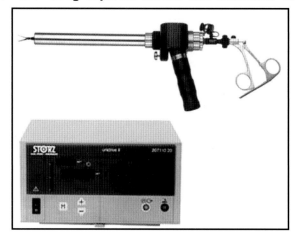

Fig. 10.13: Electrical morcellator

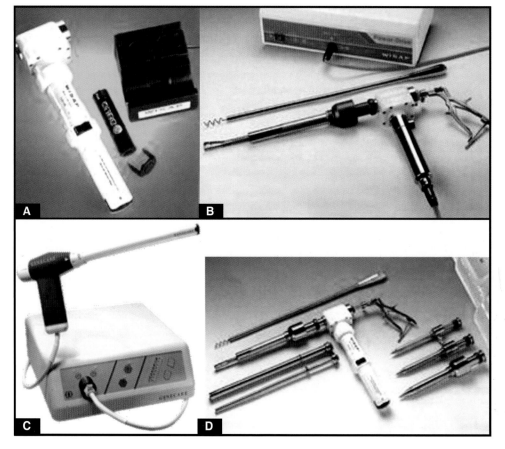

Figs 10.14A to D: Different type of morcellator

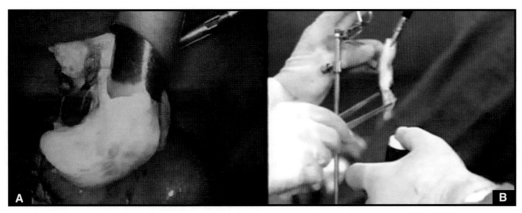

Figs 10.15A to B: Morcellation of tissue

cancer cells. Because of these concerns, tissue morcellation, a technique commonly used in noncancer laparoscopic surgery in which the tissue is divided into pieces so that it can be removed more easily should not be used for oncologic procedures. All the 10 mm or greater than 10 mm chord should be closed properly to prevent any future possibility of hernia (Figs 10.15A and B).

The suture passer should be used to pass the thread and then it should be tied externally.

Especially designed port closure instruments are also available commercially.

If port is suddenly taken out, the chances of port site hernia and adhesion is much higher. It is a good practice to insert some blunt instrument while removing the last port out, to prevent entrapment of omentum or bowel content.

After closing the rectus sheath the skin can be closed by intradermal, skin stapler or by any of the surgical skin glues available.

BIBLIOGRAPHY

1. Bach PB, Cramer LD, Warren JL, Begg CB. Racial differences in the treatment of early-stage lung cancer. N Engl J Med. 1999;341:1198-1205.
2. Ballesta-Lopez C, Bastida-Vila X, Catarci M, Mato R, Ruggiero R. Laparoscopic Billroth II distal subtotal gastrectomy with gastric stump suspension for gastric malignancies. Am J Surg. 1996;171:289-92.
3. Begg CB, Cramer LD, Hoskins WJ, Brennan MF. Impact of hospital volume on operative mortality for major cancer surgery. JAMA. 1998;280:1747-51.
4. Bouvy ND, Marquet RL, Jeekel H, Bonjer HJ. Impact of gas(less) laparoscopy and laparotomy on peritoneal tumor growth and abdominal wall metastases. Ann Surg. 1996;224:694-701.
5. Callery MP, Strasberg SM, Doherty GM, Soper NJ, Norton JA. Staging laparoscopy with laparoscopic ultrasonography: optimizing resectability in hepatobiliary and pancreatic malignancy. J Am Coll Surg. 1997;185:33-9.
6. Charlson ME, Pompei P, Ales KL, MacKenzie CR. A new method of classifying prognostic comorbidity in longitudinal studies: development and validation. J Chron Dis. 1987;40:373-83.
7. Chew DK, Borromeo JR, Kimmelstiel FM. Peritoneal mucinous carcinomatosis after laparoscopic-assisted anterior resection for early rectal cancer: report of a case. Dis Colon Rectum. 1999;42:424-6.
8. Cox DR. Regression models and life-tables. J R Stat Soc (Ser B). 1972;34:187-220.
9. Cubiella J, Castells A, Fondevila C, et al. Prognostic factors in nonresectable pancreatic adenocarcinoma: a rationale to design therapeutic trials. Am J Gastroenterol. 1999;94:1271-8.
10. DeMeester TR, Wang CI, Wernly JA, Pellegrini CA, Little AG, Klementschitsch P, Bermudez G, Johnson LF, Skinner DB. Technique, indications, and clinical use of 24 hour esophageal pH monitoring. J Thorac Cardiovasc Surg 1980;79:656–70.
11. Dieter Jr RA, Kuzycz GB. Complications and contra-indications of thoracoscopy. Int Surg 1997;82:232–9.
12. Dorrance HR, Oien K, O'Dwyer PJ. Effects of laparoscopy on intraperitoneal tumor growth and distant metastases in an animal model. Surgery. 1999;126:35-40.
13. Drouard F, Delamarre J, Capron JP. Cutaneous seeding of gallbladder cancer after laparoscopic cholecystectomy. N Engl J Med. 1991;325:316.
13. Eadie LH, Seifalian AM, Davidson BR. Telemedicine in surgery. Br J Surg 2003;90:647–58.
14. Fleshman JW, Nelson H, Peters WR, et al. Early results of laparoscopic surgery for colorectal cancer: retrospective analysis of 372 patients treated by Clinical Outcomes of Surgical Therapy (COST) Study Group. Dis Colon Rectum. 1996; 39:S53-S58.
15. Forde KA, Hulten L. Laparoscopy in colorectal surgery. Surg Endosc. 1996;10:1039-40.

16. Forster R, Storck M, Schafer JR, Honig E, Lang G, Liewald F. Thoracoscopy versus thoracotomy: a prospective comparison of trauma and quality of life. Langenbecks Arch Surg 2002;387:32–6.

17. Freedman LS. Tables of the number of patients required in clinical trials using the logrank test. Stat Med. 1982;1:121-9.

18. Geer RJ, Brennan MF. Prognostic indicators for survival after resection of pancreatic adenocarcinoma. Am J Surg. 1993;165:68-72.

19. Giulianotti PC, Coratti A, Angelini M, Sbrana F, Cecconi S, Balestracci T, Caravaglios G. Robotics in general surgery: personal experience in a large community hospital. Arch Surg 2003;138: 777–84.

20. Jacobi CA, Sabat R, Bohm B, et al. Pneumoperitoneum with carbon dioxide stimulates growth of malignant colonic cells. Surgery. 1997;121:72-78.

21. Jacobi CA, Wildbrett P, Volk T, Muller JM. Influence of different gases and intraperitoneal instillation of antiadherent or cytotoxic agents on peritoneal tumor cell growth and implantation with laparoscopic surgery in a rat model. Surg Endosc. 1999;13:1021-25.

22. Jones DB, Guo LW, Reinhard MK, et al. Impact of pneumoperitoneum on trocar site implantation of colon cancer in hamster model. Dis Colon Rectum. 1995; 38:1182-88.

23. Kalbfleisch JD, Prentice RL. The Statistical Analysis of Failure Time Data. New York, NY: John Wiley; 1980.

24. Kaplan EL, Meier P. Nonparametric estimation from incomplete observations. Am Stat Assoc. 1958;53:457-81.

25. Kumar A, Kumar S, Aggarwal S, Khilnani GC. Thoracoscopy: the preferred approach for the resection of selected posterior mediastinal tumors. J Laparoendosc Adv Surg Tech A 2002;12:345–53.

26. Lacy AM, Garcia-Valdecasas JC, Pique JM, et al. Short-term outcome analysis of a randomized study comparing laparoscopic vs open colectomy for colon cancer. Surg Endosc. 1995;9:1101-05.

27. Mack MJ. Video-assisted thoracoscopy thymectomy for myasthenia gravis. Chest Surg Clin N Am 2001;1:389–05.

28. Masaoka A, Yamakawa Y, Niwa H, Fukai I, Kondo S, Kobayashi M, Fujii Y, Monden Y. Extended thymectomy for myasthenia gravis patients: a 20-year review. Ann Thorac Surg 1996;62:853–9.

29. Melfi FM, Menconi GF, Mariani AM, Angeletti CA. Early experience with robotic technology for thoracoscopic surgery. Eur J Cardiothorac Surg 2002;21:864–8.

30. Milsom JW, Bohm B, Hammerhofer KA, et al. A prospective, randomized trial comparing laparoscopic versus conventional techniques in colorectal cancer surgery: a preliminary report. J Am Coll Surg. 1998;187:46-54.

31. Morgan JA, Ginsburg ME, Sonett JR, Morales DL, Kohmoto T, Gorenstein LA, Smith CR, Argenziano M. Advanced thoracoscopic procedures are facilitated by computer-aided robotic technology. Eur J Cardiothorac Surg 2003;23: 883–7.

32. Nagahiro I, Andou A, Aoe M, Sano Y, Date H, Shimizu N. Pulmonary function, postoperative pain, and serum cytokine level after lobectomy: a comparison of VATS and conventional procedure. Ann Thorac Surg 2001;72:362–5.

33. Nifong LW, Chu VF, Bailey BM, Maziarz DM, Sorrell VL, Holbert D, Chitwood Jr WR. Robotic mitral valve repair: experience with the da Vinci system. Ann Thorac Surg 2003;75:438–42.

34. Onnasch JF, Schneider F, Falk V, Mierzwa M, Bucerius J, Mohr FW. Five years of less invasive mitral valve surgery: from experimental to routine approach. Heart Surg Forum 2002;5:132–5.

35. Onoda N, Ishikawa T, Yamada N, Okamura T, Tahara H, Inaba M, Takashima T, Sakate Y, Chung KH. Radioisotope-navigated videoassisted thoracoscopic operation for ectopic mediastinal parathyroid. Surgery 2002;132:17–19.

36. Potosky AL, Riley GF, Lubitz JD, Mentnech RM, Kessler LG. Potential for cancer related health services research using a linked medicare-tumor registry database. Med Care. 1993;31:732-48.

37. Poulin EC, Mamazza J, Schlachta CM, Gregoire R, Roy N. Laparoscopic resection does not adversely affect early survival curves in patients undergoing surgery for colorectal adenocarcinoma. Ann Surg. 1999;229:487-92.

38. Ramshaw BJ. Laparoscopic surgery for cancer patients. CA Cancer J Clin. 1997; 47:327-50.

39. Romano PS, Mark DJ. Bias in the coding of hospital discharge data and its implications for quality assessment. Med Care. 1994;32:81-90.

40. Roviaro GC, Varoli F, Vergani C, Maciocco M. State of the art in thoracospic surgery: a personal experience of 2000 videothoracoscopic procedures and an overview of the literature. Surg Endosc 2002;16:881–92.

41. Schmid T. Editorial to: main topics: robotic surgery. Eur Surg 2002; 34:155–7.

42. Schurr MO, Arezzo A, Buess GF. Robotics and systems technology for advanced endoscopic procedures: experiences in general surgery. Eur J Cardiothorac Surg 1999;16(2):S97–S105.

43. SEER Cancer Statistics Review, 1973-1997. Bethesda, Md: National Cancer Institute; 2000.

44. Sener SF, Fremgen A, Menck HR, Winchester DP. Pancreatic cancer: a report of treatment and survival trends for 100,313 patients diagnosed from 1985-1995, using the National Cancer Database. J Am Coll Surg. 1990;189:1-7. 1094–9.

45. Soper NJ, Brunt LM, Kerbl K. Medical progress: laparoscopic general surgery. Engl J Med. 1994;330:409-19.

46. Takiguchi S, Matsuura N, Hamada Y, et al. Influence of CO2 pneumoperitoneum during laparoscopic surgery on cancer cell growth. Surg Endosc. 2000;14:41-4.

47. Tewari A, Peabody J, Sarle R, Balakrishnan G, Hemal A, Shrivastava A, Menon M. Technique of da Vinci robot-assisted anatomic radical prostatectomy. Urology 2002;60:569–72.

48. Volz J, Koster S, Schaeff B, Paolucci V. Laparoscopic surgery: the effects of insufflations gas on tumor-induced lethality in nude mice. Am J Obstet Gynecol. 1998;178:793-5.

49. Wetscher GJ, Glaser K, Wieschemeyer T, Gadenstaetter M, Prommegger R, Profanter C. Tailored antireflux surgery for gastroesophageal reflux disease: effectiveness and risk of postoperative dysphagia. World J Surg 1997;21:605–10.

50. Wexner SD, Cohen SM. Port site metastases after laparoscopic colorectal surgery for cure of malignancy. Br J Surg. 1995;82:295-98.

51. Whelan RL, Allendorf JD, Gutt CN, et al. General oncologic effects of the laparoscopic surgical approach: 1997 Frankfurt international meeting of animal laparoscopic researchers. Surg Endosc. 1998;12:1092-1095.

52. Whelan RL, Lee SW. Review of investigations regarding the etiology of port site tumor recurrence. J Laparoendosc Adv Surg Tech A. 1999;9:1-16. 22. Bouvy ND, Giuffrida MC, Tseng LN, et al. Effects of carbon dioxide pneumo-peritoneum, air pneumoperitoneum, and gasless laparoscopy on body weight and tumor growth. Arch Surg. 1998;133:652-656.

53. Wittich P, Marquet RL, Kazemier G, Bonjer HJ. Port-site metastases after CO(2) laparoscopy: is aerosolization of tumor cells a pivotal factor? Surg Endosc. 2000; 14:189-192.

54. Wykypiel H, Wetscher GJ, Klaus A, Schmid T, Gadenstaetter M, Bodner J, Bodner E. Robot-assisted laparoscopic partial posterior fundoplication with the DaVinci system: initial experiences and technical aspects. Langenbecks Arch Surg 2003;387:411–6.

55. Yim AP. Thoracoscopic thymectomy: which side to approach? Ann Thorac Surg 1997;64:584–5.

Section One

11 Laparoscopic Port Closure Technique

Minimally invasive laparoscopic surgery has revolutionized the way surgery is performed for an increasing number of patients. Incisional hernia can occur after any abdominal surgery and laparoscopic surgery is not immune to this complication. The hernia that follow laparoscopy usually occur through the larger ports (size greater than 10 mm), especially the umbilicus.

Predisposing factors include:
1. Previous laparoscopies
2. Extensive manipulation during surgery
3. Increased intra-abdominal pressure
4. Obesity
5. Use of sharp cutting-tip trocars
6. Rapid abdominal deflation at the end of surgery
7. Poor port removal techniques and defective closure of the abdominal fascia
8. Wound extension
9. Male sex
10. Infection of the wound
11. Pre-existing umbilical defects
12. Postoperative chest infections
13. Pre-existing diseases such as diabetes mellitus
14. Connective tissue disorders
15. Job profile of the patient (Weight lifting).

Among all these factors, the single most important factor remains the improper closure of the fascial defects at the port sites (Figs 11.1 and 11.2). The diagnosis is often delayed because most cases present late, and treatment might be instituted along other lines. Computed tomography scans are helpful in its

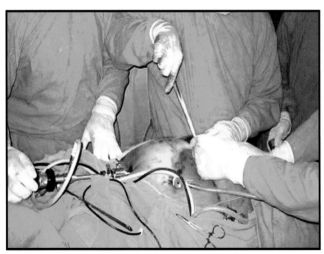

Fig. 11.1: Proper closure of port greater than 10 mm is essential to prevent hernia

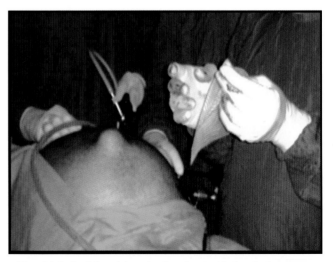

Fig. 11.2: Incisional hernia development due to improper closure of port should be repaired later by mesh

Section One

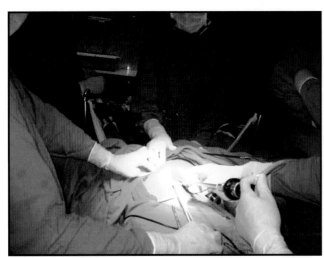

Fig. 11.3: The tip of telescope should be introduced in and cannula is pulled over telescope to prevent suction of omentum or bowel

diagnosis and will facilitate prompt treatment to avoid the grave consequence of bowel gangrene.

The hernia may become evident at any time following laparoscopic surgery and the patient may either have an uncomplicated hernia, or may be afflicted with a variety of complications such as evisceration of the bowel or omentum and it may become a cause of significant morbidity Meticulous closure of the fascia, avoidance of unnecessary wound extension, the use of non-absorbable sutures when faced with defects more than 2 cm in size, completely defining the extent of any pre-existing hernia and repairing this at the time of port site closure, are recommended to minimize the incidence of port site hernia after laparoscopic surgery.

Whilst surgical techniques and instrumentation have made significant advances, it is usual that the surgical incision is closed using invasive suturing techniques or by the use of tapes or by the use of topical cyanoacrylate skin adhesives (TCAs) for closure of surgical wounds. The incidence of incisional hernia occurring at the port sites after laparoscopic surgery, lies between 0.02 to 3.6 % and usually remains unreported, until the development of complications.

Any port closure technique should have following characteristics:
1. Effective (strong and secure) surgical wound closure
2. Faster wound closure
3. Better scar cosmesis
4. Occlusive microbial wound dressing
5. Less tissue trauma, reduced inflammatory reaction
6. No requirement for suture/staple removal
7. Easy to use/simple learning curve
8. Reduced risk of needlestick injury - safety and costs
9. Cost-effective.

WITHDRAWAL OF INSTRUMENT AND PORTS

Once the surgery is finished all the instrument should be removed carefully under vision. All the accessory port should be removed and the gas is removed by releasing the valve of 10 mm cannulas. The primary port should be taken out in the end (Fig. 11.3).

If last port is suddenly withdrawn sudden suction effect of cannula can pull the omentum or bowel inside the port wound, the chances of port site hernia and adhesion is much higher in this case. It is a good practice to insert some blunt instrument or telescope inside the abdomen while removing the last cannula out over that instrument, to prevent inadvertent entrapment of omentum or bowel.

The access technique will result in breach in continuity of abdominal wall which need to be repaired at the end of surgery. All the 10 mm or greater than 10 mm port should be repaired properly to prevent any future possibility of hernia. The rectus sheath is only necessary to suture with vicryl. Only one stitch is required in middle which will convert 10 mm wound into 5 mm. The 5 mm port wounds are not necessary to repair.

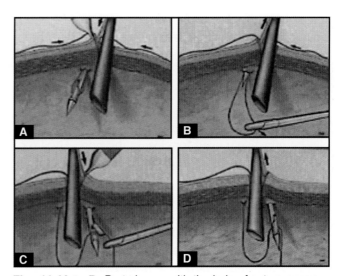

Figs 11.4A to D: Port closure with the help of suture passer

Section One

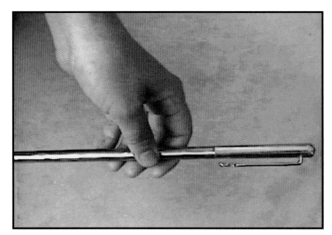

Fig. 11.5: Port closure needle

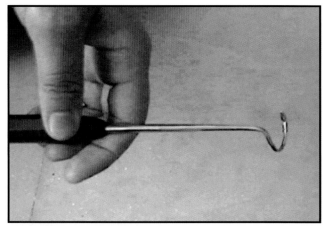

Fig. 11.6: Aneurysm needle

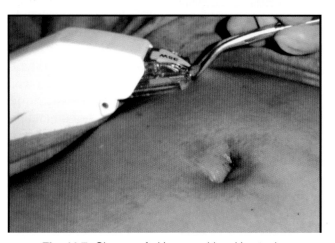

Fig. 11.7: Closure of skin wound by skin stapler

Laparoscopic Port Closure Instruments

Various types of port closure instruments are available. The suture passer is a convenient instrument for port closure. It is used to pass the thread on the side of cannula and then it is tied externally (Figs 11.4A to D).

Port Closure Needle

This is a simple instrument just like cobblers and it can be effectively used for closing the port. The tip of the instrument is blunt and the needle faces towards the fascia so the chances of injury to the bowel are less with the use of this instrument (Fig. 11.5).

Aneurysm needle can also be used for closing fascia. The advantage of this needle is that eye is at the tip and due to rigid structure there is no risk of bending or rotation of needle (Fig. 11.6).

After closing the rectus sheath the skin can be closed by intradermal, skin stapler or any of the surgical skin glues topical cyanoacrylate skin adhesives (TCAs) available (Fig. 11.7).

BIBLIOGRAPHY

1. Ahmad SA, Schuricht AL, Azurin DJ, et al. Complications of laparoscopic cholecystectomy: the experience of a university-affiliated teaching hospital. J Laparoendosc Adv Surg Tech A. 1997;7:29-35.
2. Al-Haijar N, Duca S, Molnar G, Vasilescu A, Nicolescu N. Incidents and postoperative complications of laparoscopic cholecystectomies for acute cholecystitis. Rom J Gastroenterol. 2002;11:115-19.
3. Azurin DJ, Go LS, Arroyo LR, Kirkland ML. Trocar site herniation following laparoscopic cholecystectomy and the significance of an incidental preexisting umbilical hernia. Am Surg. 1995;61:718-20.

4. Baird DR, Wilson JP, Mason EM, et al. An early review of 800 laparoscopic cholecystectomies at a university-affiliated community teaching hospital. Am Surg. 1992;58:206-10.

5. Bender E, Sell H. Small bowel obstruction after laparoscopic cholecystectomy as a result of a Maydl's herniation of the small bowel through a trocar site. Surgery. 1996;119:480.

6. Berthou JC, Charbonneau P. Elective laparoscopic management of sigmoid diverticulitis: results in a series of 110 patients. Surg Endosc. 1999;13:457-60.

7. Bhoyrul S, Payne J, Steffes B, Swanstrom L, Way LW. A randomized prospective study of radially expanding trocars in laparoscopic surgery. J Gastrointest Surg. 2000;4: 392-7.

8. Boughey JC, Nottingham JM, Walls AC. Richter's hernia in the laparoscopic era: four case reports and review of the literature. Surg Laparosc Endosc Percutan Tech. 2003;13:55-58.

9. Bowrey DJ, Blom D, Crookes PF, et al. Risk factors and the prevalence of trocar site herniation after laparoscopic fundoplication. Surg Endosc. 2001;15:663- 6.

10. Cadeddu MO, Schlachta CM, Mamazza J, Seshadri PA, Poulin EC. Soft-tissue images: trocar-site hernia after laparoscopic procedures. Can J Surg. 2002; 45:9-10.

11. Callery MP, Strasberg SM, Soper NJ. Complications of laparoscopic general surgery. Gastrointest Endosc Clin N Am. 1996;6:423-44.

12. Chevallier JM, Zinzindohoue F, Elian N, et al. Adjustable gastric banding in a public university hospital: prospective analysis of 400 patients. Obes Surg. 2002; 12:93-9.

13. Coda A, Bossotti M, Ferri F, et al. Incisional hernia and fascial defect following laparoscopic surgery. Surg Laparosc Endosc Percutan Tech. 2000;10:34-8.

14. Cottam DR, Gorecki PJ, Curvelo M, Weltman D, Angus LD, Shaftan G. Preperitoneal herniation into a laparoscopic port site without a fascial defect. Obes Surg. 2002;12:121-123.

15. Crist DW, Gadacz TR. Complications of laparoscopic surgery. Surg Clin North Am. 1993;73:265-89.

16. De Giuli M, Festa V, Denoye GC, Morino M. Large postoperative umbilical hernia following laparoscopic cholecystectomy: a case report. Surg Endosc. 1994; 8: 904-5.

17. Di Lorenzo N, Coscarella G, Lirosi F, Gaspari A. Port-site closure: a new problem, an old device. JSLS. 2002;6: 181-3.

18. Dresel A, Kuhn JA, Westmoreland MV, Talaasen LJ, McCarty TM. Establishing a laparoscopic gastric bypass program. Am J Surg. 2002;184:617-20.

19. Duron JJ, Hay JM, Msika S, et al. Prevalence and mechanisms of small intestinal obstruction following laparoscopic abdominal surgery: a retrospective multicenter study. Arch Surg. 2000;135:208-12.

20. Fear RE. Laparoscopy: a valuable aid in gynecologic diagnosis. Obstet Gynecol. 1968;31:297-309.

21. Fitzgibbons RJ Jr, Annibali R, Litke BS. Gallbladder and gallstone removal, open versus closed laparoscopy, and pneumoperitoneum. Am J Surg. 1993;165: 497-504.

22. Freedman AN, Sigman HH. Incarcerated paraumbilical incisional hernia and abscess: complications of a spilled gallstone. J Laparoendosc Surg. 1995;5:189-91.

23. Hass BE, Schrager RE. Small bowel obstruction due to Richter's hernia after laparoscopic procedures. J Laparoendosc Surg. 1993;3:421-3.

24. Horgan PG, O'Connell PR. Subumbilical hernia following laparoscopic cholecystectomy. Br J Surg. 1993;80:1595.

25. Kadar N, Reich H, Liu CY, Manko GF, Gimpelson R. Incisional hernias after major laparoscopic gynecologic procedures. Am J Obstet Gynecol. 1993;168: 1493-5.

26. Komuta K, Haraguchi M, Inoue K, Furui J, Kanematsu T. Herniation of the small bowel through the port site following removal of drains during laparoscopic surgery. Dig Surg. 2000;17:544-6.

27. Kopelman D, Schein M, Assalia A, Hashmonai M. Small bowel obstruction following laparoscopic cholecystectomy: diagnosis of incisional hernia by computed tomography. Surg Laparosc Endosc. 1994;4:325-6.

28. Kulacoglu IH. Regarding: Small bowel obstruction and incisional hernia after laparoscopic surgery: should 5-mm trocar sites be sutured? J Laparoendosc Adv Surg Tech A. 2000;10:227-8.

29. Lafullarde T, Van Hee R, Gys T. A safe and simple method for routine open access in laparoscopic procedures. Surg Endosc. 1999;13:769-72.

30. Larson GM, Vitale GC, Casey J, Voyles CR. Multipractice analysis of laparoscopic cholecystectomy in 1,983 patients. Am J Surg. 1992;163:221-6.

31. Leibl BJ, Schmedt CG, Schwarz J, Kraft K, Bittner R. Laparoscopic surgery complications associated with trocar tip design: review of literature and own results. J Laparoendosc Adv Surg Tech A. 1999;9:135-40.

32. Li P, Chung RS. Closure of trocar wounds using a suture carrier. Surg Laparosc Endosc. 1996;6:469-71.

33. Liu CD, McFadden DW. Laparoscopic port sites do not require fascial closure when nonbladed trocars are used. Am Surg. 2000;66:853-4.

34. Lumley J, Stitz R, Stevenson A, Fielding G, Luck A. Laparoscopic colorectal surgery for cancer: intermediate to long-term outcomes. Dis Colon Rectum. 2002; 45:867-72.

35. Maio A, Ruchman RB. CT diagnosis of post laparoscopic hernia. J Comput Assist Tomogr. 1991;15:1054-5.

36. Matter I, Nash E, Abrahamson J, Eldar S. Incisional hernia via a lateral 5-mm trocar port following laparoscopic cholecystectomy. Isr J Med Sci. 1996;32: 790-1.

37. Matthews BD, Heniford BT, Sing RF. Preperitoneal Richter hernia after a laparoscopic gastric bypass. Surg Laparosc Endosc Percutan Tech. 2001;11:47-9.

38. Mayol J, Garcia-Aguilar J, Ortiz-Oshiro E, De-Diego Carmona JA, Fernandez- Represa JA. Risks of the minimal access approach for laparoscopic surgery: multivariate analysis of morbidity related to umbilical trocar insertion. World J Surg. 1997;21:529-33.

39. McMillan J, Watt I. Herniation at the site of cannula insertion after laparoscopic cholecystectomy. Br J Surg. 1993;80:915.

Section One

40. McMurrick PJ, Polglase AL. Early incisional hernia after use of the 12-mm port for laparoscopic surgery. Aust N Z J Surg. 1993;63:574-5.

41. Montz FJ, Holschneider CH, Munro MG. Incisional hernia following laparoscopy: a survey of the American Association of Gynecologic Laparoscopists. Obstet Gynecol. 1994;84:881-4.

42. Morrison CP, Wemyss-Holden SA, Iswariah H, Maddern GJ. Lateral laparoscopic port sites should all be closed: the incisional "spigelian" hernia. Surg Endosc. 2002;16:1364.

43. Nakajima K, Wasa M, Kawahara H, et al. Revision laparoscopy for incarcerated hernia at a 5-mm trocar site following pediatric laparoscopic surgery. Surg Laparosc Endosc Percutan Tech. 1999;9:294-5.

44. Nassar AH, Ashkar KA, Rashed AA, Abdulmoneum MG. Laparoscopic cholecystectomy and the umbilicus. Br J Surg. 1997;84:630-3.

45. Ok E, Sozuer E. Intra-abdominal gallstone spillage detected during umbilical trocar site hernia repair after laparoscopic cholecystectomy: report of a case. Surg Today. 2000;30:1046-8.

46. Patterson M, Walters D, Browder W. Postoperative bowel obstruction following laparoscopic surgery. Am Surg. 1993;59:656-7.

47. Petrakis I, Sciacca V, Chalkiadakis G, Vassilakis SI, Xynos E. A simple technique for trocar site closure after laparoscopic surgery. Surg Endosc. 1999;13:1249- 51.

48. Plaus WJ. Laparoscopic trocar site hernias. J Laparoendosc Surg. 1993;3:567- 70.

49. Rabinerson D, Avrech O, Neri A, Schoenfeld A. Incisional hernias after laparoscopy. Obstet Gynecol Surv. 1997;52:701-03.

50. Ramachandran CS. Umbilical hernial defects encountered before and after abdominal laparoscopic procedures. Int Surg. 1998;83:171-3.

51. Reardon PR, McKinney G, Craig ES. The 2-mm trocar: a safe and effective way of closing trocar sites using existing equipment. J Am Coll Surg. 2003;196: 333-6.

52. Reardon PR, Preciado A, Scarborough T, Matthews B, Marti JL. Hernia at 5-mm laparoscopic port site presenting as early postoperative small bowel obstruction. J Laparoendosc Adv Surg Tech A. 1999;9:523-5.

53. Rosen M, Ponsky J. Minimally invasive surgery. Endoscopy. 2001;33:358-66.

54. Sanz-Lopez R, Martinez-Ramos C, Nunez-Pena JR, Ruiz de Gopegui M, Pastor- Sirera L, Tamames-Escobar S. Incisional hernias after laparoscopic vs open cholecystectomy. Surg Endosc. 1999;13:922-4.

55. Schauer PR, Ikramuddin S, Gourash W, Ramanathan R, Luketich J. Outcomes after laparoscopic Roux-en-Y gastric bypass for morbid obesity. Ann Surg. 2000; 232:515-29.

56. Schiller VL, Joyce PW, Sarti DA. Small-bowel obstruction due to hernia through the primary laparoscopic port: a complication of laparoscopic cholecystectomy. AJR Am J Roentgenol. 1994;163:480-1.

57. Susmallian S, Ezri T, Charuzi I. Laparoscopic repair of access port site hernia after Lap-Band system implantation. Obes Surg. 2002;12:682-4.

58. Velasco JM, Vallina VL, Bonomo SR, Hieken TJ. Post laparoscopic small bowel obstruction: rethinking its management. Surg Endosc. 1998;12:1043-5.

59. Voyles CR, Petro AB, Meena AL, Haick AJ, Koury AM. A practical approach to laparoscopic cholecystectomy. Am J Surg. 1991;161:365-70.

60. Wagner M, Farley GE. Incarcerated hernia with intestinal obstruction after laparoscopic cholecystectomy. WMJ. 1994;93:169-71.

61. Waldhaussen JH. Incisional hernia in a 5-mm trocar site following pediatric laparoscopy. J Laparoendosc Surg. 1996;6(1):S89-S90.

62. Wallace DH, O'Dwyer PJ. Clinical experience with open laparoscopy. J Laparoendosc Adv Surg Tech A. 1997;7: 285-8.

63. Williams MD, Flowers SS, Fenoglio ME, Brown TR. Richter hernia: a rare complication of laparoscopy. Surg Laparosc Endosc. 1995;5:419-421.

Laparoscopic General Surgical Procedures

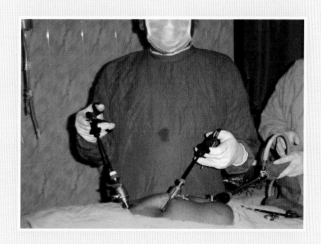

12

Laparoscopic Cholecystectomy

Laparoscopic surgery has undergone rapid development in recent years. Laparoscopic cholecystectomy was first performed in 1985. Since the introduction of laparoscopic cholecystectomy into general practice in 1990, it has rapidly become the dominant procedure for gallbladder surgery. By the end of the decade, laparoscopic cholecystectomy had spread throughout the world. The importance of laparoscopic cholecystectomy was the cultural change it engendered rather than the operation it replaced. In terms of technique, laparoscopic cholecystectomy is now the gold standard for the treatment of symptomatic gallstone disease. It is most commonly performed minimal access surgery by general surgeon's world wide. In Europe and America 98 percent of all the cholecystectomy is performed by laparoscopy. The credit of popularizing minimal access surgery goes to laparoscopic cholecystectomy. This is most popular and most accepted minimal access surgical procedure worldwide. Laparoscopic surgery has expanded from gallbladder surgery to virtually every operation in the abdominal cavity.

INDICATIONS (FIG. 12.1)

- Cholelithiasis
- Mucocele gallbladder
- Empyema gallbladder
- Cholesterosis
- Typhoid carrier
- Porcelain gallbladder
- Acute cholecystitis (calculous and acalculous)
- Adenomatous gallbladder polyps
- As part of other procedures viz. Whipple's procedure.

Contraindications

- Hemodynamic instability
- Uncorrected coagulopathy
- Generalized peritonitis
- Severe cardiopulmonary disease
- Abdominal wall infection
- Multiple previous upper abdominal procedures
- Late pregnancy.

The general anesthesia and the pneumoperitoneum required as part of the laparoscopic procedure do increase the risk in certain groups of patients. Most surgeons would not recommend laparoscopy in those with pre-existing disease conditions. Patients with

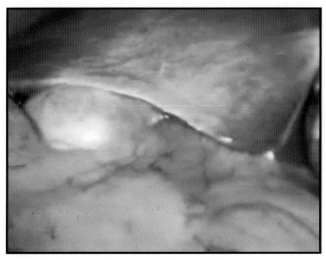

Fig. 12.1: Appearance of fundus of gallbladder in first look

severe cardiac diseases and COPD should not be considered a good candidate for laparoscopy. The laparoscopic cholecystectomy may also be more difficult in patients who have had previous upper abdominal surgery. The elderly may also be at increased risk for complications with general anesthesia combined with pneumoperitoneum.

ADVANTAGE OF LAPAROSCOPIC APPROACH

- Cosmetically better outcome
- Less tissue dissection and disruption of tissue planes
- Less pain postoperatively
- Low intraoperative and postoperative complications in experienced hand
- Early return to work.

Preoperative Investigations

Apart from routine preoperative investigations, in fit patients, the only investigations needed are ultrasound examination. Although practiced in some centers, intravenous cholangiography may not be confirmative and is attended with the risk of anaphylactic reactions.

Patient Position

Patient is operated in the supine position with a steep head-up and left tilt. This typical positioning of laparoscopic cholecystectomy should be achieved once the pneumoperitoneum has been established. The patient is then placed in reverse Trendelenburg's position and rotated to the left to give maximal exposure to the right upper quadrant.

Position of Surgical Team (Fig. 12.2)

The surgeon stands on the left side of the patient with the scrub nurse-camera holder-assistant. One assistant stand right to the patient and should hold the fundus grasping forceps.

Tasks Analysis

- Preparation of the patient
- Creation of pneumoperitoneum
- Insertion of ports
- Diagnostic laparoscopy

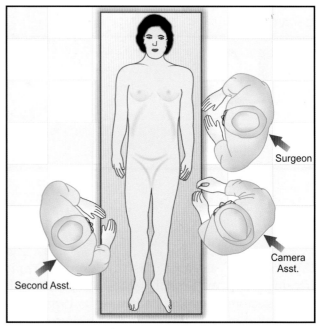

Fig. 12.2: Position of surgical team

- Dissection of visceral peritoneum
- Dissection of Calot's triangle
- Clipping and division of cystic duct and artery
- Dissection of gallbladder from liver bed
- Extraction of gallbladder and any spilled stone
- Irrigation and suction of operating field
- Final diagnostic laparoscopy
- Removal of the instrument with complete exit of CO_2
- Closure of wound.

Port Location (Figs 12.3A to C)

Four ports are used: optical (10 mm), one 5 mm and one 10 mm operating, and one 5.0 mm assisting port. The optical port is at or near the umbilicus and routinely a 30° laparoscope is used. Some surgeon who have started laparoscopy earlier is more comfortable with 0° telescope. The laparoscope is inserted through a 10 mm umbilical port and the abdominal cavity is explored for any obvious abnormalities. The secondary ports are then placed under direct visualization with the laparoscope. The surgeon places a 10 mm trocar in the midline and left to the falciform ligament at the epigastrium. Two 5 mm ports one subcostal trocar in the right upper quadrant and another 5 mm trocar, lower, near the right anterior axillary line are placed.

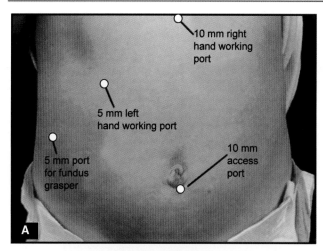

Fig. 12.3A: Ideal port position for laparoscopic cholecystectomy

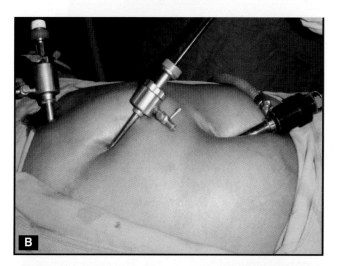

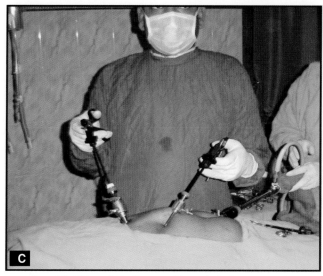

Figs 12. 3B and C: Port position of cholecystectomy

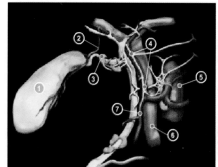

1. Gallbladder
2. Cystic artery
3. Mascagn lymph node
4. Proper hepatic artery
5. Abdominal aorta
6. Portal vein
7. Gastroduodenal artery

Fig. 12.4: Topographic anatomy of gallbladder

Laparoscopic Anatomy (Fig. 12.4)

Laparoscopic view of the right upper quadrant on first look will demonstrate primarily the subphrenic spaces, abdominal surface of diaphragm, and diaphragmatic surface of the liver. The fundus of the gallbladder can be seen popping from the inferior surface of liver. The falciform ligament is seen as a prominent dividing point between left subphrenic space and the right subphrenic space. As the gallbladder is elevated and retracted towards the diaphragm, adhesion to the omentum or duodenum and transverse colon is seen.

EXPOSURE OF GALLBLADDER AND CYSTIC PEDICLE (FIGS 12.5A TO D)

A grasper is used through the right lower 5 mm trocar to grasp the gallbladder fundus and retract it up over the liver edge to expose the entire length of the gallbladder. If there are adhesions to the gallbladder they will need to be taken down using blunt and sharp dissection. With the entire gallbladder visualized, a second grasper is inserted through the other right upper quadrant trocar to grasp the gallbladder infundibulum and retract it up and to the right to expose the triangle of Calot.

Careful evaluation of the anatomy reveals whether it is partially intrahepatic, on a mesentery, or possesses a Phrygian cap or any other odd shape. Hartmann's pouch should be identified and seen to be funnel down to continue as tubular structure, the cystic duct. It is important to identify Hartmann's pouch clearly because most of the laparoscopic surgeons clip, and divide the cystic duct, high on its termination at Hartmann's pouch, rather than attempting to trace the cystic duct's junction with the common bile duct. Dissection of the

Section Two

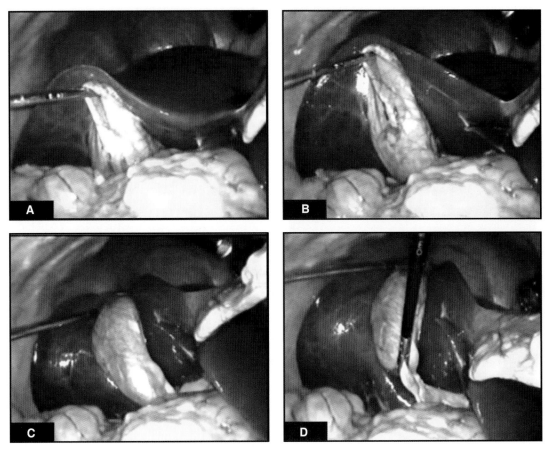

Figs 12.5A to D: Proper traction for exposure of cystic pedicle

junction of cystic duct with the CBD increases the chance of traction injury and bleeding from small vessels and lymphatic.

Cystic artery can be seen if attention is given as it runs along the surface of gallbladder. A lymph node may be seen anterior to the cystic artery. The cystic artery gives off a small artery that supplies the cystic duct. This tiny twig often avulsed and bleeds at the time of crating window between artery and duct. This bleeding stops when the cystic duct is clipped.

ADHESIOLYSIS (FIGS 12.6A TO D)

Any adhesion should be cleared from the gallbladder. The surgeon uses a dissector through the epigastric trocar to tear the peritoneal attachments from the infundibulum. The attachments are taken down from high on the gallbladder, beginning laterally in order to help avoid injury to the common bile duct. Sharp dissection may be carried out with the help of scissors

attached with monopolar current. At the time of separating adhesion, surgeon should try to be as near as possible towards gallbladder. The cystic pedicle is a triangular fold of peritoneum containing the cystic duct and artery, the cystic node and a variable amount of fat. It has a superior and an inferior leaf which are continuous over the anterior edge formed by the cystic duct (Fig. 12.7). An important consideration is the frequent anomalies of the structures contained between the two leaves (15 -20%). The normal configuration is for an anterior cystic duct with the cystic artery situated posterosuperiorly and arising from the right hepatic artery usually behind the common bile duct.

DISSECTION OF CYSTIC PEDICLE (FIGS 12.8A TO D)

The dissection of the cystic pedicle can be carried out with two handed technique. The dissection should be started with anteromedial traction by left hand grasper

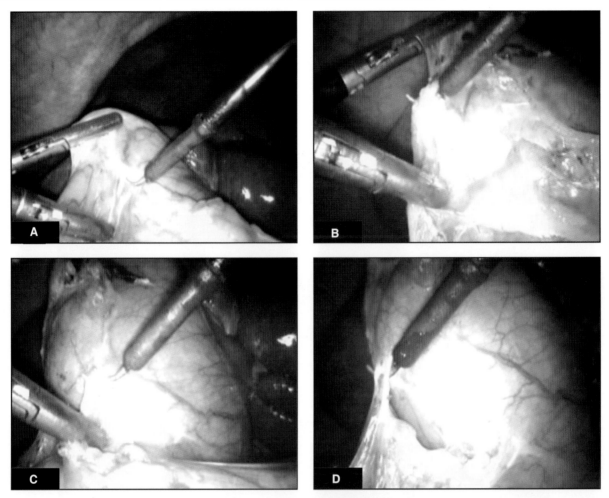

Figs 12.6A to D: Clearing adhesions by hook

placed on the anterior edge of Hartmann's pouch. The antero-medial traction by left hand will expose the posterior peritoneum. The peritoneum of the posterior leaf of the cystic pedicle is divided superficially as far back as the liver. Posterior leaf is better to dissect before anterior leaf because it is relatively less vascular and the bleeding if any, will not soil the anterior peritoneum, whereas if anterior peritoneum is tackled first, it may make the dissection area of posterior peritoneum filled with blood making dissection of this area difficult. Once the visceral peritoneum is dissected, a pledget mounted securely in a pledget holder is used for blunt dissection.

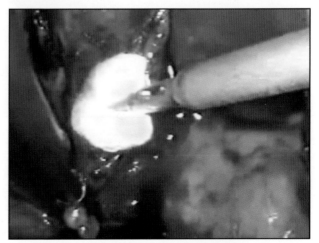

Fig. 12.7: Pledget can be used for adhesiolysis

Separation of Cystic Duct from Artery (Figs 12.9A to D)

Once the cystic duct is visualized the, dissector can be used to create a window in the triangle of Calot between the cystic duct and cystic artery. This window should be created high near the gallbladder-cystic duct junction to avoid injury to the common duct.

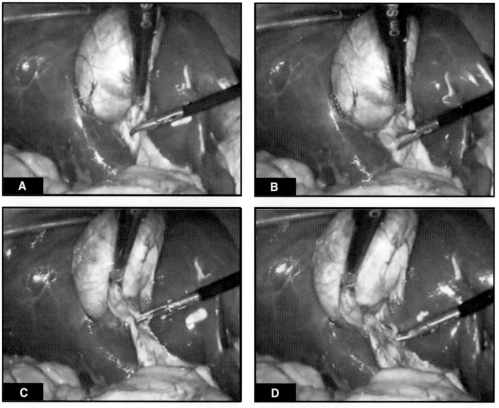

Figs 12.8A to D: Dissection of cystic pedicle

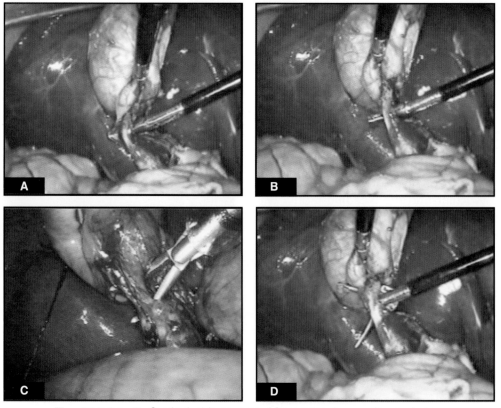

Figs 12.9 A to D: Cystic duct is separated from artery by creating a window

The separation of the cystic duct anteriorly from the cystic artery behind can be performed by a Maryland's grasper by gently opening the jaw of Maryland between the duct and artery. The opening of the jaw of Maryland dissector should be in the line of duct never at right angle to avoid injury of artery behind. Sufficient length of the cystic duct and artery on the gallbladder side should be mobilized so that three clips can be applied.

The electrosurgical hook may be inserted into the window and hooked around the cystic duct. With an up and down movement the hook is used to clear as much tissue as possible from the duct nearer to the cystic duct-gallbladder junction. Tissue that is not dissected free from the duct is retracted by the hook away from all structures and is divided using active cutting current. Depending on the length of the duct it is usually not necessary to dissect it all the way down to its junction with the common bile duct. In a similar fashion, the hook can be used to isolate the cystic artery for a length that is adequate enough to clip it.

Clipping and Division of Cystic Duct (Figs 12.10A to H)

After isolating the cystic duct and artery the clipper is introduced through the epigastric port and at least two clips are placed on the proximal side of the cystic duct. Care is taken not to place the clips too low because retraction can tent up the common bile duct or cause it to be obstructed. Another clip is placed on the gallbladder side of the cystic duct, leaving enough distance between the clips to divide it. In a similar fashion, clips are placed on the cystic artery, two proximally and one on the gallbladder side of the artery. The laparoscopic scissors are then used through the epigastric port to divide the cystic duct and artery between the clips. Both the jaw of clip applicator should be under vision.

Clipping and Division of Cystic Artery (Figs 12.11A to F)

The cystic artery is clipped and then divided by scissors. Two clips are placed proximally on the cystic artery and one clip is applied distally. The artery is then grasped with a duckbill grasper on the gallbladder wall and then divided between second and third clip.

Operative Cholangiogram (Fig. 12.12)

In many institutions routine intraoperative cholangiogram is performed. Routine cholangiogram decreases the risk of CBD injury in case of difficult anatomy. If a cholangiogram is to be performed the cystic duct is isolated and occluded with a clip which is placed high on the duct at its junction with the gallbladder. This will avoid leakage of contents from the gallbladder when the duct is opened. The scissors are used to incise the duct.

The opening in the cystic duct is made on the antero-superior aspect. Correct alignment of the cystic duct and infusion of saline facilitates insertion of ureteric catheter to perform cholangiography. Insertion is difficult if the opening in the cystic duct is made too close to the gallbladder. The dissector is used to spread the incision to adequately dilate it for introduction of the cholangiogram catheter. The catheter is introduced through one of the 5 mm port. It is secured by either inflating a balloon or placing a clip to hold it in place. The catheter is then flushed with saline to insure appropriate placement. All instruments are removed and a dynamic cholangiogram with real time fluoroscopy is performed. The contrast medium should be injected slowly during screening and the patient should be in a slight Trendelenburg's position with the table rotated slightly to the right. It is essential that the entire biliary tract is outlined.

When the cholangiogram is completed the catheter is removed, and two clips are placed proximally on the duct. The duct is then divided. Surgeon should ligate or clip cystic duct when he is sure up to the point of absolute certainness.

The main advantages of intraoperative cholangiography during cholecystectomy are:
- Detection of common bile duct stone
- Reduction of the incidence of residual common bile duct stone
- Delineation of the biliary anatomical variations at risk for bile duct injury.

Intraoperative cholangiogram is a highly sensitive tool for detecting choledocholithiasis, with an overall accuracy of 95 percent. Routine intraoperative cholangiography can diagnose unsuspected common bile duct stone in 1 to 14 percent (average 5%) of patients without indications for ductal exploration.

Section Two

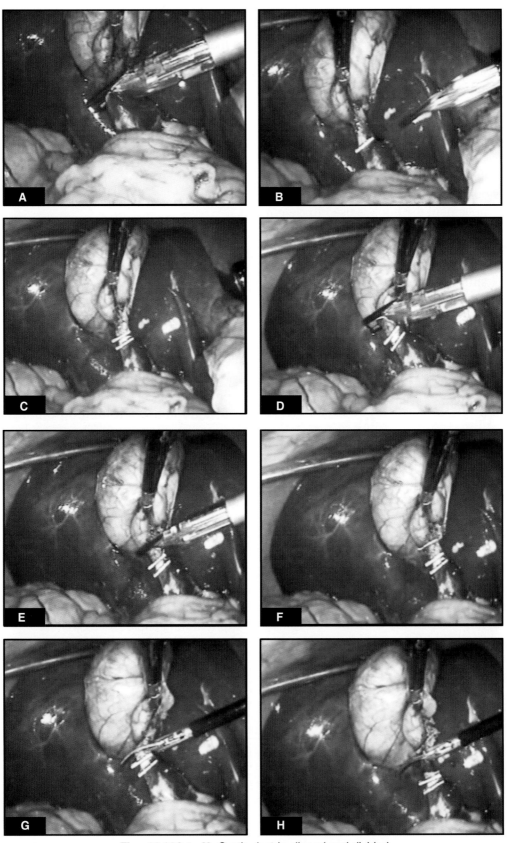

Figs 12.10A to H: Cystic duct is clipped and divided

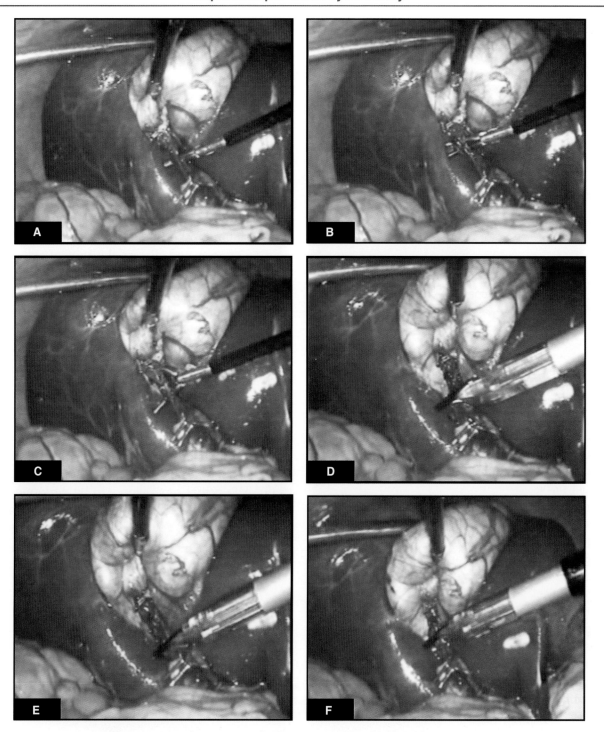

Figs 12.11A to F: Cystic artery is clipped and divided

The failure of laparoscopic intraoperative cholangiogram is due to:
- The narrowness of the cystic duct
- Cystic duct rupture
- Obstructive cystic valves
- Impacted cystic stones
- Dye extravasation from cystic duct perforation.

With increased experience successful laparoscopic intraoperative cholangiogram can be achieved in 90-99 percent of cases, a rate similar to that of

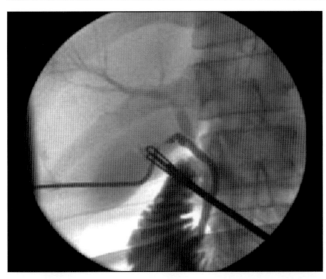

Fig. 12.12: Intraoperative cholangiogram

intraoperative Cholangiogram during open cholecystectomy.

INTRAOPERATIVE ULTRASONOGRAPHY

Many studies focused on the role of intraoperative ultrasonography in laparoscopic cholecystectomy. Intraoperative ultrasonography is technically demanding but is as accurate as intraoperative cholangiogram (88 to 100%) for screening common bile duct stone.

The advantages of intraoperative ultrasonography over intraoperative cholangiogram are:
• Speedy
• Safer
• Multiple time use
• Economical.

The greater sensitivity of intraoperative ultrasonography examination concerned mainly small stones or debris in the CBD.

The disadvantages of intraoperative ultrasonography is that it is impossible to provide extended views of the intrahepatic and extrahepatic biliary tree, difficult to show passage of contrast into the duodenum and to identify bile duct injuries.

Ligation of Cystic Duct

Although the majority of surgeons opt for clipping the cystic duct, before dividing it, this technique though quick, is intrinsically unsound, as internalization of the metal clip inside the common bile duct over the ensuing

months is well documented. There is report of internalization of clip and subsequent stone formation after many years. The internalized clip becomes covered with calcium bilirubinate pigment. For this reason, to tie the cystic duct using a catgut Roeder external slip knot should be done.

Dissection of Gallbladder from Liver Bed (Fig. 12.13)

The electrosurgical hook is used with cautery through the epigastric port to dissect the gallbladder bed of the liver. Using a grasper the gallbladder is first retracted right to expose and dissect the medial side of the attachment. The gallbladder is then retracted to the left and the lateral side is dissected. Using this back and forth action. The hook is used to dissect the gallbladder off the bed from inferior to superior until it is 90 percent removed from the liver. Holding the remaining portion of the gallbladder attached to the liver, the dissection bed and the clipped structures are evaluated and any active bleeding is stopped using heal of the hook or spatula.

Gallbladder should be separated from the liver through the areolar tissue plane binding the gallbladder to the Glisson's capsule lining the liver bed (Figs 12.14A to G). The actual separation can be performed with scissors with electrosurgical attachment or electrosurgical hook knife. Pledget can be used to

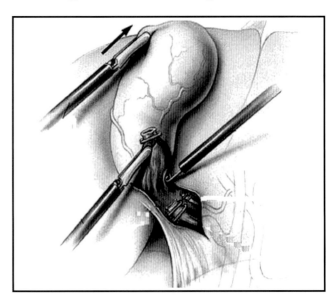

Fig. 12.13: Separation of gallbladder from GB bed

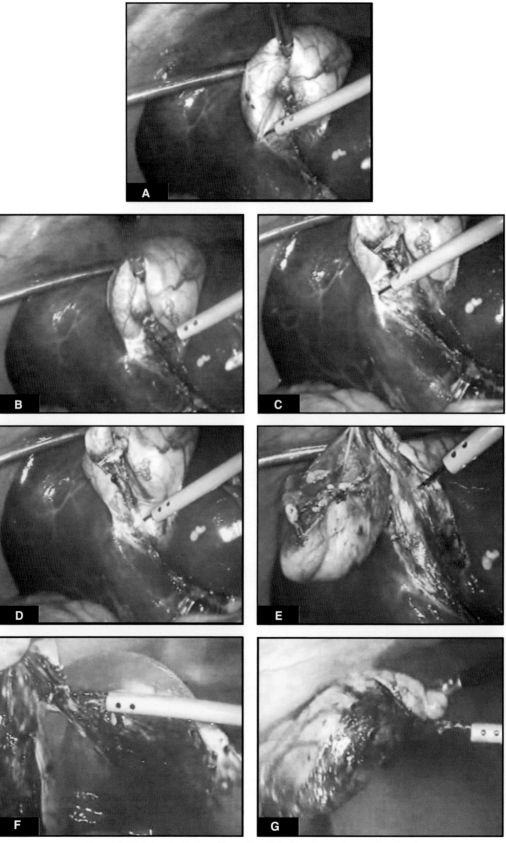

Figs 12.14A to G: Separation of gallbladder from liver using hook

remove the gallbladder from liver bed once a good plane of dissection is found. Perforation of the gallbladder during its separation is a common complication which is encountered in 15 percent of cases.

One should be careful at the time of dissection and if there is spillage of stone each stone should be removed from the peritoneal cavity to avoid abscess formation in future.

Extraction of Gallbladder (Figs 12.15A to D)

The gallbladder is now freed from the liver and placed on top of the liver. The patient is returned to the supine position and the area of dissection and the upper right quadrant are irrigated and suctioned until clear. The gallbladder is extracted through the 11 mm epigastric operating port with the help of gallbladder extractor.

Many surgeons use umbilical port for withdrawal of gallbladder. If gallbladder is removed through the umbilical port the laparoscope is placed through the epigastric port and the gallbladder is visualized on the dome of the liver. A large grasper with teeth is placed through the umbilical port and used to grasp the gallbladder along the edge of the clipped cystic duct stump. The gallbladder is then exteriorized through the umbilical incision where it is held into position with a clamp (Fig. 12.17).

First the neck of the gallbladder should be engaged in the cannula and then cannula will withdraw together with neck of gallbladder held within the jaw of gallbladder extractor (Fig. 12.16).

Once the port with the neck of the gallbladder is out, the neck is grasped with the help of a blunt hemostat and it should be pulled out with screwing.

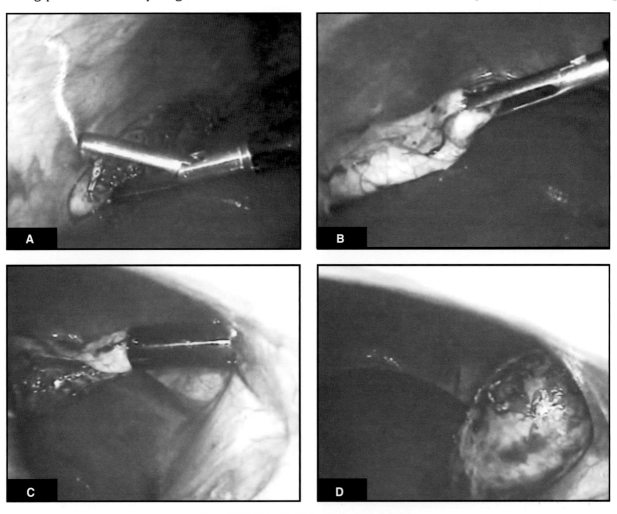

Figs 12.15A to D: Extraction of gallbladder

Section Two

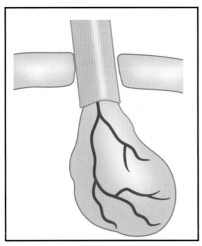

Fig. 12.16: Extraction of gallbladder by hiding the neck in cannula

If gallbladder is of small size, it will come without much difficulty, otherwise small incision should be given over the neck of the gallbladder and suction irrigation instrument should be used to suck all the bile to facilitate easy withdrawal (Figs 12.18 and 12.19).

Sometimes big stones will not allow easy passage of gallbladder and in these situation ovum forceps should be inserted inside the lumen of gallbladder through the incision of its neck and all the stone should be crushed (Fig. 12.20).

When ovum forceps is used to remove the big stones from the gallbladder, care should be taken that gallbladder should be held loose to have room for forceps otherwise it will perforate and all the stone may spill out (Figs 12.21A and B).

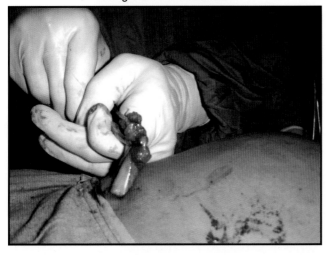

Fig. 12.17: Extraction of gallbladder by gentle pull from outside

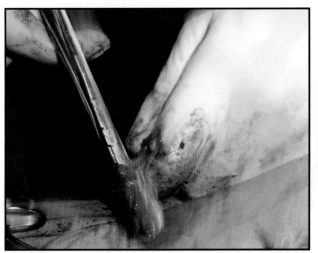

Fig. 12.19: Stone should be taken out to reduce volume of gallbladder

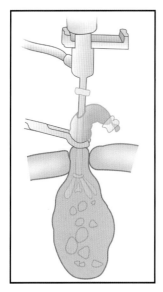

Fig. 12.18: Suction of bile to extract gallbladder

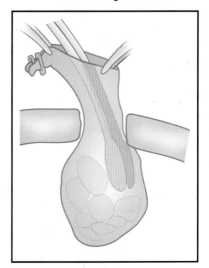

Fig. 12.20: Stone may be crushed to reduce volume of gallbladder

Section Two

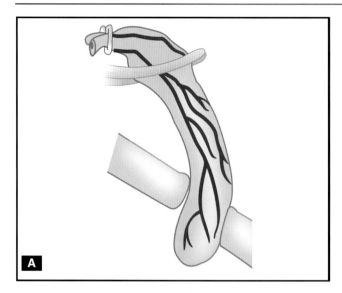

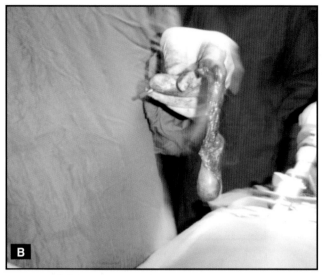

Figs 12.21A and B: Once the gallbladder is empty gentle pull from outside will facilitate its extraction

Extraction inside a bag is recommended as a safeguard against stone loss and contamination of the exit wound (Figs 12.22 and 12.23).

Three Port Cholecystectomy

Since the first laparoscopic cholecystectomy was performed, it has met with widespread acceptance as a standard procedure using four trocars. The fourth (lateral) trocar is used to grasp the fundus of the gallbladder so as to expose Calot's triangle. It has been argued that the fourth trocar is not necessary in most cases. The three-port technique is as safe as the standard four-port. The main advantages of the three-port technique are that it causes less pain, is less expensive, and leaves fewer scars. The three port cholecystectomy should be performed by experienced laparoscopic surgeon because left hand movement is very important in this surgery. Bimanual skill and correct interpretation of anatomy is must before proceeding for this technique. Three ports cholecystectomy is possible by the experienced laparoscopic surgeons.

Ending of the Operation

The instrument and then ports are removed. Telescope should be removed leaving gas valve of umbilical port open to let out all the gas. At the time of removing umbilical port, telescope should be again inserted and umbilical port should be removed over the telescope

to prevent any entrapment of omentum. The wound is then closed with suture. Vicryl should be used for rectus and unabsorbable intradermal or stapler for skin. A single suture is used to close the umbilicus and upper midline fascial opening. Many laparoscopic surgeons routinely leave this fascial defect without ill defect. Some surgeon likes to inject local anesthetic agent over port site to avoid post operative pain. Sterile dressing over the wound should be applied.

Laparoscopic Cholecystectomy in Acute Cholecystitis

Impaction of a stone in the cystic duct will result in bile stasis in the gallbladder. Acute cholecystitis results from inflammation of the mucosa of the gallbladder which may secondarily become infected. This inflammation can then evolve to hydrops of the gallbladder and gallbladder abscess. Complications such as necrosis, perforation, phlegmon or peritonitis can result if surgical intervention is not done in timely manner.

In certain cases, acute cholecystitis can be acalculous, especially in diabetic patients or in the immediate postoperative period following other surgical interventions. In the elective setting, a laparoscopic cholecystectomy has become the standard of care; the laparoscopic approach to acute cholecystitis remains controversial. In past publications, acute cholecystitis was considered as a relative or absolute contraindication to a laparoscopic approach. The

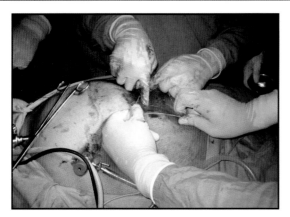

Fig. 12.22: The spilled stone and torn gallbladder can be taken out with the help of endobag

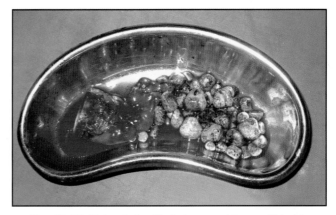

Fig. 12.23: Extracted spilled stone and torn gallbladder

laparoscopic approach to acute cholecystitis is preferred in practice by a large number of experienced teams. Nowadays, laparoscopic approach is considered safe if the intervention is performed in a timely fashion. If laparoscopy is considered in acute attack a conversion rate of 20 percent demonstrates that the procedure is only pursued when felt to be safe.

- Acute cholecystitis is distinguished from biliary colic by the presence of at least 2 of the following signs
    (a) Right upper quadrant pain lasting for more than 24 hours
    (b) Fever more than 37°C
- The presence of a palpable distended tender gallbladder
- Elevation of the WBC count greater than 11.000/mm^3
- Ultrasonographic findings demonstrating thickening of the gallbladder wall >4 mm
- Pericholecystic fluid collection in ultrasound.

The studies have concluded that the ideal time for the surgical intervention is within 48 to 72 hours of the appearance of symptoms.

Laparoscopic cholecystectomy, when performed early, leads to reduction in:
- Operative difficulty
- Conversion rate
- Operative time

One of the major determining factors is the conversion rate, an indicator of the actual difficulty of the procedure. Numerous studies have demonstrated a significantly lower conversion rate when the laparoscopic cholecystectomy is performed within the first 72 hours of the onset of symptoms as opposed to

a delayed procedure after this period. In case of an interval cholecystectomy following medical therapy, it must be performed within a period of 8 to 12 weeks. It is demonstrated that interval cholecystectomy is associated with a higher morbidity rate than in early intervention.

Laparoscopic Cholecystectomy During Pregnancy

Laparoscopic cholecystectomy is relatively contraindicated during pregnancy due to the potentially adverse side effects on the fetus. However, when complications arise, a surgical intervention becomes mandatory. This intervention should be ideally performed during the second trimester of pregnancy where the operative risks are considered to be the lowest. Laparoscopic cholecystectomy during pregnancy has been reported in many series of randomized controlled trials, with no specific complications related to the laparoscopic approach.

Postoperative Care

Most of the patients can be discharged next day of surgery. The patient who has urinary retention, prolonged nausea, more pain or difficulty in walking can be discharged after bowel sound. Threedose broad spectrum antibiotic should be administered. First dose infused 1 hour before surgery, second and third should be administered on consecutive days. Few patients may complain pain over tip of shoulder after laparoscopic surgery. This is due to irritation of diaphragm from CO_2. Tramadol hydrochloride is advised in these patients. Most of the patients are able to resume there

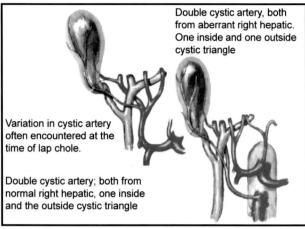

Fig. 12.24A

normal day-to-day activity within 48 to 72 hour after surgery. Generally the patient can return to their sedentary work within a week. The variation in cystic artery and hepatic duct shown in Figures 12.24A to D.

COMPLICATIONS OF LAPAROSCOPIC CHOLECYSTECTOMY

Early Complication

- Common bile duct injury
- Bile leak
- Injury to viscera
- Hemorrhage
- Retained stones and abscess formation.

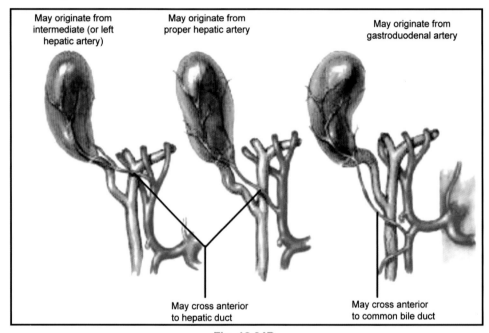

Fig. 12.24B

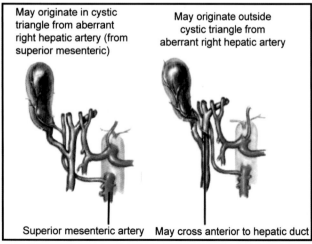

Fig. 12.24C

Late Complication

- Biliary strictures
- Cystic duct clip stones.

LAP CHOLE AND CBD INJURY

Incidence of iatrogenic CBD injury is 0.12 and 0.55 percent during open and laparoscopic cholecystectomy respectively.

Common Cause of CBD Injury

- Misinterpretation of anatomy-70 percent
- Technical errors

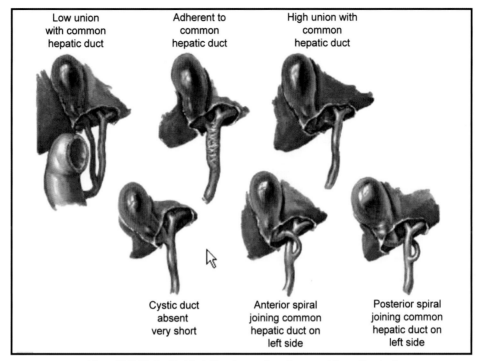

Low union
with common
hepatic duct

Adherent to
common
hepatic duct

High union with
common
hepatic duct

Cystic duct
absent
very short

Anterior spiral
joining common
hepatic duct on
left side

Posterior spiral
joining common
hepatic duct on
left side

Figs 12.24A to D: Variation in cystic artery and hepatic duct

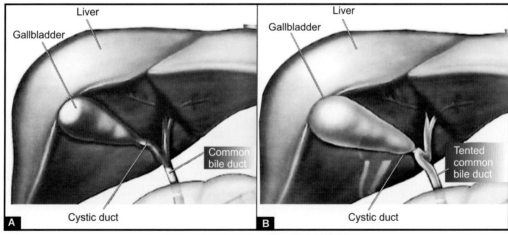

Figs 12.25A and B: Testing of CBD

- Risk factors
- Surgeon operates on image rather than reality.

Visual psychological studies has shown that laparoscopic surgeon works on snap interpretation by brain and success or disaster depends on whether snaps are right or wrong. Snap interpretation will be wrong if there is eye ball degradation. Surgeon should not dissect the cystic duct if there is lack of initial identification and memory of key structure to the point of absolute certainty (Figs 12.25A and B). Most important technical error is hilar bleeding and frantic attempts are made to control bleeding by electrosurgery. This frantic attack can catch the CBD and will be injured.

In case of bleeding surgeon should first apply pressure and if it does not stop he should take suction irrigation and atraumatic grasper to find out exact point of bleeding. Electrosurgery should be used only when bleeding point is identified.

TYPE OF CBD INJURY

Bismuth Classification

- Type 1 – CHD stump > 2 cm
- Type 2 – CHD stump < 2 cm
- Type 3 – Hilar, right and left duct confluence intact
- Type 4 – Hilar, separation of right and left ducts
- Type 5 – Injury to aberrant right duct ± CBD injury.

If complication of CBD injury is recognized intraoperatively reconstructive surgery should be performed same time if surgeon has sufficient experience. For high complete transaction Roux-en-Y hepaticojejunostomy is preferred. For lower complete injuries primary suture repair over T tube is better but long end of T tube must not be exteriorized from same site. For partial injuries insertion of T tube and Roux-en-Y serosal patch should be thought.

Strategy to Handle Complication Recognized Postoperatively

- USG + ERCP + MRCP
- Fluid + electrolyte + systemic antibiotic
- Conservative treatment and biliary drainage for 6 weeks by ERCP stent insertion or
- PTBD (Percutaneous transhepatic biliary drainage) if endoscopic stent application is not possible
- After several weeks: Reconstructive surgery
- Roux-en-Y choledocoduodenostomy or hepatojejunostomy.

All the variation of cystic duct and artery should be memorized to avoid inadvertent injury of CBD.

HOW TO AVOID INJURY

- Try to memorize initial anatomy of Calot's triangle
- A large distended gallbladder should be aspirated and lifted rather than grasped
- Anterolateral traction is better than fundus pull to avoid tenting of CBD
- Avoid meticulous dissection by energized instrument
- Better to do skeletonization through pledget
- During detachment of gallbladder from liver bed maintain plane of adipose tissue
- Use suction irrigation frequently.

Tenting of the CBD should always kept in mind at the time of dissection to avoid injury.

BIBLIOGRAPHY

1. Airan M, Appel M, Berci G, Coburg AJ, et al. Retrospective and prospective multi-institutional laparoscopic cholecystectomy study by the Society of American Gastrointestinal Endoscopic Surgeons. Surg Endosc 1992; 6: 169-76.
2. Barkum AN, Barkun JS, Fried GM, Ghitulescu G, Steinmetz O, Pham C, et al. Useful predictors of bile duct stones in patients undergoing laparoscopic cholecystectomy. Ann Surg 1994; 220: 32-9.
3. Bartlett DL, Fong Y, Fortner JG, et al: Long-term results after resection for gallbladder cancer: Implications for staging and management. Ann Surg 1996;224:639- 46.
4. Berci G, Morgenstern L Laparoscopic management of common bile duct stones. Surg Endosc 1994; 8: 1168-75.
5. Berrevoet E, Biglari M, Sinove Y, De Baardemaeker L, Troisi R, de Hemptinne B. Outpatient laparoscopic cholecystectomy in Belgium: what are we waiting for? Acta Chir Belg 2006;106: 537–40 [PMID: 17168265].
6. Branum G, Schmitt C, Baillie J, Suhoclri P, Baker M, Davidoff A, et al. Management of major biliary complications after laparoscopic cholecystectomy. Ann Surg 1993; 217: 532-41.
7. Calik A, Topaloglu S, Topcu S, Turkyilmaz S, Kucuktulu U, Piskin B. Routine intraoperative aspiration of gallbladder during laparoscopic cholecystectomy. Surg Endosc 2007;7:[Epub ahead of print] [PMID: 17285368].
8. Callagham J. Twenty-five years of gallbladder surgery in a small rural hospital. Am J Surg 1995; 169: 313-5.
9. Champault A, Vons C, Dagher I, Amerlinck S, Franco D. Low-cost laparoscopic cholecystectomy. Br J Surg 2002;89: 1602–7 [PMID: 12445073].
10. Chijiiwa K, Nakano K, Ueda J, et al: Surgical treatment of patients with T2 gallbladder carcinoma invading the subserosal layer. J Am Coll Surg 2001;192:600-7.
11. Clavies PA, Sanabria JR, Strasberg SM. Proposed classification of complications of surgery with examples of utility in cholecystectomy. Surgery 1992; 111: 518-6.
12. Cleary SP, Dawson LA, Knox JJ, et al: Cancer of the gallbladder and extrahepatic bile ducts. Curr Probl Surg 2007;44:396-482.
13. Coburn NG, Cleary SP, Tan JCC, et al: Surgery for gallbladder cancer: A population-based analysis. J Am Coll Surg 2008;207:371-82.
14. Cullen DJ, Apolone G, Greenfiled S, Guadagnoli E, Cleary P. ASA physical status and age predict morbidity after three surgical procedures. Ann Surg 1994; 220: 3-9.
15. Davies MG, O'Broin E, Mannion C, McGinley J, Gupta S, Shine MF, Lennon F. Audit of open cholecystectomy in a district general hospital. Br J Surg 1992; 79: 314-6.
16. de Aretxabala XA, Roa IS, Burgos LA, et al: Curative resection in potentially resectable tumours of the gallbladder. Eur J Surg 163:419-426, 1997 33. Fong Y, Heffernan N, Blumgart LH: Gallbladder carcinoma discovered during laparoscopic cholecystectomy: Aggressive reresection is beneficial. Cancer 1998;83:423-7.

17. Deziel DJ, Millikan KW, Economou SG, Doolas A, Ko ST, Airan MC. Complications of laparoscopic cholecystectomy: a national survey of 4292 hospitals and an analysis of 77,604 cases. Am J Surg 1993;165:9–14 [PMID: 8418705].

18. Deziel DJ, Millikan WK, Economou SG, Doolas A, Kb ST, Airan MC. Complications of laparoscopic cholecystectomy of 4,292 hospitals and an analysis of 77,604 cases. Am J Surg 1993;165:9-14.

19. Deziel DJ. Complications of cholecystectomy. Surg Clin N Am 1994;74: 809-23.

20. Dixon E, Vollmer CM Jr, Sahajpal A, et al: An aggressive surgical approach leads to improved survival in patients with gallbladder cancer: A 12-year study at a North American Center. Ann Surg 2005;241:385-94.

21. Driessen PJHA, Pradhan GN. Laparoscopic cholecystectomy in a small rural hospital. CJRM 2000;5:70–3.

22. Escarce JJ, Shea JA, Chen W, Qian Z, Schwartz JS. Outcomes of open cholecystectomy in the elderly: a longitudinal analysis of 21,000 cases in the prelaparoscopic era. Surgery 1995; 117: 156-64.

23. Fried GM, Clas D, Meakins JL. Minimally invasive surgery in the elderly patient. Surg din N Am 1994; 74: 375-87.

24. Galandiuk S, Mahid SS, Polk Jr HC, Turina M, Rao M, Lewis JN. Differences and similarities between rural and urban operations. Surgery 2006;140:589–96 [PMID: 17011906].

25. Ganey JB, Johnson PA Jr, Prillaman PE, McSwain GR. Cholecystectomy: clinical experience with a large series. Am J Surg 1986; 151: 352-7.

26. Gilliland TM, Traverso LW. Modern standards for comparison of cholecystectomy with alternative treatments for symptomatic cholelithiasis with emphasis on long term relief of symptoms. Surg Gynecol Obst 1990; 170: 39- 44.

27. Gupta A, Agarwal PN, Kant R, Malik V. Evaluation of fundusfirst laparoscopic cholecystectomy. JSLS 2004;8:255–8 [PMID: 15347114].

28. Hainsworth PJ, Rhodes M, Gompertz RHK, Armstrong CP, Lennard TWJ. Imaging of the common bile duct in patients undergoing laparoscopic cholecystectomy. Gut 1994; 35: 991-5.

29. Haynes JH, Guha SC, Taylor SG. Laparoscopic cholecystectomy in a rural family practice: The Vivian, LA, experience. J Fam Pract 2004;53:205–8 [PMID: 15000926].

30. Herzog U, Messmer R, Sutter M, Tondeffi R. Surgical treatment for cholelithiasis. Surg Gynecol Obstet 1992; 175: 238-42.

31. Jatzko GR, Lisborg PH, Pert! AM, Stettner HM. Multivariate comparison of complications after laparoscopic cholecystectomy and open cholecystectomy. Ann Surg 1995; 221: 381-6.

32. Kondo S, Nimura Y, Hayakawa N, et al: Extensive surgery for carcinoma of the gallbladder. Br J Surg 89:179-184, 2002.

33. Kumar TS, Saklani AP, Vinayagam R, Blackett RL. Spilled gall stones during laparoscopic cholecystectomy: a review of literature. Postgraduate Med J 2004;80:77–9 .

34. Leeder PC, Matthews T, Krzeminska K, Dehn TC. Routine day-case laparoscopic cholecystectomy. Br J Surg 2004;91: 312–6 [PMID: 14991631].

35. Macintyre IMC, Wilson RG. Laparoscopic cholecystectomy. BrJ Surg 1993; 80: 552-9.

36. Mayol J, Alvarez Femandez-Represa J. Imaging of the common bile duct [Letter]. Gut 1994; 35: 1773.

37. Mayol J, Tamayo FJ, Ortiz-Oshiro E, Ortega Lopez D, Vincent Hamelin E, Alvarez Femandez-Represa J. Resultados de la colecistectomia laparoscopica en pacientes ancianos. Or Esp 1995; 55; 45-7.

38. Mayol J, Vincent E, Martinez-Sarmiento J, Ortiz Oshiro E, Diaz Gonzalez J, Tamayo FJ, et al. Pulmonary embolism following laparoscopic cholecystectomy. Surg Endosc 1994; 8: 214-7.

39. McSherry CK, Glenn F. The incidence and causes of death following surgery for non-malignant biliary tract disease. Ann Surgl 980; 191:271-5.

40. McSherry CK. Laparoscopic management of common bile duct stone [Editorial]. Surg Endosc 1994; 8: 1161-2.

41. Mrozowicz A, Polkowski W. Initial three years' experience with laparoscopic cholecystectomy in a district hospital: evaluation of early results and operative measures. Ann Univ Mariae Curie Sklodowska [Med] 2004;59:26–31 [PMID: 16146044].

42. Muhe E. Die erste Cholezystektomie durch das Laparoskop. Langeb Arch Klin Chir 1986; 369: 804.

43. Nakamura S, Sakaguchi S, Suzuki S, et al: Aggressive surgery for carcinoma of the gallbladder. Surgery 1989;106: 467-73.

44. Nakeeb A, Tran KQ, Black MJ, et al: Improved survival in resected biliary malignancies. Surgery 2002;132:555-63.

45. Nimura Y, Hayakawa N, Kamiya J, et al: Hepato-pancreatoduodenectomy for advanced carcinoma of the biliary tract. Hepatogastroenterology 1991;38:170-5.

46. Parkar RB, Thagana NG, Baraza R, Otieno D. Experience with laparoscopic surgery at the Aga Khan Hospital, Nairobi. East Afr Med J 2003;80:44–50 [PMID: 12755241].

47. Patel SC, Bhatt JR. Laparoscopic cholecystectomy at the Aga Khan Hospital, Nairobi. East Afr Med J 2000;77:194–8 [PMID: 12858902].

48. Reddick EJ, Olsen DO. Laparoscopic laser cholecystectomy. Surg Endosc 1989; 3: 131-3.

49. Shirai Y, Yoshida K, Tsukada K, et al: Inapparent carcinoma of the gallbladder. An appraisal of a radical second operation after simple cholecystectomy. Ann Surg 1992;215:326-31.

50. Smith N, Max MH. Gallbladder surgery in patients over 60: Is there an increased risk? South Med J 1987; 80: 472-4.

51. Southern Surgeons group. A prospective analysis of 1518 laparoscopic cholecystectomies. N Engl J Med N 1991; 324: 1073-8.

52. Tan JT, Suyapto DR, Neo EL, Leong PS. Prospective audit of laparoscopic cholecystectomy experience at a secondary referral centre in south Australia. ANZ J Surg 2006;76:335–8 [PMID: 16768693].

53. Taylor OM, Sedman PC, Jones BM, Royston CM, Arulampalam T, Wellwood J. Laparoscopic cholecystectomy without operative cholangiogram: 2038 cases over 5-year period in two district general hospitals. Ann R Coll Surg Engl 1997;79:376–80 [PMID: 9326132].

Section Two

54. Todoroki T, Kawamoto T, Takahashi H, et al: Treatment of gallbladder cancer by radical resection. Br J Surg 1999;86:622-7.

55. Vagenas K, Karamanakos SN, Spyropoulos C, Panagiotopoulos S, Karanikolas M, Stavropoulos M. Laparoscopic cholecystectomy: a report from a single center. World J Gastroenterol 2006;12:3887–90 [PMID: 16804976].

56. Voyles CR, Sanders DL, Hogan R. Common bile duct evaluation in the era of laparoscopic cholecystectomy. 1050 cases later. Ann Surg 1994; 219: 744-52.

57. Wakai T, Shirai Y, Hatakeyama K: Radical second resection provides survival benefit for patients with T2 gallbladder carcinoma first discovered after laparoscopic cholecystectomy. World J Surg 2002;26:867-71.

58. Wang SJ, Fuller CD, Kim JS, et al: Prediction model for estimating the survival benefit of adjuvant radiotherapy for gallbladder cancer. J Clin Oncol 2008;26:2112-7.

59. Wherry DC, Marohn MR, Malanoski MP, Hetz SP, Rich NM. An external audit of laparoscopic cholecystectomy in the steady Articles Tropical Doctor October 2008;38 215 state performed in medical treatment facilities of the Department of Defense. Ann Surg 1996;224:145–54 [PMID: 8757377].

60. Williams Jr LF, Chapman WC, Bonau RA, McGee Jr EC, Boyd RW, Jacobs JK. Comparison of laparoscopic cholecystectomy with open cholecystectomy in a single center. Am J Surg 993;165:459–65 [PMID: 8480882]

61. Wittgen CM, Andrus JP, Andrus CH, Kaminski DL. Cholecystectomy. Which procedure is best for the high-risk patient? Surg Endosc 1993;7:395–9 [PMID: 8211615].

62. Yamaguchi K, Chijiiwa K, Shimizu S, et al: Anatomical limit of extended cholecystectomy for gallbladder carcinoma involving the neck of the gallbladder. Int Surg 1998;83:21-23.

63. Yamashita Y, Kurohiji T, Kakegawa T. Evaluation of two training programs for laparoscopic cholecystectomy: incidence of major complications. World J Surg 1994;18: 279-85.

Section Two

Laparoscopic CBD Exploration

Laparoscopic exploration of the common bile duct is performed either for the diagnosis or the treatment of common bile duct (CBD) stones. CBD stones demonstrated by laparoscopic intraoperative cholangiography, or laparoscopic ultrasonography are extracted either through the cystic duct or through choledochotomy. An alternative for the treatment of CBD stones is to perform an endoscopic sphincterotomy either before, during or after laparoscopic cholecystectomy.

The main advantages of intraoperative cholangiography during cholecystectomy are:

• Detection of common bile duct stone
• Reduction of the incidence of residual common bile duct stone
• Delineation of the biliary anatomical variations at risk for bile duct injury.

Intraoperative cholangiogram is a highly sensitive tool for detecting choledocholithiasis, with an overall accuracy of 95 percent. Routine intraoperative cholangiography can diagnose unsuspected common bile duct stone in 1 to 14 percent (average 5%) of patients without indications for ductal exploration.

INTRAOPERATIVE CHOLANGIOGRAPHY (IOC)

Techniques of Cholangiography

Cholangiograms obtained during laparoscopy are usually performed after catheterization of the cystic duct through a cholangioclamp (Storz Endoscopy, USA), or inserting a catheter through a hollow gasketed needle pinned through the abdominal wall along the right subcostal margin. Difficulties in catheterization of the small cystic duct have led to consider cholecysto-cholangiography by direct puncture of the gallbladder as an alternative to cystic duct cholangiography. Cystic duct cholangiography is clearly better than cholecystocholangiography, and fluoroscopic imaging should be the standard for IOC. Until now, no specific clinically significant complications directly attributable to laparoscopic IOC have been reported.

Expected success rates for laparoscopic IOC are in a 90 to 100 percent range. Inability to cannulate a narrow cystic duct is the main cause of failure. When performed after clipping (but not cutting) the anatomical structures identified by careful dissection such as the cystic artery and the cystic duct, a correctly interpreted IOC allows the detection of the most frequently reported cause of CBD injury, i.e. mistaken identification of a narrow main bile duct in place of the cystic duct.

LAPAROSCOPIC ULTRASONOGRAPHY (LUS)

Several studies on LUS have been published and conclusions of these studies favor LUS as compared to IOC. LUS is performed with a higher success rate, in less time, with better specificity, but with less precision with regard to the delineation of biliary tree anatomy. LUS is of little, if any, help in the diagnosis or prevention of bile duct injuries. While detection of smaller stones by LUS should increase its sensitivity, most of these stones are reputed to be flushed out through the sphincter and therefore the question arises if such small stones require any treatment at all. Specificity of LUS is higher (less false positives) than of IOC. When IOC and LUS were combined, there is chance of less than 1 percent of false-positives. The question that comes to mind is whether LUS should be a screening test, and IOC performed only in case of doubt or should IOC be the screening test, and LUS used only when IOC is of doubtful value? IOC performs better than LUS to delineate the entire biliary tree, from the intrahepatic tree to the pancreatic portion of the CBD. Injection of saline into the biliary tree enhanced the images obtained by LUS, especially in the distal portion of the bile duct.

Criteria for Routine Intraoperative Cholangiography

Preoperative Factors

1. Endoscopic retrograde cholangiography +/- sphincterotomy
2. Ultrasonographic findings
3. Common bile duct size (> 6 mm)
4. Choledocholithiasis
5. History of jaundice or pancreatitis
6. Elevated bilirubin, alkaline phosphatase, transaminases.

Intraoperative Factors

1. Unclear anatomy
2. Conversion to open cholecystectomy
3. Dilated cystic duct over 4 mm.

LAPAROSCOPIC EXTRACTION OF COMMON BILE DUCT STONES

Once detected during laparoscopic IOC, laparoscopic extraction of CBD stones is a logical extension of the procedure. Laparoscopic exploration of the CBD can be performed either through the cystic duct or by laparoscopic choledochotomy. A critical evaluation of the retrospective and prospective series on laparoscopic CBD exploration published since 1989 shows that both procedures are feasible and safe. Any comparisons between the two techniques would be fallacious because of their obviously different indications. Nonetheless, whenever feasible, laparoscopic transcystic CBD exploration best fulfills the expectancy of mini-invasive approach. Laparoscopic management of CBD stones is considered as technically difficult and demanding, requiring advanced laparoscopic skills as

well as expensive endoscopic and radiological equipment. Endoscopic sphincterotomy is commonly proposed preoperatively as the alternative to surgery for CBD stones. Endoscopic sphincterotomy is indicated in patients with severe cholangitis for urgent drainage of infected bile, and in patients with retained stones after cholecystectomy. In open conventional surgery, controlled studies have not shown that ES, performed either prior to surgery or in patients with gallbladder *in situ,* was superior to single-step surgical management.

In case of preoperative diagnosis of common bile duct stone, options for management include:

- Preoperative ERCP and endoscopic sphincterotomy followed by laparoscopic cholecystectomy
- Conventional open common bile duct exploration
- Laparoscopic common bile duct exploration.

Today, most of the laparoscopic surgeons prefer the "single-stage" laparoscopic approach to choledocholithiasis. None of the randomized trials published to date concluded superiority of endoscopic treatment alone or associated with surgery as compared to first-line surgical treatment. Immediate postoperative mortality was 2.6 percent in the endoscopic group as opposed to 1 percent in the surgical group. In global analysis, the rate of major and minor complications were respectively 8 and 10 percent after endoscopy followed by surgery, and 8 and 15 percent after surgery alone.

Study of European Association for Endoscopic Surgery (EAES)

	LCBDE	(ERC +/- ES) + LC	p
Patients (N)	133	136	
with CBD (%)	109 (82)	99 (73)	
Failed ERCP +/- ES		23 (17)	
Stone clearance		82/98 (84)	ns
Successful LCBDE (%)	92/109 (84)	12/17 (71)	
Conversions (%)	14 (13)	5 (5)	ns
Postoperative ES	3		
Complications	21/133	17/136	ns
Deaths	0	2	
Hospital stay (range)	6.4 (4.2-12)	9 (5.5-14)	< 0.05

ES: Endoscopic sphincterotomy
LC: Laparoscopic cholecystectomy
ERC: Endoscopic retrograde cholangiopancreaticography

Choledocholithiasis is found in approximately 10-20 percent of patients who undergo open cholecystectomies. In the era of laparoscopic cholecystectomies, the prevalence of CBD stones averages 6 percent (range; 3 to 10%). The incidence of choledocholithiasis increases over the age of 60. To achieve a maximal benefit to risk ratio, radiological investigations of the CBD should be restricted to patients with high suspicion of CBD stones, as determined by preoperative predictive scoring.

Diagnostic and therapeutic choices in cholelithiasis must be considered conjointly. Data gathered from randomized trials have demonstrated that endoscopic sphincterotomy, as an additional procedure to surgery, does not improve the clinical results in patients fit for primary single-stage surgical treatment, whether performed laparoscopically or not. Discussions regarding the optimal way to treat patients with demonstrated CBD stones could lead to endless debate. Due to marginal differences between the endoscopic and surgical techniques, the number of patients needed to show any significant difference in terms of morbidity, mortality or clearance rates would be enormous and therefore unrealistic. Cholangitis, jaundice, and CBD stones, as demonstrated on percutaneous ultrasonography, are the only reliable preoperative indicators available with predictive value of CBD stones better than 50 percent. Severe cholangitis is an unquestionable indication for urgent endoscopic drainage, regardless of whether the CBD can be cleared of associated stones or not. The notorious insufficiencies of all other preoperative indicators for CBD stones should lead to a requiem for preoperative invasive diagnostic procedures, both in terms of risk, benefits and costs.

All surgeons undertaking laparoscopic cholecystectomy must be able to perform an IOC. When IOC demonstrates CBD stones, appropriate treatment is decided according to available equipment and skills. Transcystic clearance of CBD stones is successful in at least two of three patients. In case of large (more than 20 mm) stones or other potential difficulties as regards postoperative endoscopic sphincterotomy such as a periampullary diverticulum, conversion to open surgery is indicated in case of failed laparoscopic CBD exploration. In the other cases, the available data do not allow any formal conclusions regarding the alternative between advanced laparoscopic biliary explorations and postoperative endoscopic sphincterotomy. The potential risk of reoperation in case of failed postoperative endoscopic sphincterotomy might be more theoretical than practical. In one decision analysis, assessing different approaches to using ERC in patients undergoing laparoscopic cholecystectomy, postoperative ERC was associated with less costs and morbidity, but laparoscopic CBD exploration was not considered in the study design. Last, before embarking on a more invasive laparoscopic CBD exploration policy for small stones, irretrievable by the transcystic approach, surgeons must remember that asymptomatic migration does exist, even if the definitive fate of small CBD stones remains unknown at the present time. The potential security afforded by temporary biliary drainage still has to be balanced with its unavoidable morbidity.

PROCEDURE

Patient Position

Patient is operated in the supine position with a steep head-up and left tilt. This typical positioning of laparoscopic choledochotomy should be achieved once the pneumoperitoneum has been established (Fig. 13.1).

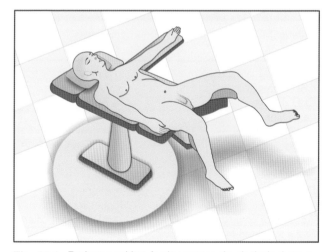

Fig. 13.1: Patient position for laparoscopic choledochotomy

Port Position

The standard 4-port configuration for laparoscopic cholecystectomy is used. A fifth port should be used later between the right midclavicular and epigastric port just below the subcostal margin for inserting the choledochoscope.

The fundus of the gallbladder should be retracted towards the right shoulder and the Hartmann's pouch should be retracted anterolaterally towards right anterior superior iliac spine. Dissection began on to the neck of the gallbladder and continued proximally until the junction of gallbladder with the cystic duct is clearly defined. Dissection should be continued proximally on to the cystic duct until there was adequate length to perform cholangiogram.

Cystic duct should be milked towards the gallbladder to dislodge any cystic duct stone into the gallbladder. Single titanium clip should be applied on the gallbladder side of cystic duct to prevent any back slippage of gallstone into the CBD and to prevent biliary spillage into the operative field.

A small nick in the cystic duct should be given with the help of hook scissors or microscissors. Intraoperative cholangiogram should be performed using a ureteric catheter (4-5 Fr) or an infant feeding tube (no 5-6), which is passed through the cystic duct into the CBD. After the insertion of the catheter, a titanium clip should be applied loosely to prevent any back

leakage of the contrast medium. Digital C-arm fluoroscopy provided the real time imaging of the biliary tree. In cases where the cystic duct could not be cannulated, contrast was directly injected into the CBD through a 24 Fr lumbar puncture needle percutaneously.

On cholangiogram, surgeon must look for any filling defect—its size, site, number of bile duct stones, and free passage of contrast into the duodenum and for any anatomical variation of the biliary tree.

Transcystic or transcholedochal approach to remove CBD stones should be decided on the following factors (Table 13.1).

CBD stone should be extracted with the help of Dormia basket / balloon catheter, irrigation/suctioning or by simply manipulating bile duct using blunt forceps. After retrieving the stones, the cystic duct stump was closed with clips or extracorporeal knots and the gallbladder was removed in the usual manner.

For transcholedochal exploration after opening up of the Calot's triangle, the anterior surface of the CBD should be dissected carefully and choledochotomy should be performed by a longitudinal incision with the help of endoscopic knife just below the insertion of the cystic duct into the bile duct (Figs 13.3A to D). Before giving incision with knife mild coagulation of serosal surface of CBD can help in prevent oozing (Figs 13.2A to D). The single large

Table 13.1: Transcystic versus transcholedochal approach for removal of CBD stone

Criteria	Findings	Transcystic approach	Transcholedochal approach	Any of these approach
Diameter of cystic duct	< 3 mm		Recommended	
CBD diameter	< 7 mm	Recommended		
CBD diameter	> 7 mm	Recommended	Recommended	Recommended
Large stone			Recommended	
Number of stone	Less than 4	Recommended	Recommended	Recommended
Number of stone	More than 4		Recommended	
Stone location	Proximal		Recommended	
Stone location	Distal			Recommended
Diameter of cystic duct	> 3 mm	Recommended	Recommended	Recommended
Junction of cystic duct with CBD	Right lateral			Recommended
Junction of cystic duct with CBD	Left lateral or posterior		Recommended	
Stone impacted in ampulla	Yes			Recommended
Severe inflammation of CBD	Yes	Recommended		
Laparoscopic suturing	Good			Recommended

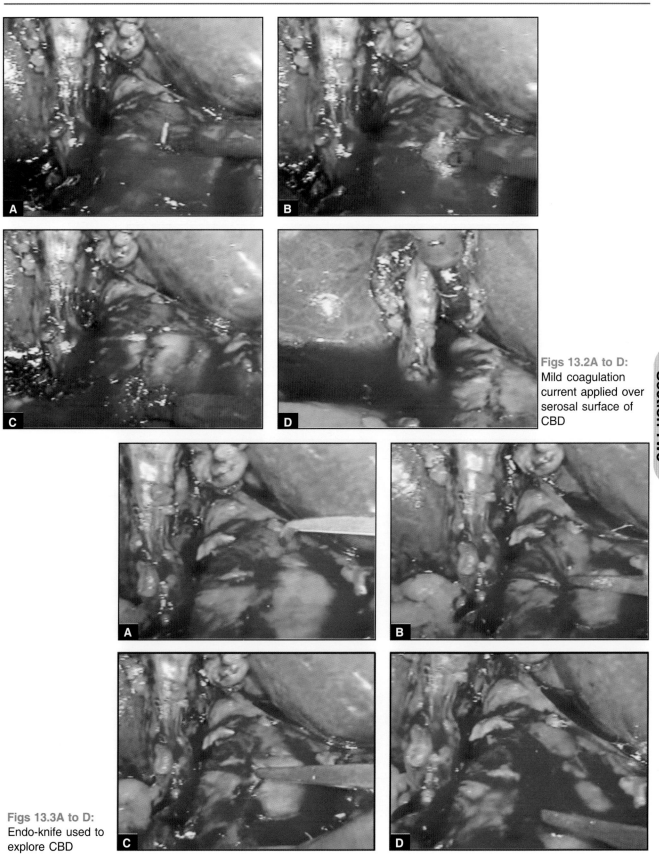

Figs 13.2A to D: Mild coagulation current applied over serosal surface of CBD

Figs 13.3A to D: Endo-knife used to explore CBD

Section Two

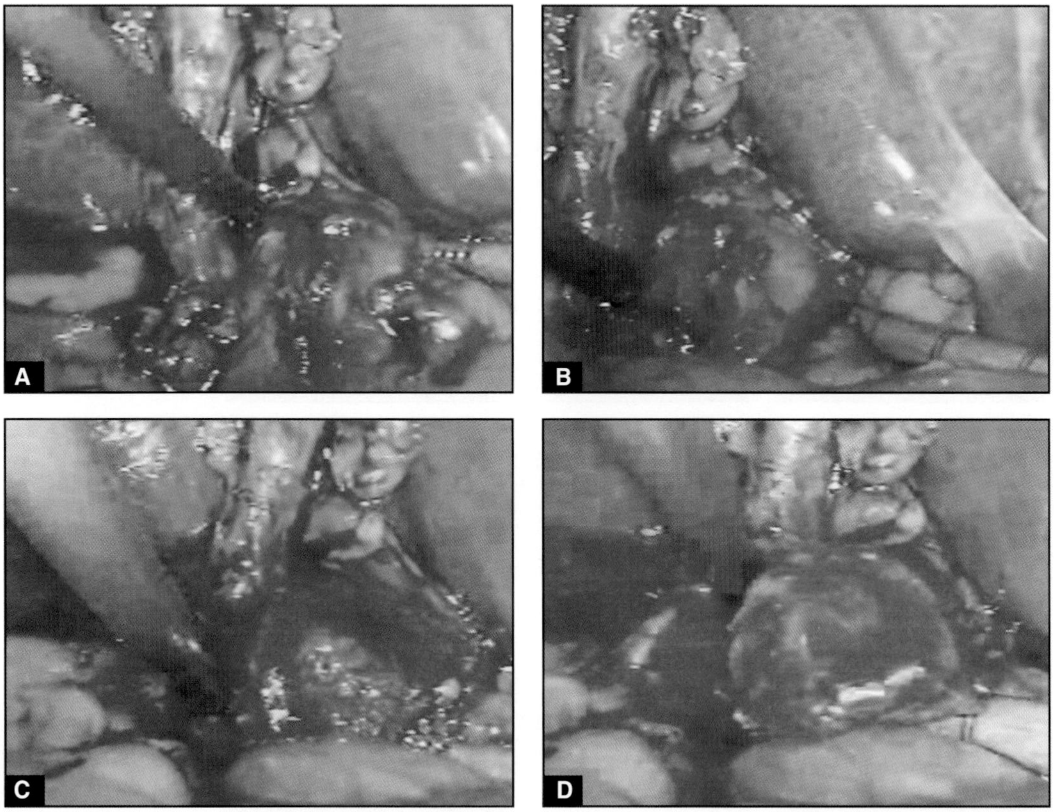

Figs 13.4A to D: Bigger single stone can be extracted by milking

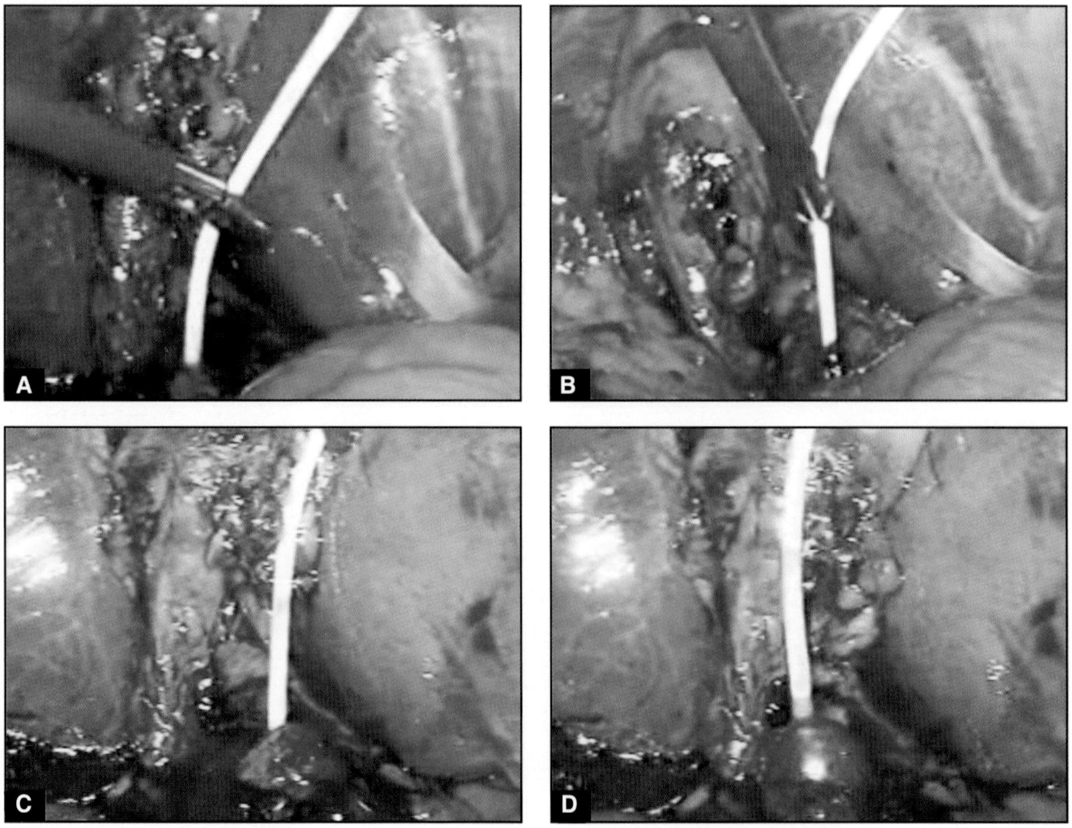

Figs 13.5A to D: Forgety catheter used to extract stone

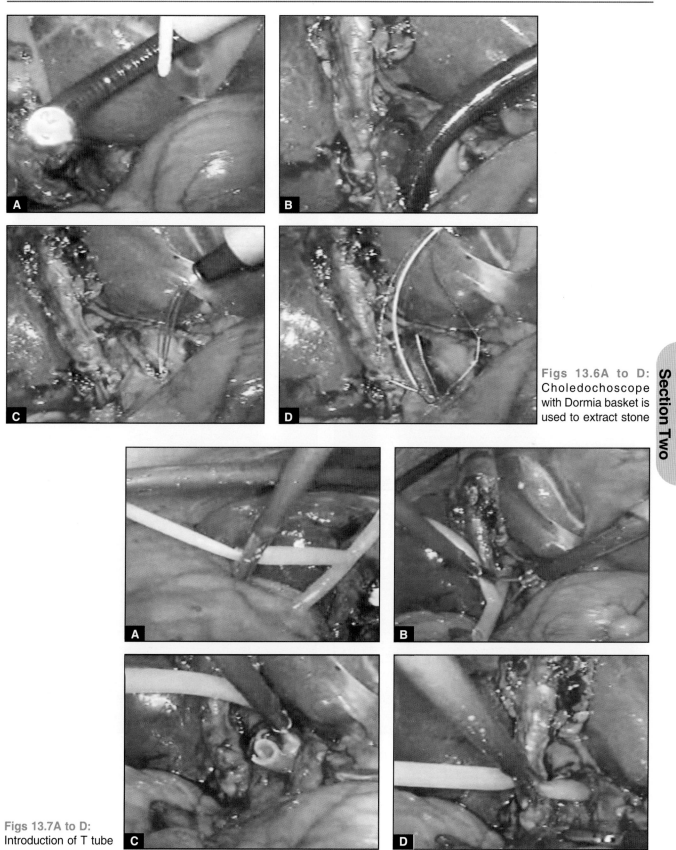

Figs 13.6A to D:
Choledochoscope
with Dormia basket is
used to extract stone

Figs 13.7A to D:
Introduction of T tube

Section Two

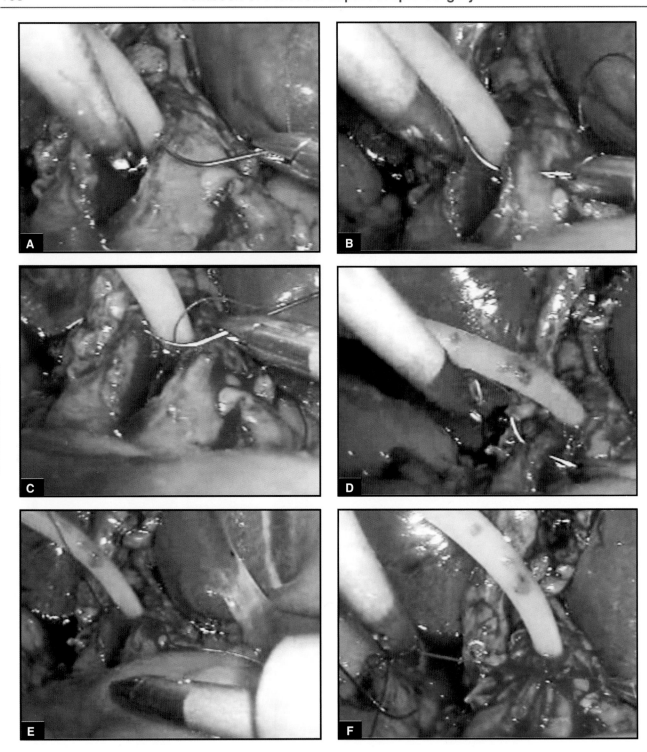

Figs 13.8A to F: T tube is fixed with intracorporeal interrupted surgeons knot

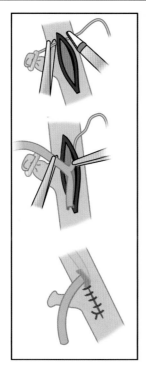

Fig. 13.9: Diagrammatic representation of T tube fixation with intracorporeal interrupted surgeons knot

stone can be retrieved by spontaneous evacuation while incising the bile duct, blunt instrumental pressure with atraumatic forceps can facilitate its easy removal (Figs 13.4A to D).

In the case of multiple stones Dormia basket, Fogarty balloon catheter or irrigation and suction can be used to remove the stone (Figs 13.5A to 13.6D).

Completion cholangiography or choledochoscopy should must be performed to assess any remaining stone. Some surgeon use 5.5 Fr bronchoscope for this purpose but ideally choledochoscope will give more flexibility.

Once all the stone is removed choledochotomy should be closed over a T tube with interrupted vicryl suture (Figs 13.7A to 13.9). In case of single stone primary closure of CBD after assessing the clearance of the CBD can be tried. After bile duct closure, cholecystectomy should be performed in the usual manner. An infrahepatic nasogastric tube drain should be use routinely is this surgery which is usually removed on day 3-4 as the output decreased below 30 ml/day.

BIBLIOGRAPHY

1. Altman DG. Practical Statistics for Medical Research. London, England: Chapman and Hall; 1992.
2. Anciaux ML, Pelletier G, Attali P, Meduri B, Liguory C, Etienne JP. Prospective study of clinical and biochemical features of symptomatic choledocholithiasis. Dig Dis Sci. 1986;31:449-53.
3. Barkun AN, Barkun JS, Fried GM, et al. Useful predictors of bile duct stones in patients undergoing laparoscopic cholecystectomy. Ann Surg. 1994;220:32-9.
4. Bates T, Ebbs SR, Harrison M, A'Hern RP. Influence of cholecystectomy on symptoms. Br J Surg. 1991;78:964-7.
5. Behan M, Kazam E. Sonography of the common bile duct: value of the right anterior oblique view. AJR Am J Roentgenol. 1978;130:701-9.
6. Bhargava S, Vashisht S, Kakaria A, Tandon RK, Berry M. Choledocholithiasis: an ultrasonic study with comparative evaluation with ERCP/PTC. Australas Radiol. 1988;32:220-6.
7. Clemets D, Aslan S, Wilkins WE. Common bile duct gallstones, anicteric presentation in the elderly: under-recognized but important. Postgrad Med J. 1990; 66:878-9.
8. Cooperberg PL, Li D, Wong P, Cohen MM, Burhenne HJ. Accuracy of common hepatic duct size in the evaluation of extrahepatic biliary obstruction. Radiology. 1980;135:141-4.
9. Cotton PB. Endoscopic retrograde cholangio-pancrea-tography and laparoscopic cholecystectomy. Am J Surg. 1993;165:474-8.
10. Cuscheri A, Croce E, Faggioni A, et al. EAES ductal stone study. Surg Endosc. 1996;10:1130-5.
11. DePaula AL, Hashiba K, Bafatto M. Laparoscopic management of choledocholithiasis. Surg Endosc. 1994;8:1399-1403.
12. Diehl AK, Sugarek NJ, Todd KH. Clinical evaluation for gallstone disease: usefulness of symptoms and signs in diagnosis. Am J Med. 1990;89:29-33.
13. Dorman JP, Franklin ME Jr, Glass JL. Laparoscopic common bile duct exploration by choledochotomy: an effective and efficient method of treatment of choledocholithiasis. Surg Endosc. 1998;12:926-8.
14. Edwin B, Rosseland ARR, Trondsen E. Prophylactic endoscopic sphincterotomy as treatment.
15. Ferzli GS, Hurwitz JB, Massaad AA, Piperno B. Laparoscopic common bile duct exploration: a review. J Laparoendosc Surg. 1996;6:413-19.
16. Gigot JF, Navez B, Etienne J, et al. A stratified intraoperative surgical strategy is mandatory during laparoscopic common bile duct exploration for common bile duct stones. Surg Endosc. 1997;11:722-8.
17. Gilliland TM, Traverso LW. Modern standards for comparison of cholecystectomy with alternative treatments for symptomatic cholelithiasis with emphasis on long-term relief of symptoms. Surg Gynecol Obstet. 1990;170:39-44.

Section Two

18. Graham SM, Flowers JL, Scott TR. Laparoscopic cholecystectomy and common bile duct stones. Ann Surg. 1993;1:61-7.
19. Gross BH, Harter LP, Gore RM, et al. Ultrasonic evaluation of common bile duct stones: prospective comparison with endoscopic retrograde cholangiography. Radiology. 1983;146:471-4.
20. Hand DJ. Discrimination and Classification. New York, NY: John Wiley and Sons; 1976.
21. Hauer-Jensen M, Ka°resen R, Nygaard K, et al. Consequences of routine preoperative cholangiography during cholecystectomy for gallstone disease: a prospective, randomized study. World J Surg. 1986;10:996-1002.
22. Hauer-Jensen M, Ka°resen R, Nygaard K, et al. Predictive ability of choledocholithiasis indicators: a prospective evaluation. Ann Surg. 1985;202:64-8.
23. Houdart R, Perniceni T, Darne B, Salmeron M, Simon JF. Predicting common bile duct lithiasis: determination and prospective validation of a model predicting low risk. Am J Surg. 1995;170:38-43.
24. Hunt DR, Reiter L, Scott AJ. Preoperative ultrasound measurement of bile duct diameter: basis for selective cholangiography Aust N Z J Surg. 1990;60: 189-92.
25. Hunt DR, Scott AJ. Changes in bile duct diameter after cholecystectomy: a 5-year prospective study. Gastroenterology. 1989;97:1485-8.
26. Hunter JG. Laparoscopic transcystic common bile duct exploration.Am J Surg. 1992;163:53-8.
27. Jennrich RI. Stepwise discriminant analysis. In: Enslein K, Ralston A, Wilf H, eds.Statistical Methods for Digital Computers. New York, NY: John Wiley and Sons;1979.
28. Jorgensen T. Abdominal symptoms and gallstone disease: an epidemiological investigation. Hepatology. 1989;9:856-60.
29. Kelly TR. Gallstone pancreatitis: the timing of surgery. Surgery. 1980;88:345-50.
30. Lacaine F, Corlette MB, Bismuth H. Preoperative evaluation of the risk of common bile duct stones. Arch Surg. 1980;115:1114-6.
31. Larson GM, Vitale GC, Casey J, et al. Multi-practice analysis of laparoscopic cholecystectomy in 1,983 patients. Am J Surg. 1991;163:221-6.
32. Liberman MA, Phillips EH, Carroll BJ, Fallas MJ, Rosenthal R, Hiatt J. Costeffective management of complicated choledocholithiasis: laparoscopic transcystic duct exploration or endoscopic sphincterotomy. J Am Coll Surg. 1996; 182:488-94.
33. Liberman MA, Phillips EH, Carroll BJ, Fallas MJ, Rosenthal R, Hiatt J. Costeffective management of complicated choledocholithiasis: laparoscopic transcystic duct exploration or endoscopic sphincterotomy. J Am Coll Surg. 1996; 182:488-94.
34. Mja°aland O, Raeder J, Aaseboe V, Trondsen E, Buanes T. Outpatient laparoscopic cholecystectomy, patient satisfaction and safety: prospective study of 200 patients. Br J Surg. In press.
35. Naude GP, Stabile BE, Bongard FS. Antegrade laparoscopic common bile duct stone removal using a balloon-tipped embolectomy catheter. J Am Coll Surg. 1997;184:655-7.
36. Neoptolemos JP, Carr-Locke DL, Fossard DP. Prospective randomized study of preoperative endoscopic sphincterotomy versus surgery alone for common bile duct stones. BMJ. 1987;294:470-4.
37. Neuhaus H, Feussner H, Ungeheuer A, Hoffmann W, Siewert JR, Classen M. Prospective evaluation of the use of endoscopic retrograde cholangiography prior to laparoscopic cholecystography. Endoscopy. 1992;24:745-9.
38. Niederau C, Sonnenberg A, Mueller J. Comparison of the extrahepatic bile duct size measured by ultrasound and by different radiographic methods. Gastroenterology. 1984;87:615-21.
39. O'Connor HJ, Bartlett RJ, Hamilton I, et al. Bile duct calibre: the value of ultrasonic and cholangiographic measurement in the postcholecystectomy patient. Gut. 1984;25: A576.
40. Onken J, Brazer S, Eisen G, et al. Accurate prediction of choledocholithiasis. In: Program and abstracts of the American Association for the Study of Liver Disease, American Gastroenterological Association, American Society for Gastrointestinal Endoscopy, and Society for Surgery of the Alimentary Tract group conference; May 15-18, 1994; New Orleans, La. Abstract 699.
41. Pasanen P, Partanen K, Pikkarainen P, Alhava E, Pirinen A, Janatuinen E. Ultrasonography, CT, and ERCP in the diagnosis of choledochal stones. Acta Radiol. 1992;33:53-56.
42. Patwardhan RV, Smith OJ, Farmelant MH. Serum transaminase levels and cholescintigraphic anomalies in acute biliary tract obstruction.Arch Intern Med. 1987; 147:1249-53.
43. Petelin JB. Clinical results of common bile duct exploration. Endosc Surg Allied Technol. 1993;1:125-9.
44. Petelin JB. Laparoscopic approach to common duct pathology.Am J Surg. 1993; 165:487-91.
45. Phillips E, Daykhovsky L, Carroll B, Gershman A, Grundfest WS. Laparoscopic cholecystectomy: instrumentation and technique. J Laparoendosc Surg. 1990; 1:3-15.
46. Phillips EH, Berci G, Carroll B, Daykhovsky L, Sackier J, Paz-Partlow M. The importance of intraoperative cholangiography during laparoscopic cholecystectomy. Am Surg. 1990;56:792-5.
47. Phillips EH, Rosenthal RJ, Carroll BJ, Fallas MJ. Laparoscopic transcystic-duct common bile duct exploration. Surg Endosc. 1994;81:389-94.
48. Phillips EH, Rosenthal RJ, Carroll BJ, Fallas MJ. Laparoscopic transcystic common bile duct exploration. Surg Endosc. 1994;8:1389-94.
49. Reiss R, Deutsch AA, Nudelman I, Kott I. Statistical value of various clinical parameters in predicting the presence of choledochal stones. Surg Gynecol Obstet. 1984;159: 273-6.
50. Robertson GSM, Jagger C, Johnson PRV, et al. Selection criteria for preoperative endoscopic retrograde cholangiography in the laparoscopic era. Arch Surg. 1996;131:89-94.

Section Two

51. Ros E, Zambon D. Postcholecystectomy symptoms: a prospective study of gall stone patients before and two years after surgery. Gut. 1987;28:1500-04.

52. Roslyn JJ, Binns GS, Hughes EF, Saunders-Kirkwood K, Zinner MJ, Cates JA. Open cholecystectomy: a contemporary analysis of 42,474 patients. Ann Surg. 1993;218:129-137.

53. Rosseland AR, Osnes M. Biliary concrements: the endoscopic approach. World J Surg. 1989;13:178-85.

54. Rosseland AR, Solhaug JH. Early or delayed endoscopic papillotomy (EPT) in gallstone pancreatitis. Ann Surg. 1984;199:165-7.

55. Roush TS, Traverso LW. Management and long-term follow-up of patients with positive cholangiograms during laparoscopic cholecystectomy. Am J Surg. 1995; 169: 484-7.

56. Saltzstein EC, Peacock JB, Thomas MD. Preoperative bilirubin, alkaline phosphatase and amylase levels as predictors of common duct stones. Surg Gynecol Obstet. 1982;154:381-4.

57. Santo PD, Kazarian KK, Rogers JF, Bevins PA, Hall JR. Prediction of operative cholangiography in patients undergoing elective cholecystectomy with routine liver function chemistry. Surgery. 1985;98:7-11.

58. Sauerbrei EE, Cooperberg PL, Gordon P, Li D, Cohen MM, Burhenne HJ. The discrepancy between radiographic and sonographic bile duct measurements. Radiology. 1980;137:751-5.

59. Schultz LS, Kamel M, Graber JN, Hickok DF. Four-year outcome data for 400 laparoscopic cholecystectomy patients: recognition of persistent symptoms. Int Surg. 1994;79: 205-8.

60. Stefanini P, Carboni M, Patrassi N, Loriga P, De Bernardinis G, Negro P. Factors influencing the long-term results of cholecystectomy. Surg Gynecol Obstet. 1974; 139:734-8.

61. Stiegman GV, Goff JS, Mansour A, Pearlman N, Reveille RM, Norton L. Precholecystectomy endoscopic cholangiography and stone removal is not superior to cholecystectomy, cholangiography, and common bile duct exploration. AmJ Surg. 1992;163:227-30.

62. Stoker ME. Common bile duct exploration in the era of laparoscopic surgery. Arch Surg. 1995;130:265-9.

63. Stoker ME. Common bile duct exploration in the era of laparoscopic surgery. Arch Surg. 1995;130:265-926.

64. Taylor TV, Armstrong CP, Rimmer S, Lucas SB, Jeacock J, Gunn AA. Prediction of choledocholithiasis using a pocket microcomputer. Br J Surg. 1988;75:138- 40.

65. Trondsen E, Edwin B, Reiertsen O, Fagertun H, Rosseland AR. Selection criteria for endoscopic retrograde cholangiography (ERCP) in patients with gallstone disease. World J Surg. 1995;19:852-7.

66. Vander Velpen GC, Shimi SM, Cuschieri A. Outcome after cholecystectomy for symptomatic gall stone disease and effect of surgical access: laparoscopic vs open approach. Gut. 1993;34:1448-51.

67. Voyles CR, Petro AB, Meena AL, Haick AJ, Koury AM. A practical approach to laparoscopic cholecystectomy. Am J Surg. 1991;161:365-70.

68. Wegge C, Kjaergaard J. Evaluation of symptoms and signs of gallstone disease in patients admitted with upper abdominal pain. Scand J Gastroenterol. 1985; 20:933-6.

69. Welbourn CRB, Mehta D, Armstrong CP, Gear MWL, Eyre-Brook IA. Selective preoperative endoscopic retrograde cholangiography with sphincterotomy avoids bile duct exploration during laparoscopic cholecystectomy. Gut. 1995;37:576- 9.

Section Two

14 Laparoscopic Appendicectomy

Appendicitis was first recognized as a disease entity in the sixteenth century and was called perityphlitis. McBurney described the clinical findings in 1889. Laparoscopic appendectomy in expert hands is now quite safe and effective. It is an excellent alternative for patients with acute appendicitis. First successful laparoscopic appendicectomy was performed by Semm in 1982. Although laparoscopic appendicectomy can be performed in all group of patients, surgeons agree that for women of child bearing age, laparoscopic appendectomy is unquestionably the method of choice.

LAPAROSCOPIC ANATOMY

The appendix is derived from a cecal diverticulum of the fetus. The appendix is generally within 1.7 cm of the ileocecal junction. Its length varies from 2 to 20 cm, average 9 cm (Fig. 14.1). Most of the time when

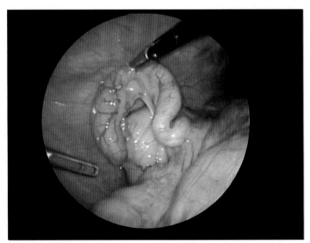

Fig. 14.1: Normal laparoscopic view of appendix

telescope is introduced through umbilicus, appendix is hidden behind the cecum.

The anterior tinea coli of the cecum are an important landmark which leads to cecum (Figs 14.2A to 14.3). The triangular mesoappendix tethers the appendix posteriorly which contains appendicular artery and veins. The appendicular artery is a branch of the ileocolic artery. Laparoscopic exposure of the appendix is facilitated by gently pulling the cecum upward.

The base of the appendix must be visualized to avoid leaving a remnant of appendix at the time of laparoscopic appendicectomy. Exposures of retrocecal appendix require mobilization of right colon. The peritoneal reflection is incised, and the cecum is pulled medially to visualize retrocecal appendix.

ADVANTAGE OF LAPAROSCOPIC APPENDECTOMY

Thorough exposure of the peritoneal cavity is possible.

Indications

Laparoscopic appendectomy	Open appendectomy
Female of reproductive age group	Complicated appendicitis
Female of pre-menopausal group	COPD or cardiac disease
Suspected appendicitis	Generalized peritonitis
High working class	
Previous lower abdominal surgery	
Obese patients	Hypercoagulable sites
Disease conditions like cirrhosis	Stump appendicitis after
of liver and sickle cell disease	previous incomplete
	appendicectomy
Immune-compromised patients	

1. Ascending colon
2. Ileocecal junction
3. Uterus

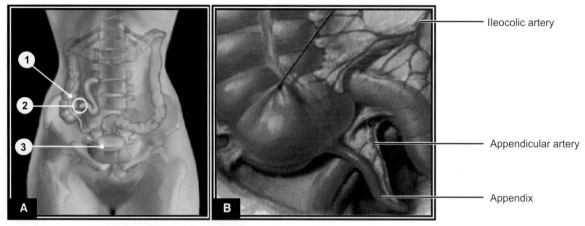

Ileocolic artery

Appendicular artery

Appendix

Figs 14.2A and B: Anatomic position of appendix

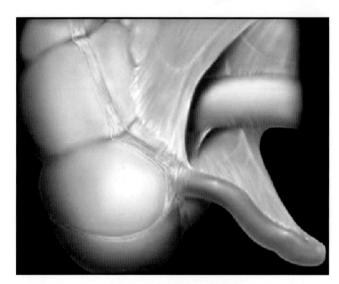

Fig. 14.3: Normal appendix

Relative Contraindications

- Complicated appendicitis
- Stump appendicitis (develops after previous incomplete appendectomy)
- Poor risk for general anesthesia
- Some cases of previous extensive pelvic surgery.

The general anesthesia and the pneumoperitoneum required as part of the laparoscopic procedure do increase the risk in certain groups of patients. Most surgeons would not recommend laparoscopic appendectomy in those with pre-existing disease conditions. Patients with moderate cardiac diseases and COPD should not be considered a good candidate for laparoscopy. The laparoscopic appendectomy may also be more difficult in patients who have had previous lower abdominal surgery. The elderly may also be at increased risk for complications with general anesthesia combined with pneumoperitoneum.

Patient Position

The patient is in supine position, arms tucked at the side. The surgeon stands on the left side of the patient with the camera holder-assistant (Fig. 14.4). For maintaining co-axial alignment surgeon should stand near left shoulder and monitor should be placed near right hip facing towards surgeon. In female, the lithotomic position should be used because it may be necessary to use uterine manipulator in difficult diagnosis (Fig. 14.5A).

Port Position

- Total 3 trocar should be used
- Two 10 mm, umbilical and left lower quadrant trocar
- One 5 mm right upper quadrant trocar
- The right upper quadrant trocar can be moved below the Bikini line in females.

ALTERNATIVE PORT AND THEATER SETUP

In beauty conscious female for cosmetic reason the base ball diamond concept of port position can be altered and three ports should be placed in such a way so that the two 5 mm port will be below Bikini line. Access should be performed by 10 mm umbilical port. Once the telescope is inside one 5 mm port should be placed in left iliac fossa below the Bikini line under vision. Second 5 mm port should be placed in right

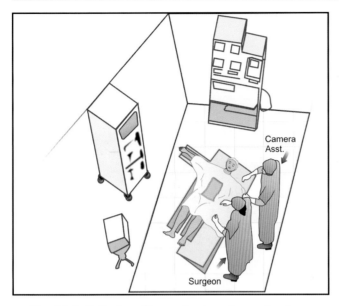

Fig. 14.4: Patient position and setup of operating team

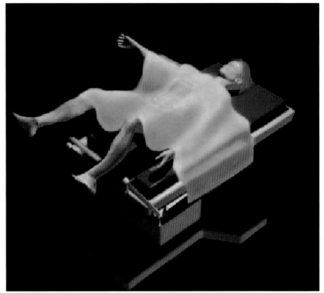

Fig. 14.5A: Patient position in female

iliac fossa, just mirror image of left port. After fixing all the ports in position, one another 5 mm telescope is introduced through left iliac fossa and surgery should be performed through umbilical port (for right hand) and left iliac fossa port (for left hand) (Fig. 14.6). In this alternative port position 60° manipulation angle cannot be achieved and it is ergonomically difficult for surgeon, but patient will get cosmetic benefit.

This alternative port position for laparoscopic appendicectomy should not be performed in case of retrocecal appendix or perforated appendix (Fig. 14.5B). Alternative port position in beauty conscious female (Fig. 14.7)

Operative Technique

Pneumoperitoneum is created in the usual fashion. Three ports are used in atraumatic grasper (Endo Babcock or Dolphin Nose Grasper) is inserted via the right upper quadrant trocar. The cecum is retracted upward toward the liver. In most cases, this maneuver will elevate the appendix in the optical field of the telescope.

Retraction of Appendix

The appendix is grasped at its tip with a 5 mm claw grasper via the RUQ trocar. It is held in upward position. After the pelvis is inspected the appendix is

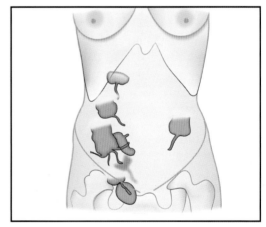

Fig. 14.5B: Variation in position of appendix

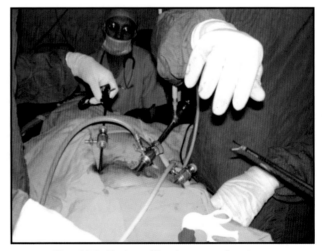

Fig. 14.6: Port position in appendicectomy

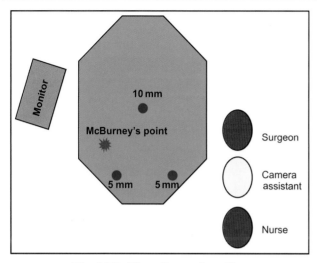

Fig. 14.7: Alternative port position

Fig. 14.8: Retraction of appendix

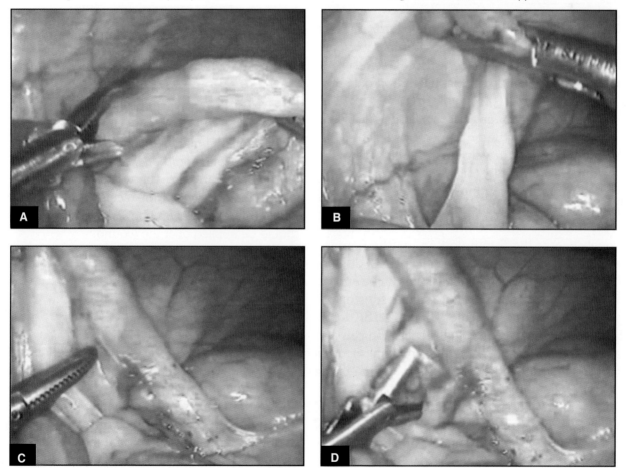

Figs 14.9A to D: Retraction of appendix and creation of a window over mesoappendix

identified, mobilized and examined properly (Figs 14.8 to 14.9D). Periappendiceal or pericecal adhesion is lysed using either bipolar or harmonics and scissors. Left lower quadrant (LLQ) grasper is used to create a mesenteric window behind the base of the appendix.

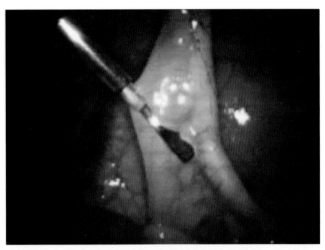

Fig. 14.10: Window in mesoappendix

A dolphin nose grasper is used to create a mesenteric window under the base of the appendix. The window should be made as close as possible to the base of the appendix and should be approximately 1 cm in size (Fig. 14.10).

The mesoappendix may be coagulated using bipolar or harmonics, it can be or clipped or stapled. It can also sutured and cut with laparoscopic scissors to skeletonize the appendix (Figs 14.11A to 14.12B).

Extracorporeal knotting performed (Meltzer or Tayside knot) for mesoappendix as well as appendix. Two endoloop sutures are passed sequentially through one of the 5 mm port and pushed around the base of appendix on top of each other at a distance of 3 to 5 mm. A third endoloop suture can be applied 6 mm distal to the second suture so that surgeon will cut between second and third (Figs 14.13A to F). Hulka tubal clips used for tubal sterilization can also be used sometime to secure the proximal or distal portion of the appendix. The luminal portion of the appendiceal stump is sterilized with electrosurgery to prevent spillage and contamination of peritoneal cavity. Betadine can be applied over the stump of appendix and thorough suction and irrigation is performed either by normal saline or Ringer's lactate solution.

After extracting the appendix out of abdominal cavity surgeon should examine the abdomen for any possible bowel injury or hemorrhage.

Stapler Appendicectomy

The stapling devices make laparoscopic appendectomy simpler and faster. The multifire stapler is introduced though a 12 mm port. The appendix may be transacted by inserting an ENDO GIA instrument via the RUQ trocar (blue cartridge, 3.5), closing it around the base of the appendix and firing it. For perforated appendicitis with or without an intra-abdominal abscess, a drain is left in the RLQ and pelvis (Fig. 14.19A to C).

Extra-corporeal knot (Meltzer, Roader or Tayside knot) should be preferred over stapler, depending on the surgeon's expertise.

Extraction of Appendix

The appendix can be removed from the abdomen with the help of grasping forceps placed through one of the 10 mm port. However, this may contaminate both the cannula and instrument. Alternatively, an endoloop suture which was tied last can be used instead of grasping forceps to pull the appendix out.

Abdomen should be examined for any possible bowel injury or hemorrhage. All the instrument should be removed carefully. The wound should be closed with suture. Use Vicryl for rectus and Unabsorbable intradermal or stapler for skin. Adhesive sterile dressing should be applied over the wound.

RISK FACTORS IN LAPAROSCOPIC APPENDECTOMY

Missed Diagnosis

There is report also of mucinous cystadenoma of the cecum missed at laparoscopic appendectomy. Less than 1 percent of all patients with suspected acute appendicitis are found to have an associated malignant process. During conventional appendectomy, through a laparotomy incision, the cecum and the appendix are easily palpated, and an obvious mass can be detected and properly managed at the time of appendectomy. The inability to palpate any mass is an inherent inadequacy of laparoscopic surgery.

Section Two

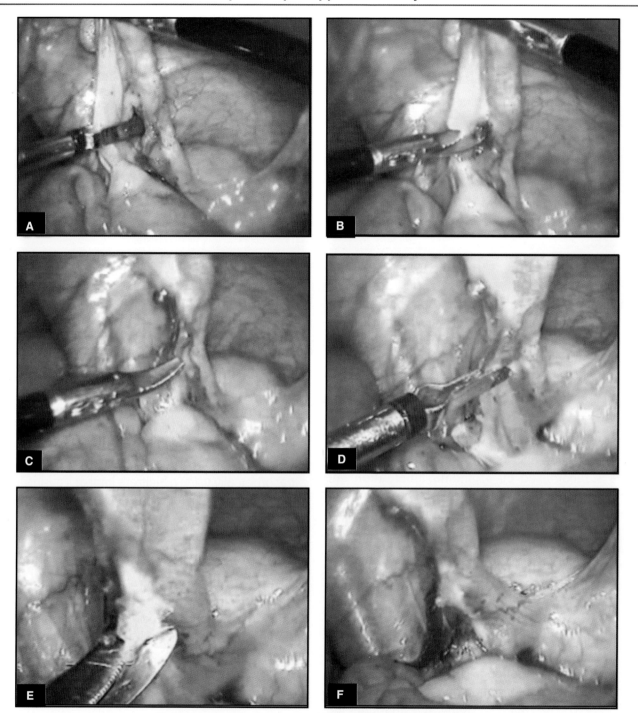

Figs 14.11A to F: Successive bipolar desiccation and cutting

Bleeding

Bleeding may occur from the mesoappendix, omental vessels or retroperitoneum. Bleeding is usually recognized intraoperatively via adequate exposure, lighting and suction. It is recognized postoperatively by tachycardia, hypotension, decreased urine output, anemia or other evidence of hemorrhagic shock.

Visceral Injury

Risk of accidental burns is higher with monopolar system because electricity seeks the path of least

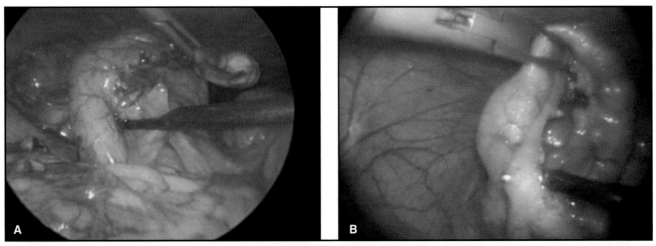

Figs 14.12A and B: Dissection of mesoappendix by monopolar hook

resistance which may be adjacent bowel. In a bipolar system since the current does not have to travel through the patient, there is little chance of injury to remote viscera. In laparoscopic appendectomy, only bipolar current should be used. Laparoscopists should also routinely explore the rest of the abdomen.

Wound Infection

Proper tissue retrieval technique is required to prevent wound infection after appendectomy.

It is recognized by erythema, fluctuation and purulent drainage from port sites. The absence of wound infections after laparoscopic appendectomy can be attributed to the practice of placing the appendix in a sterile bag or into the trocar sleeve prior to removal from the abdomen. The regular use of retrieval bag is a very good practice for preventing infection of the wound.

Incomplete Appendectomy

If surgeon is not experienced, the stump of the appendix may be too long. There is a report of intra-abdominal abscess formation due to retained fecolith after laparoscopic appendectomy. It is important that the surgeons performing laparoscopic appendectomy should remove fecolith if found, and the stump of appendix should not be big enough to contain any remaining fecolith. Incomplete appendectomy is a result of ligation of the appendix too far from the base. It may lead to recurrent appendicitis, which presents with symptoms and signs of appendicitis even after laparoscopic appendectomy.

Some surgeons prefer stapling of the appendiceal stump for laparoscopic appendectomy for the treatment of all forms of appendicitis (Figs 14.19A to 14.20). But most of the surgeons now agree that ligation of the appendectomy stump is the best approach (Figs 14.14 to 14.16C). There is report of slippage of clip, residual appendicitis followed by abscess formation after using clip for appendiceal stump. The ligation should be preformed by using endoloop, an intracorporeal surgeon's knot, or done extracorporeally using a Meltzer's knot or Tayside knot. The security of the knot is essential. It is influenced by the proper port location and experience of the surgeon.

Leakage of Purulent Exudates

It is usually seen intraoperatively while dissecting appendix. Copious irrigation and suction followed by continued antibiotics can prevent this complication until patient is afebrile with a normal white blood cell count. Retrieval bag should be used to prevent the spillage of infected material from the appendiceal lumen.

Intra-abdominal Abscess

This postoperative morbidity is recognized by prolonged ileus, sluggish recovery, rising leukocytosis, spiking fevers, tachycardia and rarely a palpable mass. After confirmation of the intra-abdominal abscess drainage of pus followed by antibiotic therapy is essential. Sometimes, laparotomy may be required.

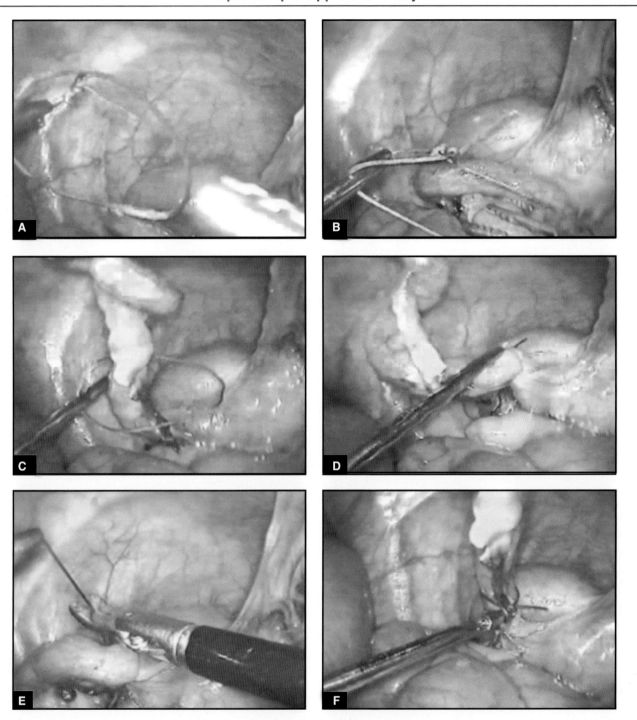

Figs 14.13A to F: Tying Roader's or Meltzer's knot over appendix

Hernia

Trocar site hernia as visible or palpable bulge is sometime encountered. Possible occult hernia is manifested by pain or symptoms of bowel obstruction.

Laparoscopic Assisted Appendectomy

It has been described for cases in which the proper endoscopic instruments and sutures are unavailable. The laparoscope facilitates the diagnosis of acute

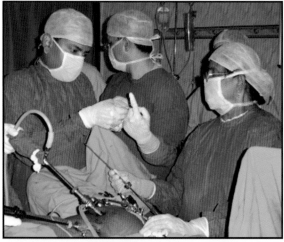

Fig. 14.14: Tying Roader's knot at the time of appendicectomy

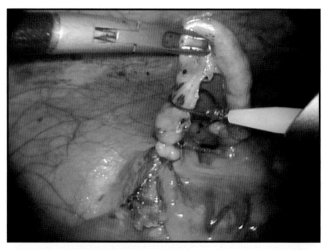

Fig. 14.15: Three Roader's or Meltzer's knot over appendix

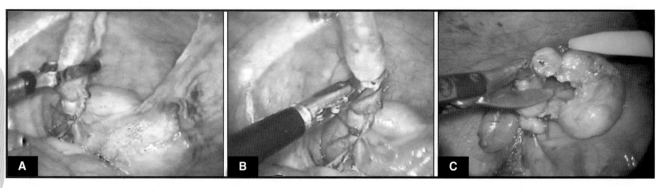

Figs 14.16A to C: Amputation of appendix

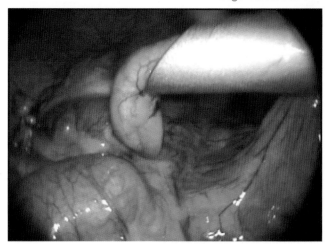

Fig. 14.17: Amputated appendix inside the cannula

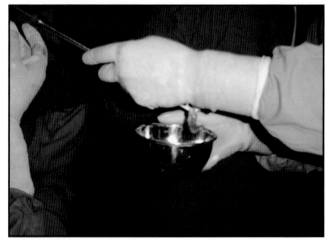

Fig. 14.18: Appendix hidden in cannula is ejected out

appendicitis and a grasper is passed through an accessory trocar located just over the McBurney's point. The tip of the appendix is grasped and then pulled along with cannula and grasper (Figs 14.17 and 14.18). Once the appendix is exteriorized the routine appendectomy is performed through this small abdominal incision. This procedure usually takes less time than total laparoscopic appendectomy but it has more incidence of incomplete appendectomy.

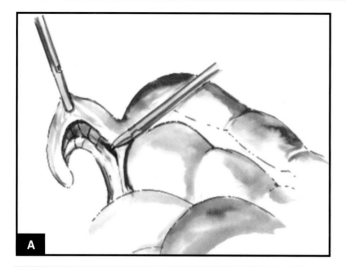

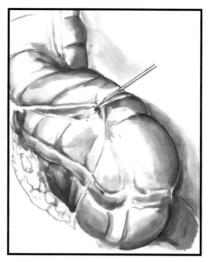

Fig. 14.20: Retrocecal appendix

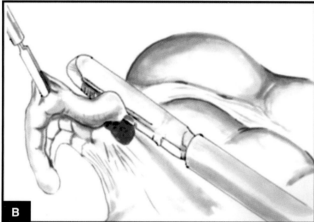

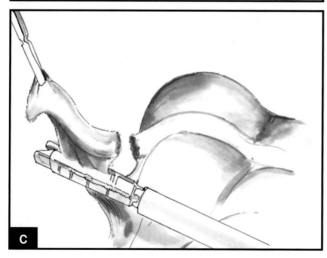

Figs 14.19A to C: Stapler appendicectomy

Discussion

Laparoscopic appendectomy has gained lot of attention around the world. However, the role of laparoscopy for appendectomy, one of the commonest indications, remains controversial. Several controlled trials have been conducted, some are in favor of laparoscopy, others not. There is also diversity in the quality of the randomized controlled trials. The main variable in these trials are following parameters:

- Number of patients in trial
- Withdrawal of cases
- Exclusion of cases
- Blinding
- Intention to treat analysis
- Publication biases
- Local practice variation
- Prophylactic antibiotic used
- Follow-up failure.

Without proper attention to the detail of all the parameters it is very difficult to draw a conclusion. It has been found among the surgeons that there is a hidden competition between laparoscopic surgeons and the surgeons who are still doing conventional surgery, and this competition influences the result of study. One should always think of laparoscopic surgery and open procedures as being complimentary to each other.

A successful outcome requires greater skills from the operator. The result of many comparative studies have shown that outcome of laparoscopic appendectomy was influenced by the experience and technique of the operator. Minimal access surgery requires different skills and technological knowledge.

Section Two

With a clear diagnosis of complicated appendicitis, the skill and experience of the surgeon should be considered for the selection of operating method. Surgeons should perform the procedure with which they are more comfortable.

Laparoscopic appendectomy is equally safe and can provide less postoperative morbidity in experienced hands, as in open appendectomy. Most cases of acute appendicitis can be treated laparoscopically. Laparoscopic appendectomy is a useful method for reducing hospital stay, complications and return to normal activity. With better training in minimal access surgery now available, the time has arrived for it to take its place in the surgeon's repertoire.

BIBLIOGRAPHY

1. Addiss DG, Shaffer N, Fowler BS, Tauxe RV. The epidemiology of appendicitis and appendectomy in the United States. Am J Epidemiol. 1990;132:910-25.
2. Alexander F, Magnuson D, DiFiore J, Jirousek K, Secic M. Specialty versus generalist care of children with appendicitis: an outcome comparison. J Pediatr Surg. 2001;36:1510-13.
3. Azzie G, Salloum A, Beasley S, Maoate K. The complication rate and outcomes of laparoscopic appendicectomy in children with perforated appendicitis. Pediatr Endosurgery Innovative Techniques. 2004;8:19-23. http://www.liebertonline.com/doi/abs/10.1089/1092641047-73513098.
4. Banieghbal B, Al-Hindi S, Davies MRQ. Laparoscopic appendectomy with appendix mass in children. Pediatr Endosurgery Innovative Techniques. 2004; 8:25-30. http://www.liebertonline.com/doi/abs/10.1089/109264-104773513106.
5. Beldi G, Muggli K, Helbling C, Schlumpf R. Laparoscopic appendectomy using endoloops: a prospective, randomized clinical trial. Surg Endosc. 2004;18: 749-50.
6. Blewett CJ, Krummel TM. Perforated appendicitis: past and future controversies. Semin Pediatr Surg. 1995;4:234-8.
7. Bratton SL, Haberkern CM, Waldhausen JH. Acute appendicitis risks of complications: age and medical insurance. Pediatrics. 2000;106:75-8.
8. Chen C, Botelho C, Cooper A, Hibberd P, Parsons SK. Current practice patterns in the treatment of perforated appendicitis in children. J Am Coll Surg. 2003; 196:212-21.
9. David IB, Buck JR, Filler RM. Rational use of antibiotics for perforated appendicitis in childhood. J Pediatr Surg. 1982;17:494-500.
10. Heiss K. Victim or player: pediatric surgeons deal with quality improvement and the information age. Semin Pediatr Surg. 2002;11:3-11.
11. Himal HS. Minimally invasive (laparoscopic) surgery. Surgical Endosc 2002;16:1647–52
12. Horwitz JR, Custer MD, May BH, Mehall JR, Lally KP. Should laparoscopic appendectomy be avoided for complicated appendicitis in children? J Pediatr Surg. 1997;32:1601-3.
13. Ikeda H, Ishimaru Y, Takayasu H, Okamura K, Kisaki Y, Fujino J. Laparoscopic vs open appendectomy in children with uncomplicated and complicated appendicitis. J Pediatr Surg. 2004;39:1680-85.
14. Kokoska ER, Silen ML, Tracy TF, Dillon PA, Cradock TV, Weber TR. Perforated appendicitis in children: risk factors for the development of complications. Surgery. 1998;124:619-26.
15. Krisher SL, Browne A, Dibbins A, Tkacz N, Curci M. Intra-abdominal abscess after laparoscopic appendectomy for perforated appendicitis. Arch Surg. 2001; 136:438-41.
16. Lintula H, Kokki H, Vanamo K, Antila P, Eskelinen M. Laparoscopy in children with complicated appendicitis. J Pediatr Surg. 2002;37:1317-20.
17. Lintula H, Kokki H, Vanamo K, Valtonen H, Mattila M, Eskelinen M. The costs and effects of laparoscopic appendectomy in children. Arch Pediatr Adolesc Med. 2004;158:34-7.
18. Lintula H, Kokki H, Vanamo K. Single-blind randomized clinical trial of laparoscopic vs open appendicectomy in children. Br J Surg. 2001;88:510-4.
19. Lund DP, Murphy EU. Management of perforated appendicitis in children: a decade of aggressive treatment. J Pediatr Surg. 1994;29:1130-4.
20. Martin LC, Puente I, Sosa JL, et al. Open vs laparoscopic appendectomy: a prospective randomized comparison. Ann Surg. 1995;222:256-62.
21. Merhoff AM, Merhoff GC, Franklin ME. Laparoscopic vs open appendectomy. Am J Surg. 2000;179:375-8.
22. Moraitis D, Kini SU, Annamaneni RK, Zitsman JL. Laparoscopy in complicated pediatric appendicitis. JSLS. 2004;8:310-13.
23. Nathaniel J, Soper L, Brunt M, Kerbl K. Laparoscopic general surgery. N Eng J Med 1994;330:409–19.
24. Newman K, Ponsky T, Kittle K, et al. Appendicitis 2000: variability in practice, outcomes, and resource utilization at thirty pediatric hospitals. J Pediatr Surg. 2003;38:372-9.
25. Nguyen NT, Zainabadi K, Mavandadi S, et al. Trends in the utilization and outcomes of laparoscopic vs open appendectomy. Am J Surg. 2004;188: 813-20.
26. Phillips S, Walton JM, Chin I, Farrokhyar F, Fitzgerald P, Cameron B. Ten year experience with pediatric laparoscopic appendectomy: are we getting better? J Pediatr Surg. 2005;40:842-5.
27. Pittman-Waller VA, Myers JG, Stewart RM, et al. Appendicitis: why so complicated? Analysis of 5755 consecutive appendectomies. American Surgeon. 2000; 66:548-54.
28. Reich H. Laparoscopic bowel injury. Surg Laparosc Endosc. 1992;2:74-8.

29. Schrenk P, Woisetschlager R, Rieger R, Wayand W. Mechanism, management, and prevention of laparoscopic bowel injuries. Gastrointest Endosc. 1996;43: 572-4.

30. Simpson J, Humes D, Speake W, Appendicitis. Clin Evid BMJ 2006; See www.clinicalevidence.com/ceweb/conditions/dsd/ 0408/0408_keymessages.jsp

31. Tang E, Ortega AE, Anthone GJ, Beart RW Jr. Intraabdominal abscesses following laparoscopic and open appendec-tomies. Surg Endosc. 1996;10:327-8.

32. Utpal De. Laparoscopic versus open appendicectomy: an Indian perspective. J Minimal Access Surg 2005;1:15–20

33. Vernon AH, Georgeson KE, Harmon CM. Pediatric laparoscopic appendectomy for acute appendicitis. Surg Endosc. 2003;18:75-9.

34. Voyles C, Tucker R. A better understanding of monopolar electrosurgery and laparoscopy. In: Brooks D, ed. Current Techniques in Laparoscopy. Philadelphia, Pa: Current Medicine; 1994:1-10.

35. Voyles CR, Tucker RD. Education and engineering solutions for potential problems with laparoscopic monopolar electrosurgery. Am J Surg. 1992;164:57-62.

36. Wagner M, Aronsky D, Tschudi J, Metzger A, Klaiber C. Laparoscopic stapler appendectomy: a prospective study of 267 consecutive cases. Surg Endosc. 1996; 10:895-9.

37. Yong JL, Law WL, Lo CY, Lam CM. A comparative study of routine laparoscopic versus open appendectomy. JSLS 2006;10:188–92

15 Laparoscopic Repair of Inguinal Hernia

Inguinal hernia results from a hole or defect in the muscles, through which the peritoneum protrudes, forming the sac (Figs 15.1 and 15.5). Inguinal herniorrhaphy is one of the most common operations that general surgeons perform. Laparoscopic herniorrhaphy is being done at a time when laparoscopic cholecystectomy has shown definite benefits over the open technique. But unlike laparoscopic cholecystectomy, laparoscopic hernia repair is an advanced laparoscopic procedure and has a longer learning curve. In addition, TEP requires higher technical expertise for successful results.

Ger in 1982 attempted minimal access groin hernia repair by closing the opening of an indirect inguinal hernial sac using Michel clips. Bogojavlensky in 1989 modified the technique by intracorporeal suture of the deep ring after plugging a PPM into the sac. Toy and Smoot in 1991 described a technique of intraperitoneal onlay mesh (IPOM) placement, where an intra-

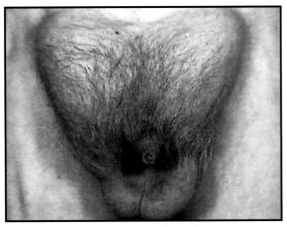

Fig. 15.1: Bilateral direct hernia

abdominal piece of polypropylene or e-PTFE was stapled over the myopectineal orifice without dissection of the peritoneum.

The present day techniques of laparoscopic hernia repair evolved from Stoppa's concept of pre-peritoneal reinforcement of fascia transversalis over the myopectineal orifice with its multiple openings by a prosthetic mesh. In the early 1990's Arregui and Doin described the transabdominal pre-peritoneal (TAPP) repair, where the abdominal cavity is first entered, peritoneum over the posterior wall of the inguinal canal is incised to enter into the avascular preperitoneal plane which is adequately dissected to place a large (15 × 10 cm) mesh over the hernial orifices. After fixation of the mesh, the peritoneum is carefully sutured or stapled. TAPP approach has the advantage of identifying missed additional direct or femoral hernia during the first operation itself.

Around the same time Phillips and McKernan described the totally extraperitoneal (TEP) technique of endoscopic hernioplasty where the peritoneal cavity is not breached and the entire dissection is performed bluntly in the extraperitoneal space with a balloon device or the tip of the laparoscope itself. An advanced knowledge of the posterior anatomy of the inguinal region is imperative. Once the dissection is complete, a 15 × 10 cm mesh is stapled in place over the myopectineal orifice. It appears to be the most common endoscopic repair today.

In both these repairs, the mesh in direct contact with the fascia of the transversalis muscle in the pre-peritoneal space, allows tissue ingrowths leading to the fixation of the mesh (as opposed to being in contact

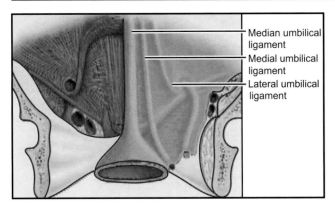

Fig. 15.2: Diagrammatic representation of ligaments

to the peritoneum as in IPOM repair where it is prone to migrate).

LAPAROSCOPIC ANATOMY

In the lower abdomen there are five peritoneal folds or ligaments which are seen through the laparoscope in umbilicus. These ligaments are generally overlooked at the time of open surgery.

One Median Umbilical Ligament

In the midline there is median umbilical ligament extends from the mid of urinary bladder up to the umbilicus. Median umbilical ligament is obliterated urachus (Fig. 15.2).

Two Medial Umbilical Ligament
One on Either Side

The paired medial umbilical ligament is obliterated umbilical artery except where the superior vesical arteries are found in the pelvic portion. The medial umbilical ligaments are the most prominent fold of the peritoneum. Sometimes, it hangs down and obscure the vision of lateral pelvic wall. These ligaments are important landmark for the lateral extent of the urinary bladder (Figs 15.3A and B).

Two Lateral Umbilical Ligaments

Lateral to the medial umbilical ligament, the less prominent paired lateral umbilical fold contains the Inferior epigastric vessels. The inferior epigastric artery is lateral border of Hesselbach's triangle and hence is useful landmark for differentiating between direct and indirect hernia. Any defect lateral to the lateral umbilical ligament is indirect hernia and medial to it is direct inguinal hernia (Fig. 15.4).

The femoral hernia is below and slightly medial to the lateral inguinal fossa, separated from it by the medial end of the iliopubic tract internally and the inguinal ligament externally.

Important landmarks for extraperitoneal hernia dissection include the musculoaponeurotic layers of the abdominal wall, the bladder, coopers ligament and the iliopubic tract. The inferior epigastric artery and vein, the gonadal vessels and vas deferens should also be recognized. The space of Retzius lies between the vesicoumbilical fascia posteriorly and the posterior rectus sheath and pubic bone, anteriorly. This is the space first entered in extraperitoneal repair of hernia.

Three dangerous areas where stapling and electrosurgery should be avoided:

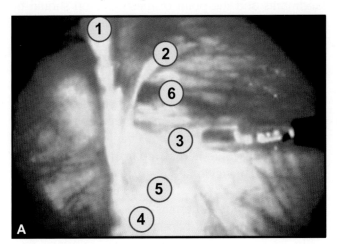

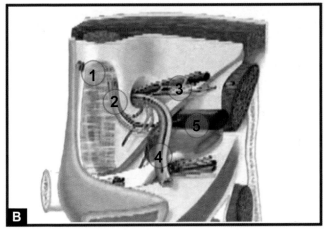

Figs 15.3A and B: Important landmarks in laparoscopic hernia repair, 1. Medial umbilical ligament, 2. Inferior epigastric vessels, 3. Spermatic vessels, 4. Vas deferens, 5. External iliac vessels in "Triangle of doom", 6. Indirect defect

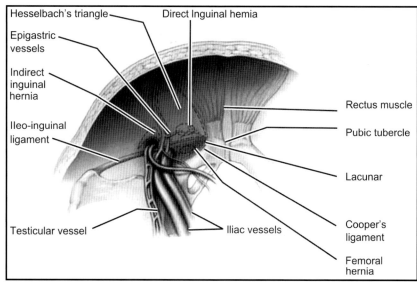

Fig. 15.4: Triangle of doom

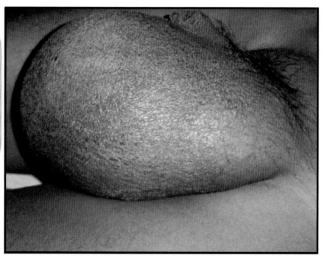

Fig. 15.5: Left side indirect hernia

Triangle of Doom

The triangle of doom is defined be vas deferens medially, spermatic vessels laterally and external iliac vessels inferiorly. This triangle contains external iliac artery and vessels, the deep circumflex iliac vein, the genital branch of genitofemoral nerve and hidden by fascia, the femoral nerve. Staple should not be applied in this triangle otherwise; chances of mortality are there if these great vessels are injured.

Triangle of Pain

Triangle of pain is defined as spermatic vessel medially, the iliopubic tract laterally and inferiorly the inferior edge of skin incision. This triangle contains lateral femoral cutaneous nerve and anterior femoral cutaneous nerve of thigh. The staple in this area should be less because nerve entrapment can cause neuralgia.

Circle of Deth

This is also called as corona mortis and refers to vascular ring form by the anastomosis of an aberrant artery with the normal obturator artery arising from a branch of the internal iliac artery. At the time of laparoscopic hernia this vessel is torn both end of vessel can bleed profusely, because both arise from a major artery.

The surgeon should remember these anatomic landmarks and the point of mesh fixation should be selected superiorly, laterally and medially.

INDICATIONS OF LAPAROSCOPIC REPAIR OF HERNIA

The indications for performing a laparoscopic hernia repair are essentially the same as repairing the hernia conventionally. There are, however, certain situations where laparoscopic hernia repair may offer definite benefit over conventional surgery to the patients. These include:
- Bilateral inguinal hernias
- Recurrent inguinal hernias.

In recurrent hernia, surgery failure rate is as high as 25 to 30 percent, if again repaired by open surgery.

The distorted anatomy after repeated surgery makes it more prone to recurrence and other complications like ischemic orchitis. In recurrent hernia, the laparoscopic approach offers repair through the inner healthy tissues with clear anatomical planes and thus, a lower failure rate. In laparoscopic bilateral repair with three ports technique, there is simultaneous access to both sides without any additional trocar placement. Even in patients with clinically unilateral defect after entering inside the abdominal cavity, there is 20-50 percent incidence of a contralateral asymptomatic hernia being found which can be repaired, simultaneously, without any additional morbidity of the patient.

Contraindications of Laparoscopic Repair of Hernia

- Non-reducible, incarcerated inguinal hernia
- Prior laparoscopic herniorrhaphy
- Massive scrotal hernia
- Prior pelvic lymph node resection
- Prior groin irradiation.

ADVANTAGES OF LAPAROSCOPIC APPROACH

- Tension free repair that reinforces the entire myopectoneal orifice
- Less tissue dissection and disruption of tissue planes
- Three ports are adequate for all type of hernias
- Less pain postoperatively
- Low intraoperatively and postoperative complications
- Early return to work.

DISADVANTAGES OF OPEN METHOD

- Requires 4 to 6 inches of incision at the groin
- Generally very painful, because of muscle spasm
- Considerable postoperative swelling of tissues in groin, around the wound.
- Requires cutting through the skin, fat, and good muscles in order to gain access for repair, which in itself causes damage.
- Frequent complications of wound hematomas, wound infection, scrotal hematomas and neuroma.
- Usually takes 6 to 8 weeks for recovery.

- Sometimes long-term disability, may follow, e.g. neuralgia, neuroma and testicular ischemia.
- Whether a flat mesh or a plug is used from the front, they don't hold themselves in place; what holds them in place are stitches, so the strength of the repair still depends on the stitches, not so much on the mesh or plug.
- Bilateral inguinal hernias require 2 incisions, doubling the pain; or 2 operations.
- Recurrent inguinal hernias are very difficult to operate open, and more liable to complications.
- The size of mesh used in open methods is limited by natural fusion of muscles.
- All meshes and plugs shrink with time, and this works against all open methods.

Any method of repair must achieve 2 fundamental goals, removal of the sac from the defect and durable closure of the defect. In addition the ideal method should achieve these with the least invasion, pain or disturbance of normal anatomy. Laparoscopic repair in expert hands is now quite safe and effective, and is an excellent alternative for patients with inguinal hernia. It is confusion that laparoscopic repair is more complex and is not widely available. The public needs to be educated as to its advantages. All surgeons agree that for bilateral or recurrent inguinal hernias, laparoscopic repair is unquestionably the method of choice. The argument against its use for unilateral or primary inguinal hernias is unfounded if it is the best for bilateral or recurrent hernias.

Types of Laparoscopic Hernia Repair

Many techniques were used to repair hernia like:
- Simple closure of the internal rings
- Plug and patch repair
- Intraperitoneal onlay mesh repair
- Transabdominal preperitoneal mesh repair (TAPP)
- Total extraperitoneal repair (TEP).

The technique of transabdominal preperitoneal repair was first described by Arregui in 1991. In the transabdominal preperitoneal (TAPP) repair, the peritoneal cavity is entered, the peritoneum is dissected from the myopectineal orifice, mesh prosthesis is secured, and the peritoneal defect is closed. This technique has been criticized for exposing intra-abdominal organs to potential complications, including small bowel injury and obstruction.

The totally extraperitoneal (TEP) repair maintains peritoneal integrity, theoretically eliminating these risks while allowing direct visualization of the groin anatomy, which is critical for a successful repair. The TEP hernioplasty follows the basic principles of the open preperitoneal giant mesh repair, as first described by Stoppa in 1975 for the repair of bilateral hernias.

Patient Selection

The general anesthesia and the pneumoperitoneum required as part of the laparoscopic procedure do increase the risk in certain groups of patients. Most surgeons would not recommend laparoscopic hernia repair in those with pre-existing disease conditions. Patients with cardiac diseases and COPD should not be considered a good candidate for laparoscopy. The laparoscopic hernia repair may also be more difficult in patients who have had previous lower abdominal surgery. The elderly may also be at increased risk for complications with general anesthesia combined with pneumoperitoneum.

If the patient is young or the hernia small, it does not matter how the hernia is repaired. Many surgeons agree that for bilateral or recurrent inguinal hernias, laparoscopic repair is unquestionably the method of choice.

Laparoscopic surgery is not recommended for big irreducible and incarcerated hernia. Hernia repair should not be performed under local anesthesia. Small direct hernia can be performed under spinal Anesthesia if TEP is planned but best anesthesia for laparoscopic hernia repair is GA.

TRANSABDOMINAL PREPERITONEAL REPAIR OF INGUINAL HERNIA

Position of Surgical Team

Surgeon stands towards the opposite side of the shoulder. Camera assistant should stand either right to the patient or on the opposite side of the patient (Fig. 15.6).

Port Position

The position of port is laparoscopic repair of transabdominal hernia repair should be again according to base ball diamond concept (Figs 15.7A to C).

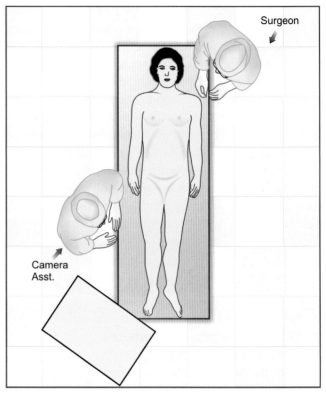

Fig. 15.6: Position of surgeon in right sided hernia

The telescopic port should be in umbilicus. A 10 mm umbilical port is used. Two other ports, usually 10 mm for dominant hand and 5 mm for non-dominant hand, are placed lateral to the umbilicus (Figs 15.8A to C). In a left sided hernia the right lateral port should be in left iliac fossa and left port in left hypochondrium so that both the instrument should make a manipulation angle of 60°. In right sided hernia surgery right port should move up towards hypochondrium and left port will come down to make the triangle.

PROCEDURE OF TAPP

After access, diagnostic laparoscopy is performed to rule out any adhesion or other intra-abdominal lesion. All the important anatomical landmark of hernia surgery is identified with the help of telescope and one atraumatic grasper. The defect should be seen carefully and if any content is present inside the sac it should be reduced gently. A sliding hernia of colon should be carefully reduced because chances of perforation of large bowel are more than other viscus. Any adhesion between bowel and omentum should be divided carefully using bipolar and scissors.

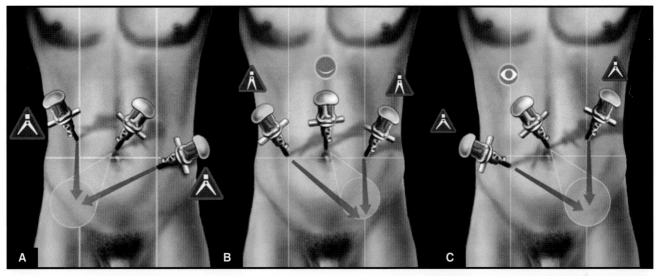

Figs 15.7A to C: (A) Port position of right sided hernia, (B) Port position of bilateral hernia, (C) Port position of left sided hernia

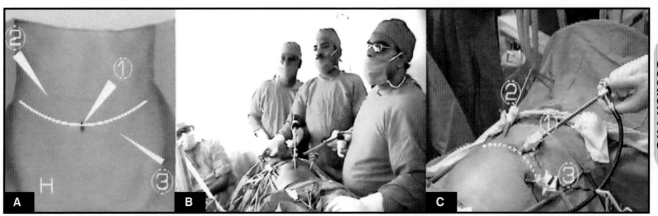

Figs 15.8A to C: (1 Camera, 2,3–Instrument) (A) Port position of right sided hernia
(B) Port position of surgical team, (C) Port position right hernia

The next step of transabdominal preperitoneal repair of hernia is creation of preperitoneal space. Many surgeons like to do hydrodissection to create this preperitoneal space but it is easy to create with sharp dissection as well. The peritoneum is cut 4 cm lateral to the outer margin of deep ring (Fig. 15.9). The flap of peritoneum is separated from above downward as soon as it will reach at the site of internal ring the hernia sac will be encountered.

Dissection should be started with opening the peritoneum lateral to the medial umbilical fold in order to identify Cooper's ligament. Stoppa's parietalization technique should be used for dissection of the spermatic cord from the peritoneum by separating the elements of the spermatic cord from the peritoneum and peritoneal sac (Fig. 15.10).

In case of indirect defect the hernial sac has to be either gently dissected free or inverted or if it is completely adhered with the transversalis fascia and cord structure it can be transected. The important landmarks of laparoscopic hernia repair are the pubic bone and inferior epigastric vessels. Surgeons should use both blunt and sharp dissection and the sac is dissected off the anterior abdominal wall. After being reduced partially it is ligated using an endo-loop and then transected with scissors. In case of bilateral hernias, the procedure is repeated on the other side. The vas and spermatic vessels has been separated from sac. Once the sac is separated, the next step is separation of sac from cord structures and dissection for creation of proper lateral space for placement of mesh. Lateral limit of dissection is the anterosuperior

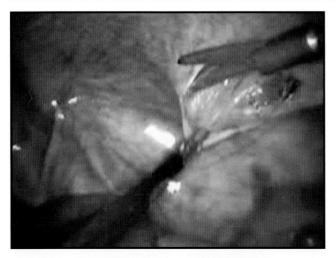

Fig. 15.9: Incision over peritoneum

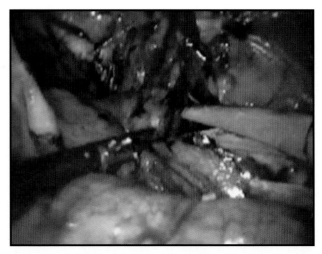

Fig. 15.10: Creation of preperitoneal space

iliac spine while inferior limit laterally is the psoas muscle. Dissection should be avoided in the "triangle of doom" which is bounded medially by the vas deferens and laterally by the gonadal vessels. A large hernial sac creates multiple planes and it is easy for the beginners to get disoriented with sac vas and vessel. The best way to avoid this confusion is that surgeon should keep himself as close as possible to the outer surface of peritoneum. If the spermatic vessels are injured accidentally it can be clipped. Even if the testicular vessel is injured, the testes will get the blood supply from collateral vessels developed through cremasteric.

In direct hernias the creation of preperitoneal space is comparatively easy as there is no chance of injury of spermatic vessels and vas. The bulge in the transversalis fascia may be repaired by suturing or stapling.

The tacker application and application of electrosurgery should be very careful at the triangle of doom, triangle of pain and trapezoid of disaster. In case of massive complete indirect scrotal hernias, no attempt should be made to reduce the sac completely as it may increase the risk of testicular nerve injury and hematoma formation.

Placement of the Mesh

Criteria for laparoscopic mesh
- Non-absorbable
- Adequate size
- Adequate memory.

A proline mesh of appropriate size, usually 15 × 15 cm should be taken and one corner of Mesh should be tailored (Fig. 15.11). Mesh should be rolled and loaded backward in one of the port. Mesh is placed inside the abdominal cavity through 12 mm port. If surgery is being performed by 10 mm port only the port should be removed and rolled mesh should be introduced though the port wound directly (Figs 15.12A and B). After introduction of mesh it is unrolled when it reaches in peritoneal cavity. The mesh is fixed medially over the Cooper's ligament and pubic bone using a tacker or anchor (Fig. 15.13). The tailored corner of mesh should be positioned inferomedially. No lateral slit should be made in the mesh and it should not be fixed lateral to cord structures to prevent injury to lateral cutaneous nerve of thigh. The mesh in this

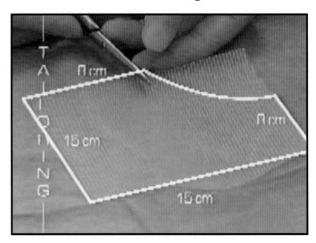

Fig. 15.11: Cutting the corner of mesh

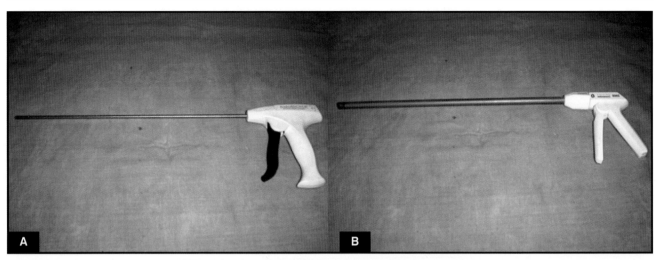

Figs 15.12A and B: (A) Hernia anchor, (B) Hernia tacker

Table 15.1: Comparison of ESS endoanchor, tyco protack, tyco tacker

Feature	ESS Endoanchor	Tyco Protack	Tyco Tacker
Number of implants	20	30	20
Geometry of implant	Anchor	Helical fastener	Helical fastener
Implant material	Nitinol	Titanium	Titanium
Implant length	5.9 mm	3.8 mm	3.6 mm
Implant width	6.7 mm	4 mm	3.4 mm
Port size required	5 mm	5 mm	5 mm
Shaft length	360 mm	356 mm	356 mm
Trigger fire orientation	Release to deploy	Depress to deploy	Depress to deploy

position covers the direct, indirect and femoral defects. It is essential that mesh should extend below the pubic tubercle so that it covers the femoral orifice. Mesh should also extend medially to cover all the possible orifices of hernia. Laterally mesh should project at least 2 to 3 cm beyond the margin of deep ring. If mesh is not of appropriate size, the chance of recurrence is high. Sometime, surgeon may be disoriented and mesh is placed with its long axis vertical instead of transverse. If mesh is cut at one of the corner chances of this disorientation is minimum.

Implant for Fixing Mesh

Many preloaded devices are available for fixing mesh in hernia surgery. Mesh is fixed medially over the Cooper's ligament and pubic bone using an implant.

Currently three popular brands of implants to fix the mesh are available. These are Tacker, Protack or Anchor. The comparative chart of these implant is shown in Table 15.1.

After adjusting the mesh properly it should be fixed by stapling first its middle part three figure above the superior limit of the internal ring. With mesh duly stapled pneumoperitoneum is reduced to 9 mm Hg. It is important to avoid pricking of the inferior epigastric artery or the testicular vessels. Intracorporeal suturing can also be used for fixation of mesh if surgeon has sufficient suturing skill.

After fixing the mesh properly the peritoneum flap is replaced over the mesh and it is closed either by staples or suture (Fig. 15.14). It is important that mesh should be completely covered by the peritoneum. Ideally peritoneum should be opposed by overlap fashion and peritoneum defect is closed either by staples or by continuous suturing and Aberdeen termination.

Repair of Bilateral Inguinal Hernia

In laparoscopic surgery postoperative recovery of bilateral hernia is same as that of unilateral hernia.

Section Two

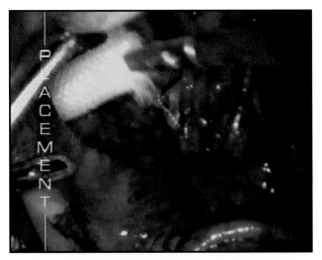

Fig. 15.13: Introduction of mesh in preperitoneal space

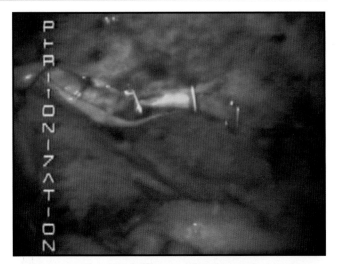

Fig. 15.14: Closure of peritoneum

The technique of bilateral laparoscopic repair of hernia is same as that of unilateral hernia. Patients with bilateral hernia are good candidate of laparoscopy. The two sides may be repaired using two meshes but single long mesh also can be used and is pushed across from one side behind the bladder, and across the inguinal orifice on the opposite side. The size of the mesh for bilateral hernia should be 30 × 15 cm (Fig. 15.15). Surgeon should avoid twisting of mesh. After placing the mesh in bilateral hernia surgery it should look just like a bow tie.

Repair of Recurrent Inguinal Hernia

Recurrent laparoscopic hernia after open surgery is better to repair laparoscopically, because external anatomy is disrupted and open repair have more chance of recurrence. Laparoscopy is method of choice for recurrent hernia. The defect is usually direct and more than one in recurrent hernia. The result of laparoscopic repair is excellent even in case of multiple hernias.

Laparoscopic Hernia in Children

Laparoscopy has been tried in little children. Only closure of ring and herniotomy is possible in pediatric age group. The sac is simply inverted and tied internally. Care should be taken that the vas or vessels should not be caught in the ligature (Figs 15.16A and B).

Ending of the Operation

At the end of surgery, the abdomen should be examined for any possible bowel injury or hemorrhage.

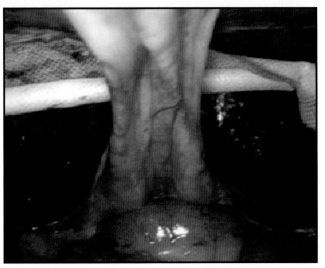

Fig. 15.15: Introduction of mesh for bilateral hernia

The entire instrument should be removed and then all the port. Each port should be removed under direct observation through telescope. Ports larger then 10 mm should be sutured. Telescope should be removed at last after releasing all the gas keeping in mind that last port should not be pulled without putting telescope or any blunt instrument in, to prevent entrapment of bowel or omentum and formation of adhesion or intestinal adhesion. Wound should be closed with suture, especially 10 mm wound.

Totally Extraperitoneal Hernia Repair

The technique of totally extraperitoneal (TEP) repair of inguinal hernia was described even before the TAPP technique; however, technical difficulties of working in closed space and anatomy with the limited working

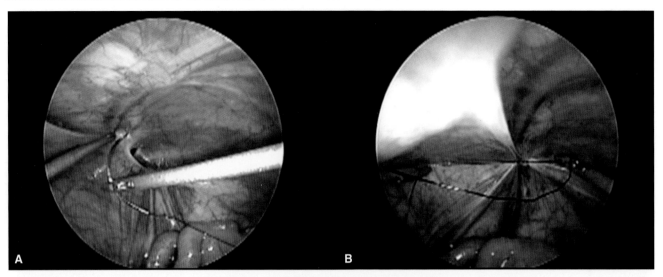

Figs 15.16A and B: Closure of defect with intracorporeal suturing in pediatric age

space hindered its popular acceptance. The effectiveness of this type of repair has been well established by the open operation of Stoppa.

ADVANTAGE OF TEP

- Pneumoperitoneum is not required
- Less chance of dangerous vessel injury or bowel injury
- The view of groin is better for dissection around the neck of sac
- Continuity of peritoneum is not breached so it may not be closed.

DISADVANTAGE OF PREPERITONEAL REPAIR

- The identification of correct plane of dissection is difficult
- The landmarks of hernia dissection can only be identified when they are encountered
- Reduction of content of sac is difficult to ensure
- Sliding hernia is difficult to recognize from outside of sac
- If the sac is cut it is difficult to close it again
- In recurrent hernia extensive adhesion make the dissection difficult because peritoneum may be adherent to the under surface of scar
- There is always a chance of breach of peritoneum continuity and this will reduce the view

- Four ports generally are necessary for bilateral hernia surgery. Whereas, in TAPP only three ports are sufficient.

Preparation of the Patient

Preparation of the patient in totally preperitoneal hernia repair is same as of the transabdominal hernia repair. Knowledge of the anatomy of the abdominal wall muscle and recognition of the transition zone that occur at the arcuate line of Douglas is very important for totally preperitoneal hernia repair.

Approach to Preperitoneal Space

In totally extraperitoneal repair of hernia, the main concern is to make an extraperitoneal space. The extraperitoneal space is made possible by the fact that the peritoneum in suprapubic region can easily be separated from anterior abdominal wall, thereby creating enough space for dissection.

A 2 cm longitudinal skin incision is made just below the umbilicus 1 cm lateral to the midline on the side of hernia (Figs 15.17A and B). The incision is deepened down to reach up to the anterior rectus sheath. All the subcutaneous fat is cleared and the rectus is opened under direct vision. Two-stay suture on each leaf of rectus sheath is placed and the rectus muscle is retracted by two retractors downward towards symphysis pubis in an oblique fashion; we should never

Section Two

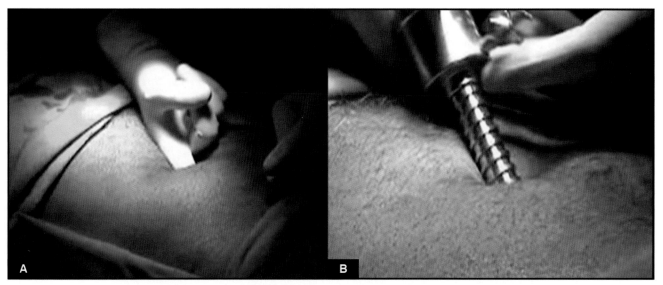

Figs 15.17A and B: Access technique of totally extraperitoneal hernia repair

cross the posterior fascia of the rectus muscle while dissecting.

By finger or swab towards the hernia, dissection should perform carefully, preperitoneal space will be found below the arcuate line of Douglas.

Insertion of Port

A balloon dissector should be introduced with telescope and balloon is inflated for further dissection of the pre-peritoneal space. A 11 mm port is introduced without its sharp tip with a laparoscope in 30°. A small preperitoneal pocket is created by manipulating laparoscope in sweeping manner.

If balloon dissector is not available the glove finger can be tied around the suction irrigation instrument and can be used to create some preperitoneal space (Figs 15.18A and B).

Sweeping Movement of Telescope

Once the telescope is placed properly a 10 mm port is inserted under direct view approximately halfway between the symphysis pubis and the umbilicus (Figs 15.19A and D). Another 5 mm port should be placed two fingers below and medial to the right anterior iliac spine. If the secondary port site is not seen clearly through the telescope one can infiltrate the port site with local anesthetic and look for the tip of the needle internally (Fig. 15.20). This will insure the exact placement of port and allow the tip of trocar to be seen by telescope at the time of insertion.

Dissection of Preperitoneal Space and Cord Structures in TEP

In totally extraperitoneal repair of hernia Stoppa's parietalization technique is used for dissection of the spermatic cord from the peritoneum by separating the elements of the spermatic cord from the peritoneum and peritoneal sac should be done (Fig. 15.21). The dissection is started by tracing the inferior epigastric vessels towards the deep ring. The upper border of the hernia sac readily recognized because indirect hernia is lateral to the inferior epigastric vessels and direct hernia is medial to that.

As the inguinal region is approached, the dissection is continued all around the sac to encircle the neck. The surgeon should try to remain close to peritoneum and dissection continues medially to separate vas from the sac. Under the neck of the sac care should be taken to avoid injury of iliac vessels.

In case of direct inguinal hernia the dissection is carried out from above downwards and progressed medially to the inferior epigastric vessels. The direct sac is freed from the transversalis fascia. Dissection should be continued until the peritoneum has reached the iliac vessels inferiorly.

Care should be taken that any hole in peritoneum should not form otherwise it will be difficult to have good working space because the gas will escape into abdominal cavity. If the hole is made anyway it should be identified and enlarged this will equalize the pressure on both side of peritoneum and allows the peritoneum

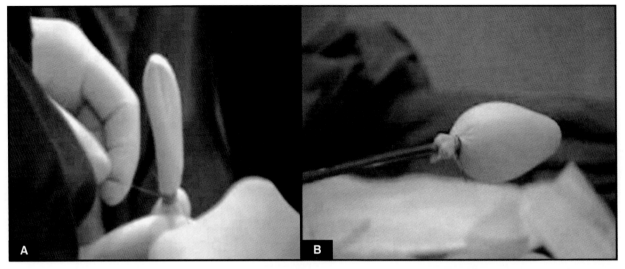

Figs 15.18A and B: Making balloon dissection with finger of gloves

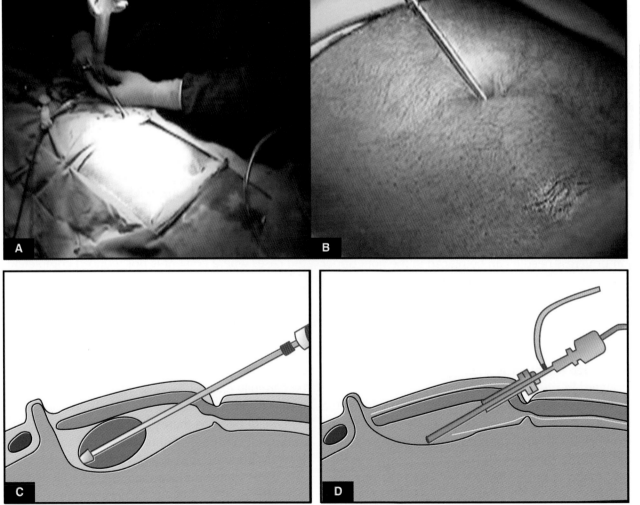

Figs 15.19A to D: Balloon dissection

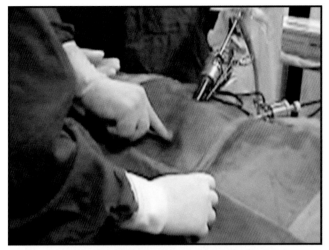

Fig. 15.20: Introduction of secondary port

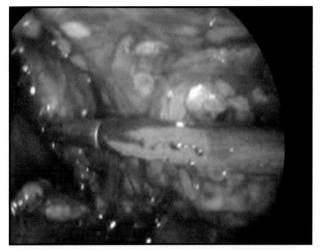

Fig. 15.21: Dissection of preperitoneal space

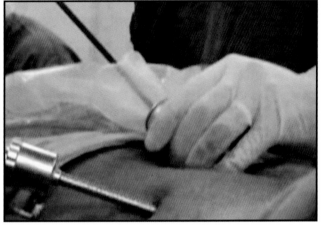

Fig. 15.22: Introduction of mesh

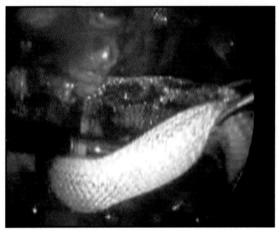

Fig. 15.23: Placement of mesh

to drop back down due to gravity. A venting 5 mm port or veress needle can be placed in the right upper quadrant at Palmer's point to decompress the abdominal cavity.

The technique of insertion of mesh in totally extraperitoneal repair of hernia is same as that of transabdominal preperitoneal. Mesh of appropriate size usually 15 × 15 cm is used and rolled and loaded backward in one of the port.

Mesh should be fixed by stapling first in its middle part three finger above the superior limit of the internal ring (Figs 15.22 and 15.23). In totally extraperitoneal repair some surgeon do not use staple, because peritoneum is not breached and once the gas from preperitoneal space is removed, it will place the mesh in its proper position. In 1 to 2 percent of cases of TEP conversion to open or TAPP may be necessary due to

large peritoneal tear making the vision difficult or in the cases where content is not reduced completely.

Laparoscopic Repair of Femoral Hernia

Laparoscopic repair of femoral hernia is same as that of laparoscopic direct or indirect hernia. It can be performed by both TAPP and TEP methods. In case of laparoscopic femoral hernia repair the sac should be carefully excised because rigid femoral ring make it difficult to mobilize the sac. The dissection should be careful because there is increased risk of injury of abnormal obturator artery on lateral to the sac. If femoral hernia defect is between the iliopubic tract and pubic ramus and can be easily identified. Repair of the femoral canal should be done by approximating iliopubic tract to the Cooper's ligament by proline stitches.

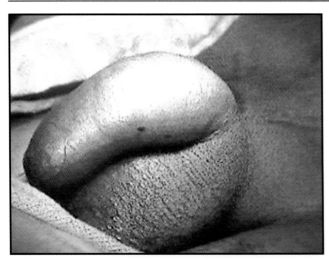

Fig. 15.24: Postoperative scrotal hematoma

ENDING OF THE OPERATION

At the end of surgery the abdomen should be examined for any possible bowel injury or hemorrhage. The entire instrument should be removed and then all the port. Generally vicryl is used for rectus and unabsorbable intradermal and stapler for skin. Adhesive sterile dressing should be applied over the wound.

COMPLICATIONS OF LAPAROSCOPIC HERNIA REPAIR

Like any other laparoscopic procedures, complications have been recorded during the learning curve. The major problems include:
• Recurrence
• Neurovascular injury
• Urinary tract injury
• Injury to vas
• Testicular complications
• Problems due to mesh.

The mechanism of recurrence can be related to lack of understanding of the difficult laparoscopic anatomy, wrong hernia repair technique or the wrong prosthesis. These include incomplete dissection without proper pocket formation, missed sac, migration of mesh due to small sized mesh which may be prone to displaced once fixed, inadequate fixation with rolling up of the mesh and hematoma formation leading to infection.

The complication of laparoscopic hernia repair can be summarized as follows:
• *Immediate:* Visceral injury, vascular injury, injury to vas, spermatic vessels (Fig. 15.24)

• *Late:* Bowel adhesions to mesh, intestinal obstruction, fistulization, orchitis, testicular atrophy, nerve entrapment, incisional hernia recurrence (Fig. 15.26).

Relative Contraindication for Laparoscopic Approach

A. Obesity with BMI >30
B. Significant chest disease
C. Patient on anticoagulants
D. Adhesions
E. Massive hernias
F. Pregnancy
G. Unfit for GA.

Inguinal Hernia Repair in Pediatric Patients

Small children gain little benefit from laparoscopic hernia repair as inguinal skin crease incision used in the herniotomy is one of best incisions as far as cosmesis is concerned. It is hardly visible after a few months. Also, it is covered by underwear. Compared to this three stab incisions, however small, are in the visible area.

Inguinal Hernia Repair in Obese Patients

Operations in patients with BMI above 27 may be difficult for less experienced surgeons, particularly when trying to encircle an indirect sac. Patients with BMI of above 30 should be encouraged to loose weight or should even be turned down for the laparoscopic approach. They are incidentally more likely to develop recurrence after an open hernia repair. It is also easy for the laparoscopic surgeon to become disoriented when the patient is very obese.

Inguinal Hernia Repair in Recurrence

Generally, the short-term recurrence rate of laparoscopic inguinal hernia repair is reported to be less than 5%. In both the open and laparoscopic repair procedures, the aim is to cover the whole inguino-femoral area by a preperitoneal prosthetic mesh, and recurrences should not occur. When they do occur, recurrences must be regarded as technical failures. Recurrences after laparoscopic repair most often result from using too small a mesh, or not using staples to fix the mesh. Most recurrences after laparoscopic hernia repair occurred medially, and the technique was

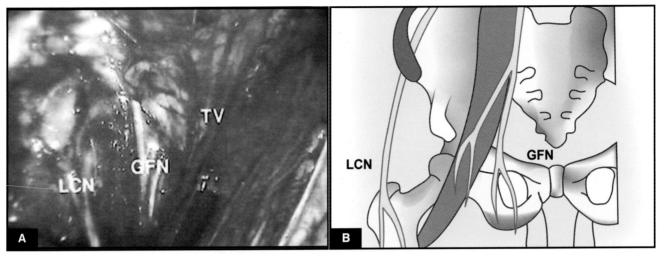

Figs 15.25A and B: Anatomical landmarks, TV–Testicular vessel, GFN–Genitofemoral nerve, LCN–Lateral cutaneous nerve of high

adjusted. The mesh is now placed at least until the midline, and occasionally hernia staples are used when an adequate overlap (2 cm) cannot be achieved medially. The totally extraperitoneal technique is now used more often, allowing for better visual control in the medial part of the operating field.

Operating Time

Operating times of surgical techniques varies between surgeons and also vary considerably between centers. It reduces with experience and comparison between laparoscopic and open surgery is subject to bias due to pre-existing familiarity with open techniques. It is less important to the patient than a successful operation; the time taken to perform the surgery can have cost implications. The operative time to perform unilateral primary inguinal repair has frequently been reported as longer for laparoscopic compared to open repair, however, the mean difference in 36 of 37 randomized trials is 14.81 minutes. These differences disappear in bilateral and recurrent hernia repairs.

Postoperative Pain and Amount of Narcotics Used

The open tension-free mesh repair is found to cause less postoperative pain than open non-mesh repairs, however, most randomized trials assessing post-operative pain between open tension-free repairs and laparoscopic repairs, report less pain in the

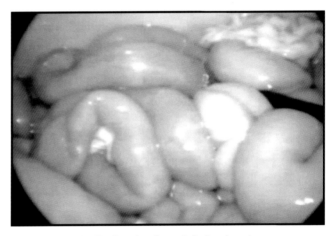

Fig. 15.26: Perforation bowel during hernia surgery

laparoscopic groups. In many cases, this also results in less analgesia being consumed by the patient.

Complication Rates

Complications in endoscopic inguinal hernia surgery are more dangerous and more frequent than those of open surgery, especially in inexperienced hands and hence are best avoided. It is possible to avoid most of these complications if one follows a set of well-defined steps and principles of endoscopic inguinal hernia surgery.

Complications of laparoscopic repair of inguinal hernia can be divided into:
• Intraoperative
• Postoperative.

INTRAOPERATIVE COMPLICATIONS AND PRECAUTION

During Creation of Preperitoneal Space

This is the most important step for beginners.
- A wide linea alba may result in breaching the peritoneum; in such a situation, it is best to close the rectus and incise the sheath more laterally.
- Improper placement of balloon trocar causing dissection of muscle fibers.
- Entry into peritoneum causing pneumoperitoneum
- Rupture of balloon in preperitoneal space.
- The Hassan's trocar must snugly fit into the incision to avoid CO_2 leak.

To avoid these, one must ensure that the balloon is made properly and the correct space is entered by retracting the rectus muscle laterally to visualize the posterior rectus sheath. Also the balloon trocar is inserted gently, parallel to the abdominal wall, to avoid puncturing the peritoneum. The balloon must be inflated slowly with saline to ensure smooth and even distension and prevent its rupture.

Precautions During Port Placement

The trocars should be short and threaded in proportion to less workspace and to ensure a snug fit respectively. The skin incisions should be just adequate to grip the trocar and prevent its slipping. The patient should empty their bladder before surgery as the suprapubic trocar could injure a filled bladder. The pressure in the preperitoneal space must be such as to offer sufficient resistance during trocar insertion to avoid puncturing the peritoneum.

Correct Identification of the Anatomical Landmarks

The next most important and crucial step in any hernia surgery is the correct identification of anatomical landmarks. This is difficult for beginners as the anatomy is different from that seen in open surgery. The first most important step is to identify the pubic bone. Once this is seen, the rest of the landmarks are traced keeping this as reference point. One is advised to keep away from the triangle of doom, which contains the iliac vessels and to avoid placing tacks in the triangle of pain laterally.

Bladder Injuries

Bladder injury most commonly occurs during port placement, dissecting a large direct sac or in a sliding hernia. It is mandatory to empty the bladder prior to an inguinal hernia repair to avoid a trocar injury. It is advisable that beginners catheterize the bladder during the initial part of their learning curve. The diagnosis is evident when one sees urine in the extraperitoneal space. Repair is done with vicryl in two layers and a urinary catheter inserted for 7-10 days.

Bowel Injuries

Bowel injury is rare during hernia surgery. It can occur when reducing large hernias, inadvertent opening of peritoneum causing the bowel to come into the field of surgery and in reduction of sliding hernias. Injury is best avoided in such circumstances by opening the hernial sac as close as possible to the deep ring. The initial studies showed a higher incidence, especially with TAPP, but it decreased over time.

Vascular Injury

This is one of the commonest injuries occurring in hernia repair and often a reason for conversion. The various sites where it can occur is rectus muscle vessel injury during trocar insertion; inferior epigastric vessel injury; bleeding from venous plexus on the pubic symphysis; aberrant obturator vein injury; testicular vessel injury; and the most disastrous of all, iliac vessels, which requires an emergency conversion to control the bleeding and the immediate services of a vascular surgeon to repair the same. Most of the other bleeding can be controlled with cautery or clips. Careful dissection and adherence to the principles of surgery will help in avoiding most of these injuries.

Injury to Vas Deferens

Injury occurs while dissecting the hernia sac from the cord structures. The injury causes an eventual fibrotic narrowing of the vas. A complete transaction of the vas needs to be repaired in a young patient. An injury to the vas is best avoided and this may be done by identifying before dividing any structure near the deep ring or floor of the extraperitoneal space. Also, the separation of cord structures from the hernial sac must be gentle and direct; grasping of vas deferens with forceps must be avoided.

Pneumoperitoneum

It is a common occurrence in TEP which every surgeon should be prepared to handle. Putting the patient in Trendelenburg's position and increasing the insufflation pressures to 15 mm Hg helps. If the problem still persists, a Veress needle can be inserted at Palmer's point.

POSTOPERATIVE COMPLICATIONS

Seroma/Hematoma Formation

It is a common complication after laparoscopic hernia surgery, the incidence being in the range of 5-25% (Fig. 15.24). They are especially seen after large indirect hernia repair. Most resolve spontaneously over 4-6 weeks. A seroma can be avoided by minimizing dissection of the hernia sac from the cord structures, fixing the direct sac to pubic bone and fenestrating the transversalis fascia in a direct hernia. Some surgeons put in a drain if there is excessive bleeding or after extensive dissection.

Urinary Retention

This complication after hernia repair has a reported incidence of 1.3 to 5.8%. It is usually precipitated in elderly patients, especially if symptoms of prostatism are present. These patients are best catheterized prior to surgery and catheter removed the next day morning.

Neuralgias

The incidence of this complication is reported to be between 0.5 and 4.6% depending on the technique of repair. The intraperitoneal onlay mesh method had the highest incidence of neuralgias in one study and was hence abandoned as a form of viable repair. The commonly involved nerves are lateral cutaneous nerve of thigh, genitofemoral nerve and intermediate cutaneous nerve of thigh (Figs 15.25A and B). They are usually involved by mesh-induced fibrosis or entrapment by a tack. The complication is prevented by avoiding fixing the mesh lateral to the deep inguinal ring in the region of the triangle of pain, safe dissection of a large hernial sac and no dissection of fascia over the psoas.

Testicular Pain and Swelling

It occurs due to excessive dissection of a sac from the cord structures, especially a complete sac. The reported incidence is of 0.9 to 1.5% ,most are transient. Orchitis was found in a small number of patients but did not lead to testicular atrophy.

Mesh Infection and Wound Infection

Wound infection rates are very low. Mesh infection is a very serious complication and care must be taken to maintain strict aseptic precautions during the entire procedure. Any endogenous infection must be treated with an adequate course of antibiotics prior to surgery.

Recurrence

It is the most important endpoint of any hernia surgery. It requires a proper and thorough knowledge of anatomy and a thorough technique of repair to help keep the recurrence in endoscopic repair to a minimum.

POSTOPERATIVE RECOVERY

Marked variations are seen in postoperative recovery due to patient motivation, postoperative advice, and definition of "normal activity", existing co-morbidity and local "culture". Nevertheless all trials reporting this as an endpoint of study show a significant improvement in the laparoscopic group, with no real difference between the TAPP and TEP groups. This is estimated to equate to an absolute difference of about 7 days in terms of time off work.

RECURRENCE

Recurrence rates are low with the use of mesh and not significantly different between open or laparoscopic techniques.

CAUSES OF RECURRENCE IN LAPAROSCOPIC INGUINAL HERNIA REPAIR

The factors involved in mesh dislocation or failure are insufficient size, wrong/defective material, incorrect placement, immediate or very early displacement by folding, lifting by a hematoma or urinary retention, missed cord lipomas and herniation through the keyhole (mesh slit) late displacement by insufficient scar tissue ingrowth, mesh protrusion, collagen disease or pronounced shrinkage. Despite the correct and stable mesh position, there is still a limited risk of a late sliding of the retroperitoneal fat under/ in front of the mesh into the enlarged inner ring.

Leibl in 2000 advised to avoid slitting of the mesh and increase its size to reduce the recurrence rate. Generous dissection of preperitoneal space is required to eliminate potential herniation through the slit or strangulation of the cord structures completely and reduces the risk of genitofemoral neuropathy.

Mesh Size

The mesh size should be adequate to cover the entire myopectineal orifice. The established size in 2006 is 15 × 10 cm per unilateral hernia, with minor deviations.

Mesh Material

The mechanical strength of available meshes exceeds the intra-abdominal peak pressures and by far even the lightweight meshes are strong enough for inguinal repair. Aachen group made an important contribution for understanding the interaction of the living tissue with the implanted mesh material. The negative impact of pronounced shrinkage of the traditional heavy weight meshes was recognized as an important factor promoting recurrence. Schumpelick introduced the logical trend of the use of light weight meshes. The new macroporous compound meshes present both the successful reduction of the overall foreign body amount and the preservation of mesh elasticity after the scar tissue ingrowths, due to very limited shrinkage and reduced bridging effect.

Fixation of the Mesh

In the early years of laparoscopic hernia repairs, a strong fixation seemed to be the most important factor in prevention of recurrence. With growing size of the mesh and true macroporous materials being used, the belief in strength reduced and gave way to the concern of acute/chronic pain possibly caused by fixation. The controversy of fixing or nonfixing the mesh is currently under scrutiny.

Technical Experience

The long learning curve of endoscopic repairs presents the potential risk of technical errors leading to unacceptable rise of recurrence rate. This fact highlights the need for structured well-mentored teaching, a high level of standardization of the procedure and rigorous adherence to the principles of laparoscopic hernia repair. The impact of experience on the recurrence rate was in both extremes well documented.

Collagen Status

Inborn or acquired abnormalities in collagen synthesis are associated with higher incidence of hernia formation and recurrences.

Other Factors

The negative effect on healing in hernia repair is often related with malnutrition, obesity, steroids, type II diabetes, chronic lung disease, jaundice, radiotherapy, chemotherapy, oral anticoagulants, smoking, heavy lifting, malignancy and anemia. Laparoscopic inguinal hernia repair offers excellent results in experienced hands.

Bilateral Assessment and Treatment

Up to 30 percent of patients with a unilateral hernia will subsequently develop a further hernia on the contralateral side. Also, when examined at operation, 10-25 percent is found to have an occult hernia on the contralateral side. Both laparoscopic approaches allow assessment and treatment of the contralateral side at the same operation without the need for further surgical incisions, very little further dissection and minimal additional postoperative pain. In open surgery a further large incision is required in the opposite groin. This considerably impairs postoperative mobility and increases the likelihood of admission to hospital. Some surgeons advocate routine repair of the contralateral side during laparoscopic repair.

Cost Effectiveness

It is suggested that laparoscopic hernia repair is more expensive to perform than open hernia repair. The primary reason for this relates to the cost of extra

Section Two

equipment used for the laparoscopic repair with secondary costs attributed to perceived increases in operating time for the laparoscopic procedure. From the Indian perspective, various factors come into play when analyzing the cost implications of laparoscopic repair of inguinal hernia. In most hospitals, except the larger corporate ones, the theatre time is charged on a per-case basis rather than by the hour. Thus, increase in the operating time, particularly during the learning curve, does not necessarily mean additional expense for the patient. If the surgeon were to adopt cost-containment strategies such as use of reusable laparoscopic instruments (which is more or less the norm in India) as against disposable ones, use of indigenous balloons devices rather than commercially available ones, sparing use of fixation devices and reliance on sutures for fixation of the mesh, the cost of the laparoscopic hernia repair should be comparable to the open repair. It is likely that many surgeons are already practicing these strategies and passing on the benefits of laparoscopic repair to their patients.

Learning Curve

This period represents the developmental and learning curve for the consultant and the senior registrars. There have been some modifications of the technique as difficulties have been recognized. There is steep learning curve for laparoscopic repair. Initially everyone used to fix mesh with staples, but nowadays many surgeons are using sutures for it. As experience increases, our ability to recognize finer structures and to keep within the correct tissue planes, improves. This has been associated with lower minor-complication rates and higher percentage of pain-free recoveries.

RECOMMENDATION

The important points to be kept in mind during the surgery are:
  i. After dissecting direct sac, all peritoneal adhesions around the margin of the defect should be meticulously lysed.
  ii. Always search for an indirect sac, even if a direct hernia has been reduced.
  iii. Reflect the peritoneum off the cord completely.
  iv. Place an adequate size mesh to cover the myopectineal orifice completely, preferably the size of 15 × 15 cm.
  v. The lower margin of the mesh must be comfortably placed - medially in the retropubic space and laterally over the psoas muscle.
  vi. Perform a 2-point fixation of the mesh on the medial aspect over the Cooper's ligament.
  vii. Avoid cutting of the mesh over the cord. This weakens the mesh and provides a potential site for recurrence.
  viii. Ensure adequate hemostasis prior to placing the mesh.
  ix. The most important factor is the adequate training and learning of the right technique.

Vascular Injury

The incidence of vascular injury has been documented to be about 0.5-1 percent and inferior epigastric artery is the one most commonly traumatized.
- *Injury to iliac vessels:* Chances of mortality
- *Inferior epigastric vessel:* Hematoma
- *Iliopubic vein and artery which traverse the lacunar ligament:* Hematoma
- *Injury to Spermatic vessels:* Postoperative scrotal hematoma.

Nerve Entrapment and Injury

The lateral cutaneous nerve of thigh and the femoral branch of genitofemoral nerve are the two nerves vulnerable to trauma due to indiscriminate placement of staplers lateral to the spermatic cord on the iliopubic tract.
- Injury of lateral cutaneous nerve injury.
- *Most common nerve injured is lateral femoral cutaneous nerve (2%):* Hyperesthesia or paresthesia of upper aspect of thigh and hip.
- If pain starts days after surgery, it will recover within 2-4 weeks (or percutaneous steroid).
- If pain starts within 24 hours of surgery there is permanent nerve damage.
- Cryotherapy with destruction of sensory branch is indicated.
- Lifelong numbness.

Nerve entrapment should be avoided in laparoscopic repair of hernia:
- Genitofemoral nerve injury.
- *Genitofemoral nerve injury (1%):* Hyperesthesia or Paresthesia of scrotum.

- Not significant.
- With time it will subside.

Other Complications

- Migration of mesh.
- Rejection of mesh (Rare).
- Bowel adhesion.

Complete transaction of vas requires immediate anastomosis. Other complications include testicular pain, orchitis, epididymitis, swelling due to seromas or hematoma. The treatment is supportive and incidence of all these complications is similar to that in conventional surgery.

After some experience most cases of inguinal hernia can be treated laparoscopically. Several prospective randomized trials comparing open versus laparoscopic repair have reported. Reduced postoperative pain, earlier return to work and fewer complications and less chance of recurrences for the laparoscopic approach are some of the crucial advantages. Although the procedural cost for laparoscopic hernia repair is more compared to conventional repair but overall expense for open repair is high if we calculate number of working days lost and medication is taken into consideration. Data is now available which documents the totally extraperitoneal repair to have distinct advantage over the transabdominal preperitoneal repair in terms of lesser postoperative complications and lower recurrence rate. TAPP has been stated to violate the peritoneal cavity with all its known possible complication of pneumoperitoneum, vessel or bowel injury. There is no doubt that the laparoscopic hernia repair is a proven technique and will become more popular over a period of time.

Perforation

The first important step after access to the abdomen has been gained, is to check for damage caused by trocar insertion. A second 5 mm port may then be inserted under vision in an appropriate quadrant to take a palpating rod.

The usual site of insertion of the trocar/cannula for diagnostic laparoscopy is below or to the side of the umbilicus. This position may require to be altered in the presence of abdominal scars. The use of a 30° forward oblique telescope is preferable for viewing the surface architecture of organs. By rotation of the telescope, different angles of inspection can be achieved.

A systematic examination of the abdomen must be performed just as in laparotomy. We begin at the left lobe of the liver but any scheme can be used as long as it is consistent. Next, check around the falciform ligament to the right lobe of liver, gallbladder and hiatus. After checking the stomach, move on to the cecum and appendix and check the terminal ileum. Follow the colon round to the sigmoid colon, and then check the pelvis. Surgeon should be conversant with sampling and biopsy techniques, the use of position and manipulation to aid vision.

When performing a diagnostic laparoscopy to confirm appendicitis, a 5 mm port is placed in the left iliac fossa to facilitate manipulation. The patient is placed headdown and rotated to the left to displace the small bowel from the pelvis and allow the uterus and ovaries to be checked. This, however, should be limited to avoid contamination of subphrenic spaces, if this is not already present.

At the time of diagnostic laparoscopy all the abdominal organs are inspected for any gross anatomical abnormalities. Abdominal cavity is inspected for excess of fluids. Samples are taken if free fluid is present for laboratory tests (chemistry, cytology or bacteriology). Peritoneal lavage and adhesiolysis may need to be performed to improve visualization of organs. At the time of peritoneal lavage when fluid is sucked from the cul-de-sac, it is important to keep all the holes of the suction-irrigator beneath the level of the fluid to avoid removing pneumoperitoneum. If the suction-irrigator is positioned improperly, the CO_2 gas will be removed preferentially. However, with high-flow insufflators, pneumoperitoneum rarely is lost and quickly restored.

Ending of the Operation

At the end of surgery, abdomen should be re-examined for any possible bowel injury or hemorrhage. The entire accessory, instrument and then the port is removed. The telescope should be removed leaving gas valve of umbilical port open to let out all the gas. Once the complete gas is out, for removing primary cannula telescope or any blunt instrument should be introduced again and cannula should be pulled over that instrument to prevent pull of omentum or bowel. Wound should be closed with suture. Vicryl should be used for rectus and Unabsorbable intradermal or stapler for skin. Only 10 mm port wound is necessary to repair. Adhesive sterile dressing over the wound should be applied.

At the end of diagnostic laparoscopy surgeon can perform therapeutic laparoscopy if indicated and consent from patients relative can be obtained.

Patient may be discharged on the same day after operation if every thing goes well. The patient may have slight pain initially but usually resolves. Diagnostic laparoscopic is a useful method for reducing hospital stay, complications and return to normal activity if carried on in proper manner.

COMPLICATIONS

Complications may occur during access, trocar insertion, or the diagnostic manipulation of viscera. These complications include, cardiac arrhythmias, hemodynamic instability due to decreased venous return, bleeding, bile leak, perforation of a hollow viscus, laceration of a solid organ, vascular injury, gas embolism, and subcutaneous or extraperitoneal dissection of the insufflation gas. If proper sterilization of instrument is not done, wound infection or leakage of ascites may occur postoperatively. Failure to accurately diagnose the extent of intra-abdominal pathology is another potential complication for which patient may have to go for other surgery.

CONCLUSION

Diagnostic laparoscopy is one of the very important method of investigation for patients in whom the diagnosis or extent of the disease is unclear or the abdominal findings are equivocal. It can be performed safely in an inpatient or outpatient setting, potentially expediting diagnosis and treatment.

Laparoscopic hernia repair is safe and provide less postoperative morbidity in experienced hands and definitely have many advantages over open repair. For bilateral and recurrent inguinal hernias, laparoscopic approach is recommended. Nowadays, it is recommended also for primary inguinal hernia. For sliding hernia also TAPP is the preferred approach.

"The final word on hernia will probably never be written. In collecting, assimilating and distilling the wisdom of today we must provide a base from which further advances may be made."

BIBLIOGRAPHY

1. Aasvang E, Kehlet H. Chronic postoperative pain: the case of inguinal herniorrhaphy. Br J Anaesth 2005;95(1): 69–76.
2. Abrahamson J. Etiology and pathophysiology of primary and recurrent groin hernia formation. Surg Clin North Am 1998;78: 953–972 22. Barkun JS, et al. Laparoscopic verus open inguinal herniorrhaphy: preliminary results of a randomized controlled trial. Surgery 118: 703–10.
3. Amid PK, Shulman AG, Lichtenstein IL. Open "tensionfree" repair of inguinal hernias: the Lichtenstein technique. Eur J Surg 1996;162(6): 447–53.
4. Bay-Nielsen M, Nilsson E, Nordin P, Kehlet H. Chronic pain after open mesh and sutured repair of indirect inguinal hernia in young males. Br J Surg 2004;91(10): 1372–6.
5. Bay-Nielsen M, Perkins FM, Kehlet H. Pain and functional impairment 1 year after inguinal herniorrhaphy: a nationwide questionnaire study. Ann Surg 2001;233(1): 1–7
6. Beets GL, et al. Open or laparoscopic pereperitoneal mesh repair for recurrent inguinal hernia: a randomized controlled trial. On the repair of inguinal hernia University of Maastricht, Maastricht, The Netherlands, 108.
7. Bessel JR, et al. A randomized controlled trial of laparoscopic extraperitoneal hernia repair as a day surgical procedure. Surg Endosc 1996;10: 495–500.
8. Burney RE, et al. Core outcomes measures for inguinal hernia repair. J Am Coll Surg 185: 509–15.
9. Callesen T, Bech K, Kehlet H. Prospective study of chronic pain after groin hernia repair. Br J Surg 1999;86(12): 1528–31.
10. Champault G, et al. Inguinal hernia repair: totally preperitoneal laparoscopic approach versus Stoppa operation. Randomized trial of 100 cases. Surg Laparosc Endosc 7: 445–50.
11. Cunningham J, et al. Cooperative hernia study: pain in the postrepair patient. Ann Surg 224: 598–602.
12. Cunningham J, Temple WJ, Mitchell P, Nixon JA, Preshaw RM, Hagen NA. Cooperative hernia study. Pain in the postrepair patient. Ann Surg 1996;224(5): 598–602
13. Damamme A, et al. Evaluation me´dico-e´conomique de la cure de hernie inguinale: Shouldice vs laparoscopie. Ann Chir 52: 11–16 29. Fuchsja¨ger N, Feichter A, Kux M. Die Lichtenstein-Plug Methode sur Reparation von Rezidivleistenhernien: Indikation, Technik und Ergebnisse. Chirurg 1995;66: 409–412.
14. EU Hernia Trialists Collaboration. Repair of groin hernia with synthetic mesh: meta-analysis of randomized controlled trials. Ann Surg 2002;235(3): 322–32.
15. Gerber S, Hammerli PA, Glattli A. Laparoscopic transabdominal preperitoneal hernioplasty. Evaluation of complications due to transabdominal approach. Chirurg 2000;71(7): 824–8.

16. Glassow F. Inguinal hernia repair. Am J Surg 1976;131: 306–311 .

17. Grant AM (2002) Open mesh versus non-mesh repair of groin hernia: meta-analysis of randomised trials based on individual patient data [corrected]. Hernia 6(3): 130–136.

18. Heikkinen T, et al. Total costs of laparoscopic and Lichtenstein inguinal hernai repairs: a randomized prospective study. Surg Laparosc Endsoc 7:1–5

19. Helbling C, Schlumpf R (2003) Sutureless Lichtenstein: first results of a prospective randomised clinical trial. Hernia 7(2): 80–84 23. Hidalgo M, Castillo MJ, Eymar JL, Hidalgo A. Lichtenstein inguinal hernioplasty: sutures versus glue. Hernia 2005;9: 242–244 24. Topart P, Vandenbroucke F, Lozac_h P. Tisseel versus tack staples as mesh fixation in totally extraperitoneal laparoscopic repair of groin hernias: a retrospective analysis. Surg Endosc 2005;19(5): 724–727 133.

20. Herzog U, Kocher T. Leistenhernienchirurgie in der Schweiz 1994: eine Umfrage an 142 Ausbildungskliniken in der Schweiz [Surgery ofinguinal hernia in Switzerland in 1994: a survey of 142 teaching clinics in Switzerland]. Chirurg 1996;67:921–6.

21. Hofbauer C, et al. Late mesh rejection as a complication to transab- 1064 dominal preperitoneal laparoscopic hernia repair. Surg Endosc 12: 1164–5.

22. Hyryla ML, Sintonen H. The use of health services in the management of wound infection. J Hosp Infect 1994;26:1–14.

23. International Association for the Study of Pain. Classification of chronic pain. Descriptions of chronic pain syndromes and definitions of pain terms. Prepared by the International Association for the Study of Pain Subcommittee on Taxonomy. Pain Suppl 1986;3: S1–S226.

24. Kald A, et al. Surgical outcome and cost-minimisation-analysis of laparoscopic and open hernia repair: a randomised prospective trial with one year follow-up. Eur J Surg 163: 505–10.

25. Kingsnorth AN, Gray MR, Nott DM (1992) Prospective randomized trial comparing the Shouldice and plication darn for inguinal hernia. Br J Surg 79: 1068–70.

26. Kumar S, Wilson RG, Nixon SJ, Macintyre IM. Chronic pain after laparoscopic and open mesh repair of groin hernia. Br J Surg 2002;89(11): 1476–1479 21. Canonico S, Santoriello A, Campitiello F, Fattopace A, Corte AD, Sordelli I, Benevento R. Mesh fixation with human fibrin glue (Tissucol) in open tension-free inguinal hernia repair: a preliminary report. Hernia 2005;9: 330–333.

27. Lawrence K, et al. Randomised controlled trial of laparoscopic versus open repair of inguinal hernia repair: early results. Br Med J 311: 981–5.

28. Lichtenstein IL, Shulman AG, Amid PK. The tension-free repair of groin hernias. In: Nyhus LM (ed) Hernia Lippincott, Philadelphia, 1995;237–249.

29. Liem MSL, et al. Comparison of conventional anterior surgery and laparoscopic surgery for inguinal hernia repair. N Engl J Med 336: 1541–7.

30. Liem MSL, et al. Cost-effectiveness of extraperitoneal laparoscopic inguinal hernia repair: a randomized comparison with conventionalherniorrhaphy. Ann Surg 336: 668–76.

31. Lorenz H, Trede M. Oral communication at the surgical week in Mexico City. TAPP vs Shouldice. Surg Week, August 1997.

32. Lowham AS, et al. Mechanisms of hernia recurrence after preperitoneal mesh repair: traditional and laparoscopic. Ann Surg 225: 422–431.

33. Maddern GJ, et al. A comparison of laparoscopic and open hernia repair as a day surgical procedure. Surg Endosc 8: 1404–08.

34. McCormack K, Scott NW, Go PM, Ross S, Grant AM. Laparoscopic techniques versus open techniques for inguinal hernia repair. Cochrane Database Syst Rev 2003;(1): CD001785.

35. Memon MA, Cooper NJ, Memon B, Memon MI, Abrams KR. Meta-analysis of randomized clinical trials comparing open and laparoscopic inguinal hernia repair. Br J Surg 2003;90(12): 1479–92.

36. Mikkelsen T, Werner MU, Lassen B, Kehlet H. Pain and sensory dysfunction 6 to 12 months after inguinal herniotomy. Anesth Analg 2004;99(1): 146–151.

37. Mixter CG, Meeker LD, Gavin TJ. Preemptive pain control in patients having laparoscopic hernia repair: a comparison of ketorolac and ibuprofen. Arch Surg 1998;133: 432–7.

38. MRC Laparoscopic Groin Hernia Trial Group Laparoscopic versus open repair of groin hernia: a randomised comparison. The MRC Laparoscopic Groin Hernia Trial Group. Lancet 1999;354(9174): 185–90.

39. Nilsson E, et al. Methods of repair and risk for reoperation Swedish hernia surgery from 1992 to 1996. Br J Surg 85: 1686–1691.

40. Nordin P, Bartelmess P, Jansson C, Svensson C, Edlund G Randomized trial of Lichtenstein versus Shouldice hernia repair in general surgical practice. Br J Surg 2002;89(1): 45–9.

41. Nyhus LM, Klein MS, Rogers FB. Inguinal hernia. Curr Probl Surg 1991;38: 28.

42. Payne JH Jr, et al. Laparoscopic or open inguinal herniorraphy? A randomized prospective trial. Arch Surg 129: 973–81.

43. Poobalan AS, Bruce J, King PM, Chambers WA, Krukowski ZH, Smith WC. Chronic pain and quality of life following open inguinal hernia repair. Br J Surg 2001;88(8): 1122–6.

44. Poobalan AS, Bruce J, Smith WC, King PM, Krukowski ZH, Chambers WA. A review of chronic pain after inguinal herniorrhaphy. Clin J Pain 2003;19(1): 48–54.

45. Rotman N, et al. Prophylactic antibiotherapy in abdominal surgery: first vs third-generation cephalosporins. Arch Surg 124: 323–7.

46. Rutkow IM. The recurrence rate in hernia surgery: how important is it? Arch Surg 1995;130: 575–6.

47. Salcedo-Wasicek MD, Thirlby RC. Postoperative course after herniorrhaphy: a case-controlled comparison of patients receiving workers compensation vs patients with commercial insurance. Arch Surg 1995;130: 29–32.

48. Sales JP, Lorand I, Gayral F. Pratiques Franc¸aises enmatie're de cure de hernie inguinale. Etude des donne´es. PMSI National 1997. In: Congre's de l'Association Franc¸aise de Chirurgie. Paris., October 1999;4-5:2000.

Section Two

49. Schrenk P, et al. Prospective randomized trial comparing postoperative and return to physical activity after transabdominal preperitoneal, total preperitoneal and Shouldice techniques for inguinal hernia repair. Br J Surg 83: 1563–1566.

50. Shulman AG, Amid PK, Lichtenstein IL. The safety of mesh repair for primary inguinal hernia. Am Surg 1992;58: 255–7.

51. Simons MP, Hoitsma HFW, Mullan FJ. Primary inguinal hernia repair in the Netherlands. Eur J Surg 1995;161: 345–8.

52. Southern Surgeons Club A prospective analysis of 1518 laparoscopic cholecystectomies. N Engl J Med 324: 1073–78.

53. Stoker DL, et al. Laparoscopic versus open inguinal hernia repair: randomized prospective trial. Lancet 343: 1243–5.

54. Striffeler H, Zufferey S, Schweizer W (1993) Quality control after introduction of a new hernia technique. Barwell transversal fasciaplasty. Helv Chir Acta 59(5–6): 771–4.

55. Taylor SG, O'Dwyer PJ. Chronic groin sepsis following tension- free inguinal hernioplasty. Br J Surg 1999;86: 562–5.

56. Vogt DM, et al. Preliminary results of a prospective randomized trial of laparoscopic only versus conventional inguinal herniorrhaphy. Am J Surg 169: 84–90.

57. Vrijland WW, van den Tol MP, Luijendijk RW, Hop WC, Busschbach JJ, de Lange DC, van Geldere D, Rottier AB, Vegt PA, JN IJ, Jeekel J. Randomized clinical trial of nonmesh versus mesh repair of primary inguinal hernia. Br J Surg 2002;89(3): 293–7.

58. Wellwood J, et al. Randomised controlled trial of laparscopic versus open mesh repair for inguinal hernia: outcome and cost. Br Med J 317: 103–10.

59. Wilson MS, Deans GT, Brough WA. Prospective trial comparing Lichtenstein with laparoscopic tension-free mesh repair of inguinal hernia. Br J Surg 1995;82: 274–7.

60. Wright DM, et al. Early outcome after open versus extra-peritoneal tension-free hernioplasty: a randomized clinical trial. Surgery 119: 552–7.

61. Zieren J, Zieren HU, Jacobi CA, Wenger FA, Muller JM. Prospective randomized study comparing laparoscopic and open tensionfree inguinal hernia repair with Shouldice's operation. Am J Surg 1998;1065;175: 330–3.

Section Two

16 Laparoscopic Repair of Ventral Hernia

INTRODUCTION

Ventral hernias refer to fascial defects of the anterolateral abdominal wall through which intermittent or continuous protrusion of abdominal tissue or organs may occur (Fig. 16.1). They are either congenital or acquired. In adults, more than 80% of ventral hernias result from previous surgery hence the term incisional hernias. They have been reported to occur after 0-26% of abdominal procedures. Although these hernias mostly become clinically manifest between 2 to 5 years after surgery, studies have shown that, the process starts within the first postoperative month. They are said to occur as a result of a biomechanical failure of the acute fascial wound coupled with clinically relevant impediments to acute tissue repair and normal support function of the abdominal wall.

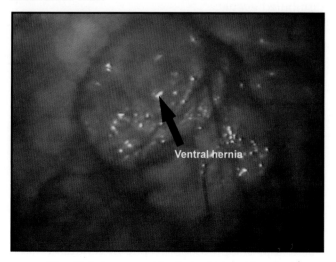

Fig. 16.1: Laparoscopic view of ventral hernia

Historically, incisional hernias have been repaired with either primary suture techniques or placement of a variety of prosthetic materials. Before the 1960's, most ventral hernias were repaired primarily with suture and a few with metallic meshes. Even with some modifications, recurrence rates with the primary suture repair ranged from 24-54%. The introduction of polypropylene mesh repair by Usher in 1958 opened a new era of tension-free herniorrhaphy. Recurrence rates with prosthetic mesh decreased to 10-20%. Subsequently, it was realized that the placement and fixation of the mesh was more crucial in determining the outcome of the repair. The placement of the mesh in the preperitoneal, retromuscular position with a wide overlap of at least 5 cm over the hernia defect in all directions was introduced in the late 1980's. The refinement of this method decreased the recurrence rates to as low as 3.5% making it to be declared the standard of care of ventral hernias. However, implantation of the mesh by open techniques requires wide dissection of soft tissue contributing to an increase in wound infection and wound-related complications.

Ventral hernia results from a weakness in the musculo-aponeurotic layer of the anterior abdominal wall. This type of hernia has root of development during the period of development like; omphalocele, gastroschisis and congenital umbilical hernia.

Recently, the ventral hernias are reported more due to iatrogenic factor. Even after laparoscopic surgery, if the 10 mm port is not repaired properly there is always a chance of ventral hernia (Incisional hernia) development. Obviously the initial closure is the most important, since faulty technique will universally lead to development of herniation. There are other associated co-morbid conditions, which may encourage the creation of incisional herniation. These include intra-abdominal or wound infection, morbid obesity, steroid use, previous use of the incision, hematoma formation and respiratory compromise with increased cough. Other factors include duration of the operation, crossing incisions, ineffective wound drainage, and excessive wound tension. Two other important variables include nutritional aspects as well as presence of cancer which overall reduce the ability for wound healing and collagen deposition in the wound.

The repair of incisional and ventral hernias continues to be a surgical challenge. Reports published in the medical literature indicate 3 to 13 percent of laparotomy patients develop incisional hernias. Moreover, clinical studies indicate that the traditional, or open, technique to repair large abdominal wall defects is associated with recurrence rates ranging from 25-49 percent.

Among the non-iatrogenic ventral hernias, divarication of rectus abdominis, umbilical, para-umbilical, spigelian and epigastric are more common. In 1992, a successful series of laparoscopic incisional hernia repairs was reported in the medical literature. Since then, the technique has been refined and has grown in acceptance within the surgical community.

The laparoscopic technique for ventral hernia repair involves the placement of a tension free prosthetic bridge across the musculofacial defect rather than attempting to approximate the edge of defect. The hernia defect is covered by appropriate size of mesh once the content of the sac is reduced. Most of the time sac content is omentum. Sometime omentum is adhered so tightly that electrosurgical dissection with the help of bipolar is essential. Recently, many newer type of mesh is available in which PTFE and polypropylene is more popular. There was always a fear of bowel adhesion and fistulization with use of polypropylene mesh but the clinical evidence of thousands of surgery has suggested that the omental adhesion is expected but bowel adhesion is not common and intraperitoneal placement of poly-propylene mesh is quite safe.

Almost all type of ventral hernia can be repaired by minimal access surgical approach. Hernias like multiple defects (Swiss cheese hernias) are greatly benefited by this approach as all defects get directly visualized and appropriately covered by single mesh.

Contraindication of laparoscopic repair of ventral hernia are very large hernia with huge protrusion of skin which is thin enough and skin fold is necessary to correct by abdominoplasty. Dense intra-abdominal adhesions are also a relative contraindication of laparoscopic repair of ventral hernia.

LAPAROSCOPIC ANATOMY

Ventral hernia develops due to structural weakness of the abdominal wall. The muscle and fascia that span the space between costal margin superiorly, the spine and muscles of the back posteriorly, and the pelvis inferiorly support the abdominal wall by giving strength. The parietal peritoneum in ventral hernia extends into the defect to form the sac. Adhesions to adjacent viscera must be divided to define the defect.

OPERATIVE PROCEDURE

Patient should be clearly informed that laparoscopic repairs will not help cosmetically if the skin is lax and hanging loosely. Bowel preparation is a good practice to have more room inside the abdominal cavity to handle instrument. After anesthesia, nasogastric tube is must to deflate the stomach completely because in most of the cases access should be through left hypochondria. Splenohepatomegaly is absolute contraindication of the access through left hypochondrium. Patient is placed in supine position without any tilt of the operation table so that bowel is distributed evenly.

Position of Surgical Team

Surgeon stands left to the patient with camera operator on his left or right side depending upon the location of ventral hernia (Fig. 16.2). If ventral hernia is below the umbilicus, the camera operator stands right to the patient. If the defect is above umbilicus, camera operator should stand left to the patient. Monitor should be placed opposite to surgeon and instrument trolley should be towards the leg of the patient.

Port Position

Technique of laparoscopic repair of ventral hernia is quite simple. First pneumoperitoneum is created at

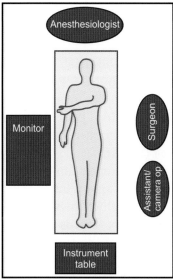

Fig. 16.2: Operating room setup in ventral hernia repair

a site away from the defect. Three port techniques are used for laparoscopic repair of ventral hernia. The first step in performing laparoscopic repair of ventral hernia is gaining access to the free peritoneal cavity. A site distant from any prior incision and the hernia defect is chosen. Typically this is in the right upper quadrant (RUQ) or left upper quadrant (LUQ) (Figs 16.3 to 16.7). The absence of incisions in these locations does not necessarily guarantee the absence of adhesions to viscera. While many approaches for access to the peritoneal cavity have been described, including blind insufflation and specialty trocars, open access in the fashion of Hasson is by far the safest alternative.

Once the pneumoperitoneum is created all other port is placed according to base ball diamond concept.

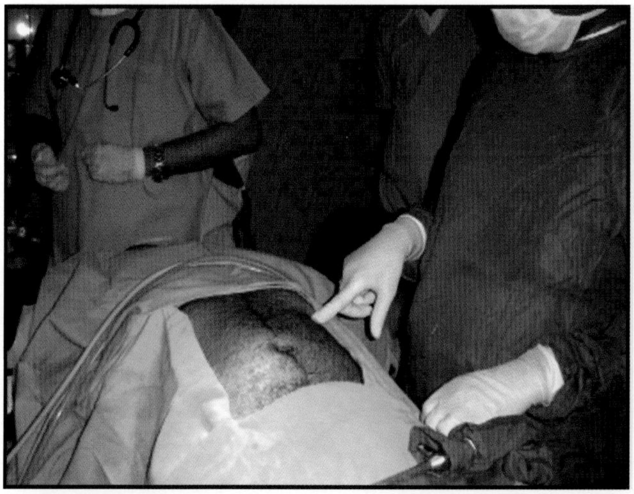

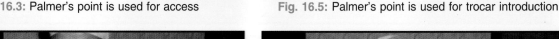

Fig. 16.3: Palmer's point is used for access

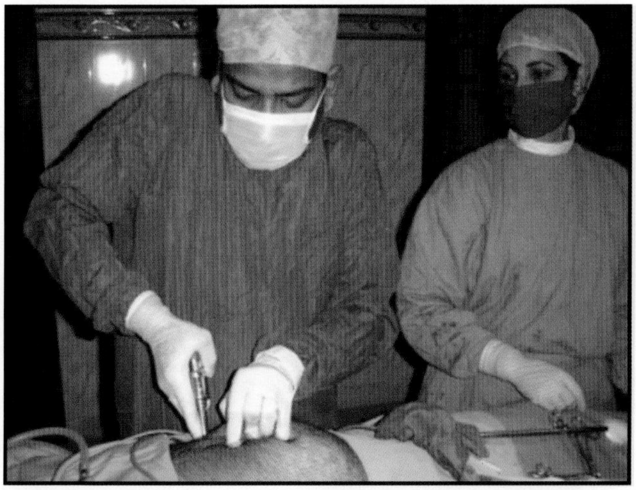

Fig. 16.5: Palmer's point is used for trocar introduction

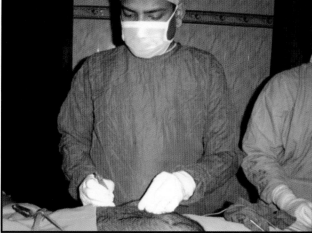

Fig. 16.4: Veress needle introduction through Palmer's point

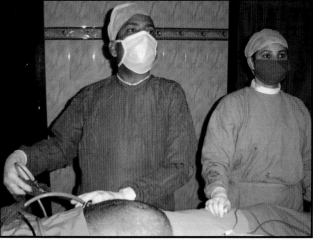

Fig. 16.6: Telescope is introduced to check any adhesion

The most preferred site of access is left hypochondrium in most midline and lower abdominal defect.

First access should be preferably through left hypochondria if Veress needle technique is used and

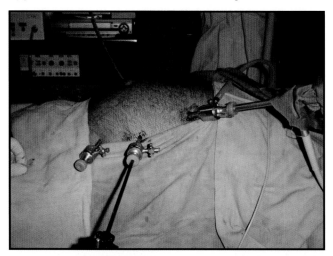

Fig. 16.7: Secondary ports are introduced

then two other ports should be made so that proper triangle is formed. The distance between two ports should not be less than 5 cm (Fig. 16.3).

The telescope will first enter through left hypochondriac port but once dissection starts the telescope will come in the middle, so that the angle between two working port will become 60°. The 10 mm 30° telescope is better to view anterior abdominal wall (Fig. 16.7).

The ventral hernia repair can be performed by two techniques. First technique is intraperitoneal or onlay mesh technique in which mesh is placed without dissecting peritoneum. This is also called as onlay method. All content of the sac is reduced and any adhesion (if present) is cleared. Appropriate size of mesh is then inserted.

After free access to the peritoneal cavity is obtained. This also represents the greatest risk to the patient. The difficulty of adhesiolysis is unpredictable, although

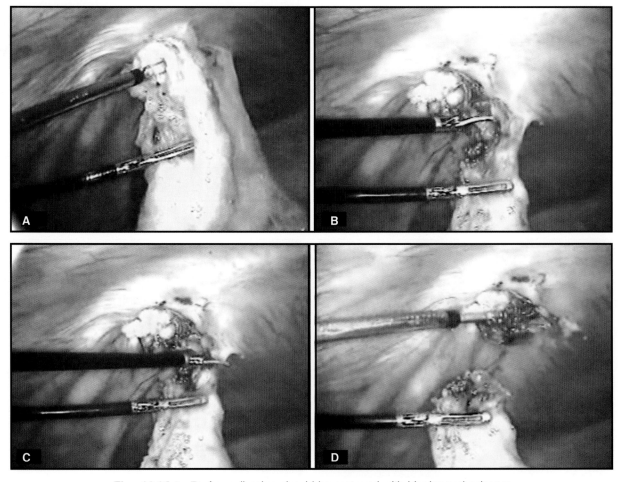

Figs 16.8A to D: Any adhesion should be removed with bipolar and scissors

the presence of polypropylene mesh should be a red flag indicating the potential for the presence of dense and difficult to dissect adhesions, often involving the bowel. All maneuvers performed as part of the lysis of adhesions must be done under direct vision. This is best carried out by sharp dissection utilizing bimanual palpation of the anterior abdominal wall, placing the adhesions under variable degrees of tension (Figs 16.8 and 16.9). There is significant risk in extensive blunt dissection, as the bowel may be fixed at several points placing it at risk for unrecognized perforation with the tip of dissecting instruments. In spite of the enthusiasm

for different energy sources, these are best avoided. As in open cases, dissection should be carried out at the avascular junction of the adhesions and the anterior abdominal wall. Ligating clips or the limited application of an energy source can be used when significant bleeding or vessels are encountered. In the majority of cases, even this is unnecessary. The risk of monopolar cautery is well known, but there is also risk of thermal injury by direct contact with ultrasonic or radio frequency dissection instruments. This is particularly true in the poorly visualized area behind adhesions.

If omentum is adhered with the anterior abdominal wall it should be dissected after applying bipolar or extracorporeal knot (Figs 16.10A and B). It is critical that all adhesions to the anterior abdominal wall be released to allow adequate patch placement and fixation.

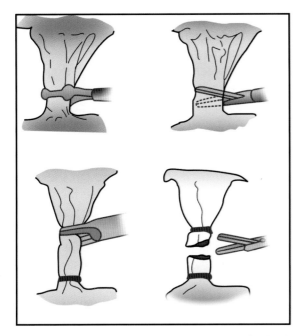

Fig. 16.9: Bipolar can be used safely in case of adhesion with omentum

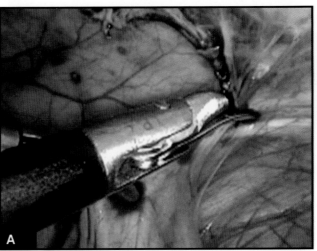

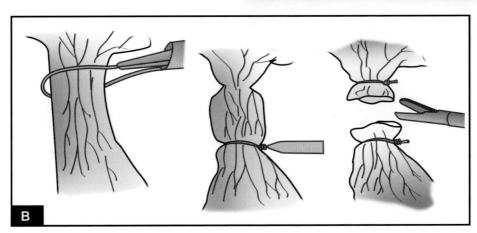

Figs 16.10A and B: Extracorporeal knot can be used in case of adhesion with omentum

Section Two

Once adhesiolysis has been completed, the exact extent of the defect can be directly evaluated. The defects are carefully drawn onto the skin of the anterior abdominal (Fig. 16.11). In the case of multiple defects, the area drawn should include all of the defects. We have progressed to repairing the entire area of a previous incision as opposed to simply repairing a single defect. There have been a number of patients who have presented later in follow-up and are discovered to have a new hernia, outside the area of previous repair. In open surgery these may have simply been considered recurrences. If there is any difficulty in delineating the margins of the defect, a spinal needle can be passed perpendicular to the anterior abdominal wall and through the margins of the defect.

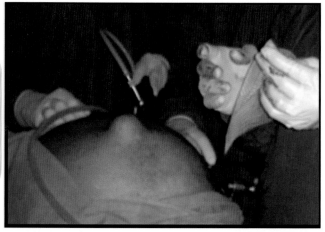

Fig. 16.11: Appropriate size of mesh should be used to prevent recurrence

The selection of size of mesh is important to prevent recurrence of hernia and it should be sufficiently big so that approximately 4 cm healthy margin of defect of hernia should be covered all around. Recently new hybrid mesh has been introduced with absorbable material on one side and unabsorbable proline on the other. These meshes are better than proline because adhesion is less likely to develop due to absorbable material towards the bowel.

The mesh is fixed along margins and around the ring of defect of rectus to ensure a close approximation of mesh to abdominal wall. Care should be taken that mesh should not be corrugated and it should be in proper contact with anterior abdominal wall. Tacker, Protack or Endo anchor can be used to fix the mesh. After fixing the mesh greater omentum is speeded like an apron in between the bowel and mesh (Figs 16.12A and B). Some adhesion of mesh with omentum is always expected in this technique. If patient is early mobilized and newer generation of mesh is used the long-term complication of adhesion is very less with this technique.

Loosely held mesh hanging through the anterior abdominal wall will definitely increase the chance of adhesion with bowel. Tacker should be used to fix the mesh in position. Recently, a technique of using proline suture to fix the mesh with anterior abdominal wall is used with the help of suture passer or looping technique with the help of Veress needles cannula. The main idea of this method is to reduce the cost of surgery, but there is increased chance of infection and

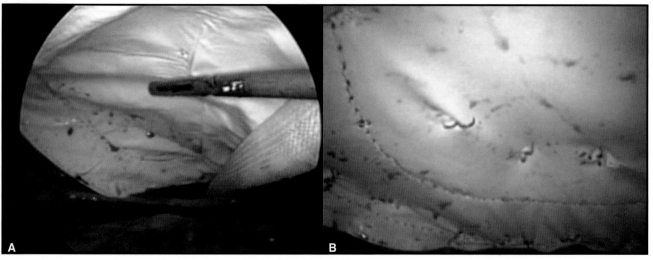

Figs 16.12A and B: Fixation of mesh can be accomplished with endoanchor

adhesion with this method. We also lack any long-term randomized controlled trial to prove the outcome of this external suture technique to fix the mesh in ventral hernia repair.

CHOICE OF MESH IN VENTRAL HERNIA

Synthetic Materials

A variety of synthetic polymeric meshes were developed in the second half of the 20th century and revolutionized hernia repair. With these meshes, abdominal wall defects could be repaired without undue tension on the sutured tissue, decreasing the high recurrence rates of abdominal wall hernia repair. Sir Francis Usher introduced woven monofilament polypropylene mesh in 1958. It was modified to a knitted mesh in 1962 so that the mesh would not unravel when it was cut. Polypropylene mesh gained widespread popularity over the next 30 years and several types of polypropylene mesh are commercially available today. Polyester mesh was also introduced in the 1950's in Europe. Rives and Stoppa employed polyester mesh in their landmark article describing a preperitoneal technique of ventral hernia repair in 1989. The technique described by Rives and Stoppa has become the standard by which all abdominal wall incisional hernia repairs are measured. Polypropylene mesh and polyester mesh revolutionized abdominal wall repair because the meshes did not deteriorate with age, were pliable, and would stretch, allowing for more even load distribution. Nevertheless, the large interstices in polypropylene and polyester mesh promoted adhesion formation when the mesh came into contact with the visceral abdominal cavity. Reported complications included small bowel obstruction, erosion, and fistulization. Expanded polytetrafluoroethylene (ePTFE), initially used as a vascular prosthesis, was adapted for abdominal wall incisional hernia repair in 1983 by WL Gore and Associates and modified several times in the 1990's. Unlike the polypropylene and polyester meshes that preceded it, ePTFE is microporous and select products are uniquely designed with pores measuring 3 microns on the visceral side facing the abdominal cavity and 22 microns facing the abdominal wall. This design promotes fibroblastic and vascular ingrowth from the abdominal wall 22 micron side, but inhibits tissue

attachment to the material on 3 micron side when exposed to the intra-abdominal cavity. There are no reports of fistulization or small bowel obstructions due to adhesions from ePTFE material.

Synthetic meshes, made of materials such as ePTFE (expanded polytetrafluoroethylene) and polypropylene is used most of the time for repair of hernia. The repair process for these materials is based on scar formation in and around the mesh. The advantage of using these materials is that they generally do not react with the human tissue. They are strong and do not tear easily, are readily available, inexpensive, and have a long history of being used for soft tissue replacements.

However, use of synthetic materials is not without problems. As a foreign material, body may react to its presence by growing around it (encapsulation) in an attempt to exclude it from body. In the process, tissue forms a capsule of rigid, fibrous scar tissue around the synthetic material. The rigid capsule could affect the function and the aesthetic outcome of the repair. Furthermore, foreign bodies such as synthetic materials increase the risk of infection when implanted in the body. As part of the foreign body response, the repair site may be subjected to inflammation, infection and pain.

SURGISIS

It is porcine intestinal submucosa and specifically designed as a surgical graft for hernia and abdominal body wall repair (Fig. 16.13). Surgisis gold combines

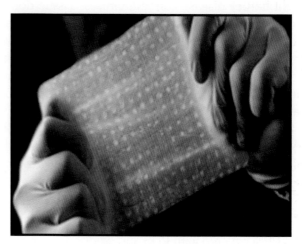

Fig. 16.13: Surgisis

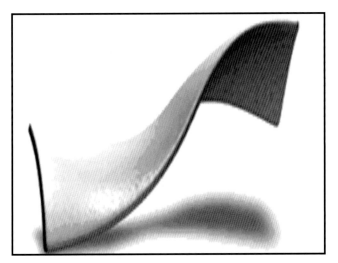

Fig. 16.14: AlloDerm

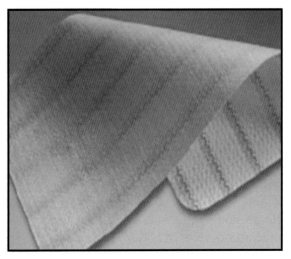

Fig. 16.15: Proceed

strength with flexibility in a naturally occurring graft material that allows for hernia repair without the need for a permanent synthetic prosthesis. Surgisis® Gold™ supports the surgical site while the body's natural healing process replaces the graft with new host tissue. It is collagen biomatrix, naturally occurring and acellular with 18 months shelf life.

ALLODERM

It is biological dermal matrix from processed donated human tissue (Fig. 16.14). AlloDerm is processed from donated human skin. The tissue goes through a cell removal process while retaining the important biochemical and structural components. AlloDerm is, thus, acellular human tissue. Since AlloDerm is derived from human tissue, there may be a concern that it might harbor disease carrying viruses. Tissue donors are screened and tested for transmissible diseases including HIV, hepatitis, and syphilis before tissue processing. AlloDerm has been utilized in more than 7,50,000 implants and grafts to date, without any reported incidence of viral disease transmission to a patient. AlloDerm repairs damaged tissue by providing a foundation for new tissue regeneration. The skin components preserved in AlloDerm contain the information that will help your own tissue to grow into the AlloDerm after placement at the repair site.

PROCEED

Soft PPM covered with PDS and oxidized regenerated cellulose fabric (Fig. 16.15).

Preperitoneal Repair of Ventral Hernia

This technique is also called inlay technique of laparoscopic ventral hernia repair. The peritoneum is incised and preperitoneal space is created in this technique. The sac of the hernia if excised nicely. It can give some extra flap of peritoneum for successful overlapping of both the edges. In this technique margin of defect is sutured intracorporeally to decrease the gap. Pressing the abdominal wall on both the side from outside will help to obliterate the space in this hernia surgery. Either intracorporeal stitches or external mattress sutures can be used to fix the mesh to the musculofacial defect. Once the mesh is fixed, the peritoneum is sutured using vicryl to cover the mesh. This method of laparoscopic ventral hernia repair is same as that of open surgery and it is supposed that formation of adhesion is less.

COMPLICATIONS

- Bowel adhesion
- Fistulization
- Nerve injury
- Vascular injury.

Multiple studies have documented that open hernioplasty has significant morbidity. Leber reported a 27 percent long-term complication rate with open repair; among them being infection, hematoma and seroma, chronic sinus tract formation, mesh extrusion, fistula formation as well as soft tissue problems such as non-healing wound. White reported 34 percent of 250 open ventral hernia repairs had wound related complications. The complications of the open repair mainly relate to the type of mesh that is most commonly used (polypropylene and polyester meshes). In addition, the wide dissection of soft tissue that is required for a Stoppa type retro-rectus repair or a Chevrel type anterior repair leads to the many wound related problems.

Some patient will develop a fluid collection, what is commonly called a seroma, between the mesh and the abdominal wall. Many of these are not apparent to the patient or the surgeon but some are evident and can be bothersome to the patient. Complications from these seromas were some time reported in many studies. Most surgeons do not aspirate these fluid collections for fear of infecting the prosthetic. However, the author has freely aspirated the seromas if they are large or if they are bothersome to the patient. The author has never seen an infection of the prosthetic from aspiration of these fluid collections if full aseptic precaution is taken.

Probably the most dreaded complication that has been seen is bowel injury. Enterotomy is a well-documented complication and commonly occurs and can be readily visualized and handled through an incision. Laparoscopy presents a whole new situation with respect to enterotomy. Prevention is the first line of defense. Lysis of adhesions is well visualized due to the magnification and high intensity light source inherent in the laparoscopic technique. It is very important that energy sources be used very sparingly if at all during lysis of adhesions. If a surgeon enters the proper planes, there is very little bleeding and thus low need for energy sources. Inappropriate use of energy sources is a common cause of unrecognized enterotomy. Monopolar cautery has the problem of current spread, and it is easy to coagulate one area and see the current spread to the adjacent area instantaneously. For this reason monopolar cautery should not be used adjacent to the bowel. The ultrasonic or radio frequency dissection instruments are "sold" with the supposed advantage that there is minimal thermal spread unlike monopolar cautery. Although this may be true, the tip remains very hot and any touching of viscera can cause a burn that may not be apparent during the operation. It is only after several hours, either that night or the next day, when the tissue sloughs, that the enterotomy presents

itself. We do not recommend the use of ultrasonic or radio frequency dissection instruments for this reason. The most important thing to remember is that if lysis of adhesions involving the intestine is not safe, i.e. the surgeon cannot see well or the surgeon cannot determine if an enterotomy has occurred, the patient should be opened! Deaths have been reported from laparoscopic incisional hernioplasty due to bowel injuries that have not been perceived during surgery and only become apparent postoperatively. By the time the diagnosis is made, the patients are septic and succumb to this complication.

DISCUSSION

Initially described in 1992, laparoscopic repair of incisional hernias has evolved from an investigational procedure to one that can safely and successfully be used to repair ventral hernias. The well-established benefits of laparoscopy repair are less postoperative pain, reduced hospital stay and recovery time, low complication and recurrence rates based on numerous reports, meta-analysis and few randomized trials. Conventionally, the laparoscopic ventral hernia repair (LVHR) entails the intraperitoneal placement and fixation of the prosthetic mesh. An alternative technique have been tried in few studies and proposed and to be an advancement of the conventional approach.

Despite its significant prevalence and associated morbidity, there is little in the way of evidence based guidelines regarding the timing and method of repair of ventral and particularly, incisional hernias. Several large studies on laparoscopic ventral hernia repair (LVHR) have been reported. This technique has proven to be a safe and feasible alternative to open mesh repair. Although many are retrospective series and a few comparative studies, only two completed randomized trials comparing open versus laparoscopic mesh repair have been published. Based on these studies, LVHR has been found to have shorter operating time depending on the surgeon's experience, shorter hospital stay, and lower complication rates especially wound and mesh infections and lower recurrence rate during the follow-up period. This evidence has led to the suggestion that now; it would be unethical to conduct a prospective randomized controlled trial comparing LVHR and open approach.

Section Two

LVHR techniques are based on the fundamental principles of the open preperitoneal repair described by Stoppa and Rives. The placement of a large mesh in the preperitoneal location allows for an even distribution of forces along the surface area of the mesh, which may account for the strength of the repair and the decreased recurrence associated with it. The repair capitalizes on the physics of Pascal's principle of hydrostatics by using the forces that create the hernia defect to hold the mesh in place. For this to attain maximum effect, there has to be a wide mesh overlap over the defect and adequate, secure fixation. In the open approach, attaining an overlap of 3-5 cm required extensive soft tissue dissection, with the resultant increase in wound complications. Larger defects should require more overlap and smaller ones theoretically less. The laparoscopic approach not only allows clear definition of the defect margins but also the identification of additional defects that may not have been clinically apparent preoperatively.

Both the inlay and onlay placements of prosthetic mesh embrace these fundamental principles of hernia repair. The onlay and the transabdominal inlay methods, allow for adequate diagnostic laparoscopy to clearly define the margins and the number of the hernia defects including the occult ones. The TEP approach has the same draw back as the open method in detecting subclinical hernias. The TAP method requires the dissection of a large flap of peritoneum with extraperitoneal fat, fascia and posterior rectus sheath where present to accommodate a suitably sized mesh. The extent of dissection will thus be proportional to the size and the number of the defects. Dissection of the peritoneum has also been found to be quite difficult in recurrent and incisional hernias. Furthermore, the minimal reduction and resection of the hernia sac has been suggested to increase the incidence of seroma formation. The TEP approach also entails considerable tissue dissection albeit with a balloon catheter. This is even more marked in the obese, with a thick layer of subcutaneous tissue fat. Any amount of dissection albeit minimal entails creation of an additional wound in tissues, which in incisional and recurrent hernias may already be unhealthy due to previous surgical insults.

In comparing these two methods therefore, two issues needs to be considered regarding the dissection. One, the ease of achieving the adequate overlap of the hernia defect of 3-5 cm. The balloon catheter allows for blind dissection while raising peritoneal flaps would require a considerable dissection especially for larger defects. Two, the wound and mesh related complications due to extensive dissection of the open repair method have been partly attributed to tissue damage hematoma formation and devascularization. Thus in as far as adequate overlap of all hernia defects and preservation of intact tissue physiology are concerned, the intraperitoneal approach is the most ideal particularly for large, incisional and recurrent hernias, as well as for the obese and other patients occult defects.

One of the critical technical points that significantly impact on any method of hernia mesh repair is adequate mesh fixation. The mesh is held in position by sutures and/or staples, clips, tacks, intra-abdominal pressure and later by fibrinous growth. The most widespread technique in onlay approach involves fixation of mesh with tacks and transabdominal permanent sutures. Some surgeons have tried to reduce the operating and possibly postoperative discomfort by reducing or eliminating the use of sutures. The physics of mesh fixation do not support the sole placement of tacks. Majority of the meshes used are about 1 mm thick. A perfectly placed tack can be expected to penetrate only 2 mm beyond the mesh thus tacks will not give the same holding strength as full thickness abdominal wall suture. Furthermore, the mesh is placed against the peritoneum, so any ingrowth is most likely into the peritoneum and not into the fascia.

Detachment of tacks has also been attributed to some recurrence of hernia. Postoperative recurrence of ventral hernia repair is reported to be as high as 13% when only a stapling, clipping or the tacking device is used for mesh fixation. Proper use of the transfascial fixation sutures in combination with staples decreased the recurrence rate to as low as 2 %. Therefore the current recommendation for mesh fixation is that a transfascial suture should be placed at a distance of 5 cm each along the perimeter of the mesh and tacking devices be used to affix the edge of the mesh at 1 cm intervals. The preperitoneal approach mesh fixation differs in that, there is immediate and continued fixation by the intact peritoneal sac and whether tacks or sutures or both are used, they fix the mesh directly onto the fascia. The primary concern of the peritoneal flap in the inlay technique is to achieve secure fixation of the mesh to the underlying fascia. The fibrinous ingrowth is from the fascia and not the peritoneum. Furthermore the preperitoneal positioning confers with the original design of Stoppa.

Perhaps the most compelling advantage of the preperitoneal placement of the mesh in the inlay approach is the avoidance of direct interaction between the mesh and the intra-abdominal viscera. Contact of the viscera with foreign material such as the prosthesis may lead to an inflammatory response and adhesion formation which can induce chronic pain, intestinal obstruction, enterocutaneous fistula and infertility. In addition, adhesions complicate any future intra-abdominal surgery. The peritoneal covering also allows the use of conventional meshes, which have been associated with intense inflammatory response and adhesion formation by some workers. The choice of the mesh used in LVHR may be the most contentious issue, particularly when financial cost is a major consideration.

The biomaterials available for ventral hernia repair have undergone many changes over the last several years. There are new products that have either been recently introduced or are in developmental stages. All seek to achieve two goals; rapid and permanent ingrowth into the body wall and diminution of the risk of intestinal adhesions while maintaining its tensile strength. The visceral side should be smooth, nonerosive antiadhesive and not easily susceptible to infection. This visceral barrier should be present for at least one week because this is the time frame in which adhesions forms. The ventral side should be macroporous allowing for fibroblast in growth and a foreign body reaction may be necessary for incorporation and high tensile strength.

Polypropylene (prolene) mesh, introduced by Sir Francis Usher in 1958 and modified in 1962 has gained widespread popularity and several types are commercially available today. Polyester mesh was introduced in Europe in the 1950s. Stoppa used the polyester mesh in their landmark article describing preperitoneal repair of ventral hernia in 1989. Prolene mesh is currently the most widely used because it is relatively inexpensive, easy to handle, has a memory and is firmly incorporated in the abdominal wall due to its ability to induce an intense inflammatory

reaction. A 2-5% fistula rate has been reported with polypropylene mesh used intra-abdominally leading to the suggestion the great care must be taken to separate it from the bowel if it has to be used at all. However, some studies do not support this view. Bingener found no association of visceral adhesion when prolene was used with adequate omental interposition between it and the bowel. In another study involving 136 patients, Vrijland concluded that enterocutaneous fistula appears to be very rare after prolene mesh repair regardless of intraperitoneal placement, omental coverage or closing the peritoneum.

A study comparing the biomaterials used in LVHR found polyester to have the highest incidence of infection, fistulization and recurrence. The expanded polytetrafluoroethylene (ePTFE) has the longest history in the use for these hernias repair. The original description of the procedure used an early generation of the ePTFE product. The current product has one smooth surface with 3 microns ePTFE interstices, while the other side has 22 microns interstices to facilitate fibroblastic ingrowth for firm fixation. Other modifications of this product involve incorporation of antimicrobials on the visceral surface. All of the composite prostheses have ePTFE and prolene or polyester but differ in the number and attachment of them together. There are no reports of intestinal fistulization or obstruction with ePTFE though it has also been found to induce inflammation and fibrosis in laboratory animals.

However, the use of synthetic materials is not without problems. As a foreign material, the repair site is subjected to inflammation, susceptibility to infection and pain as a foreign body response. Encapsulation could affect the elastic function of the abdominal wall and aesthetic outcome of the repair. This has stimulated the search for natural biological prostheses like surgisis, collagen, glycosaminoglycans from porcine intestinal submucosa and alloderm. The financial cost to clinical-benefit ratio for use of the substantially expensive composite meshes is unquantified and is likely to remain as such because, given the widespread acceptance of composite products, a randomized, clinical comparison with prolene is unlikely to occur. Therefore, in selected circumstances, it may be acceptable to use a simple

Section Two

mesh, if this can be excluded from the bowel by tissue interposition be it omentum or peritoneum. A composite mesh should be considered as the current standard of care.

The extraperitoneal placement of the prostheses would in principle diminish the intra-abdominal complications associated with formation of adhesions. It would also allow the safe use of the conventional meshes like prolene, which has high intrinsic tensile strength, good memory, and cheaper . In addition the peritoneal coverage over the entire mesh provides additional security of fixation and a better mechanical advantage. As such it can be seen as an advance over the onlay approach. However, the placement is technically demanding as evidenced by the high iatrogenic peritoneal tears in the largest series and it may not be feasible in the scarred abdomen of incisional and recurrent hernias, which constitute the bulk and seems to benefit most, from LVHR. Thus the issue of limitation of patient population amongst the technical feasibility and adequacy of defect coverage are issues of great concern before the method is accepted as an additional procedure for LVHR.

The good results and the attributed safety of LVHR are based on the large number of studies mainly utilizing the intraperitoneal approach. The generalization of the procedure has resulted in multiple variations of techniques. Overall, fewer complications are reported after LVHR than after open mesh repair especially in relation to wound and mesh infection. The efficacy of the inlay approach as an advancement of the conventional repair needs to be evaluated in terms of the several specific complications that are of particular relevance in laparoscopic procedures.

Probably the most dreaded complication is bowel injury and particularly if it is missed intraoperatively. It is a potentially lethal complication. The overall incidence of bowel injury does not differ significantly between open repair and laparoscopic repair and is generally low with either approach (1 to 5% when serosal injuries are included). Pneumoperitoneum may hinder the recognition of bowel injury at the time of operation. There have also been reports of late bowel perforation secondary to thermal injury with laparoscopic repair.

Minimizing the use of electrocauterization and ultrasonic dissection markedly reduces the risk of bowel injury. The visualization afforded by the pneumoperitoneum place adhesions between the abdominal wall and the bowel under tension. The high intensity light source and the magnification inherent in the laparoscopy facilitate identification of the least vascularized planes. As far as possible, direct grasping the bowel should be avoided preferring simply to push it or to grasp the adhesions themselves to provide counter traction. External pressure on the hernia may also help. Larger vessels in the omentum or adhesions are controlled with clips. Some degree of oozing from the dissected areas is tolerated; such oozing almost always settles down without specific hemostatic measures.

In cases of dense adhesions it is preferable to divide the sac or the fascia rather than risk injury to bowel. Densely adherent polypropylene mesh is best excised the abdominal wall rather than attempting to separate it from the serosa of the bowel. If bowel injury is suspected immediate and thorough inspection should be carried out. It may be difficult or impossible to find the exact site of injury later once the bowel has been released and freed of its attachments. Once the injury is recognized, it is the surgeon's level of comfort with laparoscopic suture repair determines the best approach. With minimal spillage of bowel contents, the injury may be treated with either laparoscopic repair or open repair; the latter usually can be carried out through a mini-laparotomy over the injured area. Whether the mesh prosthesis is put primarily or later depends on the degree of contamination. More significant bowel injuries necessitate conversion to open repair. Missed injuries manifest postoperatively mandating re-exploration with occasional removal of the mesh and immediate recurrence of the hernia.

One of the greatest benefits of LVHR is the reduction in wound and mesh infections. In a detailed analysis of wound complications from a pooled data of forty-five published series involving 5340 patients, Pierce reported wound infection rates of 4.6-8 times fold higher in open versus LVHR. The number of mesh infections was also significantly higher with open approaches. Wound problems are strongly linked with soft tissue dissection required for retromuscular

after laparoscopic repair. Laparoscopy provides better vision of peritoneal cavity, and allows early mobilization.

The incidence of peptic ulcer disease has decreased nowadays with vast improvement in medical therapy. However, minimal invasive surgery still has a significant role to play in treatment of complicated disease. It decreases hospital stay and overall recovery period as compared to open surgery regardless of the preference of the individual surgeon. Our result has shown that the laparoscopic surgery may become the gold standard for surgical treatment of complicated peptic ulcer disease. Laparoscopic closure of duodenal ulcer perforation is an attractive alternative to conventional surgery with the benefits of minimally invasive surgery such as parietal wall integrity, cosmetic benefits and early subjective postoperative comfort and rehabilitation.

BIBLIOGRAPHY

1. Andersen IB, Bonnevie O, Jorgensen T et al. Time trends for peptic ulcer disease in Denmark, 1981–1993. Analysis of hospitalization register and mortality data. Scand J Gastroenterol 1998;33:260–6.
2. Canoy DS, Hart AR, Todd CJ. Epidemiology of duodenal ulcer perforation: a study on hospital admissions in Norfolk, United Kingdom. Dig Liver Dis 2002;34:322–7.
3. Crofts TJ, Park KG, Steele RJ et al. A randomized trial of nonoperative treatment for perforated peptic ulcer. N Engl J Med 1989;320:970–973.
4. Darby CR, Berry AR, Mortensen N. Management variability in surgery for colorectal emergencies. Br J Surg 1992;79:206–210.
5. Dawson EJ, Paterson-Brown S. Emergency general surgery and the implications for specialisation. Surgeon 2004; 2:165–170.
6. Dunkley AS, Eyers PS, Vickery CJ et al. The emergency general surgeon: a new career pathway? Bull Royal Coll Surg Engl 2007;89:32–6 World J Surg 2008;32:1456–61 1461.
7. Lau JY, Sung JJ, Lam YH et al. Endoscopic retreatment compared with surgery in patients with recurrent bleeding after initial endoscopic control of bleeding ulcers. N Engl J Med 1999;340:751–6.
8. Lunevicius R, Morkevicius M. Systematic review comparing laparoscopic and open repair for perforated peptic ulcer. Br J Surg 2005;92:1195–1207.
9. Mercer SJ, Knight JS, Toh SK et al; Implementation of a specialist-led service for the management of acute gallstone disease. Br J Surg 2004;91:504–8.
10. Noguiera C, Silva AS, Santos JN et al. Perforated peptic ulcer: main factors of morbidity and mortality. World J Surg 2003;27:782–7.
11. Paimela H, Oksala NK, Kivilaakso E. Surgery for peptic ulcer today. A study on the incidence, methods and mortality in surgery for peptic ulcer in Finland between 1987 and 1999. Dig Surg 2004;21:185–91.
12. Post PN, Kuipers EJ, Meijer GA. Declining incidence of peptic ulcer but not of its complications: a nation-wide study in The Netherlands. Aliment Pharmacol Ther 2006;23:1587–93 9. Leontiadis GI, Sharma VK, Howden CW. Proton pump inhibitor treatment for acute peptic ulcer bleeding. Cochrane Database Syst Rev 2006;25(1):CD002094.
13. Qvist P, Arnesen KE, Jacobsen CD et al. Endoscopic treatment and restrictive surgical policy in the management of peptic ulcer bleeding. Five years' experience in a central hospital. Scand J Gastroenterol 1994;29:569–76.
14. Read TE, Myerson RJ, Fleshman JW et al. Surgeon specialty is associated with outcome in rectal cancer treatment. Dis Colon Rectum 2002;45:904–14
15. Ripoll C, Banares R, Beceiro I et al. Comparison of transcatheter arterial embolization and surgery for treatment of bleeding peptic ulcer after endoscopic treatment failure. J Vasc Interv Radiol 2004;15:447–50.
16. Thomsen RW, Riis A, Munk EM, et al. 30-day mortality after peptic ulcer perforation among users of newer selective COX-2 inhibitors and traditional NSAIDs: a population-based study. Am J Gastroenterol 2006;101:2704–2710. Epub 2006 Oct 6.
17. Tu JV, Austin PC, Johnston KW. The influence of surgical specialty training on the outcomes of elective abdominal aortic aneurysm surgery. J Vasc Surg 2001;33:447–52
18. Zorcolo L, Covotta L, Carlomagno N et al 2003. Toward lowering morbidity, mortality, and stoma formation in emergency 1460 World J Surg (2008) 32:1456–1461 123 colorectal surgery: the role of specialization. Dis Colon Rectum 2003;46:1461–1467.

19 Laparoscopic Fundoplication

Gastroesophageal reflux disease (GERD) is defined as the failure of the anti-reflux barrier, allowing abnormal reflux of gastric contents into the esophagus. It is a mechanical disorder which is caused by a defective lower esophageal sphincter, a gastric emptying disorder or failed esophageal peristalsis. Gastroesophageal reflux is one of the most common digestive symptoms. Exposure of the esophageal mucosa to acid, enzymes and other digestive secretions, leads to acute and chronic inflammation, with pain, and ulceration or stricture formation if untreated.

Heartburn occurs in 5 to 45 percent of adults in western countries, depending on the frequency of symptoms 30 to 45 percent suffer from symptoms once a month and 5 to 10 percent every day. The majority of patients suffering from GERD experience minor symptoms for which they do not seek medical attention. Age does not seem to have an impact on the frequency of GERD symptoms, and no causal factor has been identified. Esophagitis due to reflux occurs in approximately 2 percent of the global population. It is the most frequent form of lesion detected on upper gastrointestinal endoscopy, occurring more frequently than gastric ulcers or duodenal ulcers. GERD is often a chronic ailment. After a 5 to 10 years follow-up, about two-thirds of patients complain of persistent symptoms requiring occasional or continuous treatment.

PATHOPHYSIOLOGY

The pathophysiology of GERD is multifactorial, although it is usually due to the weakening of the anatomical or functional gastroesophageal barrier located at the esophagogastric junction. Injury to the esophageal mucosa by acid-peptic gastric secretions, while secondary to this weakening, plays a major role in the development of GERD symptoms and lesions. In fact, suppressing the gastric acid secretion, which is the usual treatment of this ailment, leads to the disappearance of symptoms and healing of lesions in almost all cases. GERD is therefore acid dependent.

Symptoms

- Heartburn (Retrosternal burning)
- Regurgitation
- Pain
- Respiratory symptoms.

Diagnostic Test

Endoscopy

- Barium swallow
- Esophageal transit +/- manometry
- pH monitoring.

Treatment of GERD

Medical therapy is the first line of management. Esophagitis will heal in approximately 90 percent of cases with intensive medical therapy. However, symptoms recur in more than 80 percent of cases within one year of drug withdrawal. Since it is a chronic condition, medical therapy involving acid suppression and/or pro-motility agents may be required for the rest of patient's life. Despite the fact that current medical management is very effective for the majority, a small number of patients do not get complete relief of symptoms. Currently, there is increasing interest in the surgical management of gastroesophageal reflux disease (GERD).

The goal of surgical therapy is to recreate an anti-reflux barrier. It is the only treatment capable of changing the natural history of GERD. There has been renewed interest in this therapy with the advent of laparoscopic surgery.

Indications for Surgical Treatment

Currently, there is increasing interest in the surgical management of gastroesophageal reflux disease (GERD). There are a number of reasons for this. Despite the fact that current medical management is very effective for the majority a small number of patients do not get complete relief of symptoms. Secondly, some patients, particularly those who are in their twenties or thirties, face the prospect of a lifetime of continuous proton pump inhibitor therapy with the possible risk of, as yet, unknown side effects. In addition, the laparoscopic approach with its benefits of reduced operative trauma and less time off work has become more common place. As a consequence, general practitioners and gastro-enterologists are more ready to refer patients with disabling symptoms for surgical treatment. The gold standard anti-reflux operation is undoubtedly the Nissen type of total fundoplication and many studies have affirmed its effectiveness in controlling acid reflux. However, new symptoms after fundoplication such as gas bloat and dysphagia, which probably result from a hyper-competent lower esophageal sphincter produced by the Nissen operation, are common.

Concerning the indication for surgery, a distinction between heartburn and regurgitation symptoms is considered important (medical treatment appears to be more effective for heartburn than for regurgitation). Even after successful medical acid suppression, the patient can have recurrent symptoms of epigastric pain and retrosternal pressure as well as food regurgitation due to an incompetent cardia, insufficient peristalsis, or a large hiatal hernia.

Surgical therapy should be considered in individuals with documented GERD who:
- Refractory to medical management
- Associated with hiatus hernia
- Intolerance to PPH or H_2 receptors
- Not compliant to medical therapy
- Have complications of GERD, e.g. Barrett's esophagus, stricture, grade 3 or 4 esophagitis
- Atypical symptoms like: Asthma, hoarseness, cough, chest pain and aspiration.

Study has shown those patients resistant to anti-secretory treatment are not a good candidate for antireflux surgery.

Methods of Fundoplication

- The classical open methods
- The modern laparoscopic techniques.

Laparoscopic fundoplication is a safe procedure, and can provide less postoperative morbidity in experienced hands. This is a surgical procedure done for gastroesophageal reflux disease (GERD). Fundus of the stomach which is on the left of the esophagus and main portion of the stomach is wrapped around the back of the esophagus until it is once again in front of this structure. The portion of the fundus that is now on the right side of the esophagus is sutured to the portion on the left side to keep the wrap in place. The fundoplication resembles a buttoned shirt collar. The collar is the fundus wrap and the neck represents the esophagus imbricated into the wrap. This has the effect of creating a one way valve in the esophagus to allow food to pass into the stomach, but prevent stomach acid from flowing into the esophagus and thus prevent GERD.

Laparoscopic fundoplication is a useful method for reducing hospital stay, complications and return to normal activity.

Types of Fundoplication Surgery

Laparoscopic fundoplication has become the standard surgical method of treating gastroesophageal reflux disease. Although Nissen total fundoplication is the most commonly performed procedure, partial fundoplication, either anterior or posterior, is becoming more acceptable because of a suggested lower risk of long-term side effects (Fig. 19.3).

Section Two

The 360° Nissen fundoplication (NF) has been the standard operation for gastroesophageal reflux, but is associated with substantial rates of, "gas bloat," gagging and dysphasia (Fig. 19.1).

Toupet fundoplication (TF), a 270° posterior wrap, has fewer complications, and its outcome in compared with Nissen fundoplication is favorable both in children as well as adults (Fig. 19.2).

Although Nissen total fundoplication is the most commonly performed procedure, partial fun-doplication, either anterior or posterior, is becoming more acceptable because of lower risk of long-term complication. Dor in 1962 described anterior fundoplication as an anti-reflux operation for patients who had a Heller's myotomy for achalasia. In the 1970s, Watson developed an operation for patient suffering from GERD.

Most surgeon believe that the Toupet fundoplication (TF), a 270° posterior wrap originally described in conjunction with myotomy for achalasia, has fewer

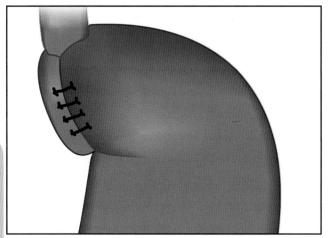

Fig. 19.1: Nissen fundoplication (NF)

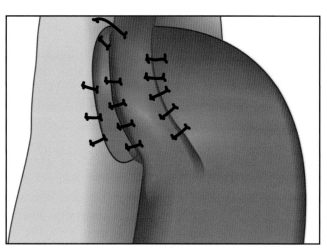

Fig. 19.2: Toupet fundoplication (TF), a 270° wrap

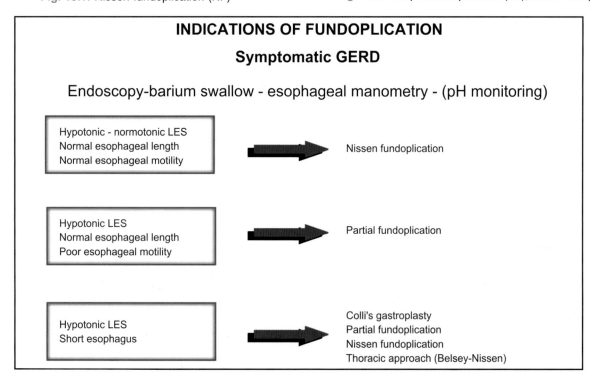

Fig. 19.3: Selection of type of fundoplication

Section Two

complications, and its long-term outcome in compared with Nissen fundoplication is favorable both in children as well as adults. This article describes a technique of laparoscopic posterior Toupet fundoplication.

The main tasks of this operation consist of:
1. Preparation of the patient.
2. Creation of pneumoperitoneum. Insertion of port.
3. Diagnostic laparoscopy and dissection of visceral peritoneum.
4. Mobilization of 5 cm intra-abdominal esophagus.
5. Fundus pull from below the esophagus.
6. Insertion of posterior sutures to tighten the crural opening.
7. Fixation of fundus to the left crura.
8. Fixation of the fundus with the right crura.
9. Fixation of the fundus with esophagus. Inspection of tightness of fundoplication.
10. Irrigation and suction of operating field.
11. Final diagnostic laparoscopy for any bowel injury or hemorrhage.
12. Removal of the instrument with complete exit of CO_2. Closure of wound.

Patient Selection

Many patients have symptoms palliated by lifestyle like diet and exercise, others by simple medication, and some by strong medication like, proton pump inhibitors. A certain proportion of patient has refractory or long-term symptoms, and operation can be considered in this group of patients. As reflux symptoms are frequent and variable, it is wise to obtain both ambulatory 24 pH-metry and esophageal motility studies prior to surgery. Upper GI endoscopies should be performed in all patients.

OPERATIVE TECHNIQUE

Patient Position

The patient is placed on the operating table with the legs in stirrups, the knees slightly bent and the hips flexed approximately 10°. The operating table is tilted head up by approximately 15°. Compression bandage are used on leg during the operation to prevent thromboembolism. The surgeon stands between the patient's legs. The first assistant, whose main task is to position the video camera, sits on the patient's left side.

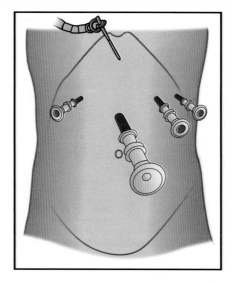

Fig. 19.4: Laparoscopic fundoplication port position

The instrument trolley is placed on the patient's left allowing the scrub nurse to assist with placing the appropriate instruments in the operating ports.

Television monitors are positioned on either side of the top end of the operating table at a suitable height for surgeon, anesthetist and assistant to see the procedure.

Port Position

The 10 mm camera (port 1) is placed in the mid-line approximately 5 cm above the umbilicus; this position will vary depending on the build of the patient (Fig. 19.4). After inserting the camera, a 5 mm port (2) is inserted in the right upper quadrant 8-10 cm from the mid-line. A port (3), with a variable 5-10 mm diaphragm, is placed in the left upper quadrant - a mirror image of the one on the patient's right. This allows both 5 mm and 10 mm instruments to be used through the same cannula without changing ports. A further 5 mm port (4) is positioned in the left anterior axillary line immediately below the costal margin. This port is mainly used for a forceps which will hold the tape encircling the esophagus (Fig. 19.5). Liver retraction used to be one of the more problematic aspects of laparoscopic fundoplication. In our experience these difficulties have been largely overcome by the use of the Nathanson liver retractor. Alternate port position in laparoscopic fundoplication show in Figures 19.6A and B.

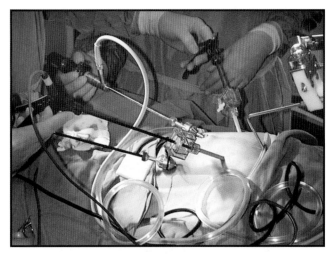

Fig. 19.5: Port position in fundoplication

POSITION

Tissue Dissection and Mobilization

Dissection starts at the avascular portion of the lesser omentum above the hepatic branch of the vagus. The dissection is continued carefully up to the hiatus, which can be seen through the defect created. An opening is created in the lesser omentum, below the hepatic branch of vagus to allow better access to the hiatus (Figs 19.7A to D).

The right crus is dissected using electrosurgery and scissors to identify the plane between the crus and surrounding loose areolar tissues. The loose areolar tissue around the esophagus is exposed and secures the bleeding from any blood vessels visible during mobilization of esophagus. Always remember not to injure the esophageal wall and vagal fibers when dissecting this area around esophagus. The space between the hiatus and the anterior aspect of esophagus is developed using fine dissection by scissors to divide blood vessels crossing this space.

Lesser Sac Opened

The posterior aspect of the left crus is identified as it meets the right crus and dissection of its surface commences especially the peritoneal covering over the margin of right crus is dissected down to the fundus from the diaphragm known as Rosetti dissection technique. Dissection of the posterior aspect of the left crus is done by lifting the intra-abdominal esophagus forwards with a blunt instrument. A sling is fed into the jaws of the grasping forceps and then pulled round behind the esophagus (Fig. 19.8).

Sling is passed through a separate punctured wound from abdominal wall without port. A grasping forceps is inserted through one of the port to hold the sling so that the esophagus can be manipulated. Dissection surroundings of esophagus in the posterior mediastinum should for approximately 5 to 6 cm. Mobilization of the esophagus and stomach should be sufficient enough to have a good floppy fundus for wrap (Figs 19.9A to F).

• The next step is to pull the fundus from behind the esophagus to form a wrap.

Fundus Pull

After mobilizing the fundus nicely the tip of the fundus is pulled by one of the grasper introduced through

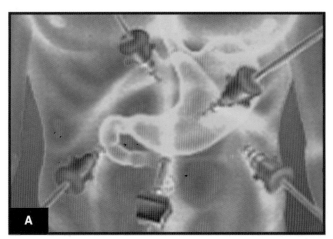

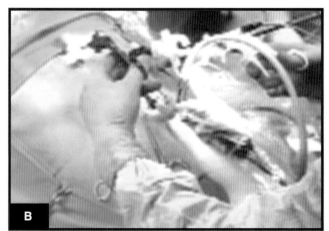

Figs 19.6A and B: Alternative port position in laparoscopic fundoplication

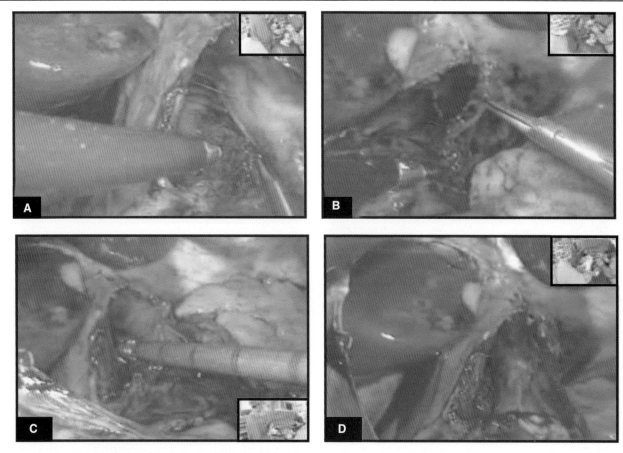

Figs 19.7A to D: Mobilization of esophagus

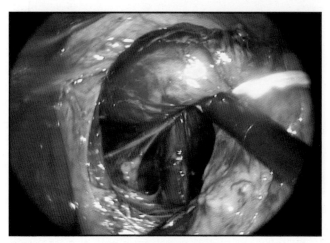

Fig. 19.8: Sling insertion

below and right side of the esophagus (Figs 19.10 to 19.11B).

The mobilization of stomach should be adequate to give a floppy fundus for plication otherwise patient may develop dysphagia. One stay suture may be applied to the fundus to hold it in place or one of the grasper may be used to keep it pulled. The next step is crural repair.

Crural Approximation

Crura should be approximated behind the esophagus using two or three sutures of 2/0 braided polyamide on a 30 mm needle using Tumble Square Knot. A further one or two sutures are inserted in the same way, at about 1 cm intervals and tied using Tumble square knot. It is important not to make the crural opening too tight since this will produce dysphagia (Figs 19.12A and B).

Fundoplication

Suture is applied which involves a 1 cm bite of the seromuscular layer of gastric fundus, which is sutured to the anterior aspect of the left crus. Since the fundus lays some way from the left crus, the slip reef knot or Tumble square knot is particularly valuable for this suture. After this, a further suture is placed between

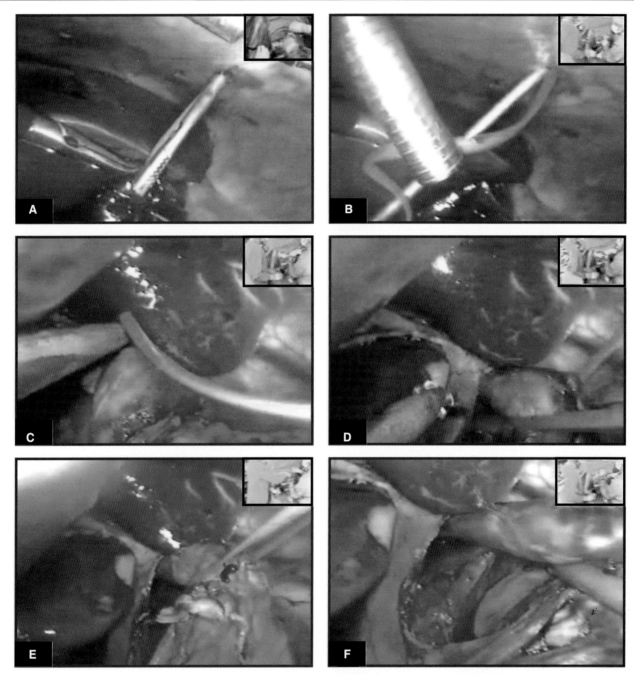

Figs 19.9A to F: Sling application around esophagus for proper exposure of crura

the fundus and the left anterior aspect of the hiatus. The next suture is placed between the fundus and the right anterior aspect of the hiatus (Figs 19.13A to C).

Further three sutures are then positioned at approximately 1 cm intervals to the posterior fundus and the right crus. The sling used for esophageal retraction is removed. One or two suture may be placed to fix the side of the esophagus with the wrapped portion of the stomach (Figs 19.14A and B). But always remember the wrap is not in place due to these sutures. The suture of fundus with crura actually holds the wrap in position. Never take a full thickness bite on the oesophagus with Endoski needle otherwise there is always a chance of perforation of esophagus.

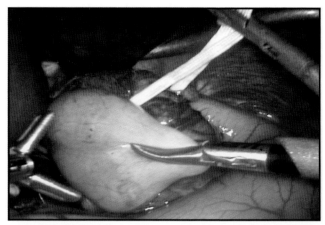

Fig. 19.10: Mobilized fundus of stomach is pulled from behind the esophagus

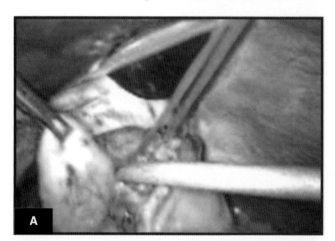

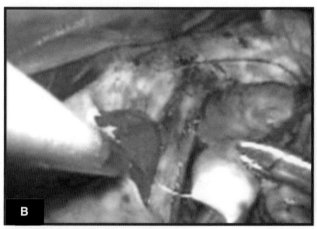

Figs 19.11A and B: Fundus of stomach is pulled from behind the esophagus

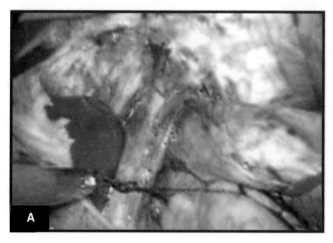

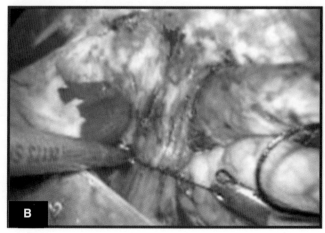

Figs 19.12A and B: Approximation of crura

Ending of the Operation

Abdomen should be examined for any possible bowel injury or hemorrhage. The instrument and then port should be removed carefully. Remove telescope leaving gas valve of umbilical port open to let out all the gas. Close the wound with suture. Use vicryl for rectus and unabsorbable intradermal or stapler for skin. Apply adhesive sterile dressing over the wound.

Section Two

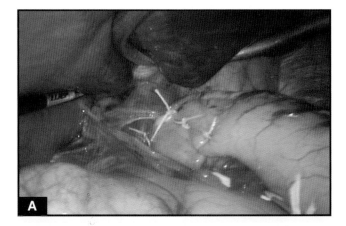

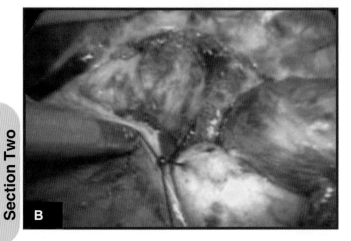

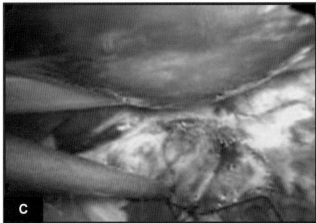

Figs 19.13A to C: Fixation of wrap by intracorporeal sutures

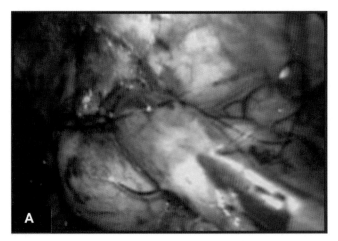

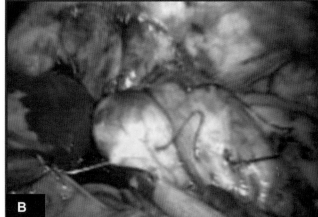

Figs 19.14A and B: Fixation of fundus with esophagus

Patient may be discharged 2 days after operation if every thing goes well. The patient may have slight dysphagia initially but usually resolves after 6 weeks. The patient having any complain of dysphagia should be examined endoscopically after 3 to 4 weeks of operation.

BIBLIOGRAPHY

1. Akinola E, Rosenkrantz TS, Pappagallo M, McKay K, Hussain N. Gastroesophageal reflux in infants <32 weeks gestational age at birth: lack of relationship to chronic lung disease. Am J Perinatol 2004;21: 57–62.

2. Anvari M, Bamehriz F. Outcome of laparoscopic Nissen fundoplication in patients with body mass index e" 35. Surg Endosc 2006;20:230–4.

3. Augood C, MacLennan S, Gilbert R, Logan S. Cisapride treatment for gastroesophageal reflux in children. Cochrane Database Syst Rev 2003;CD002300.

4. Boyce PM, Talley NJ, Burke C, Koloski NA. Epidemiology of the functional gastrointestinal disorders diagnosed according to Rome II criteria: an Australian population-based study. Int Med J 2006;36:28–36.

5. Bredenoord AJ, Weusten BL, Smout AJ. Symptom association analysis in ambulatory gastro-esophageal reflux monitoring. Gut 2005;54:1810–7.

6. Cameron BH, Blair GK, Murphy JJ III, Fraser GC. Morbidity in neurologically impaired children after percutaneous endoscopic versus Stamm gastrostomy. Gastrointest Endosc 1995;42:41–4.

7. Cezard JP. Managing gastroesophageal reflux disease in children. Digestion 2004;69(1): 3–8.

8. Chicella MF, Batres LA, Heesters MS, Dice JE. Prokinetic drug therapy in children: a review of current options. Ann Pharmacother 2005;39: 706–711.

9. Chitkara DK, Fortunato C, Nurko S. Esophageal motor activity in children with gastroesophageal reflux disease and esophagitis. J Pediatr Gastroenterol Nutr 2005;40: 70–5.

10. Chung DH, Georgeson KE. Fundoplication and gastrostomy. Semin Pediatr Surg 1998;7: 213–19. 173.

11. Colletti RB, Di Lorenzo C. Overview of pediatric gastroesophageal reflux disease and proton pump inhibitor therapy. J Pediatr Gastroenterol Nutr 2003;37(1): S7–S11.

12. Costantini M, Crookes PF, Bremner RM, Hoeft SF, Ehsan A,n Peters JH, Bremner CG, DeMeester TR. Value of physiologic assessment of foregut symptoms in a surgical practice. Surgery 1993;114:780–86.

13. Craig WR, Hanlon-Dearman A, Sinclair C, Taback S, Moffatt M. Metoclopramide, thickened feedings, and positioning for gastroesophageal reflux in children under two years. Cochrane atabase Syst Rev 2004;CD003502.

14. Curry JI, Lander TD, Stringer MD. Review article: erythromycin as a prokinetic agent in infants and children. Aliment Pharmacol Ther 2001;15: 595–603.

15. D'Alessio MJ, Arnaoutakis D, Giarelli N, Villadolid DV, Rosemurgy AS. Obesity is not a contraindication to laparoscopic fundoplication. J Gastrointest Surg 2005;9:949–54.

16. Davidson GP, Omari TI. Pathophysiological mechanisms of gastroesophageal reflux disease in children. Curr Gastroenterol Rep 2001;3: 257–62.

17. Esposito C, Langer JC, Schaarschmidt K, Mattioli G, Sauer C, Centonze A, Cigliano B, Settimi A, Jasonni V. Laparoscopic antireflux procedures in the management of gastroesophageal reflux following esophageal atresia repair. J Pediatr Gastroenterol Nutr 2005;40: 349–351 44. Farrell TM, Richardson WS, Halkar R, Lyon CP, Galloway KD, Waring JP, Smith CD, Hunter JG. Nissen fundoplication improves gastric motility in patients with delayed gastric emptying. Surg Endosc 2001;15: 271–274.

18. Eubanks TR, Omelanczuk P, Richards C, Pohl D, Pellegrini CA. Outcomes of laparoscopic antireflux procedures. Am J Surg 2000; 179:391–5.

19. Franco MT, Salvia G, Terrin G, Spadaro R, De Rosa I, Iula VD, Cucchiara S. Lansoprazole in the treatment of gastroesophageal reflux disease in childhood. Dig Liver Dis 2000;32: 660–666.

20. Fraser J, Watson DI, O'Boyle CJ, Jamieson GG. Obesity and its effect on outcome of laparoscopic Nissen fundoplication. Dis Esophagus 2001;14:50–53.

21. Galvani C, Fisichella PM, Gorodner MV, Perretta S, Patti MG. Symptoms are a poor indicator of reflux status after fundoplication for gastroesophageal reflux disease. Arch Surg 2003;138:514–519.

22. Georgeson K (2005) Personal experience with laparoscopic fundoplication in children. Elsevier, Birmingham, AL.

23. Georgeson KE. Laparoscopic fundoplication and gastrostomy. Semin Laparosc Surg 1998;5: 25–30.

24. Gilger MA, Yeh C, Chiang J, Dietrich C, Brandt ML, El-Serag HB. Outcomes of surgical fundoplication in children. Clin Gastroenterol Hepatol 2004;2: 978–84.

25. Gold BD. Outcomes of pediatric gastroesophageal reflux disease: in the first year of life, in childhood, and in adults . . . oh, and should we really leave Helicobacter pylori alone? J Pediatr Gastroenterol Nutr 2003;37(1): S33–S39.

26. Gregersen H, Drewes AM. Functional findings in irritable bowel syndrome. World J Gastroenterol 2006;12:2830–2838.

27. Gwee K, Chua ASB. Functional dyspepsia and irritable bowel syndrome, are they different entities and does it matter? World J Gastroenterol 2006;12:2708–2712.

28. Hassall E. Wrap session: is the Nissen slipping? Can medical treatment replace surgery for severe gastroesophageal reflux disease in children? Am J Gastroenterol 1995;90: 1212–1220.

29. Hassall E. Decisions in diagnosing and managing chronic gastroesophageal reflux disease in children. J Pediatr 2005;146: S3–S12.

30. Hatch KF, Daily MF, Christensen BJ, Glasgow RE. Failed fundoplications. Am J Surg 2004;188: 786–91.

31. Jamieson GG, Duranceau A. What is a Nissen fundoplication? Surgery 1984;159:591–3.

32. Jamieson JR, Stein HJ, DeMeester TR, Bonavina L, Schwizer W, Hinder RA, Albertucci M. Ambulatory 24-h esophageal pH monitoring: normal values, optimal thresholds, specificity, sensitivity, and reproducibility. Am J Gastroenterol 1992;87:1102–11.

33. Jesch NK, Schmidt AI, Strassburg A, Gluer S, UreBM. Laparoscopic fundoplication in neurologically impaired children with percutaneous endoscopic gastrostomy. Eur J Pediatr Surg 2004;14: 89–92.

Section Two

34. Jones R, Canal DF, Inman MM, Rescorla FJ. Laparoscopic fundoplication: a three-year review. Am Surg 1996;62: 632–6.
35. Khajanchee YS, O'Rourke RW, Lockhart B, Patterson EJ, Hansen PD, Swanstrom LL. Postoperative symptoms and failure after antireflux surgery. Arch Surg 2002;137:1008–14.
36. Klauser AG, Schindlbeck NE, Muller-Lissner SA. Symptoms in gastro-esophageal reflux disease. Lancet 1990;335: 205–8.
37. Langer JC. The failed fundoplication. Semin Pediatr Surg 2003;12: 110–17.
38. Lindquist SG, Kirchhoff M, Lundsteen C, Pedersen W, Erichsen G, Kristensen K, Lillquist K, Smedegaard HH, Skov L, Tommerup N, Brondum-Nielsen K. Further delineation of the 22q13 deletion syndrome. Clin Dysmorphol 2005;14: 55–60.
39. Liu DC, Somme S, Mavrelis PG, Hurwich D, Statter MB, Teitelbaum DH, Zimmermann BT, Jackson CC, Dye C. Stretta as the initial antireflux procedure in children. J Pediatr Surg 2005;40:148–151; discussion 151–142.
40. Lord RVN, Kaminski A, Oberg S, Bowrey DJ, Hagen JA, DeMeester SR, Sillin LF, Peters JH, Crookes PF, DeMeester TR. Absence of gastroesophageal reflux disease in a majority of patients taking acid suppression medications after Nissen fundoplication. J Gastrointest Surg 2002;6:3–10.
41. Ludemann R, Watson DI, Jamieson GG, et al. Five-year follow-up of a randomized clinical trial of laparoscopic total versus anterior 180° fundoplication. Br J Surgery 2005;92:240–3.
42. Madan A, Minocha A. Despite high satisfaction, majority of gastro-esophageal reflux disease patients continue to use proton pump inhibitors after antireflux surgery. Aliment Pharmacol Ther 2006;23:601–605.
43. Maddern GJ. The reproducibility of esophageal manometry. Dis Esophagus 1991;4:95–99.
44. Mattioli G, Sacco O, Repetto P, Pini Prato A, Castagnetti M, Carlini C, Torre M, Leggio S, Gentilino V, Martino F, Fregonese B, Barabino A, Gandullia P, Rossi GA, Jasonni V Necessityfor surgery in children with gastro-oesophageal reflux and supraoesophageal symptoms. Eur J Pediatr Surg 2004;14: 7–13.
45. Ollyo JB, Lang F, Fontolle CH, et al. Savary's new endoscopic grading of reflux esophagitis: a simple, reproducible, logical, complete and useful classification. Gastroenterology 1990;89:A100.
46. Papasavas PK, Keenan RJ, Yeaney WW, Caushaj PF, Gagne DJ, Landreneau RJ. Effectiveness of laparoscopic fundoplication in relieving the symptoms of gastroesophageal reflux disease (GERD) and eliminating antireflux medical therapy. Surg Endosc 2003;17:1200–1205.
47. Patterson EJ, Davis DG, Khajanchee Y, Swanstrom LL. Comparison of objective outcomes following laparoscopic Nissen fundoplication versus laparoscopic gastric bypass in the morbidly obese with heartburn. Surg Endosc 2003;17:1561–1565.
48. Post JC, Ze F, Ehrlich GD. Genetics of pediatric gastroesophageal reflux. Curr Opin Allergy Clin Immunol 2005;5: 5–9 60. Ravelli AM, Milla PJ. Vomiting and gastroesophageal motor activity in children with disorders of the central nervous system. J Pediatr Gastroenterol Nutr 1998;26: 56–63.
49. Quigley EMM. Changing face of irritable bowel syndrome. World J Gastroenterol 2006;12:1–5.
50. Rothenberg SS. The first decade's experience with laparoscopic Nissen fundoplication in infants and children. J Pediatr Surg 2005;40: 142–146; discussion 147.
51. Rothenberg SS. Laproscopic redo Nissen fundoplication in infants and children. Surg Endosc 2006;20(10): 1518–20.
52. Rudolph CD. Supraesophageal complications of gastroesophageal reflux in children: challenges in diagnosis and treatment. Am J Med 2003;115(Suppl 3A): 150S–6S.
53. Schier F. Indications for laparoscopic antireflux procedures in children. Semin Laparosc Surg 2002;9: 139–45.
54. Shay S, Tutuian R, Sifrim D, Vela M, Wise J, Balaji N, Zhang X, Adhami T, Murray J, Peters J, Castell D. Twenty-four hour ambulatory simultaneous impedance and pH monitoring: a multicenter report of normal values from 60 healthy volunteers. Am J Gastroenterol 2004;99:1037–1043. J Gastrointest Surg 2007;11:642–7. 647.
55. Smith CD, McClusky DA, Rajad MA, Lederman AB, Hunter JG. When fundoplication fails: redo? Ann Surg 2005;241:861–71.
56. Spechler SJ, Lee E, Ahnen D, Goyal RK, Hirano I, Ramirez F, Raufman JP, Sampliner R, Schnell T, Sontag S, Vlahcevic ZR, Young R, Williford W. Long-term outcome of medical and surgical therapies for astroesophageal reflux disease: follow-up of a randomized controlled trial. JAMA 2001;285(18):2331–38.
57. Spechler SJ. The management of patients who have "failed" antireflux surgery. Am J Gastroenterol 2004;99:552–61.
58. Spence GM,Watson DI, Jamieson GG, Lally CJ, Devitt PG. Single center prospective randomized trial of laparoscopic Nissen versus anterior 90° fundoplication. J Gastrointest Surg 2006;10:698–705.
59. Spiroglou K, Xinias I, Karatzas N, Karatza E, Arsos G, Panteliadis C. Gastric emptying in children with cerebral palsy and gastroesophageal reflux. Pediatr Neurol 2004;31: 177–82.
60. Spitz L, McLeod E. Gastroesophageal reflux. Semin Pediatr Surg 2003;12: 237–40.
61. Stylopoulos N, Rattner DW. The history of hiatal hernia surgery: from Bowditch to laparoscopy. Ann Surg 2005;241:185–193.
62. Sydorak RM, Albanese CT. Laparoscopic antireflux procedures in children: evaluating the evidence. Semin Laparosc Surg 2002;9: 133–38.
63. Thomson M, Fritscher-Ravens A, Hall S, Afzal N, Ashwood P, Swain CP. Endoluminal gastroplication in children with significant gastroesophageal reflux disease. Gut 2004;53: 1745–50.

64. Vaezi MF, Richter JE. Role of acid and duodeno-gastroeso-phageal reflux in gastroesophageal reflux disease. Gastroenterology 1996; 111:1192–9.

65. Vandenplas Y, Hassall E. Mechanisms of gastroesophageal reflux and gastroesophageal reflux disease. J Pediatr Gastroenterol Nutr 2002;35: 119–136.

66. Watson DI, Jamieson GG, Lally C, Archer S, Bessell JR, Booth M, Cade R, Cullingford G, Devitt PG, Fletcher DR, Hurley J, Kiroff G, Martin CJ, Martin IJ, Nathanson LK, Windsor JA. Multicenter prospective double blind randomized trial of laparoscopic Nissen versus anterior 90 degree partial fundoplication. Arch Surg 2004;139:1160-1167.

67. Watson DI, Jamieson GG, Pike GP, et al. Prospective randomized double-blind trial between laparoscopic Nissen fundoplication and anterior partial fundoplication. Br J Surg 1999;86:123–130.

68. Zeid MA, Kandel T, el-Shobary M, Talaat AA, Fouad A, el-Enien AA, el-Badrawy T, el-Hak NG, el-Wahab MA, Ezzat F. Nissen fundoplication in infants and children: a long-term clinical study. Hepatogastroenterology 2004;51: 697–700.

Section Two

Sleeve Gastrectomy

INTRODUCTION

Obesity has become a major health problem in the last few decades. Obesity is the most prevalent chronic disease of the 21st century. The World Health Organization (WHO) has identified obesity as one of the five leading health risks in developed countries. WHO has reported that over a billion people are overweight and that 300 million are clinically obese, with a projection of 3 million deaths annually worldwide. In the United States, 65 percent of adult Americans are overweight and 31 percent are clinically obese. Fourteen percent of American children and adolescents are obese. Bariatric surgery is now considered the only valid therapeutic option for morbidly obese patients but can be associated with significant risk, especially in patients affected by life-threatening comorbidities. Morbid obesity [defined as a body mass index (BMI) more than 40 kg/m^2] affects 4.7 percent of Americans and these numbers are rapidly rising. For these patients, surgery represents the most effective treatment. However, failure is frequent issue and selection of correct surgery is paramount of success.

The sleeve gastrectomy is a restrictive form of weight loss surgery in which approximately 85 percent of the stomach is removed leaving a cylindrical or sleeve-shaped stomach with a capacity ranging from about 60 to 150 cc, Stomach is reduced to about 15 percent of its original size, by surgical removal of a large portion of the stomach along greater curvature (Fig. 20.1). The open edges are then attached together with the help of stapler to form a sleeve or tube with a banana shape (Figs 20.2A and B). The procedure permanently reduces the size of the stomach. The procedure is performed either open or laparoscopically and is not reversible.

Laparoscopic sleeve gastrectomy is a relatively new option originally published by Marceau et al. Unlike many other forms of bariatric surgery, the outlet valve and the nerves to the stomach remain intact and, while the stomach is drastically reduced in size, its function is preserved. Again, other forms of surgery such as the Roux-en-Y gastric bypass, the sleeve gastrectomy is not reversible.

Because the new stomach continues to function normally there are far fewer restrictions on the foods which patients can consume after surgery, although the quantity of food eaten will be considerably reduced. This is seen by many patients as being one of the great

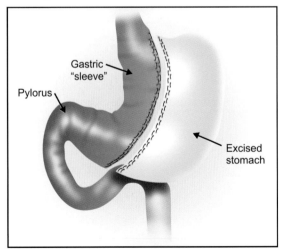

Fig. 20.1: Sleeve gastrectomy

advantages of the sleeve gastrectomy, as is the fact that the removal of the majority of the stomach also results in the virtual elimination of hormone (Ghrelin) produced within the stomach which stimulate hunger.

Ghrelin Hormone

Ghrelin got its name from the word "ghre" from the Proto-Indo-European language, meaning to grow. Scientists did not go purposefully looking for a substance that stimulated appetite. Indeed the discovery of ghrelin occurred when scientists were investigating drugs that stimulated the release of growth hormone from the anterior pituitary gland. They came across some drugs that, rather than acting on the growth hormone releasing hormone receptor, were acting on an unknown receptor located in the hypothalamus and pituitary, these drugs were called growth hormone secretagogues. It was concluded that the body had a second pathway for the induction of growth hormone secretion.

Ghrelin was identified as being the natural legend for these receptors causing secretion of growth hormone in 1999 by the Japanese scientist Masayasu Kojima (see key references). During Kojima's

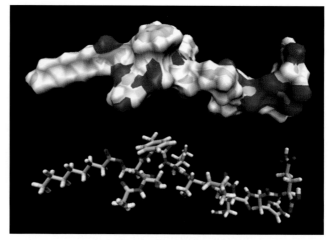

Fig. 20.2A: Ghrelin hormone

investigations, they found that although ghrelin's receptors were in the brain, ghrelin was surprisingly identified in the human stomach and circulating in the blood leading to the conclusion that it was released from the stomach where it then travelled in the blood and acted on the brain.

Ghrelin is a hormone produced mainly by P/D1 cells lining the fundus of the human stomach and epsilon cells of the pancreas that stimulates hunger

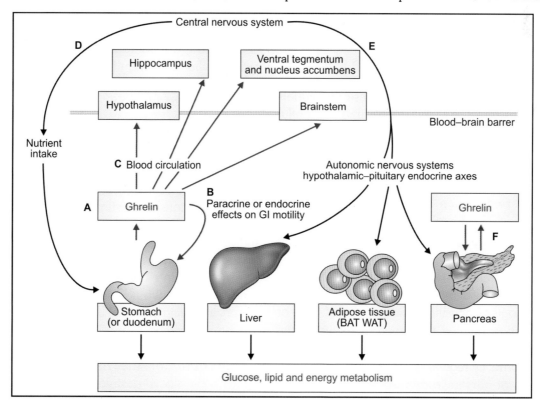

Fig. 20.2B: Role of ghrelin in glucose and lipid metabolism

(Fig. 20.2). Ghrelin levels increase before meals and decrease after meals. It is considered the counterpart of the hormone leptin, *produced by adipose tissue, which induces satiation when present at higher levels.* In some bariatric procedures, the level of ghrelin is reduced in patients, thus causing satiation before it would normally occur. Ghrelin is also produced in the hypothalamic arcuate nucleus, where it stimulates the secretion of growth hormone from the anterior pituitary gland. Receptors for ghrelin are expressed by neurons in the arcuate nucleus and the ventromedial hypothalamus. Once the high amount of ghrelin is secreted the patient feel intense hunger (Fig. 20.3). Apart from hunger Ghrelin plays a significant role in neurotrophy, particularly in the hippocampus, and is essential for cognitive adaptation to changing environments and the process of learning.

Ghrelin has emerged as the first circulating hunger hormone. Ghrelin and synthetic ghrelin mimetic increase food intake and increase fat mass by an action exerted at the level of the hypothalamus. They activate cells in the arcuate nucleus that include the orexigenic neuropeptide Y (NPY) neurons. Ghrelin-responsiveness of these neurones is both leptin- and insulin-sensitive. Ghrelin also activates the mesolimbic cholinergic-dopaminergic reward link, a circuit that communicates the hedonic and reinforcing aspects of natural rewards, such as food, as well as of addictive drugs, such as ethanol (Fig. 20.3).

Ghrelin levels in the plasma of obese individuals are lower than those in leaner individuals. Recently, Scripps research scientists have developed an anti-obesity vaccine, which is directed against the hormone ghrelin. The vaccine uses the immune system, specifically antibodies, to bind to selected targets, directing the body's own immune response against them. This prevents ghrelin from reaching the central nervous system, thus producing a desired reduction in weight gain.

Obesity is the result of multifactorial changes involving both genetic and environmental factors. The physiopathology of obesity from the point of view of intake regulation has led to numerous experimental studies aimed at identifying new forms of regulation. These new forms of regulation are not only found in the secretion of ghrelin from gastrointestinal system

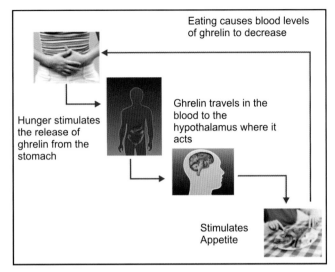

Fig. 20.3: Mode of action of ghrelin

but also in the adipose tissue (via the metabolism of leptin and insulin) and the central nervous system to finally produce the relevant orexigenic or anorexigenic effect.

Advantage of Sleeve Gastrectomy

Some authors described LSG as a stand-alone procedure with good results with respect to excessive weight loss (EWL) and lower plasma ghrelin levels. Also, there are numerous reports of morbidly obese patients who underwent LSG as a first step before an intended malabsorptive procedure and lost their excessive weight after LSG, so that further surgery was not necessary. This is important because the disadvantages of the malabsorptive procedure are avoided. Perhaps the greatest advantage of the gastric sleeve lies in the fact that it does not involve any bypass of the intestinal tract and patients do not therefore suffer the complications of intestinal bypass such as intestinal obstruction, anemia, osteoporosis, vitamin deficiency and protein deficiency. It also makes it a suitable form of surgery for patients who are already suffering from anemia, Crohn's disease and a variety of other conditions that would place them at high risk for surgery involving intestinal bypass. Sleeve gastrectomy can be performed laparoscopically without much problem in patients who are extremely overweight and this account for the rising popularity of the laparoscopic sleeve gastrectomy.

Disadvantage of Sleeve Gastrectomy

Perhaps the main disadvantage of this form of surgery is that it does not always produce the reduction in weight which people would wish for and, in the longer term, can result in weight regain. This is indeed true of any form of purely restrictive surgery, but is perhaps especially true in the case of the sleeve gastrectomy. Because the procedure requires stapling of the stomach patients do run the risk of leakage and of other complications directly related to stapling. In addition, as with any surgery, patients run the risk of additional complications such as postoperative bleeding, small bowel obstruction, pneumonia and even death. The risk of encountering any of these complications is, however, extremely small and varies from about 0.5 and 1 percent. Having said this, the risk of death from this form of surgery at about 0.25 percent is extremely small.

The risks and complications of the sleeve gastrectomy

As with all forms of weight loss surgery, the vertical gastrectomy does carry risk and these will clearly vary from one patient to the other.

Complications include:

- Gastric leakage and fistula 1.0 percent
- Deep vein thrombosis 0.5 percent
- Non-fatal pulmonary embolus 0.5 percent
- Postoperative bleeding 0.5 percent
- Splenectomy 0.5 percent
- Acute respiratory distress 0.25 percent
- Pneumonia 0.2 percent
- Death 0.25 percent.

Surgical Technique

The patient is positioned in a modified reverse Trendelenburg position with the right arm away from the body. The abdomen is prepared and draped in the customary fashion. Ports are used according to baseball diamond concept as shown in (Figs 20.5A and B).

After exploration of the abdomen and the anterior wall of the stomach, the liver is retracted via fifth port (Fig. 20.6).

Dissection should be started with dissection of the short gastric vessels to the point of the angle of His

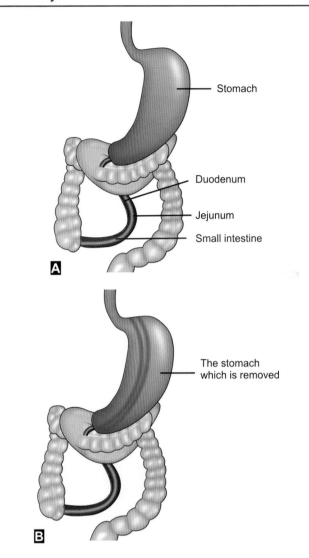

Figs 20.4A and B: Before and after sleeve gastrectomy

using either the Harmonic Scalpel (Ethicon Endo-Surgery) or Ligasure. The greater omentum is then separated from the greater curvature under protection of the gastroepiploic arcade. The endpoint of the preparation is about 7-8 cm prepyloric (Fig. 20.7).

A 34-Fr tube is then positioned along the lesser curvature of stomach as the leading structure for the stapling line to follow. After freeing the omentum, staple should be applied along the greater curvature strictly along the stomach tube using a 60-mm Endo-GIA, Ethicon Endo-Surgery or Auto Suture (Fig. 20.8). The starting point is 7-8 cm prepyloric to the point of the angle of His. Typically, four to five staple lines are needed (Figs 20.9A to C).

Section Two

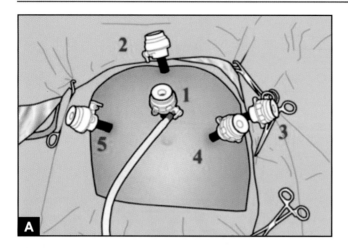

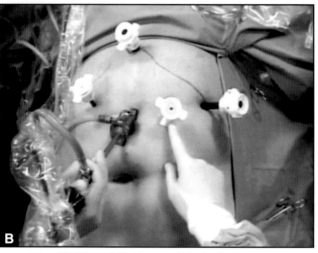

Figs 20.5A and B: Port position for laparoscopic
sleeve gastrectomy

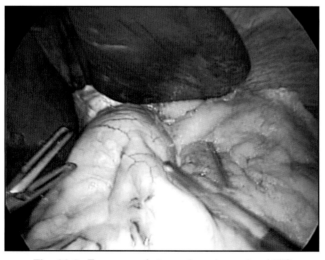

Fig. 20.6: Exposure of stomach up to angle of HIS

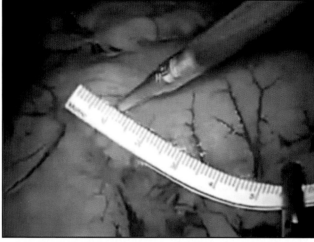

Fig. 20.7: 6 cm of stomach towards the pylorus is left

Different types of stapler are available in the market

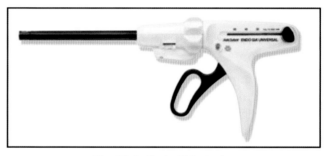

Fig. 20.8: Endo GIA stapler

The dissected part of the stomach is withdrawn from the abdomen at port no: 3 and the staple line will be overstitched by absorbable intracorporeal suturing. This is done not to prevent insufficiency in the staple line but rather to prevent staple line bleeding. It is possible to overstitch only areas of bleeding between the staples, not the whole staple line.

Like most of the bariatric surgery operations, currently there are multiple variations in the technique for the LSG. Some of these variations are: the size of bougie (determines the size of the pouch) beside which the Endo GIA Staplers are placed to divide the stomach, the level at which the surgeons start the division in the central area. Many surgeons leave most of the antrum for its pumping, emptying action and also to avoid the possibility of leak from this thick-walled tough area 1, 2, 3 and thirdly, to reinforce or not reinforce this long staple line.

Section Two

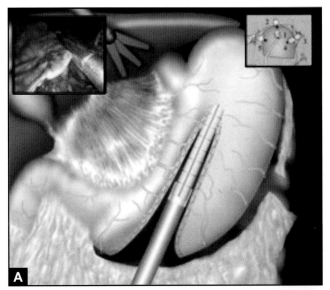

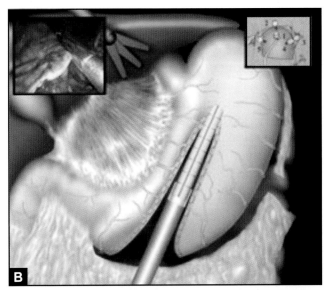

Fig. 20.9A: After dissecting the greater omentum from the greater curvature, a 34-Fr stomach tube is placed along the lesser curvature. The first staple line is then set strictly along the stomach. The starting point of the dissection of the greater curvature is about 7-8 cm prepyloric

Fig. 20.9B: The second staple line is set strictly and continued along the stomach tube

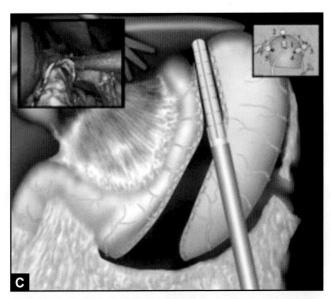

Fig. 20.9C: Finishing of the gastric sleeve with the third staple line. The greater curvature is resected to the point of the angle of His

Five or six ports are used for LSG and the surgeon standing between the patient's legs. An open technique could be used for the first port, establishing a pneumoperitoneum of 15 mm Hg. Then, two right ports, one left port, and a midline ports are usually sufficient (Fig. 20.5). The right subcostal trocar is used to insert the fan retractor for the liver. The camera should be placed high between the umbilicus and xiphoid. Initial decompression of the stomach with NGT is preferable. Some surgeons commence the laparoscopic sleeve gastrectomy with an opening through the gastrocolic ligament to lesser sac, and

Section Two

firstly cut-staple the vertical channel along the bougie. It is better to first mobilize the greater curvature outside the epiploic arcade, near to the gastric wall, which will be removed. With the patient in reverse Trendelenberg position, the posterior stomach wall is visualized and fine adhesions to the pancreas are divided and the lesser sac totally freed using harmonic scalpel, ligasure, or coagulation hook. The left side of the GE junction should be cleared off fat to avoid later compromise of the stapling during creation of the sleeve (Figs 20.10A to D). Left crus should be exposed completely.

Majority of surgeons start the dissection 5-10 cm proximal to the pylorus, but some European surgeons start the dissection closer to the pylorus. If the dissection starts too close to the pylorus, the antrum will not empty properly and its pumping mechanism will be defective, thus postoperative nausea may occur. The linear Endo-GIA stapler is generally introduced through a right trocar towards the left shoulder and leaves about 1 cm of fat pad along the lesser curvature (3 cm width). This assures adequate blood supply on the lesser curvature for the sleeve. Transaction of the stomach should be started 6 cm proximal to the pylorus and then the anesthesiologist inserts a 36-40-Fr bougie down to pylorus, if the LSG is intended as the sole operation but if as a preliminary step before duodenal switch, a 60-Fr bougie is used. Kueper, et al consider a 34-Fr bougie which results in a pouch of 100 ml. The sleeve is started at the lower end of the crow's foot. The procedure requires five to six firings of the linear cutting stapler (60 cm long, 4.8-mm staple-

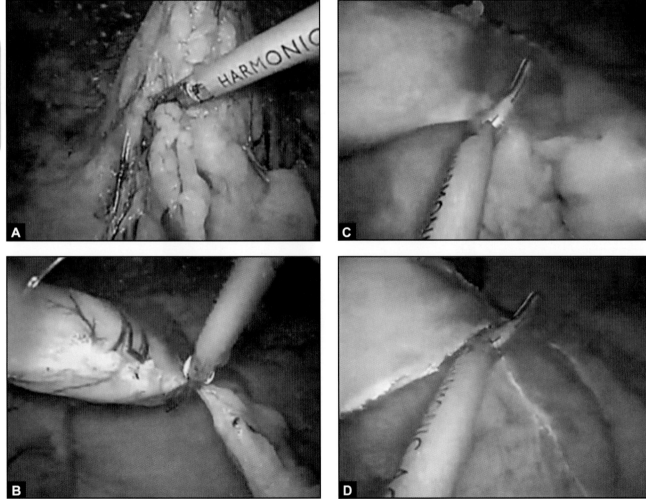

Figs 20.10A to D: Dissection and mobilization of stomach along the greater curvature outside the epiploic arcade

height, and green cartridge) to divide the entire stomach (Figs 20.11A to H). It is important to remove all fundus to avoid regain of weight. The vagus nerves anteriorly and posteriorly are preserved for normal gastric emptying.

The resected greater curvature could be extracted in a bag via epigastric or right paramedian port-site after being dilated to two-finger diameter. The typical specimen has the shape of a comma or banana with the fundus at the top. In dividing the stomach, most

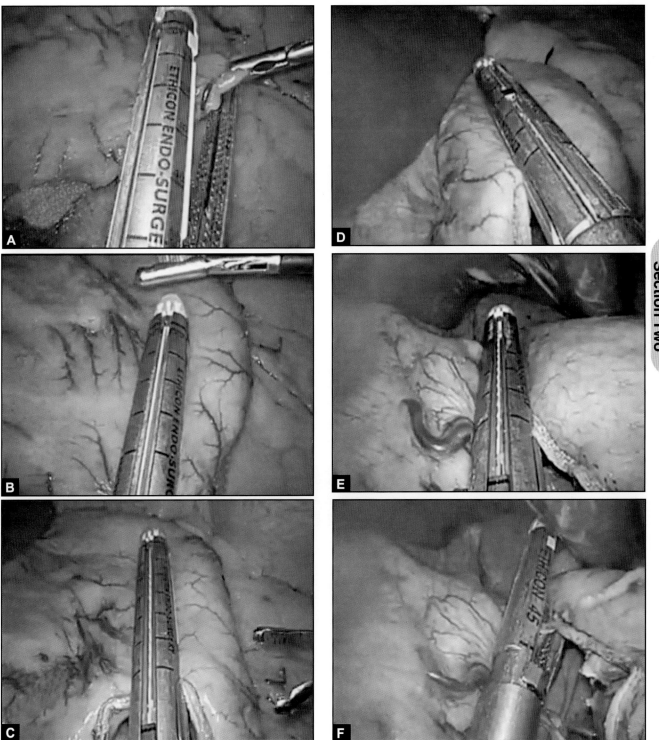

Figs 20.11A to F

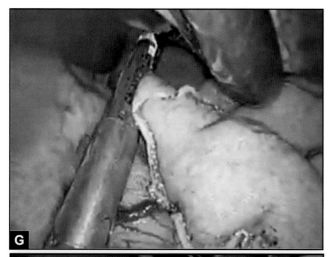

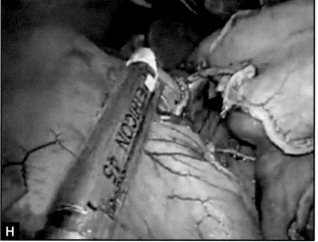

Figs 20.11G and H

Figs 20.11A to H: Gastrectomy with the help of ENDO GI stapler

surgeons use over sewing of the staple-line by continuous or interrupted absorbable sutures to prevent bleeding and leak.

Intraoperative testing through an 18-Fr Argyle tube with diluted methylene blue or air under saline using a gastroscope, with concurrent compression of prepyloric area is a complementary step. A Gastrografin® swallow is ordered by many surgeons on the second postoperative day, or others perform this study only if there is a problem. A liquid diet may be commenced on the first postoperative day.

WEIGHT LOSS

"Durable" weight loss is the one most important gain of bariatric surgery operations, and it is the parameter by which success or failure of weight-reducing techniques is measured. Success of treatment has been defined as weight loss >50 percent of excess weight, maintaining or even losing further after surgery (Table 20.1).

The percentage weight loss after LSG in 707 morbidly obese patients included in the reviewed series is 40 percent (a mean) after a mean follow up of 14 months (Table 20.1).

Effect on Associated Comorbidities

Laparoscopic sleeve gastrectomy had been carried out for super obese patients with multiple severe

	Table 20.1: Outcome of published series on sleeve gastrectomy					
S.No.	Author	No.of pts.	Average Preop BMI	Bougie (Fr)	FU (Months)	%wt. loss
1.	Weimer et al (2007)	A=25	61.6	NR	60	62% at 12 ms.
		B=32	60.8	44	60	C>B>A
		C=63	60.3	32	60	significantly
2.	Strekas (2008)	93	46.86±6.48	36	12.51±4.15	58.32±16.54%,
3.	*Dapri et al (2007)*	A=20	42.5	34	12	48.3%
		B=20	47	34	12	49.5%
4.	Lee et al (2007)	216	49±11	32		
5.	Melissas, et al (2007)	23	47.2±4.8	34	12	33.1%
6.	**Hamoui**	118	55		24	47.3%
7.	Langer, et al (2006)					
	(sleeve dilatation)	23	48.5 ± 6.9	48	12	56%
8.	Quesada (2008)	15	54	38	6	44%

Contd...

Contd...

Section Two

Contd...

S.No.	Author					
9.	**Baltasar (2006)** **(re-sleeve)**	2	46, 42			
10.	Cottam et al (2006) (initial, high-risk)	126	65.3±0.8	48	12	46%
11.	Vidal et al (2007) (effect of LSG on DM)	35		48		NR
12.	Silecchia, et al (2006)	41;supero-bese ≥ 2 major comorbidities	57.3±6.5	48	22.2± 7.1	NR
13.	DePaula et al (2008) (effect of LSG as initial to 2 diff. procedures on DM with BMId ≤ 35	39	23.4 to 34.9	NR	7	22%
14.	Madhala, et al (2008) (technique)	25	44 ± 2	50	4	22.7%
15.	Till, et al (2008) (LSG in morbid obese children)	4 (≤ 14.5 yrs.)	48.4	40	12	23%
Total		707	MEAN=57.76	MEAN=43.7Fr.	Mean=14.5 months	Mean= 40%

Table 20.2: Main complications of LSG in the reviewed published series

S.No.	Author	No.of pts.	Main complications	Recommendations
1.	Weimer (2007)	120	Reflux symptoms, severe esophagitis	
2.	Strekas (2008)	93	4 cases of gastric leak, 3 managed conservatively	More suitable for intermediate morbidly obese patients with BMI between 40 and 50 kg/m
3.	Dapri et al (2007)	20+20	1 early leak. 1 late leak, 1 stenosis	Better mobilize the stomach than resect it
4.	Lee et al (2007)	23	2 leaks	Recommended for BMI< 50 kg/m^2
5.	Melissas et al (2007)	23	8 GERD; only one persisted	The term restrictive may not be applicable to the LSG
6.	Hamoui, et al (2006)	118	One death due to gastric leakage	Out of 118 super obese patients, only 6 requested second stage duodenal switch.
7.	Langer, et al (2006)	23	One severe GERD one renal failure	Sleeve dilatation doesn't necessarily lead to weight gain
8.	Quesada (2008)	15	-	LSG is best option in the presence of adhesions
9.	Baltasar (2006)	2	-	Re-LSG is achievable with minimal complication
10.	Cottam et al (2006) (initial, high-risk)	126 (+9.3 comorbidities in each; mean)	-	Only 36 pts. (39%) Were in need of the second stage. LSG is a good initial op. in those severely combor-bid patients.
11.	Vidal et al (2007) (effect of LSG on DM)	35	-	DM resolved in 51.3 percent 4 months after LSG.
12.	Silecchia, et al (2006)	41 Superobese ≥ 2 major comorbidities	1 leakage, 1 bleeding, 1 transient renal failure	After 12 months, 57.8% of the patients were comorbidity-free

Contd...

Contd...

13.	DePaula et al (2008)	39	2 leakage, 2 renal failure	50% resolution of DM after 7 months.
14.	Madhala, et al (2007)	25	-	-
15.	Till, et al (2008) (LSG in morbid obese children)	4 ($\leq$ 14.5 yrs.)	-	Comorbidities improved significantly
	Total	707	11 gastric leaks, 1 DEATH, 4 RF, 1 stenosis = 17; 2.4%	

comorbidities and in at least 50 percent of the patients; there was marked improvement of the comorbidities specially Diabetes Mellitus which got marked benefit in 50 to 57 percent.

Complications

In one of the reviewed series (n= 707), there are 17 major complications with an incidence of 2.4 percent. One should consider the heterogeneity of the patient's population where those with high risk and multiple severe comorbidities are included. One death due to gastric leakage reported with 11 gastric leakage, 4 renal failures and 1 stenosis. GERD occurs in too many cases but most of the patients improve gradually on conservative management. Bleeding from the suture line reported rarely and could be managed conservatively in most of the cases.

LSG as Initial Step for Super Obese and High-risk Patients

In two studies LSG was used as a planned initial step for entertained other major final technique due to super obesity with poor general condition in an attempt to minimize the risk in this subgroup of patients. During the post-LSG follow-up, the authors found the second stage operation is only needed in 5 percent in one study 12 and 39 percent in the others (Table 20.2).

LSG in Morbidly Obese Children

Till et al carried-out LSG in 4 morbidly obese pediatric patients with multiple comorbidities. Marked improvements in their comorbidities and 23 percent weight loss had been achieved after 12 months follow-up.

Conclusion

As the prevalence of morbid obesity continues to escalate, the incidence of progressively complicated patients will rise. Clearly, a valid and effective strategy, beyond the current comprehensive evaluation measures, is needed for the optimal management of these patients.

Bariatric surgery is the most effective treatment for severe obesity, producing durable weight loss, improvement of comorbid conditions, and longer life. Patient selection algorithms should favor individual risk benefit considerations over traditional anthropometric and demographic limits. Bariatric care should be delivered within credentialed multidisciplinary systems. Roux-en-Y gastric bypass (RGB), adjustable gastric banding (AGB), and biliopancreatic diversion with duodenal switch (BPDDS) are validated procedures that may be performed laparoscopically. Laparoscopic sleeve gastrectomy (LSG) also is a promising procedure. Comparative data find that procedures with more dramatic clinical benefits carry greater risks, and those offering greater safety and flexibility are associated with less reliable efficacy.

Sleeve gastrectomy has been introduced and well accepted recently into the armamentarium of bariatric procedures. It was initially intended as a first step for poor-risk patients deemed too ill to undergo biliopancreatic diversion with duodenal switch or Roux-en-Y gastric bypass. Some of the patients lost significant weight and declined the proposed second stage, becoming the first patients with sleeve gastrectomy as a sole procedure. Sleeve gastrectomy has gained popularity with both bariatric surgeons and patients, mainly because of its relative operative simplicity and lower risk profile.

BIBLIOGRAPHY

1. Almogy G, Crookes PF, Anthone GJ. Longitudinal gastrectomy as a treatment for the high risk super-obese patients. Obes Surg 2004;14:492-7.
2. Angrisani L, Lorenzo M, Borrelli V, Giuffre´ M, Fonderico C, Capece G. Is bariatric surgery necessary after intragastric balloon treatment? Obes Surg 2006;16:1135-7.
3. Baltasar A, Serra C, Perez N, Bou R, Bengochea M. Re-sleeve gastrectomy. Obes Surg 2006;16:1535-8.
4. Buchwald M, Williams SE. Obesity surgery worldwide. Obes Surg 2004;14:1157-64.
5. Busetto L, Segato G, De Luca M et al. Preoperative weight loss by intragastric balloon in super-obese patients treated with laparoscopic gastric banding: a case control study. Obes Surg 2004;14:671-6
6. Cottam D, Qureshi FG, Mattar SG et al. Laparoscopic sleeve gastrectomy as an initial weight loss procedure for high risk patients with morbid obesity. Surg Endosc 2006;20:859-63.
7. Eisendrath P, Cremer M, Himpens J, Cadiere GB, Le Moine O, Deviere J. Endotherapy including temporary stenting of fistulas of the upper gastrointestinal tract after laparoscopic bariatric surgery. Endoscopy 2007;39:625-30.
8. Eynden FV, Urbain P. Small intestine gastric balloon impact on treated by laparoscopic surgery. Obes Surg 2001;11:646-8.
9. Flum DR, Salem L, Elrod JB et al. Early mortality among Medicare beneficiaries undergoing bariatric surgical procedures. JAMA 2005;294:1903-8.
10. Genco A, Bruni T, Doldi SB et al. BioEnterics Intragastric Balloon: the Italian experience with 2,515 patients. Obes Surg 2005;15:1161-4.
11. Genco A, Cipriano M, Bacci V et al. Bioenterics Intragastric Balloon (BIB): a double blind, randomised, controlled, cross-over study. Int J Obes 2006;30:129-33.
12. Gumbs A, Gagner M, Dakin G et al. Sleeve gastrectomy for morbid obesity. Obes Surg 2007;17:562-9.
13. Hamoui N, Anthone GJ, Kaufman HS, Crookes PF. Sleeve gastrectomy in the high-risk patients. Obes Surg 2006;16:1445-9.
14. Kueper MA, Kramer KM, Kirschniak A et al. Laparoscopic Sleeve Gastrectomy: standardized technique of a potential stand-alone bariatric procedure in morbidly obese patients. World J Surg 2008;32:1462-5.
15. Langer FB, Bohdjalin A, Felberbauer FX et al. Does gastric dilatation limit the success of sleeve gastrectomy as a sole operation for morbid obesity? Obes Surg 2006;16:166-171.
16. Marceau P, Biron S, Bourque RA et al. Biliopancreatic diversion with a new type of gastrectomy. Obes Surg 1993;3:29-35.
17. Melissas J, Kuokouraki S, Askoxylakis J et al. Sleeve gastrectomy—a restrictive procedure? Obes Surg 2007;17:57-62.
18. Milone L, Strong V, Gagner M. Laparoscopic sleeve gastrectomy is superior to endoscopic intragastric balloon as a first stage procedure for superobese patients. Obes Surg 2005;15:612-7.
19. O'Brien PE, McPhail T, Chaston TB et al. Systematic review of medium-term weight loss after bariatric operations. Obes Surg 2006;16:1032-40.
20. Regan JP, Inabnet WB, Gagner M. Early experience with two stage laparoscopic Roux-en-Y gastric bypass as an alternative in the super-super obese patient. Obes Surg 2003;13:861-4.
21. Roa PE, Kaidar-Person O, Pinto D et al. Laparoscopic Sleeve Gastrectomy as treatment for morbid obesity: technique ad short-term outcome. Obes Surg 2006;16:1323-6.
22. Rubin M, Yehoshua RT, Stein M et al. Laparoscopic Sleeve Gastrectomy with minimal morbidity. Early results in 120 morbidly obese patients. Obes Surg 2008.
23. Sallet JA, Marchesini JB, Paiva DS et al. Brazilian multicenter study on the intragastric balloon. Obes Surg 2004;14:991-8.
24. Marceau P, Biron S, Bourque RA et al. Biliopancreatic diversion with a new type of gastrectomy. Obes Surg 1993;3:29-35.
25. Cottam D, Qureshi FG, Mattar SG et al. Laparoscopic sleeve gastrectomy as an initial weight-loss procedure for highrisk patients with morbid obesity. Surg Endosc 2006;20:859-63.
26. Silecchia G, Boru C, Pecchia A et al. Effectiveness of laparoscopic sleeve gastrectomy (first-stage of biliopancreatic diversion with duodenal switch) on comorbidities in super-obese high-risk patients. Obes Surg 2006;16:1138-44.
27. Frezza EE. Laparoscopic vertical sleeve gastrectomy for morbid obesity. The future procedure of choice? Surg Today 2007;37:275-81.
28. Roa PE, Kaidar-Person O, Pinto D et al. Laparoscopic sleeve gastrectomy as treatment for morbid obesity: technique and short-term outcome. Obes Surg 2006;16:1323-6.
29. Mognol P, Chosidow D, Marmuse JP. Laparoscopic sleeve gastrectomy as an initial bariatric operation for high-risk patients: initial results in 10 patients. Obes Surg 2005;15:1030-33.
30. Aggarwal S, Kini SU, Herron D. Laparoscopic sleeve gastrectomy for morbid obesity: a review. Surg Obes Relat Dis 2007;3:189-94.
31. Himpens J, Dapri G, Cadiere GB. A prospective randomized study between laparoscopic gastric banding and laparoscopic isolated sleeve gastrectomy: results after 1 and 3 years. Obes Surg 2006;16:1450-6.
32. Roberts K, Duffy A, Kaufman J et al. Size matters: gastric pouch size correlates with weight loss after laparoscopic Roux-en-Y gastric bypass. Surg Endosc 2007;21:1397-1402.

Section Two

21 Laparoscopic Splenectomy

Laparoscopic splenectomy first started in early nineties but due to the lack of an acceptable conversion rate it was not accepted by most of the laparoscopic surgeons. Now due to increased proficiency in the performance of laparoscopic procedures, conversion rate is now inexistent even with large spleens. To date, this procedure continues to be associated with a steep learning curve but remains very rewarding, elegant procedure. The indications for this procedure have broadened and are now the same as with open procedures. They range from idiopathic thrombo-cytopenic purpura, unresponsive hemolytic anemia to staging procedures and to primary splenic cysts.

Only contraindication of laparoscopic splenectomy is excessively large spleens with weight over 1000 gm. We personally believe that the maneuvers used to remove such large spleens do not warrant these procedures. One should always remember that by laparoscopic approach, the spleen cannot be removed in its integral anatomical form and is usually shredded. If there is any need to preserve splenic integrity, then laparoscopic approach should not indicated.

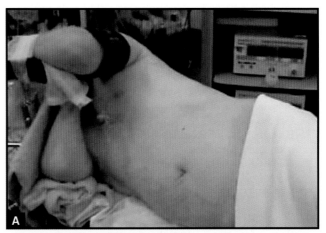

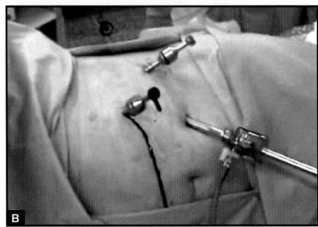

Figs 21.2A and B: Port position

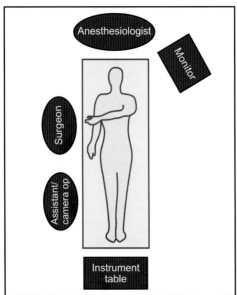

Fig. 21.1: Position of surgical team

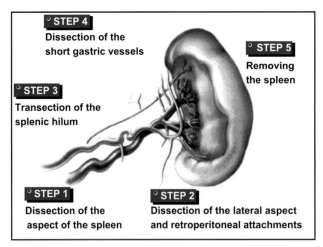

STEP 4
Dissection of the short gastric vessels

STEP 5
Removing the spleen

STEP 3
Transection of the splenic hilum

STEP 1
Dissection of the aspect of the spleen

STEP 2
Dissection of the lateral aspect and retroperitoneal attachments

Fig. 21.3: Various steps of splenectomy

OPERATING ROOM SET-UP AND PATIENT POSITION

Patient is placed in supine and semi left lateral position on the table. Surgeon stands to the right of patient (Fig. 21.1). Camera operator stands right side of the patient next to the surgeon towards right hand side of surgeon. Monitor is placed left to the patient and Mayo's stand is placed near the feet of the patient (Figs 21.2A and B). Various steps of splenectomy shown in Figure 21.3.

Port Position

Port position should be decided according to base ball diamond concept depending on the size of spleen.

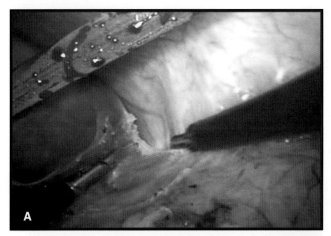

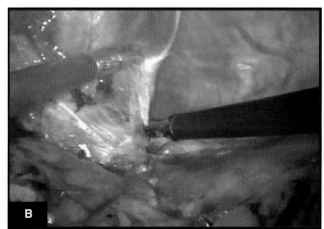

Figs 21.4A and B: Dissection of the inferior aspect of the spleen

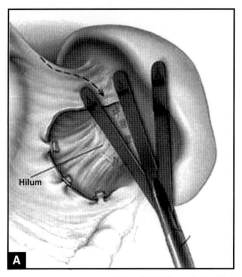

Hilum

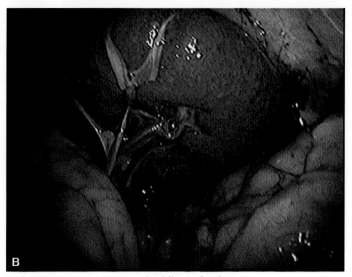

Figs 21.5A and B: Retractor is necessary to expose the hilum of spleen

Section Two

Operative Procedure

Laparoscopic splenectomy can be described in 5 steps:

Step 1: Dissection of the inferior aspect of the spleen.

Step 2: Dissection of the lateral and retroperitoneal attachments.

Step 3: Transaction of the splenic hilum.

A 10 mm fan retractor is inserted and will lift the inferior aspect spleen superiorly. The tail of the pancreas should be identified. The splenorenal and colosplenic ligaments are divided with sharp dissection. The dissection is continued superior and lateral to mobilize the entire spleen (Figs 21.4 and 21.5).

It is essential to continue our dissection posterior and inferior to the spleen as far as possible. Its purpose is to sufficiently expose the posterior aspect of the splenic hilum (Fig. 21.6). The entire anterior aspect of the hilum should also be well-visualized (Figs 21.7A to D).

Occasionally, the short gastric vessels will have to be first transacted to gain additional exposure.

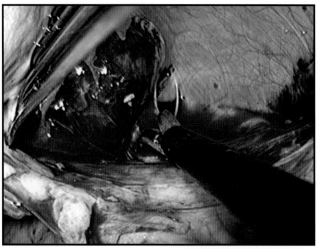

Fig. 21.6: Transaction of the splenic hilum

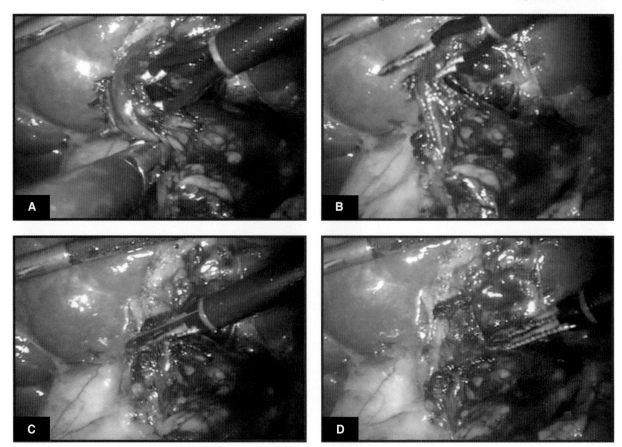

Figs 21.7A to D: Dissection of splenic hilum

Stapler is inserted and each jaw should be positioned anterior and posterior to the splenic vessels. Although this procedure appears very audacious to the neophyte, complete hemostasis of the splenic hilum is usually achieved. The instrument is fired several times in sequence (Figs 21.8A to F).

Step 4: Dissection of the short gastric vessels.

The short gastric vessels are best divided using energy like either ligasure harmonic or simple bilateral. The clip or stapler may be used also for short gastric vessels. Each time the spleen is moved superiorly, inferiorly or medially and all the attachment should be

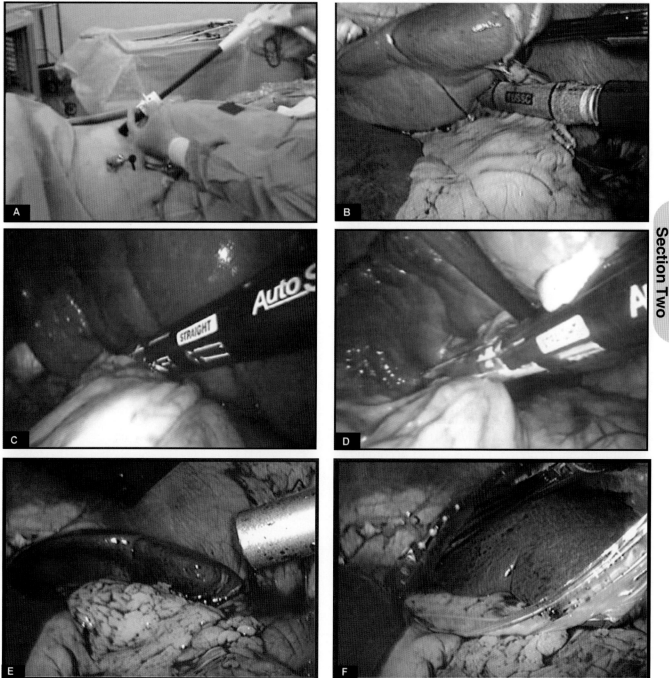

Figs 21.8A to F: Use of endo GI linear stapler or vascular stapler can make the laparoscopic splenectomy easy but many surgeon use extracorporeal knot as their main skill to secure splenic umenti

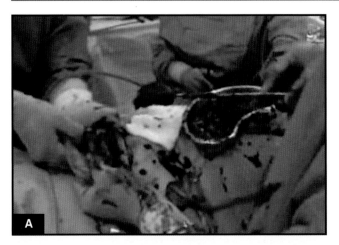
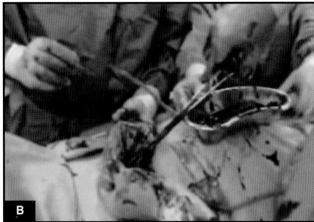

Figs 21.9A and B: Manual morcellation of the spleen inside endobag

carefully dissected. With slow and careful separation of ligaments the spleen should be entirely detached.

Step 5: Removing the spleen

The most lateral 12 mm trocar is removed; its site is enlarged and replaced by 15 mm trocar. An endobag is introduced and deployed in the intra-abdominal cavity. The spleen is placed in the specimen retrieval bag. The specimen retrieval bag is closed and brought against the anterior abdominal wall. It is open via the enlarged trocar site. The spleen is then sectioned in smaller pieces in the specimen retrieval bag and removed with a large clamp (Figs 21.9A and B).

A drain is left in the intra-abdominal cavity. The final evaluation of abdominal cavity is done and the instruments are removed. Port is closed according to need.

BIBLIOGRAPHY

1. Baccarani U, Carroll BJ, Hiatt JR, Donini A, Terrosu G, Decker R, Chandra M, Bresadola F, Phillips EH. Comparison of laparoscopic and open staging in Hodgkin disease. Arch Surg 1998;133:517–22.
2. Baccarani U, Terrosu G, Donini A, Zaja F, Bresadola F, Baccarani M. Splenectomy in hematology: current practice and new perspectives. Haematologica 1999;84:431–6. 842 Surg Endosc 2008;22:821–848 123.
3. Berends FJ, Schep N, Cuesta MA, Bonjer HJ, Kappers-Klunne MC, Huijgens P, Kazemier G. Hematological long-term results of laparoscopic splenectomy for patients with idiopathic thrombocytopenic purpura: a case-control study. Surg Endosc 2004;18:766–70.
4. Brunt LM, Langer JC, Quasebarth MA, Whitman ED. Comparative analysis of laparoscopic versus open splenectomy. Am J Surg 1996;172:596–601 Surg Endosc 2008;22:821–848 847.
5. Casaccia M, Torelli P, Squarcia S, Sormani MP, Savelli A, Troilo B, Santori G, Valente U. Laparoscopic splenectomy for hematologic diseases: a preliminary analysis performed on the Italian Registry of Laparoscopic Surgery of the Spleen (IRLSS). Surg Endosc 2006;20:1214–20.
6. Casaccia M, Torelli P, Squarcia S, Sormani MP, Savelli A, Troilo BM, Santori G, Valente U, Basso N, Silecchia G, et al. The Italian Registry of Laparoscopic Surgery of the Spleen (IRLSS): a retrospective review of 379 patients undergoing laparoscopic splenectomy. Chir Ital 2006;58:697–707.
7. Cordera F, Long KH, Nagorney DM, McMurtry EK, Schleck C, Ilstrup D, Donohue JH. Open versus laparoscopic splenectomy for idiopathic thrombocytopenic purpura: clinical and economic analysis. Surgery 2003;134:45–52.
8. Curran TJ, Foley MI, Swanstrom LL, Campbell TJ. Laparoscopy improves outcomes for pediatric splenectomy. J Pediatr Surg 1998;33:1498–1500.
9. Dagash H, Chowdhury M, Pierro A. When can I be proficient in laparoscopic surgery? A systematic review of the evidence. J Pediatr Surg 2003;38:720–4.
10. Delaitre B, Blezel E, Samama G, Barrat C, Gossot D, Bresler L, Meyer C, Heyd B, Collet D, Champault G. Laparoscopic splenectomy for idiopathic thrombocytopenic purpura. Surg Laparosc Endosc Percutan Tech 2002;12:412–9.
11. Delaitre B, Maignien B. Splenectomy by the laparoscopic approach: report of a case. Presse Med 1991;20:2263.
12. Delaitre B, Pitre J. Laparoscopic splenectomy versus open splenectomy: a comparative study. Hepatogastro- enterology 1997;44:45–9.
13. Donini A, Baccarani U, Terrosu G, Corno V, Ermacora A, Pasqualucci A, Bresadola F. Laparoscopic vs open splenectomy in the management of hematologic diseases. Surg Endosc 1999;13:1220–25.
14. Eden OB, Lilleyman JS. Guidelines for management of idiopathic thrombocytopenic purpura. The British Paediatric Haematology Group. Arch Dis Child 1992;67:1056–8.

Section Two

15. Esposito C, Corcione F, Garipoli V, Ascione G. Pediatric laparoscopic splenectomy: are there real advantages in comparison with the traditional open approach? Pediatr Surg Int 1997;12:509–510.

16. Franciosi C, Caprotti R, Romano F, Porta G, Real G, Colombo G, Uggeri F. Laparoscopic versus open splenectomy: a comparative study. Surg Laparosc Endosc Percutan Tech 2000;10:291–5.

17. Gadenstatter M, Lamprecht B, Klingler A, Wetscher GJ, Greil R, Schmid T. Splenectomy versus medical treatment for idiopathic thrombocytopenic purpura. Am J Surg 2002;184:606–10.

18. Gadner H. Management of immune thrombocytopenic purpura in children. Rev Clin Exp Hematol 2001;5:201–222.

19. George JN, Woolf SH, Raskob GE, Wasser JS, Aledort LM, Ballem PJ, Blanchette VS, Bussel JB, Cines DB, Kelton JG, et al. Idiopathic thrombocytopenic purpura: a practice guideline developed by explicit methods for the American Society of Hematology. Blood 1996;88:3–40.

20. Glasgow RE, Mulvihill SJ. Laparoscopic splenectomy. World J Surg 1999;23:384–8.

21. Jugenburg M, Haddock G, Freedman MH, Ford-Jones L, Ein SH. The morbidity and mortality of pediatric splenectomy: does prophylaxis make a difference? J Pediatr Surg 1999;34:1064– 7.

22. Katkhouda N, Grant SW, Mavor E, Friedlander MH, Lord RV, Achanta K, Essani R, Mason R. Predictors of response after laparoscopic splenectomy for immune thrombocytopenic purpura. Surg Endosc 2001;15:484–8.

23. Khan LR, Nixon SJ. Laparoscopic splenectomy is a better treatment for adult ITP than steroids—it should be used earlier in patient management: conclusions of a ten-year follow-up study. Surgeon 2007;5:3–4, 6–8.

24. Knauer EM, Ailawadi G, Yahanda A, Obermeyer RJ, Millie MP, Ojeda H, Mulholland MW, Colletti L, Sweeney JF. 101 aparoscopic splenectomies for the treatment of benign and malignant hematologic disorders. Am J Surg 2003;186:500–04.

25. Kojouri K, Vesely SK, Terrell DR, George JN. Splenectomy for adult patients with idiopathic thrombocytopenic purpura: a systematic review to assess long-term platelet count responses, prediction of response, and surgical complications. Blood 2004;104:2623–34.

26. Konstadoulakis MM, Lagoudianakis E, Antonakis PT, Albanopoulos K, Gomatos I, Stamou KM, Leandros E, Manouras A. Laparoscopic versus open splenectomy in patients with beta thalassemia major. J Laparoendosc Adv Surg Tech A 2006;16:5–8,

27. Kucuk C, Sozuer E, Ok E, Altuntas F, Yilmaz Z. Laparoscopic versus open splenectomy in the management of benign and malign hematologic diseases: a ten-year single-center experience. J Laparoendosc Adv Surg Tech A 2005;15:135–139.

28. Lozano-Salazar RR, Herrera MF, Vargas-Vorackova F, Lopez-Karpovitch X. Laparoscopic versus open splenectomy for immune thrombocytopenic purpura. Am J Surg 1998;176:366–9

29. Mantadakis E, Buchanan GR. Elective splenectomy in children with idiopathic thrombocytopenic purpura. J Pediatr Hematol Oncol 2000;22:148–53.

30. Napoli A, Catalano C, Silecchia G, Fabiano P, Fraioli F, Pediconi F, Venditti F, Basso N, Passariello R. Laparoscopic splenectomy: multidetector row CT for preoperative evaluation. Radiology 2004;232:361–7.

31. Owera A, Hamade AM, Bani Hani OI, Ammori BJ. Laparoscopic versus open splenectomy for massive splenomegaly: a comparative study. J Laparoendosc Adv Surg Tech A 2006;16:241–6.

32. Pace DE, Chiasson PM, Schlachta CM, Mamazza J, Poulin EC. Laparoscopic splenectomy: does the training of minimally invasive surgical fellows affect outcomes? Surg Endosc 2002;16:954–6.

33. Park A, Marcaccio M, Sternbach M, Witzke D, Fitzgerald P. Laparoscopic vs open splenectomy. Arch Surg 1999;134:1263–9.

34. Peters MB Jr, Camacho D, Ojeda H, Reichenbach DJ, Knauer EM, Yahanda AM, Cooper SE, Sweeney JF. Defining the learning curve for laparoscopic splenectomy for immune thrombocytopenia purpura. Am J Surg 2004;188:522–5.

35. Phillips EH, Carroll BJ, Fallas MJ. Laparoscopic splenectomy. Surg Endosc 1994;8:931–3.

36. Rattner DW, Apelgren KN, Eubanks WS. The need for training opportunities in advanced laparoscopic surgery. Surg Endosc 2001;15:1066–70.

37. Rege RV, Joehl RJ. A learning curve for laparoscopic splenectomy at an academic institution. J Surg Res 1999;81:27–32.

38. Rescorla FJ. Laparoscopic splenectomy. Semin Pediatr Surg 2002;11:226–32.

39. Rhodes M, Rudd M, O'Rourke N, Nathanson L, Fielding G. Laparoscopic splenectomy and lymph node biopsy for hematologic disorders. Ann Surg 1995;222:43–46.

40. Rothenberg SS. Laparoscopic splenectomy in children. Semin Laparosc Surg 1998;5:19–24.

41. Sampath S, Meneghetti AT, MacFarlane JK, Nguyen NH, Benny WB, Panton ON. An 18-year review of open and laparoscopic splenectomy for idiopathic thrombo-cytopenic purpura. Am J Surg 2007;193:580–584.

42. Sauerland S, Agresta F, Bergamaschi R, Borzellino G, Budzynski A, Champault G, Fingerhut A, Isla A, Johansson M, Lundorff P, Navez B, Saad S, Neugebauer EA. Laparoscopy for abdominal emergencies: evidence-based guidelines of the European Association for Endoscopic Surgery. Surg Endosc 2006;20:14–29,

43. Schlinkert RT, Mann D. Laparoscopic splenectomy offers advantages in selected patients with immune thrombocytopenic purpura. Am J Surg 1995;170:624–7.

44. Shimomatsuya T, Horiuchi T. Laparoscopic splenectomy for treatment of patients with idiopathic thrombocytopenic purpura: comparison with open splenectomy. Surg Endosc 1999;13:563–6.

Section Two

45. Smith CD, Meyer TA, Goretsky MJ, Hyams D, Luchette FA, Fegelman EJ, Nussbaum MS. Laparoscopic splenectomy by the lateral approach: a safe and effective alternative to open splenectomy for hematologic diseases. Surgery 1996;120:789–94.

46. Tanoue K, Okita K, Akahoshi T, Konishi K, Gotoh N, Tsutsumi N, Tomikawa M, Hashizume M. Laparoscopic splenectomy for hematologic diseases. Surgery 2002;131:S318–S323.

47. Targarona EM, Espert JJ, Balague C, Piulachs J, Artigas V, Trias M. Splenomegaly should not be considered a contraindication for laparoscopic splenectomy. Ann Surg 1998;228:35–39.

48. Trias M, Targarona EM, Espert JJ, Cerdan G, Bombuy E, Vidal O, Artigas V. Impact of hematological diagnosis on early and late outcome after laparoscopic splenectomy: an analysis of 111 cases. Surg Endosc 2000;14:556–60.

49. Vecchio R, Cacciola E, Lipari G, Privitera V, Polino C, Cacciola R. Laparoscopic splenectomy reduces the need for platelet transfusion in patients with idiopathic thrombocytopenic purpura. JSLS 2005;9:415–18.

50. Velanovich V. Laparoscopic vs open surgery: a preliminary comparison of quality-of-life outcomes. Surg Endosc 2000;14:16–21.

51. Waldhausen JH, Tapper D. Is pediatric laparoscopic splenectomy safe and cost effective? Arch Surg 1997;132:822–24.

52. Walsh RM, Heniford BT, Brody F, Ponsky J. The ascendance of laparoscopic splenectomy. Am Surg 2001;67:48–53.

53. Watanabe Y, Horiuchi A, Yoshida M, Yamamoto Y, Sugishita H, Kumagi T, Hiasa Y, Kawachi K. Significance of laparoscopic splenectomy in patients with hypersplenism. World J Surg 2007;31:549–55.

54. Yee LF, Carvajal SH, de Lorimier AA, Mulvihill SJ. Laparoscopic splenectomy: the initial experience at University of California, San Francisco. Arch Surg 1995;130:874–9.

55. Yuan RH, Chen SB, Lee WJ, Yu SC. Advantages of laparoscopic splenectomy for splenomegaly due to hematologic diseases. J Formos Med Assoc 1998;97:485–489 193. Diaz J, Eisenstat M, Chung R. A case-controlled study of laparoscopic splenectomy. Am J Surg 1997;173:348–50.

Laparoscopic Gynecological Procedures

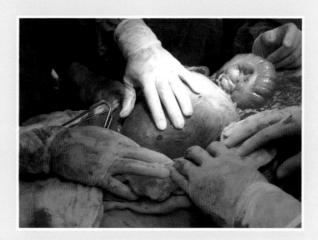

22 Laparoscopic Management of Hepatico-pancreatic Diseases

The indications and preparation for laparoscopic liver surgery remain the same as in open hepatic surgery. Visualization is excellent with the laparoscope, and the addition of laparoscopic ultrasound has been shown to help intraoperative plans in 66 percent of cases when compared to laparoscopic exploration alone. The ability of visual inspection laparoscopy to assess resectability as opposed to inoperability remains relatively low. It can be improved by extended laparoscopy combined with laparoscopic contact ultrasonography. The technique of extended laparoscopy consists of full inspection of the peritoneal cavity, liver with contact laparoscopic ultrasound scanning, entry and inspection of lesser sac, examination of porta hepatis, duodenum, transverse mesocolon, and coeliac and portal vessels. This procedure thus entails extensive dissection and is used to assess operability in patients with pancreatic cancer, hepatic neoplasms and gastroesophageal cancers where it often entails lymph node sampling. Laparoscopic hepatic surgery, while technically difficult, can be performed safely with good results with careful patient selection. Attention to the etiology of the lesion and its location is essential. Ideal candidates have a large solitary cyst or a symptomatic benign mass located superficially, laterally, or far enough from the pedicle to allow direct clamping of the liver or access to the hilum to perform a Pringle maneuver should bleeding occur. Contraindications to this technique include patients with cirrhosis, hepatocellular carcinoma, or posterior or centrally located lesions. While we have utilized this approach for solitary small metastatic disease, hydatid disease, hepatic abscess, and PCLD,

these should be viewed with a great deal of circumspection. Problems exist to varying degrees should any of these lesions be spilled. Port site recurrences remain a concern when using laparoscopy in any patient with cancer. This is of special concern when considering pairing this approach with cryoablation. With echinococcal cysts, the risk of spillage is also obvious, though less problematic with calcified cysts. If one does use a laparoscopic approach for hydatid disease, we recommend a cholangiogram to rule out a connection with the biliary system. While fenestration of polycystic liver disease has been described both by open and laparoscopic approaches, transcystic fenestration of deeper cysts makes the control of bleeding difficult.

Laparoscopic liver surgery provides advantages over open surgery for the liver since the Chevron incision is completely avoided and the surgery is performed through tiny incisions. As a consequence the duration of stay in hospital, the amount and duration of postoperative discomfort, and the length of recovery are much shorter after the laparoscopic procedure compared to open surgery. To safely perform liver surgery laparoscopically, the surgeon must be both an accomplished laparoscopist and hepatic surgeon. Few surgeons, however, are as comfortable with open hepatic surgery as they are with the gallbladder, hernia, appendix, or stomach. Furthermore, only a limited number of lesions, depending upon their location and etiology, can be approached by laparoscopy. The most commonly performed procedures are symptomatic solitary hepatic cyst, symptomatic polycystic liver disease, hydatid cyst, focal nodular hyperplasia, adenoma, abscess, metastatic breast cancer, and calcified gallbladder.

TECHNIQUE OF LAPAROSCOPIC MANAGEMENT OF HYDATID CYSTIC LIVER

The procedure is performed with the patient under general anesthesia with oro- or nasogastric decompression and a pneumoperitoneum of 12-14 mm Hg (Fig. 22.1).

The patients can be placed in the "French" position, a modified lithotomy with minimal flexion of the hips, and the primary surgeon positioned between the legs. The first assistant or second surgeon stands on the patient's left side and the scrub nurse between them. For fenestrations, use a four-trocar configuration. A 10 mm port at the umbilicus house the 30° telescope. A 5 mm trocar placed just below the xiphoid process to the right or the left of the falciform ligament, depending on the location of the cyst. This port is used to expose the liver, often using an irrigation aspiration probe. Two other 5 mm or 10 mm ports, in the right and left flank, allows the surgeon to puncture the cyst dome, aspirate its contents, and excise the cyst wall in a careful sequential fashion to facilitate hemostasis. For more extensive procedures, a strong light source (300 W xenon) and high-quality 30° scopes are required. To perform resections safely with a minimum of wasted motion, the four-hand technique is used by many surgeons. This uses four to six trocars and allows for the primary surgeon to expose and dissect the liver while second surgeon obtains control and transects the blood vessels and bile ducts. The procedure entails the same components as in open hepatic surgery. First, the patient is explored, both visually and ultra-sonographically. Mobilization of the liver and hilar dissection are performed as necessary to obtain vascular control. Division and ligation of the round ligament followed by freeing of the falciform and the right or left triangular ligaments allow access to perform thorough exploration, resection, and hemostasis. A gauge soaked with 3% saline is kept around the cyst to prevent contamination by spillage (Fig. 22.2). Spiral needle is used to administer 10% saline inside the cyst (Figs 22.3A and B). Dissection is begun by scoring Glisson's capsule with the high frequency electrosurgery. Parenchymal dissection can be performed using the ultrasonic dissector. After resection, the mass is placed in an impermeable specimen bag for removal (Figs 22.4A to D). Cholangiography is very useful to detect possible bile leaks. The raw surface of the liver is then inspected, coagulated and covered with fibrin glue. The specimen is extracted either by partial morcellation, dilatation at the umbilicus, enlarging another port site, or by a small McBurney or subcostal incision (Figs 22.5A and B).

LAPAROSCOPIC LIVER RESECTION

The most common indication for laparoscopic liver resection is a solitary liver metastasis from a colorectal cancer, but it may also be used for hepatocellular carcinoma (HCC) and for benign liver tumors or cysts.

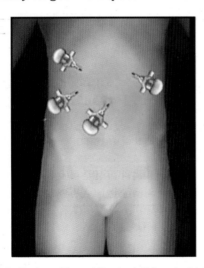

Fig. 22.1: Port position of the hydatid cyst of left lobe

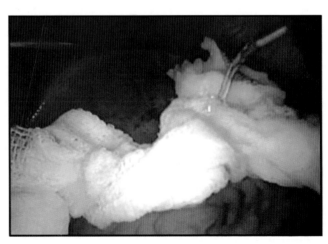

Fig. 22.2: Gauge piece introduced soaked with 3% saline

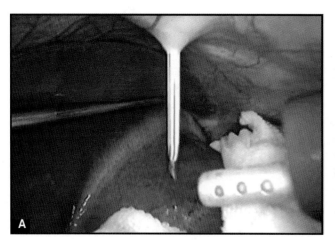
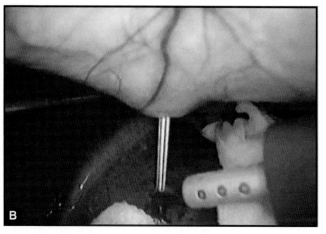

Figs 22.3A and B: Instillation of hypertonic saline inside the cyst though percutaneous spinal needle

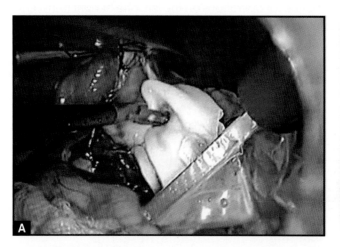
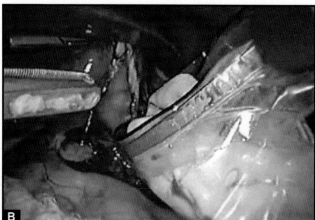
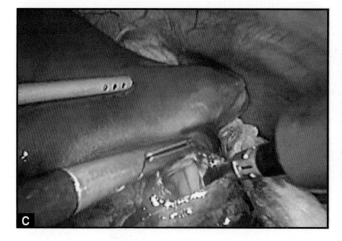
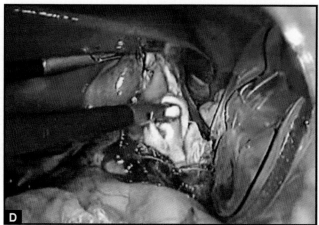

Figs 22.4A to D: Opening of the cystic wall and extraction of germinal layer

Laparoscopic liver resections, offer advantages over the conventional open approach in two important respects:

1. Reduced operative blood loss
2. Lower major postoperative morbidity.

Although laparoscopic staging for intra-abdominal cancer including primary and secondary hepatic tumors has been in established practice for many years, laparoscopic liver resections are still in the early clinical evaluation stage. Nonetheless, the results to date have been uniformly favorable especially for left lobectomy and pluri-segmentectomies although right hepatectomy has been performed by the laparoscopically assisted or the hand-assisted laparoscopic surgical (HALS) approach.

The HALS approach by facilitating these dissections and greatly increasing the safety makes quite a big difference to the uptake amongst hepatobiliary and general surgeons with an interest in liver surgery. The procedures, which are in established practice by the laparoscopic and HALS approach are:

1. Extended laparoscopic staging
2. Hepatic resections
3. Laparoscopic *in situ* thermal ablation
4. Laparoscopic cryosurgery
5. Radical de-roofing of simple hepatic cysts
6. Hepatic surgery for parasitic cysts.

Laparoscopic Staging of Tumors

Laparoscopy can nicely detect seedling metastases and small hepatic deposits missed by preoperative thin slice multi-detector CT or MRI. Some surgeons add lavage cytology to diagnostic laparoscopic visual inspection. This detects exfoliated tumors cells in gastrointestinal, pancreatic and ovarian cancers.

HEPATIC RESECTIONS

Approaches

Both the laparoscopic and the HALS approach can be used for hepatic resection. The hand-assisted approach expedites the operation and provides an effective safeguard against major hemorrhage that may be encountered during the operation. A 7.0 cm incision is necessary for the insertion of the hand access device, such as the Omniport. This may be introduced through midline for operations on the left lobe or right transverse for resections on the right liver. It is important that the optical port is placed such that it is well clear of the internal hand.

Component Tasks in Laparoscopic Hepatic Resections

These component tasks cover all the surgical technical aspects of the various hepatic resections: hepatectomy, pluri-segmentectomies, segmentectomies.

Contact Ultrasound Localization and Mapping of the Intended Resection

Contact ultrasound is indispensable for hepatic resections. The precise localization and extent of the

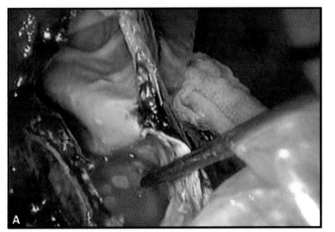 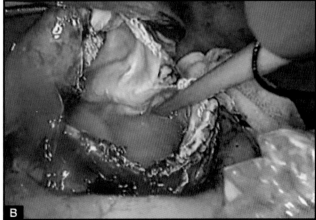

Figs 22.5A and B: Removal of cyst with the help of endobag

lesion especially when this is intrahepatic can only be determined by contact ultrasound scanning, the findings of which determine the extent of resection segments required. In contrast, the mapping of the outlines of the resection is best carried out by the argon plasma spray coagulation.

Division of Falciform Ligament, Exposure of the Suprahepatic Vena Cava and of the Main Hepatic Veins

Division of falciform ligament is needed for major right and left resections. The division of the falciform ligament close to the liver substance is best carried out with a combination of scissors and electro-coagulation and is greatly facilitated by the use of curved coaxial instruments. The round ligament Ligamentum Teres can be left undivided except in patients undergoing skeletonization for right extended hepatectomy.

Exposure of Suprahepatic Inferior Vena Cava and Main Hepatic Veins

Exposure of suprahepatic inferior vena cava and main hepatic veins are only required for major hepatectomies. The two leaves of the falciform ligament separate posteriorly to envelop the suprahepatic inferior vena cava and the three main hepatic veins. The right leaf becomes the upper leaf of the right coronary ligament of the liver and the left leaf becomes the upper layer of the left triangular ligament. These both leaves are divided after soft coagulation with the curved coaxial scissors. Ultrasonic shears may be used for this purpose, but this is more difficult as this energized device is straight.

The peritoneal division is extended in both directions to open up the retrohepatic caval space, which consists of relatively avascular loose fibroareolar tissue. The upper end of the caval canal is dissected further with a combination of blunt and sharp scissor dissection to divide fibrous bands. As the dissection precedes, about 1.5 cm of the inferior vena cava, the origin of the right hepatic vein are exposed. Further exposure of the right and middle hepatic veins is achieved beneath the liver and from the right side required for a right hepatectomy. The left hepatic vein is very easily exposed from the left side above the liver.

Exposure of Infrahepatic Inferior Vena Cava and Division of the Posterior Minor Hepatic Veins

Exposure of infrahepatic inferior vena cava and division of the posterior minor hepatic vein is necessary for the skeletonization of the right liver necessary for a right hepatectomy. It is performed by retraction of the inferior surface of the right lobe of the liver with an atraumatic flexible ring or fan retractor to put the peritoneum sweeping up from the right kidney to the liver on the stretch. This peritoneum is divided with the curved coaxial scissors and soft electrocoagulation over a wide front and close to the liver edge. There is usually little fat found underneath the peritoneum except in very obese individuals.

Once the peritoneum is divided the retractor is replaced which gently lifts the inferoposterior aspect of the liver upwards to expose the areolar tissue plane covering the vena cava and the minor retrohepatic veins which vary in number from 3 to 5. The inferoposterior aspect of the liver is lifted gently but progressively to expose the vena cava behind the liver. As minor hepatic veins are encountered draining into the inferior vena cava, they are skeletonized by the curved coaxial scissors and then clipped before they are divided. The mobilization continues upwards until the right and middle hepatic vein is reached.

Opening the Cave of Retius

Opening the cave of Retius is common to both right and left resections. The cave of Retius refers to the umbilical fissure bridged by variable amount of hepatic tissue anteriorly, which overlies the ligamentum teres containing the obliterated umbilical vein on its way to join the left branch of the portal vein at the bottom of the pit. The bridge of liver tissue is crushed and coagulated by an insulated grasping forceps, after which it is divided which will separate segment III on the left side from the quadrate lobe opening up the cave of Retius and exposing the terminal segment of the round ligament.

Hilar Dissection

The dissection of the hilum commences by division of the peritoneum along the margin of the hepatic hilum to expose the common hepatic duct and its bifurcation and the right and left branches of the common hepatic artery. Further dissection is needed to bring down the hilar plate and to skeletonize the right and left hepatic ducts, the two branches of the common hepatic artery and, more posteriorly, the two branches of the portal vein for right and left hepatectomy.

Removal of the Gallbladder

Removal of the gallbladder en block with the hepatic substance constitutes an integral part of right hepatectomy and segmentectomy involving segments IVa and V. The dissection of the cystic duct and artery is followed by ligature or clipping of the medial end of the cystic duct and clipping of its lateral end before it is divided.

Inflow Occlusion Prior to Hepatic Resection

Temporary inflow occlusion of the vascular supply to the liver is necessary for major hepatic resections and also to reduce the 'heat-sink effect' of the substantial blood flow through the liver during *in situ* ablation by cryotherapy or radiofrequency thermal ablation. Several type of clamps are available for this purpose but the most suitable are the parallel occlusion clamps, which are introduced through 5.5 mm ports by means of an applicator, which is used to engage and disengage the clamps. Thus, when the clamp is in use it does not occupy a port, which can thus be used for dissection. The application of these parallel occlusion clamps is very easy particularly with the hand-assisted approach and minimal dissection is required. The surgeon just makes a small window through an avascular area of lesser omentum just proximal to the hepatoduodenal ligament enveloping the bile duct, hepatic arteries and portal vein.

The parallel occlusion clamp is introduced from the right by means of its applicator. The jaws are opened as the hepato-duodenal ligament is reached and applied across the full width of the hepato-duodenal ligament and then released to occlude the bile duct, portal vein and hepatic arteries. It is extremely important that the period of inflow vascular occlusion to the liver does not exceed 30 minute at any one-time period.

For removal of the clamp, the introducer is inserted through the port and used to engage the clamp, which then is opened and removed through the same port by the introducer.

Transection of the Hepatic Parenchyma

The transection of the hepatic parenchyma for all the major resections should be carried in the absence of a positive-pressure pneumoperitoneum. In hand-assisted laparoscopic surgery, this translates to replacement of the hand access device with a disposable retractor that also acts as a wound protector preventing its contamination by malignant cells during the hepatic resection and removal of the specimen. The hepatic resection must also be carried out with a low patient CVP, produced by a head-up tilt and appropriate vasodilator medication by the anesthetist.

The hepatic artery to the resection area is best secured by clips or ligatures in the liver substance rather than extrahepatically. The vascular stapling or ligature and division of the main hepatic veins draining the liver during hepatectomy are carried out at the end of the parenchymal transection.

The actual technique of liver resection varies from simple finger or forceps fracture with individual clipping or ligature of bile ductules to use of energized systems like ultrasonic dissection or LigaSure. The liver parenchymal surface is first coagulated and then crushed using a long-jawed crushing laparoscopic forceps to fracture the liver parenchyma exposing sizeable vessels and ducts.

All sizeable blood vessels and bile ducts are clipped before being cut. As the cleft deepens, bands of liver tissue, which are not severed, are presumed to contain large vessels which may be obscured by adherent layer of liver parenchyma. In this situation, palpation of the bridge between the index finger and thumb of the assisting hand will identify the nature of the structure. All sizeable veins can be transected using an endolinear cutting stapler mounted with 35 mm vascular cartridge introduced through the mini-laparotomy wound.

In the case of pluri-segmentectomy, after the segment has been separated on three sides, it often remains attached to the liver by bridge of liver tissue. If this connection is no thicker than 1.0 cm, it is simply staple transected by the application of the endolinear cutting stapler to detach completely the area from the liver.

After resection, the specimen is removed through the open mini-laparotomy wound. The final stage consists in securing complete hemostasis.

Hemostasis of the Cut Liver Surface

Only minor oozing happens from the cut liver substance if the technique of hepatic transection has been performed correctly and in the presence of a low CVP of patient. Complete hemostasis is achieved by argon plasma coagulation. Application of fibrin glue or other synthetic sealants are very helpful in preventing hemostasis.

Insertion of Drains

Once the resection is complete before the retractor is removed and the wound closed using mass closure with monofilament polydioxanone the silicon drain should be introduced. It is advisable to insert two large silicon drains one above and the other below the liver. These must be sutured to the abdominal wall to prevent accidental dislodgment after the operation. Effective drainage is crucial to prevent postoperative biloma.

Postoperative Management

It is important to stress that these patients should be nursed postoperatively in a hepatobiliary unit with immediate access to high dependency and intensive care if needed. The management is the same as after any other laparoscopic surgery with daily monitoring of the liver function tests, hematology and blood urea nitrogen and serum electrolytes. Opiate medication and sedation are avoided in patients with compromised liver function. Repeated ultrasound scan should be carried out in all patients after hepatic resection. This is necessary to identify early fluid collections most usually bile, which if found are monitored by serial ultrasound studies and aspirated or drained percutaneously under radiological control if persistent.

Using right technique, necessary expertise and appropriate technology, laparoscopic and especially hand-assisted hepatic resections can be carried out safely. The data from the published reports to date indicate benefits over the open approach and these include reduced blood loss and lower postoperative morbidity.

LAPAROSCOPIC PANCREATIC SURGERY

The laparoscopic management of pancreatic disease is one of the most challenging in laparoscopic surgery. This is especially true when considering that of pancreatic resection. Well trained laparoscopic surgeons have found that operating on the pancreas, like virtually all intra-abdominal procedures, is technically feasible. Laparoscopic principles suggest that the patient will probably benefit from less postoperative pain, improved wound cosmetics, quicker return to routine activities, and shorter hospital stay. Ultimately the acceptance of many laparoscopic operations will be determined by their degree of difficulty, the operating time, the cost (both hospital and societal), and patient outcomes.

In comparison with the literature available on other laparoscopic operations, the information available on pancreatic resection is too scant to draw firm conclusions. However, leaders in the field have demonstrated that pancreatic resection is feasible, and are carefully examining their outcomes to further elucidate the role of this technically demanding procedure.

Laparoscopic procedures for the pancreas fall into four main categories:
1. Laparoscopic staging of pancreatic malignancy
2. Bilioenteric or gastroenteric bypass
3. Pancreatic resection
4. Management of pancreatic pseudocysts.

Anatomic Considerations

The majority of the pancreas lies in a retroperitoneal position, transversely oriented from the second and third portions of the duodenum to the hilum of the spleen. Anterior access to the gland (body and tail) is readily obtained by division of the gastrocolic omentum. This division may be performed by electrocautery, multiple individual clip applications or vascular stapling devices, or ultrasonic dissection.

Access may be obtained through the gastrohepatic ligament, although the exposure is usually less adequate. The patient is positioned in slight headup position to allow gravity retraction of the viscera. An oblique angle (30° or 45°) telescope is necessary for adequate visualization. Laparoscopic ultrasound is proving to be an essential tool for many aspects of pancreatic surgery.

Section Three

Laparoscopic Staging of Pancreatic Malignancy

Patients with pancreatic malignancy generally present at later stages of disease. Frequently the disease is unresectable due to tumor size or tumor metastases by the time symptoms occur. Surgical resection for pancreatic cancer still offers the only reasonable chance at a cure. Historically, many patients underwent unnecessary laparotomy in an effort to assess resectability. CT scans have helped many patients avoid the morbidity of a non-therapeutic laparotomy. However, even with this modality, unre-sectability rates at laparotomy can approach 60 percent. This is most often due to the presence of unrecognized peritoneal metastases (<1 cm) and tumor invasion not appreciated on CT scan. Spiral CT and magnetic resonance imaging (MRI) are more reliable for predicting unresectability, but are still not adequate in our opinion. Megibow and coworkers reported a sensitivity of 77 percent, a specificity of 50 percent, and an overall accuracy of 73 percent for dynamic CT scanning. Also in their study, they found no additional benefit from MRI.

Diagnostic laparoscopy further narrows patient selection for therapeutic laparotomy. Warshaw and coworkers found that an additional 35 percent of patients could avoid laparotomy with the use of diagnostic laparoscopy. Despite improving non-invasive imaging methods since Warshaw and coworker's early reports, more recent studies confirm Warshaw and coworker's initial findings that a significantly number of patients (22 to 35%) can avoid laparotomy with the use of staging laparoscopy.

Further, the sensitivity for evaluation of unresectable disease appears further enhanced with the addition of the laparoscopic ultrasound to the laparoscopic staging procedure. Callery and coworkers use a multifrequency laparoscopic ultrasound probe to search for occult metastases and assess posterior invasion into vascular structures like the portal vein. Tumors other than pancreatic were included. Fifty patients were referred for staging laparoscopy after interpretation of conventional noninvasive imaging modalities had determined the tumor to be resectable. Laparoscopic ultrasound established unresectability in 11 patients (22%) in whom staging laparoscopy alone was negative. In another study by John and coworkers

involving 40 consecutive patients with pancreatic cancer presenting for diagnostic laparoscopy, laparoscopic ultrasound found an additional 25 percent (10 patients) whose disease was unresectable when compared with laparoscopy alone. They found the use of ultrasound significantly improved specificity and accuracy as compared with laparoscopy alone (88 % and 81 % vs 50% and 60%, respectively).

Staging Laparoscopy Technique

Patients generally undergo staging laparoscopy on the same day they are scheduled for resection. Patients are placed in the supine position on an electrically equipped bed (preferably). A 10 mm trocar is placed in the infraumbilical position to serve as the camera port. The abdomen is insufflated to 15 mm Hg. A 30° laparoscope is used. A second port of 5 mm is placed in the right midclavicular line several centimeters from the subcostal margin. A four-quadrant exploration is then carried out. Grasping devices, biopsy forceps, or electrocautery instruments may be alternatively introduced through the 5 mm port. Important peritoneal surfaces to visualize for areas of metastases include the undersurface of abdomen including falciform, diaphragm, and liver. The omentum must be examined thoroughly and when possible retracted superiorly to evaluate the base of the transverse colon, its mesentery, and the ligament of Treitz (this may require an additional port).

If there is evidence of unresectability, the procedure is terminated. Otherwise laparoscopic ultrasound is carried out. A second 10 mm port is placed in the right midclavicular line at the level of the umbilicus. Laparoscopic ultrasound is then performed using a 9-mm in diameter linear array 7.5 MHz contact ultrasound probe with Doppler flow capability. The liver is systematically scanned (anterior, lateral, inferior) at penetration depths of 7 cm for evidence of metastatic spread or extent of primary tumor invasion. Frequently; biliary and pancreatic metastases to the liver have a characteristic bulls-eye appearance with an echoic rim encircling a mixed-echo tumor center. If found, biopsy for such lesions may be attempted percutaneously with laparoscopic ultrasound guidance.

Attention is then turned to ultrasonic evaluation of the portahepatic, peripancreatic, para-aortic, and celiac axis for evidence of nodal disease. Lymph nodes greater than 10 mm may be biopsied. Laparoscopic ultrasound with Doppler flow capability is then used to help locate and assess the potential for tumor extension to surrounding peripancreatic vascular structures (primarily portal vein, but also superior mesenteric vein and artery, and celiac axis).

Bilioenteric or Gastroenteric Anastomosis for Pancreatic Malignancy

Unresectable patients might be candidates for biliary or enteric bypass. The risk and benefits of bypass must be weighed against existing palliative options, the patient's condition, existing or impending obstruction, and expected length of survival based on tumor burden. For most patients with unresectable disease, life expectancy can be expected to be less than 1 year. Proper management tailored to the individual patient's needs is important so as to offer as much quality of life free from hospitalization as possible.

Commonly, patients will present with some degree of biliary obstruction or will suffer from it during the course of the disease. Most patients with obstructive jaundice are best treated by placing an endoscopic or percutaneous stent. The success rate is high (85%), with a low associated mortality (1 to 2%). Studies comparing open bypass with those stented endoscopically for obstructive jaundice found no advantage to the surgical approach . Morbidity from stent placement includes potentially frequent admission to hospital (occlusion, infection) and significant cost for endoscopic retrograde cholangiopancreatography (ERCP) and stent. However, repeat placement has become less necessary with the use of improved techniques and stent design. Patients may present or develop distorted duodenal anatomy that makes initial or subsequent stent placement impossible. This finding may be coupled with gastric outlet obstruction. In these patients, bypass procedures may be offered after evaluation of surgical risk or life expectancy.

The morbidity of open surgical bypass is substantial (19%). Laparoscopic biliary (cholecystojejunostomy) or gastric bypass (gastrojejunostomy) is feasible. There is potential for shorter recovery, shorter return to activity; and low morbidity, as evident in several small studies. Nathanson suggests that the bypass should be reserved for a later date from the diagnostic laparoscopy at such time when duodenal obstruction precludes repeat stent or there is stent failure (blockage, recurrent sepsis). For the stomach, failure would include when symptoms of gastric outlet arise. Conditions at initial laparoscopy that might argue for immediate bypass include inability to stent the biliary system in the preoperative setting, endoscopic or radiologic evidence of impending duodenal obstruction, or laparoscopic impression of large locally advanced mass with minimal to no evidence of metastatic spread.

Biliary and Gastric Bypass

Cholecystojejunostomy may be carried out if the gallbladder is present and suitable for anastomosis, and the cystic duct is patent and its junction to the common bile duct (CBD) is far from the tumor. Frequently this information is available by preoperative imaging studies (ERCP or percutaneous transluminal cholangiography). If not, patency of cystic duct and its relation to primary tumor location may be obtained by performing a cholangiogram after cannulation of the gallbladder. Similarly, laparoscopic ultrasound may be used for such an assessment.

For either anastomosis, patients are positioned supine and the port placement is the same. A 10 mm trocar is placed at the inferior umbilical region and a 30° telescope is used. Additional ports and operating room personnel are positioned.

The omentum and transverse colon are elevated with instruments introduced through the epigastric and either 12 mm port. The small bowel is traced back to the ligament of Treitz. A loop of small bowel is then chosen that will comfortably reach stomach and gallbladder without tension (note that this is true once the transverse colon and omentum are allowed to return to normal position). For the biliary bypass, a cholecystotomy is performed with electrocautery on the gallbladder fundus. The biliary contents are then aspirated. An enterotomy is performed on the antimesenteric surface of the chosen small bowel loop. A 30 mm endoscopic stapler is introduced through the right 12 mm port. The jaws of the stapler are opened and one arm of the stapler is inserted into the enterotomy. The jaws of the stapler are then closed to function as a large grasper. The stapler and small bowel contained within are then maneuvered adjacent to the cholecystotomy. The jaws of the stapler are opened again and the free arm of the stapler maneuvered into the cholecystotomy. Assistance is provided by a blunt grasping instrument inserted through the additional ports (epigastric). After proper alignment is assured, the stapler is fired to complete the anastomosis. The original sites may be closed with additional firings of the stapler. At this point the endoscopic stapler will be introduced through the left 12 mm port. Care must be taken not to narrow the anastomosis or the lumen of the small bowel significantly.

To fashion the gastric bypass, a dependent site is chosen along the greater curvature. The gastrocolic omentum is divided close to the greater curve within the gastroepiploic arcade for a distance of approximately 3 to 4 cm with the ultrasonic scalpel or by electrocautery. A gastrotomy is made on the greater curvature. The anastomosis will be formed along the greater curve but will extend into the posterior wall of the stomach. Typically, the stapled anastomosis will be created by introducing the stapler through the right 12 mm port. The anastomosis should consist of two firings of the 30 mm endoscopic linear cutter.

Ideally, the stapled anastomosis should be aligned to cross the greater curvature to the posterior surface (i.e. through the area of divided gastrocolic omentum). If fashioned in this way, the original puncture sites will be easier to close and the anastomosis more dependent.

Laparoscopic Pancreatic Resection

Indications for complete or partial pancreatic resection include:
1. Adenocarcinoma
2. Insulinoma (neuroendocrine)
3. Chronic pancreatitis.

Improved technique and postoperative care have rendered morbidity and mortality for pancreatic resection, including Whipple's procedure, to less than 5%. Laparoscopic techniques could potentially lower this rate even more or at least afford less pain and a more rapid recovery.

Laparoscopic Whipple's procedure was first carried out by Gagner in a small series of three patients with various diseases (pancreatitis, ampullary cancer, adenocarcinoma). He subsequently has reported on a pylorus-preserving technique performed in one patient with pancreatitis. The initial experience indicates that

it is technically feasible, but because of its operative time, complexity, and as yet no demonstrated improvement in outcome, this procedure must be considered investigational. Hand-assisted laparoscopic surgery may make pancreatic resection more practical.

Laparoscopic pancreatic procedures involving distal pancreatectomy appear to hold more promise at present. Soper and coworkers reponed success with his technique in the pig model. Gagner and coworkers successfully performed distal pancreatectomy for a variety of disease processes including islet cell tumors, cystadenocarcinoma, and pseudocyst. The spleen was preserved in all cases and operating times ranged from 2.5 to 5 hours. Cases were managed with the patient in the left lateral position, with pancreatic division carried out with a 60 mm linear cutter. Others are reporting initial success with distal resection.

Laparoscopic Management of Pancreatic Pseudocyst

Pancreatic pseudocysts may be defined as a collection of pancreatic secretions, serous fluid, or necrotic debris surrounded by a nonepithelialized wall made up of granulation tissue and variable degree of fibrous tissue. Pancreatic pseudocysts must be distinguished from true cysts of the pancreas, which are characterized histologically by the presence of an epithelial lining. Pseudocyst formation is the result of a post-inflammatory process arising from patients with acute or chronic pancreatitis. An understanding of the natural history of pancreatic pseudocyst is important when deciding on invasive therapy versus expectant management. Studies like those by Bradley and coworkers had a great influence in the management of pseudocystic disease. Bradley and coworkers suggested the likelihood of regression diminished and the likelihood of complications rose dramatically after a 6 weeks period. More recent data suggest that this patient population may be watched safely for longer periods. Yeo and coworkers followed asymptomatic patients with pseudocysts by CT scanning for 1 year (48% were successfully observed with only a 2.7% complication rate). The only predictor for intervention was size greater than 7.4 +/-0.6 cm.

General asymptomatic patients with pancreatic pseudocyst may be followed up for extended periods of time. This conservative approach is more likely to be successful in patients with small 6 cm pseudocysts. Other options are available for drainage procedures (e.g. percutaneous transgastric, ERCP).

Laparoscopic Pseudocyst Drainage

Preoperative decision making and subsequent laparoscopic operative approach should mimic that of open operative planning. The selection of procedure will depend on the anatomic location of the pseudocyst, pseudocyst size, and associated pancreatic duct or distal common bile duct abnormalities.

Reports by Newell and coworkers document that pseudocyst-gastrostomy is technically easier than pseudocyst-jejunostomy, while remaining equally efficacious. Laparoscopic pseudocyst-gastrostomy is technically easier, but cyst-jejunostomy is also technically feasible for the cyst not amenable to gastric drainage by standard surgical principles.

Laparoscopic pseudocyst-gastrostomy was first performed by Petelin in 1991. Principles of operative drainage include biopsy of cyst wall to rule out neoplasm, dependent drainage, and precise hemostatic technique to avoid hemorrhage.

The patient position and port placement are the same as described for the bypass procedure. The pseudocyst may often be seen pushing the stomach forward. A small gastrotomy is established with cautery over the most prominent portion of the pseudocyst. Ultrasound may be helpful in locating the pseudocyst and the site of the initial gastrotomy. The gastrotomy is then extended for several centimeters with electrocautery.

A small window is developed through the posterior wall of the stomach with electrocautery. One must remember that the posterior wall of stomach and cyst capsule will be fused and that this requires a deeper dissection with cautery than felt comfortable by the surgeon. Ultrasound may be helpful to plan dissection where the stomach wall or cyst is thinnest. The window is made large enough to accommodate the endoscopic stapler. A biopsy of the wall may be carried out at this time. Two firings of the stapler are used to create a substantial anastomosis (stapler insertion through the more comfortable 12 mm pon, usually the right). Hemostasis at the staple line should be assured. The gastrotomy is closed with either sutures or staples.

CONCLUSION

The laparoscopic approach to hepatic and pancreatic surgery has rapidly been shown to be of considerable value. The laparoscopic approach to the pancreas has value with respect to staging, bypass procedures, and pseudocyst drainage. Pancreatic resection is feasible, but must still be considered investigational.

BIBLIOGRAPHY

1. Adamson GD, Cuschieri A. Multimedia article: laparoscopic infracolic necrosectomy for infected pancreatic necrosis. Surg Endosc. 2003;17:1675.
2. American Joint Commission on Cancer. Exocrine pancreas. In: Greene FL, Page DL, Fleming ID, et al., eds. AJCC Cancer Staging Manual, 5th ed. New York: Springer-Verlag, 2002, pp 157–64.
3. Andren-Sandberg A, Lindberg CG, Lundstedt C, Ihse I. Computed tomography and laparoscopy in the assessment of the patient with pancreatic cancer. J AmColl Surg 1998;186:35–40.
4. Ashley SW, Perez A, Pierce EA, et al. Necrotizing pancreatitis: contemporary analysis of 99 consecutive cases. Ann Surg. 2001;234:572-80.
5. Baril NB, Ralls PW, Wren SM, et al. Does an infected peripancreatic fluid collection or abscess mandate operation? Ann Surg. 2000;231:361-7.
6. Beger HG, Rau B, Isenmann R. Prevention of severe change in acute pancreatitis: prediction and prevention. J Hepatobiliary Pancreat Surg. 2001;8:140-7.
7. Birkmeyer JD, Stukel TA, Siewers AE, Goodney PP, Wennberg DE, Lucas FL. Surgeon volume and operative mortality in the United States. N Engl J Med. 2003; 349:2117-27.
8. Birkmeyer JD, Warshaw AL, Finlayson SR, Grove MR, Tosteson AN. Relationship between hospital volume and late survival after pancreaticoduodenectomy. Surgery. 1999;126:178-83.
9. Buchler MW, Gloor B, Muller CA, Friess H, Seiler CA, Uhl W. Acute necrotizing pancreatitis: treatment strategy according to the status of infection. Ann Surg. 2000;232:619-26.
10. Carter R. Management of infected necrosis secondary to acute pancreatitis: a balanced role for minimal access techniques. Pancreatology. 2003;3:133-8.
11. Castellanos G, Serrano A, Pinero A, et al. Retroperitoneoscopy in the management of drained infected pancreatic necrosis. Gastrointest Endosc. 2001;53:514-15.
12. Clancy TE, Ashley SW. Current management of necrotizing pancreatitis. Adv Surg. 2002;36:103-21.
13. Conlon KC, Dougherty E, Klimstra DS, et al. The value of minimal access surgery in the staging of patients with potentially resectable peripancreatic malignancy. Ann Surg 1996; 223:134–40.
14. Connor S, Alexakis N, Raraty MGT, et al. Early and late complications after pancreatic necrosectomy. Surgery. 2005;137:499-505.

15. Connor S, Ghaneh P, Raraty M, et al. Minimally invasive retroperitoneal pancreatic necrosectomy. Dig Surg. 2003;20:270-7.

16. Connor S, Neoptolemos JP. Surgery for pancreatic necrosis: "whom, when and what." World J Gastroenterol. 2004;10:1697-8.

17. Connor S, Raraty MGT, Howes N, et al. Surgery in the treatment of acute pancreatitis: minimal access pancreatic necrosectomy. Scand J Surg. 2005;94:135-42.

18. Cuschieri A, Hall AW, Clark J. Value of laparoscopy in the diagnosis and management of pancreatic carcinoma. Gut 1978;19:672–7.

19. Cuschieri A. Laparoscopic hand-assisted surgery for hepatic and pancreatic disease. Surg Endosc. 2000;14:991-6.

20. Cuschieri A. Pancreatic necrosis: pathogenesis and endoscopic management. Semin Laparosc Surg. 2002;9:54-63.

21. Dugernier TL, Laterre P-F, Wittebole X, et al. Compartmentalization of the inflammatory response during acute pancreatitis: correlation with local and systemic complications. Am J Respir Crit Care Med. 2003;168:148-57.

22. Fernandez-del Castillo C, Rattner DW, Makary MA, Mostafavi A, McGrath D, Warshaw AL. Debridement and closed packing for the treatment of necrotizing pancreatitis. Ann Surg. 1998;228:676-84.

23. Finlayson EVA, Goodney PP, Birkmeyer JD. Hospital volume and operative mortality in cancer surgery: a national study. Arch Surg. 2003;138:721-6.

24. Gupta A, Watson DI. Effect of laparoscopy on immune function. Br J Surg. 2001; 88:1296-1306.

25. HALS Study Group. Hand-assisted laparoscopic surgery vs standard laparoscopic surgery for colorectal disease: a prospective randomized trial. Surg Endosc. 2000;14:896-901.

26. Hamad GG, Broderick TJ. Laparoscopic pancreatic necrosectomy. J Laparoendosc Adv Surg Tech A. 2000;10:115-18.

27. Horvath KD, Kao LS, Ali A, Wherry KL, Pellegrini CA, Sinanan MN. Laparoscopic assisted percutaneous drainage of infected pancreatic necrosis. Surg Endosc. 2001;15:677-82.

28. Horvath KD, Kao LS, Wherry KL, Pellegrini CA, Sinanan MN. A technique for laparoscopicassisted percutaneous drainage of infected pancreatic necrosis and pancreatic abscess. Surg Endosc. 2001;15:1221-5.

29. Jimenez RE, Warshaw AL, Rattner DW, Willett CG, McGrath D, Fernandez-del Castillo C. Impact of laparoscopic staging in the treatment of pancreatic cancer. Arch Surg 2000;135:409–14.

30. Kamei H, Yoshida S, Yamasaki K, Tajiri T, Shirouzu K. Carbon dioxide pneumoperitoneum reduces levels of TNF-a mRNA in the brain, liver, and peritoneum in mice. Surg Endosc. 2001;15:609-13.

31. Kim WW, Jeon HM, Park SC, Lee SK, Chun SW, Kim EK. Comparison of immune preservation between CO_2 pneumoperitoneum and gasless abdominal lift laparoscopy. JSLS. 2002;6:11-5.

32. Lau ST, Simchuk EJ, Kozarek RA, Traverso LW. A pancreatic ductal leak should be sought to direct treatment in patients with acute pancreatitis. Am J Surg. 2001;1:411-5.

33. Laveda R, Martinez J, Munoz C, et al. Different profile of cytokine synthesis according to the severity of acute pancreatitis. World J Gastroenterol. 2005;11: 5309-13.

34. Lempinen M, Puolakkainen P, Kemppainen E. Clinical value of severity markers in acute pancreatitis. Scand J Surg. 2005;94:118-23.

35. Liu R, Traverso LW. Laparoscopic staging of unresectable pancreatic cancer. Surg Endosc 2004;18:S256.

36. Louvet C, Andre T, Lledo G, et al. Gemcitabine combined with oxaloplatin in advanced pancreatic adenocarcinoma: Final results of a GERCOR multicenter phase II study. J Clin Oncol 2002;20:1512–8.

37. Papachristou GI, Whitcomb DC. Predictors of severity and necrosis in acute pancreatitis. Gastroenterol Clin North Am. 2004;33:871-90.

38. Pooran N, Indaram A, Singh P, Bank S. Cytokines (IL-6, IL-8, TNF): early and reliable predictors of severe acute pancreatitis. J Clin Gastroenterol. 2003; 37:263-6.

39. Ramudo L, Manso MA, De Dios I. Biliary pancreatitis-associated ascitic fluid activates the production of tumor necrosis factor-alpha in acinar cells. Crit Care Med. 2005;33:143-8.

40. Raraty MGT, Neoptolemos JP. Compartments that cause the real damage in severe acute pancreatitis. Am J Respir Crit Care Med. 2003;168:141-2.

41. Targarona EM, Gracia E, Garriga J, et al. Prospective randomized trial comparing conventional laparoscopic colectomy with hand-assisted laparoscopic colectomy: applicability, immediate clinical outcome, inflammatory response, and cost. Surg Endosc. 2002;16:234-9.

42. Targarona EM, Gracia E, Rodriguez M, et al. Hand-assisted laparoscopic surgery. Arch Surg. 2003;138:133-41.

43. Traverso LW, Kozarek RA. Pancreatic necrosectomy: definitions and technique. J Gastrointest Surg. 2005;9: 436-9.

44. Tzovaras G, Parks RW, Diamond T, Rowlands BJ. Early and long-term results of surgery for severe necrotising pancreatitis. Dig Surg. 2004;21:41-7.

45. Warshaw AL. Pancreatic necrosis: to debride or not to debride, that is the question. Ann Surg. 2000;232: 627-9.

46. West MA, Baker J, Bellingham J. Kinetics of decreased LPS-stimulated cytokine release by macrophages exposed to CO2. J Surg Res. 1996;63:269-274. Downloaded from www.archsurg.com on March 28, 2009

47. Wu FPK, Sietses C, von Blomberg BME, van Leeuwen PAM, Meijer S, Cuesta MA. Systemic and peritoneal inflammatory response after laparoscopic or conventional colon resection in cancer patients: a prospective, randomized trial. Dis Colon Rectum. 2003;46:147-55.

48. Zengin K, Taskin M, Sakoglu N, Salihoglu Z, Demiroluk S, Uzun H. Systemic inflammatory response after laparoscopic and open application of adjustable banding for morbidly obese patients. Obes Surg. 2002;12:276-9.

Section Three

23

Diagnostic Laparoscopy

Diagnostic laparoscopy is a minimally invasive surgical procedure that allows the visual examination of intra-abdominal organs in order to detect pathology. The procedure allows the direct visual examination of intra-abdominal organs including large surface areas of the liver, gallbladder, spleen, peritoneum, pelvic organs, and retroperitoneum. Biopsies, aspiration, and cultures can be obtained, and laparoscopic ultrasound may be used.

Diagnostic laparoscopy is safe and well tolerated and can be performed in an outpatient or inpatient setting under general anesthesia. There may also be unique circumstances where office based diagnostic laparoscopy may be considered under local anesthesia. These circumstances should include only procedures where complications and the need for therapeutic procedures through the same access are extremely unlikely. Manipulation and biopsy of the viscera is possible through additional ports. Diagnostic laparoscopy is the most commonly performed gynecological procedure today. Its greatest advantage is that it has replaced exploratory laparotomy.

Diagnostic laparoscopy was first introduced in 1901, when Kelling, performed a peritoneoscopy in a dog and was called ''celioscopy''. A Swedish internist named Jacobaeusc is credited with performing the first diagnostic laparoscopy on human in 1910. He described its application in patients with ascites and for the early diagnosis of malignant lesions.

In last ten years laparoscopy has made a great difference to the diagnosis of abdominal acute and chronic pain. It has evolved as an informative important method of diagnosing a wide spectrum of both benign and malignant diseases. Elective diagnostic laparoscopy refers to the use of the procedure in chronic intra-abdominal disorders. Emergency diagnostic laparoscopy is performed in patients presenting with acute abdomen.

INDICATIONS

The indications for diagnostic laparoscopy can be divided into two main groups.

Non-traumatic, Non-gynecological Acute Abdomen Like

- Appendicitis
- Diverticulitis
- Duodenal perforation
- Mesenteric adenitis
- Intestinal adhesion
- Omental necrosis
- Intestinal infarction
- Complicated Meckel's diverticulum
- Bedside laparoscopy in the ICU
- Torsion of intra-abdominal testis.

Gynecological Abdominal Emergencies Like

- Ovarian cysts
- Pelvic inflammatory diseases
- Acute salpingitis
- Ectopic pregnancy
- Endometriosis
- Perforated uterus due to criminal abortion
- Salpingitis.

One of the important uses for diagnostic laparoscopy is the investigation of female infertility. Tubal causes of infertility are found in 15 percent of couple. In these patients laparoscopy not only allows tubal patency to be assessed but also enables other features in the pelvis to be examined. Most important findings related to infertility is kinking of the tube, fimbrial damage or ovarian adhesions. The presence of corpus luteum is considered as good evidence of current ovulation.

If tubal recanalization surgery is planned, it is good idea to perform a preliminary laparoscopy to asses the prospect of successful anastomosis. If the length of remaining tube is less than 2 cm the recanalization surgery should not be attempted and IVF should be tried.

Ovarian biopsy can also be taken at the time of diagnostic laparoscopy to diagnose the cause of amenorrhea and infertility. Although the functional test of ovarian stimulation by gonadotropin releasing hormone is more in use but it can be still of help if the presence of primordial follicles is in doubt in primary amenorrhea or premature ovarian failure.

CONTRAINDICATIONS

Contraindications may include:
- Hemodynamic instability
- Mechanical or paralytic ileus
- Uncorrected coagulopathy
- Generalized peritonitis
- Severe cardiopulmonary disease
- Abdominal wall infection
- Multiple previous abdominal procedures
- Late pregnancy.

However, the final decision is determined not only by the clinical condition of patients, but also by the surgeon's judgment.

Choice of Anesthesia

Diagnostic laparoscopy can be performed under local anesthesia. Sedation with diazepam and pethidine can be used to make patient unaware of procedure because unpleasant sensation of stretching of peritoneum due to pneumoperitoneum cannot be abolished by local anesthesia.

Local anesthetic 4 percent Xylocain can be injected subcutaneously over inferior crease of umbilicus (Fig. 23.1).

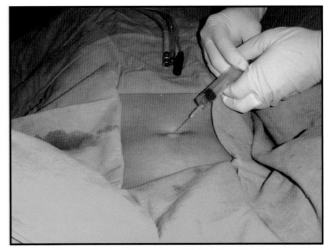

Fig. 23.1: Local anesthesia can be used for diagnostic laparoscopy

Epidural anesthesia is not liked by many anesthetists because to anesthetize the entire peritoneum high block is necessary and it would interfere with intercostals nerves and respiration will be affected. General anesthesia with good muscle relaxation is ideal in laparoscopic surgery.

LAPAROSCOPIC ANATOMY

Diagnostic laparoscopy can be necessary for many undiagnosed surgical problem and knowledge of laparoscopic anatomy of whole abdomen is necessary. However, most common indication of diagnostic laparoscopy is gynecological and especially infertility.

From anterior to posterior, following important tubular structures are found crossing the brim of true pelvis. The round ligament of the uterus, the infundibulopelvic ligament, which contains the gonadal vessels and the ureter. The ovaries and fallopian tube is found between the round ligament and the infundibulopelvic ligament (Fig. 23.2).

The fallopian tubes arise from the superior portion of the uterus just above the attachment points of the round ligament. Laparoscopically, the round ligaments overhang the fallopian tube because of uterine manipulation and can be easily mistaken for them. The fallopian tubes towards its lateral end encircle the ovaries partially with their fimbriated ends.

If the uterus is deviated to the contralateral side with the help of uterine manipulator infundibulopelvic ligament is spread out and a pelvic side wall triangle is created. The base of this triangle is the round ligament,

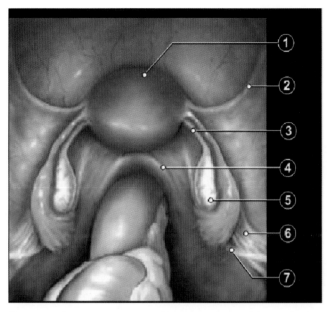

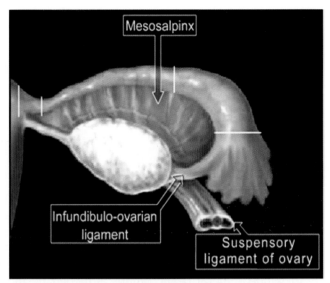

Fig. 23.3: Anatomy of adenexa

Fig. 23.2: Laparoscopic anatomy of normal pelvis, 1-Uterus, 2- Round ligament, 3-Utero-ovarian ligament (proper ovarian ligament), 4- Uterosacral ligament, 5-Ovary, 6-Suspensory ligament of the ovary, 7-Ureter

the medial side is the infundibulopelvic ligament, and the lateral side is the external iliac artery. The apex of this triangle is the point at which the infundibulopelvic ligament crosses the external iliac artery (Fig. 23.3).

Patient Position

The anesthetized patient is placed on the operating table with the legs straight or lithotomy position if female. The lithotomy position will allow the gynecologists and assistant to work simultaneously and uterine manipulation would be possible. The thighs must not be flexed onto the abdominal wall as they would be in the full lithotomy position used for other open surgical gynecological procedures. The operating table is tilted headup or down by approximately 15° depending on the main area of examination. Compression bandage may be used on leg during the operation to prevent thromboembolism especially if patient is in lithotomy position.

Position of the Surgical Team

Before starting diagnostic laparoscopy a best guess is made about the quadrant in which pathology is likely to be found. The surgeon should stand opposite to this quadrant to allow direct view into this quadrant. If

the pathology is more likely in pelvic cavity the surgeon stands on left side of the patient. The first assistant, whose main task is to position the video camera, is also on the patient's left side. The instrument trolley is placed on the patient's left, allowing the scrub nurse to assist with placing the appropriate instruments in the operating ports. Television monitors are positioned on either side of the top end of the operating table at a suitable height for surgeon, anesthetists, as well as assistant to see the procedure.

Port Position

Generally one optical port in umbilicus and one 5 mm port in left iliac fossa are required. Some gynecologist put their second port in suprapubic region in midline. In our opinion, left iliac fossa port is better because it gives elevation angle of 30° and manipulation angle of 60°, which is ergonomically better. With suprapubic port elevation angle of instrument and tubal structure is 90° and hence lifting up of ovary and tube may be difficult without grasping it (Fig. 23.4).

During diagnostic laparoscopy it is advisable that both telescope and probing instrument is held by surgeon himself as he knows better what he wants to see and where he want to concentrate more and which structure he wants to see in magnified close-up view. At the time of diagnostic laparoscopy surgeon should try to be very gentle with the tubal structure and bowel so that adhesion will not form and stricture of tube will not occur.

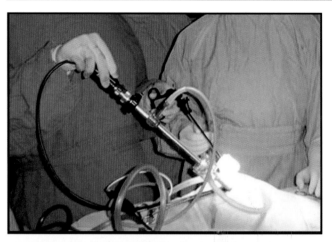

Fig. 23.4: Port position for diagnostic laparoscopy

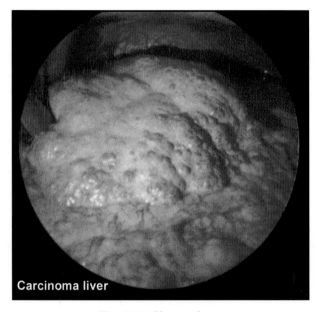

Carcinoma liver

Fig. 23.5: Hemangioma

Viewing of lateral pelvic organs is helped by the manipulation of mobile structure with a solid port introduced through the left iliac fossa port. Many gynecologists introduce the second port in suprapubic region but the elevation angle of the instrument is 90° and the mobilization of organs is difficult.

A three-port approach should be used if there is any difficulty in manipulation with two ports especially in case of extensive adhesion.
• 10 mm umbilical (optical)
• 5 mm suprapubic
• 5 mm right hypochondrium.

A 30° telescope is employed in most instances, as this facilitates easier inspection of the deeper peritoneal cavity and abdominal organs. The secondary ports are inserted under laparoscopic vision. The selected site on the abdominal wall is identified by finger indentation of the parietal peritoneum.

The optimum incision is in the subumbilical region. The open technique for trocar insertion is recommended if patient presents with severe abdominal distension. Nitrous oxide is used if diagnostic laparoscopy is performed in local anesthesia because nitrous oxide has its own analgesic effect. Carbon dioxide is the preferred gas if diagnostic laparoscopy is performed under general anesthesia. Insufflation should be very slow and with care taken not to exceed 12.0 mm Hg.

Operative Procedure

The first step in diagnostic laparoscopy is thorough exploration, just as during exploratory laparotomy. A systematic approach to exploration is essential to ensure that nothing is missed.

Systemic Plan of Inspection in Mid Abdomen

Positioning is the primary means of displacing the bowel and exposing peritoneal surfaces. In women with a deep pelvis, the bowel should be displaced gently into the upper abdomen, using a blunt probe or closed blunt grasping instrument to avoid laceration of the bowel or mesentery. An additional port with a blunt tipped instrument may be used. Occasionally, fan retractor should be used to retract full sigmoid colon. This instrument can be inserted through a 5-mm trocar sleeve and fanned out in the abdomen to retract the bowel. Some common findings (Figs 23.5 to 23.11).

Inspection of Pelvis

Patient should again positioned in steep Trendelenburg's position.

After assessing the genital organs, the gynecologist may wish to view areas outside the pelvis. This should be done by tilting the table head up or laterally to examine the paracolic or sub-diaphragmatic spaces. Systematic plan of inspection of pelvis in shown in Figures 23.9A to C.

Section Three

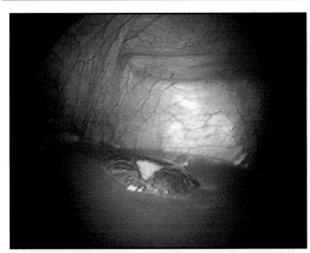

Fig. 23.6: Carcinomatosis

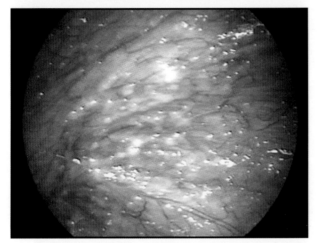

Fig. 23.7: Endometriosis

ROLE OF LAPAROSCOPY IN ASCITES

Although the determination of the etiology of ascites is usually straight forward by history, physical examination, and analysis of ascitic fluid, the diagnosis of tuberculous or carcinomatous ascites may be elusive. In such cases, laparoscopy with biopsy is highly accurate. Peritoneal mesothelioma is frequently missed on ascitic fluid by cytology and by blind biopsy. This entity is readily diagnosed by laparoscopy with peritoneal biopsy. Laparoscopy may be useful in the evaluation of hepatic malignancy (either primary or metastatic). Eighty percent to 90% of these lesions are present on the hepatic surface and up to 2/3 of the liver surface may be inspected by laparoscopy. When surgical resection is a therapeutic option, laparoscopy

may reveal small (1 cm or less) metastatic lesions, peritoneal metastases, or cirrhosis, which represent contraindications to resection and are frequently missed on CT, MRI, and US. The use of laparoscopic ultrasound allows detection of deeper lesions and vascular infiltration.

In studying the role of laparoscopy in the diagnosis and differential diagnosis of ascites out of 2,500 patients who underwent laparoscopy 30.89% had ascites; liver cirrhosis underlay it in 57.78%, peritoneal carcinosis in 26.29%, primary and metastatic carcinoma in 12.95%, tuberculous peritonitis in 1.42%, more rarely other diseases. Liver cirrhosis, malignant tumors and the other hepatic affections with concomitant ascites in their course can certainly be diagnosed laparoscopically. Laparoscopy with oriented biopsy of peritoneum and liver is of decisive importance in differentiating peritoneal carcinosis from tuberculosis. In peritoneal carcinosis the diagnosis (as based in clinical and laboratory findings) coincided perfectly with the laparoscopic and histologic one in 24.5%, partially in 45.5%. In 30% there was no congruence at all. Laparoscopy and the test methods associated with it contributed to the accurate diagnosis of peritoneal carcinosis in 75.5% of the patients. Ovarian carcinoma (20.9%) and cancer of the stomach (16.3%) underlay peritoneal carcinosis most frequently, other diseases by far more seldom.

Diagnostic peritoneoscopies was performed in 226 patients with ascites. Satisfactory examination was possible in 220 patients. Clinical diagnosis was confirmed at peritoneoscopy in 82.7% of patients. Peritoneoscopic examination corrected the clinical diagnosis in 13.7%, was inconclusive in 2.6% and was incorrect in 0.8% of cases. It was 100% diagnostic in malignant peritonitis and 89.5% in patients with tuberculous peritonitis. Pseudomyxoma peritoneal and mesothelioma were suspected in one patient each at peritoneoscopy and was confirmed histologically. The utility of routine ascitic fluid examination was reviewed in all patients. The ascitic fluid was transudative in 81.9%, exudative in 8.6% and indeterminate in 9.5% of patients with cirrhosis of liver. Patients with tuberculous peritonitis had exudative, transudative and indeterminate ascites in 71.8%, 3.2% and 25% respectively. The ascites in patients with malignant peritonitis was either exudative (80%) or indeterminate (20%). There was considerable overlap in the nature

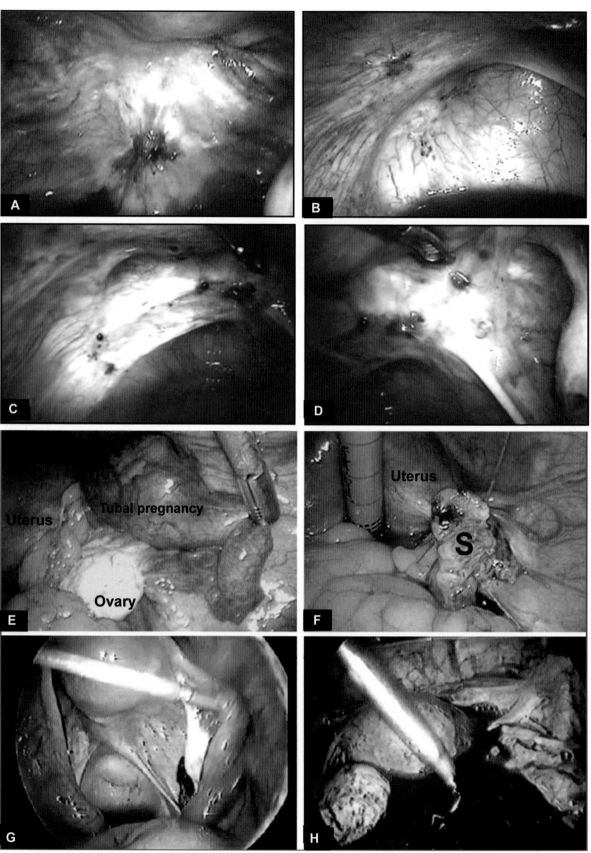

Figs 23.8A to H: Ectopic pregnancy

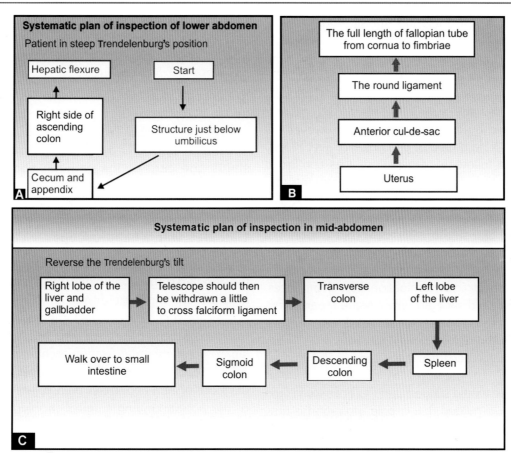

Figs 23.9A to C: Systematic plan of inspection of pelvis

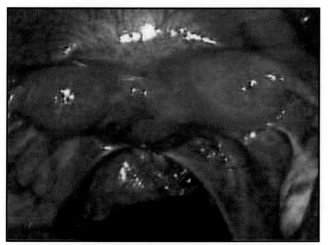

Fig. 23.10: Bicornuate uterus

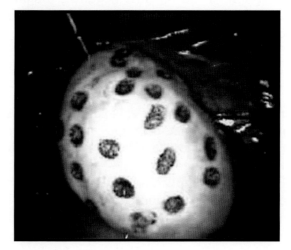

Fig. 23.11: Polycystic ovary

of ascites present in the three groups of patients. We therefore conclude that peritoneoscopy is the most valuable investigation in the diagnosis of ascites, particularly in exudative and indeterminate types.

The Value of Laparoscopic Diagnosis of TB

The laparoscopic and pathological diagnoses of 43 patients who underwent abdominal laparoscopy for various indications are presented. Major indications for the laparoscopy included hepatomegaly in 32 patients, ascites in 28, and pyrexia of unknown origin (PUO) in 18 patients. A combination of two or more of these indications was a more common feature. The most frequently encountered laparoscopic diagnoses were tuberculosis and chronic liver disease (16 patients each), followed by cancer (9 patients). However, on pathological examination of peritoneal or liver biopsy tissue and on follow-up, tuberculosis was confirmed in 12 patients, chronic liver disease in 14 patients and hepatocellular carcinoma in 11 patients. No complications were encountered during the laparoscopy. Our findings indicate that abdominal laparoscopy is a safe, quick and inexpensive diagnostic tool, particularly when appropriate and adequate tissue is taken for pathological examination. In such instances, laparoscopy would save an unnecessary laparotomy, especially where tuberculosis and cancer are considered in the differential diagnosis.

Due to its high accuracy some suggest PCR before laparoscopy. In the light of our accumulated experience, we would suggest that PCR of ascetic fluid obtained by US-guided fine needle aspiration is now the investigation of choice for patients with the described clinical and radiological presentations and should at least be attempted before surgical intervention. If the result is negative, diagnostic laparoscopy or, if this is not feasible, laparotomy should be performed.

Pretherapeutic Gastric Carcinoma Assessment

A pretherapeutic staging system to design operative or neoadjuvant treatments in gastric cancer is needed. It can be done under local anesthesia sensitive predictor of peritoneal recurrence.

Regarding complications of dialysis catheter insertion Tiong reported surgical early and late complications of dialysis catheter. Of open Tenckhoff catheter insertion under local anesthesia in a single institution. A review was carried out on 164 insertions in 139 patients over a three-year period. Tenckhoff catheter insertion for CAPD is a procedure associated with significant surgical morbidity. Patients with diabetes mellitus, glomerulonephritis and ongoing sepsis are at greater risk of early complications, and hence, must have their conditions stabilized or treated

before surgery. In addition, prolonged surgical time and patients with previous abdominal surgery are at increased risk. The rate of complications may be improved by early consideration of patients with poor tolerance of local anesthetic surgery or with previous abdominal surgery for laparoscopic insertion under general anesthesia. To prevent late complications dominated by CAPD peritonitis, patients' nutritional status and care of the catheter should both be optimized.

New Technique for Dialysis Catheter using Laparoscopy

Open insertion of peritoneal dialysis (PD) catheters is the standard surgical technique, but it is associated with a relatively high incidence of catheter outflow obstruction and dialysis leak. Omental wrapping is the most common cause of mechanical problem; laparoscopic omental fixation technique is of higher value in addition to laparoscopic surgery also enabled diagnosis of intra-abdominal pathologies and treatment of the accompanying surgical problems during the same operation.

The risk of port-site metastases in those undergoing laparoscopy for gynecologic malignancy was highest in those with ascites in a study of 82 patients. The study participants underwent 87 procedures that involved 330 trocar sites. The overall risk of port-site metastases per procedure was 2.3%, and per port site was 2.4%, Dr Nimesh Nagarsheth, at an international congress sponsored by the Society of Laparoendoscopic Surgeons reported 39 patients with endometrial cancer, 29 with ovarian cancer, and 14 with cervical cancer. Twenty of those were treated for recurrent cancer, and 10 had ascites. They were followed for an average of 361 days. Port-site metastases occurred in two patients. The first developed metastases at five sites, and was diagnosed 13 days after second-look laparoscopy for stage IIIB ovarian cancer. The second had metastases at three sites, and was diagnosed 46 days after second-look laparoscopy for stage IIIC primary peritoneal cancer. Both patients had ascites.

Laparoscopy in ascites is a safe and cost effective diagnostic modality and its rules extended the diagnostic procedure providing in unexplained cause of ascites definitive diagnosis.

In such instances, laparoscopy would save an unnecessary laparotomy; especially where tuberculosis and cancer are considered in the differential diagnosis staging laparoscopy with peritoneal lavage cytology is a safe, effective tool in patients with locally advanced gastric cancer, especially in patients receiving neoadjuvant chemotherapy. The ability of minimally invasive surgeons and endoscopists to diagnose and palliate unrespectable pancreatic cancer is likely to continue to improve and these techniques will play an increasingly important role in the care of patients with pancreatic cancer. Likewise, the accuracy of radiological imaging techniques to detect unrespectable disease will also continue to advance and further decrease the incidence of nontherapeutic laparotomies. It is valuable in many therapeutic uses as in staging of tumor, catheter placement in nephrogenic ascites.

DIAGNOSTIC LAPAROSCOPY

The first important step after access to the abdomen has been gained, is to check for damage caused by trocar insertion. A second 5 mm port may then be inserted under vision in an appropriate quadrant to take a palpating rod.

The usual site of insertion of the trocar/cannula for diagnostic laparoscopy is below or to the side of the umbilicus. This position may require to be altered in the presence of abdominal scars. The use of a 30° forward oblique telescope is preferable for viewing the surface architecture of organs. By rotation of the telescope, different angles of inspection can be achieved.

A systematic examination of the abdomen must be performed just as in laparotomy. We begin at the left lobe of the liver but any scheme can be used as long as it is consistent. Next, check around the falciform ligament to the right lobe of liver, gallbladder and hiatus. After checking the stomach, move on to the caecum and appendix and check the terminal ileum. Follow the colon round to the sigmoid colon, and then check the pelvis. Surgeon should be conversant with sampling and biopsy techniques, the use of position and manipulation to aid vision.

When performing a diagnostic laparoscopy to confirm appendicitis, a 5 mm port is placed in the left iliac fossa to facilitate manipulation. The patient is placed head down and rotated to the left to displace the small bowel from the pelvis and allow the uterus and ovaries to be checked. This, however, should be limited to avoid contamination of subphrenic spaces, if this is not already present.

At the time of diagnostic laparoscopy all the abdominal organs are inspected for any gross anatomical abnormalities. Abdominal cavity is inspected for excess of fluids. Samples are taken if free fluid is present for laboratory tests (chemistry, cytology or bacteriology). Peritoneal lavage and adhesiolysis may need to be performed to improve visualization of organs. At the time of peritoneal lavage when fluid is sucked from the cul-de-sac, it is important to keep all the holes of the suction-irrigator beneath the level of the fluid to avoid removing pneumoperitoneum. If the suction-irrigator is positioned improperly, the CO_2 gas will be removed preferentially. However, with high-flow insufflators, pneumoperitoneum rarely is lost and quickly restored.

Laparoscopy for Abdominal Trauma

The diagnostic laparoscopy of various organs is shown in Figures 23.12 to 23.17.

Trauma is the leading cause of death between 1 and 44 years. In all age groups, it is surpassed only by cancer and atherosclerosis in mortality. The evaluation and treatment of abdominal injuries are critical components in the management of severely injured trauma patients. Because missed intra-abdominal injuries are a frequent cause of preventable trauma deaths, a high index of suspicion is warranted. Multiple factors, including the mechanism of injury, the body region injured, the patient's hemodynamic and neurological status, associated injuries, and institutional resources influence the diagnostic approach and the outcome of abdominal injures.

Laparoscopy was first used for a trauma patient in 1956 by Lamy, who observed two cases of splenic injury. Since then, Gazzaniga noted that laparoscopy is useful for determining the need for laparotomy. In 1991, Berci reported that he had reduced the number of non-therapeutic laparotomies performed for hemoperitoneum by 25% through the use of laparoscopy in 150 patients with blunt abdominal trauma.

Data shows that laparoscopy is a useful modality for evaluating and managing hemodynamically stable

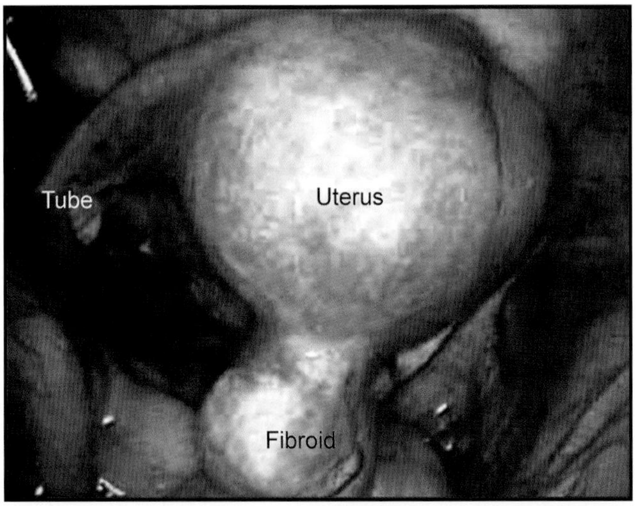

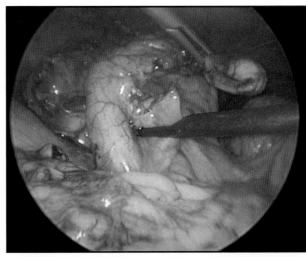

Fig. 23.12: Fibroid

Fig. 23.13: Adhesion of appendix

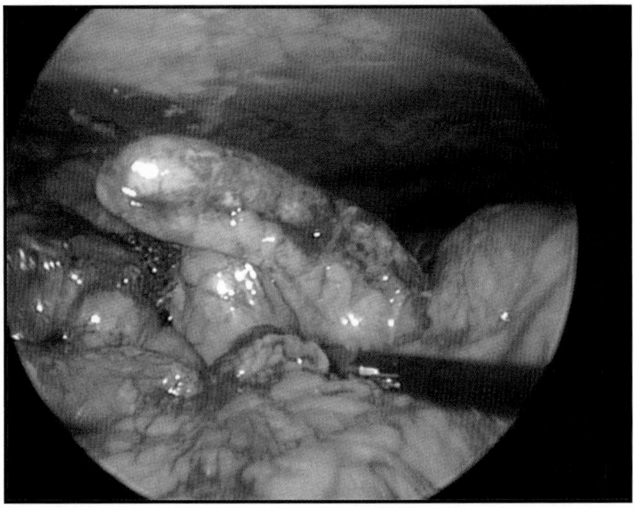

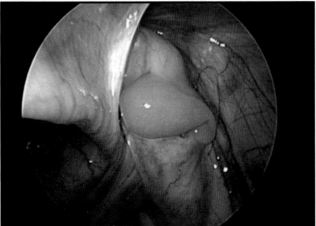

Fig. 23.14: Acute appendicitis

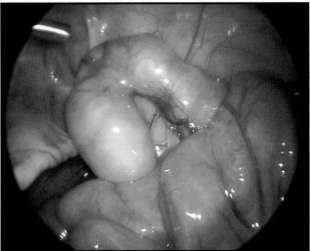

Fig. 23.15: Diverticulum

Fig. 23.16: Impalpable testes

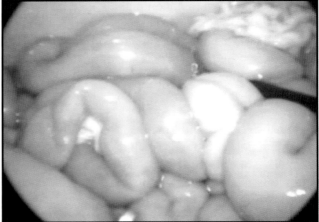

Fig. 23.17: Perforation of small bowel

trauma patients with penetrating injuries. Increased use of laparoscopy in select patients with penetrating abdominal trauma will decrease the rate of negative and nontherapeutic laparotomies, thus lowering morbidity, decreasing length of hospitalization, and provide for more efficient utilization of available resources. As technology and expertise among surgeons continues to improve, more standard therapeutic interventions may be done laparoscopically in the future. Mandatory surgical exploration for gunshot wounds to the abdomen has been a surgical dictum for the greater part of this century. Although non-operative management of blunt solid organ injuries and low-energy penetrating injuries such as stab wounds is well established, the same is not true for gunshot wounds. The vast majority of patients who sustain a gunshot injury to the abdomen require immediate laparotomy to control bleeding and contain contamination. Non-operative treatment of patients with a gunshot injury is gaining acceptance in only a highly selected subset of hemodynamically stable adult patients without peritonitis. Although the physical examination remains the cornerstone in the evaluation of patients with gunshot injury, other techniques such as computed tomography, diagnostic peritoneal lavage, and diagnostic laparoscopy allows accurate diagnosis of intra-abdominal injury. The ability to exclude internal organ injury non-operatively avoids the potential complications of unnecessary laparotomy. Clinical data to support selective non-operative management of certain gunshot injuries to the abdomen are accumulating, but the approach has risks and requires careful collaborative management by emergency physicians and surgeons experienced in the care of penetrating injury. Sosa reported 121 consecutive abdominal gunshot wounds managed with laparoscopy. Seventy-nine (65%) had negative laparoscopy, and these patients were managed without laparotomy. Another 7.2% avoided nontherapeutic laparotomy.

It is very important to determine the presence, location, and severity of intra-abdominal injury to decide the surgical intervention; and to thoroughly evaluate intra-abdominal organs for associated injuries in the trauma patient. For stab wounds, serial physical examination is supplemented by local wound exploration, diagnostic peritoneal lavage (DPL),

abdominal US, abdominal CT, Magnetic resonance imaging (MRI), and in some cases, angiography to maximize the value of surgical intervention and to reduce negative and non-therapeutic laparotomy. Despite their many positive qualities, these diagnostic methods have some drawbacks. DPL is an invasive but sensitive procedure; it may result in non-therapeutic laparotomy with its attendant morbidity. The use of CT is limited to the hemodynamically stable patient. There has been increasing interest in the use of abdominal US because it is portable, noninvasive, rapid, and easily repeatable. However, it is less accurate for diagnosis of diaphragmatic and hollow viscera. With experience in laparoscopic cholecystectomy and the advent of improved and readily accessible laparoscopic equipment and devices, laparoscopic surgery became widespread for intra-abdominal operations, setting the stage for renewed interest in its applications for the diagnosis of traumatic abdominal injuries and examination of their therapeutic potential.

In the evaluation and management of the abdominal injury, current diagnostic methods have a defined sensitivity, specificity, and accuracy, but none of these represents a gold standard. Thus, abdominal exploration by laparotomy should not be discarded as a worthy diagnostic and therapeutic procedure for patients with equivocal and unreliable findings. It is associated with complication rates as high as 40% including a 10 to 40% negative laparotomy rate, a 20% morbidity rate, a 0 to 5% mortality rate, and a 3% long-term risk of bowel obstruction secondary to adhesions.

Laparoscopy has been reported infrequently as a therapeutic tool in selected trauma patients. Examples of therapeutic laparoscopy include repair of diaphragmatic lacerations with sutures, staples, or prosthetic mesh; suturing of gastrointestinal perforations; hemostasis of low-grade liver and splenic lacerations; resection of small bowel and colon; cholecystectomy; splenectomy; and distal pancreatectomy. Autotransfusion of collected blood from the hemoperitoneum is another potential application. Fabian in a large study of 182 trauma patients, reported one suture repair of diaphragmatic injury. Successful laparoscopic repair of small bowel, colon, and rectal injuries, and laparoscopic repair of a small gastric stab wound using hernia stapler have been

Section Three

reported recently. For the repair of solid visceral injuries, there are three methods that merit investigation: The totally laparoscopic procedure, the laparoscopically assisted procedure, hand-assisted laparoscopic surgery (HALS). The argon beam coagulator, fibrin glue, topical hemostatic agent, and absorbable mesh may be beneficial for hepatic and splenic lacerations. Laparoscopic repair of bowel injuries can be performed using suture or staples. Primary suture repair of a small bowel injury would be amenable by a totally laparoscopic procedure. Using a porcine model, Pietrafitta and Soperet described a technique for an intraperitoneal functional end-to-end anastomosis of the small intestine. Milsom and Bohm modified these techniques and reported that their technique for intracorporeal intestinal anastomosis has been proven safe in dozens of animal and human procedures, but that it had some drawbacks. It requires a long operating time and needs two or three 30 mm Endo-GIAs and a skin incision for specimen retrieval. Recently, animal research has assessed the potential for hand-assisted laparoscopic exploration to detect traumatic injuries. Asbun reported that hand-assisted laparoscopic exploration is more accurate than laparoscopic exploration alone in detecting injuries (63 vs. 38%), but that it still resulted in an unacceptable rate of missed injuries.

Hand-assisted laparoscopic surgery allows for the application of minimally invasive surgical techniques to complex intra-abdominal operations, particularly when specimen removal is required. The rationale for this approach is that the hand offers the surgeon some advantage in terms of tactile feedback, exposure, retraction, and orientation, enabling the surgeon to perform with greater safety and efficiency. Most trauma surgeons consider omental herniation through an anterior abdominal stab wound an indication for laparotomy because frequently there are significant intra-abdominal injuries. As an alternative to laparotomy, the herniated omentum was evaluated and managed, with laparoscopy performed through the abdominal stab wound or accessory trocar. If there are no significant injuries, the wound can be managed without further treatment. Depending on the surgeon's preference, therapeutic laparoscopy can be continued.

The complications of laparoscopy for trauma include not only the usual complications of anesthesia and laparoscopy, but also some that are unique to the trauma patient. Fabian independently reported the development of tension pneumothorax in patients with diaphragmatic injury from positive-pressure pneumoperitoneum. If suspected, induction of pneumoperitoneum is stopped, and an immediate needle thoracocentesis is performed, followed by a tube thoracostomy if needed. However, routine prophylactic tube thoracostomy is not indicated. The risks of gas embolism in patients with intra-abdominal venous injuries, especially liver lacerations, are another problem. Among 133 laparoscopic examinations of trauma, Smith did encounter this complication in two patients with injuries of the inferior vena cava tamponaded by clot.

This potential problem of laparoscopy has stimulated interest in "gasless" laparoscopy based on expansion of the peritoneal cavity by mechanical retractors. In addition to averting the risks of tension pneumothorax and gas embolism, it facilitates the use of conventional instruments such as hemostats, needles, sutures, and electrocautery, resulting in significant cost savings. The major disadvantage of gasless laparoscopy, however, is the excessive cost of the powered mechanical arm and the poor exposure in the lateral gutters. Less expensive apparatus to lift the abdominal wall is expected. The transperitoneal absorption of carbon dioxide may cause metabolic and hemodynamic changes such as acidosis, cardiac suppression, atelectasis, subcutaneous emphysema, and increased intracranial pressure, resulting in more profound consequences for the trauma patient. Joseph demonstrated that carbon dioxide (CO_2) pneumoperitoneum causes significantly increased intracranial pressure in a porcine model of head injury.

The results of this study led them to recommend the avoidance of CO_2 pneumoperitoneum for the evaluation of patients with head injuries. Undoubtedly, gasless laparoscopy could replace CO_2 pneumoperitoneum in these cases. Missed intra-abdominal injuries are among the most frequent causes of potentially preventable trauma deaths. The evaluation and management of abdominal trauma is dependant on multiple factors, including mechanism of injury, location of injury, hemodynamic status of the patient, neurological status of the patient, associated injuries, and institutional resources. Therefore careful selection, high index of suspicion, and a low threshold for laparotomy will provide the patient the benefits of minimal invasive surgery and reducing the rates and morbidity of unnecessary laparotomy.

Ending of the Operation

At the end of surgery, abdomen should be re-examined for any possible bowel injury or hemorrhage. The entire accessory instrument and then port is removed. The telescope should be removed leaving gas valve of umbilical port open to let out all the gas. Once the complete gas is out, for removing primary cannula telescope or any blunt instrument should be introduced again and cannula should be pulled over that instrument to prevent pull of omentum or bowel. Wound should be closed with suture. Vicryl should be used for rectus and un-absorbable intradermal or stapler for skin. Only 10 mm port wound is necessary to repair. Adhesive sterile dressing over the wound should be applied.

At the end of diagnostic laparoscopy surgeon can perform therapeutic laparoscopy if indicated and consent from patients relative can be obtained.

Patient may be discharged on the same day after operation if every thing goes well. The patient may have slight pain initially but usually resolves. Diagnostic laparoscopic is a useful method for reducing hospital stay, complications and return to normal activity if carried on in proper manner.

Complications

Complications may occur during access, trocar insertion, or the diagnostic manipulation of viscera. These complications include, cardiac arrhythmias, hemodynamic instability due to decreased venous return, bleeding, bile leak, perforation of a hollow viscus, laceration of a solid organ, vascular injury, gas embolism, and subcutaneous or extraperitoneal dissection of the insufflation gas. If proper sterilization of instrument is not done then wound infection or leakage of ascites may occur postoperatively. Failure to accurately diagnose the extent of intra-abdominal pathology is another potential complication for which patient may have to go for other surgery.

CONCLUSION

Diagnostic laparoscopy is one of the very important method of investigation for patients in whom the diagnosis or extent of the disease is unclear or the abdominal findings are equivocal. It can be performed safely in an inpatient or outpatient setting, potentially expediting diagnosis and treatment.

Section Three

24 Laparoscopic Small Bowel Surgery

Since the first reports of laparoscopic surgery for inflammatory bowel disease from Peters in 1992, several literatures have subsequently shown the potential advantage of Minimal Access surgery for small bowel surgery. The increased use of laparoscopy in the management of gastrointestinal problems continues to expand. Procedures such as jejunostomies, diagnosis of intestinal obstruction or ischemia, resection of the small bowel, and lysis of adhesions can be managed with this technique.

Laparoscopic Resection of Small Bowel

The role of laparoscopy in resection of small bowel has increased in last 5 year. Laparoscopic small bowel resection can be performed safely in the setting of benign as well as malignant disease and imparts many of the benefits of minimally invasive surgery. The affected small bowel and mesentery can be thoroughly inspected and resected laparoscopically and bowel continuity restored through an entirely intracorporeal technique or laparoscopic assisted technique.

Indications

A small bowel resection is the surgical removal of one or more segments of the small intestine. Laparoscopic small bowel resection with primary anastomosis is most frequently indicated for benign diseases.

The most common indications are:
- Isolated Crohn's disease
- Gastrointestinal stromal tumors
- Benign strictures, and
- Vascular malformations.

Malignant conditions represent relative contra-indications in that they are rare and if diagnosed or suspected, laparoscopic method should not be considered as method of choice. The conduct of the laparoscopic operation should be in a manner very similar to that of a conventional small bowel resection.

Patient Positioning and Operating Room Setup

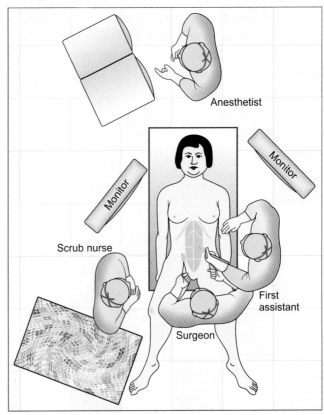

Fig. 24.1: Position of the surgical team for ileal resection

The patient is placed supine in a modified lithotomy position using Dan Allen stirrups. Surgery is begun in the Trendelenburg position (20° head-down tilt) and, after cannula insertion, the patient is tilted left side down for ileal surgery or the right side down for jejunal surgery Figure 24.1.

After insertion of port, the surgeon stands between the legs. The scrub nurse should stand on the right side near the knee. Assistant stand on the right side, one monitor is placed close to the patient's right shoulder, the second monitor is placed near the left shoulder, the best location for viewing by the nurse.

Port Position

Port should be positioned according to base ball diamond concept and should be opposite to the site of pathology Figure 24.2.

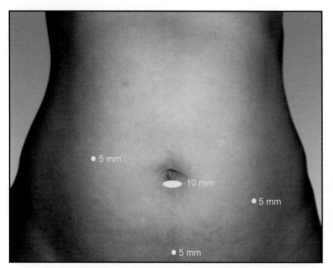

Fig. 24.2: Position of the cannulae for ileal resection

For jejunal surgery, the left- and right-sided cannulae may suffice. For ileal surgery, it may be preferable to use the suprapubic cannula.

Operative Technique

Once the preoperative diagnosis is confirmed and the surgeon has confirmed that laparoscopic procedure appears feasible, the pathology is located by Walk Over the entire length of the small intestine and placing a suture just upstream of the pathology.

Walk Over the small bowel is accomplished from proximal to distal by placing the patient on the left

side up, in slight reverse Trendelenburg position until the mid small bowel is reached, then adjusting the patient to the right side up with Trendelenburg position to run the distal half of the small intestine.

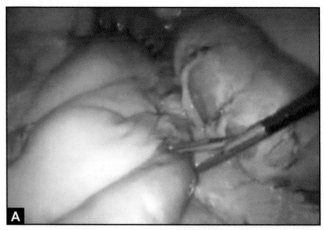

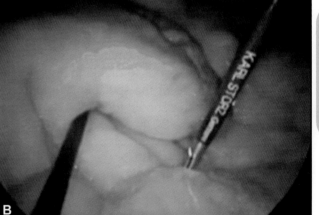

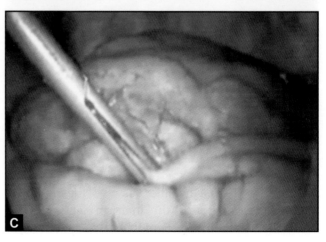

Figs 24.3A to C

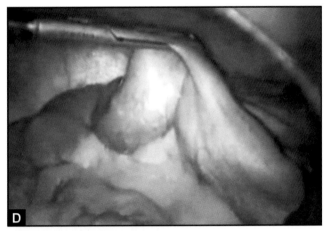

Fig. 24.3D

Figs 24.3A to D: Walk over to small intestine in order to detect pathology

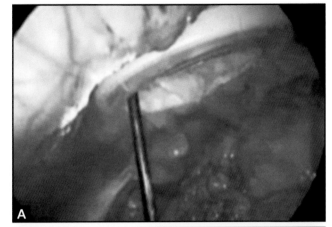

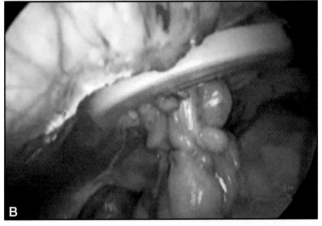

Figs 24.5A and B: Loop of intestine to be resected is drawn out through wound protector

The surgeon should start the "Walk Over" from between the legs then switch to the left side of the patient for the distal half. The technique of inspection should be "hand-over-hand" or "hand-to-hand" (Figs 24.3A to D) based on the degree of freedom present within the abdominal cavity.

If it will be advantageous to divide the mesenteric vessels before delivery of the specimen through the abdominal incision, this should ideally be done using ideally LigaSure Figure 24.4.

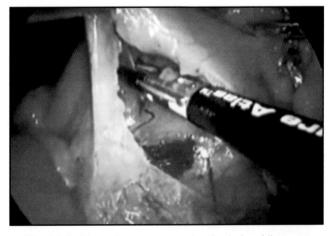

Fig. 24.4: Dissection mesentery by the help of ligasure

Main vessel supplying the affected segment can also be ligated, and leave the other vessels of the mesentery to be divided through the incision. This may be especially helpful in a patient with a thick abdominal wall. Once the specimen is fully mobilized, a port site is enlarged to 3-5 cm. For small incisions, a transverse incision is preferred. The anterior rectus sheath is transversely incised, the rectus muscles retracted, and the posterior sheath also transversely incised. If the incision has to be larger because of a bulky tumor, a longitudinal incision in the midline is accomplished above and below the umbilicus.

The wound is protected using a plastic sheath and the loop of intestine to be resected is drawn out through the enlarged incision Figures 24.5A and B. Wound protection is important to reduce any contamination by tumor cells or intestine and it may also facilitate the specimen extraction. The resection and anastomosis are then made in a standard manner extracorporeally, either by a hand-sewn or stapled method. The mesenteric defect is usually closed with a running absorbable suture through the incision (Figs 24.6A and B).

After performing the anastomosis, the abdomen is copiously irrigated with warm sterile saline solution

Section Three

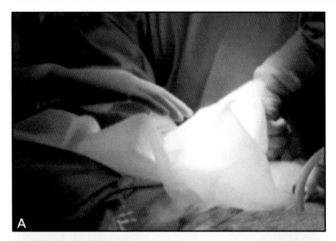

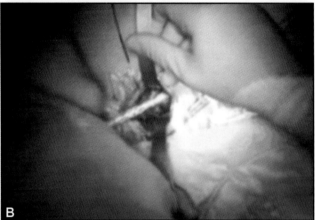

Figs 24.6A and B: Resection and anastomosis in a standard manner extracorporeally

through the incision. The fluid is removed by placing the patient in the head-up position and passing a sump suction cannula into the pelvis. After irrigation of the peritoneal cavity, the abdominal wall is closed with a running suture or a series single suture.

The most important steps of laparoscopically assisted small bowel surgery are to localize and mobilize the diseased segment and deliver it through a small incision of hand port. The laparoscopic technique has become procedure of choice for isolated benign small diseases. Intracorporeal anastomosis can also be attempted but extracorporeal anastomosis is more popular at this time because most of the dissection and anastomosis can safely be performed using conventional techniques through a small incision used to remove the specimen.

The role of this approach in cancer surgery is limited. If there is diffuse spread of the disease, then it may be reasonable to consider a laparoscopic localization of the tumor in order to minimize the incision, or to consider only biopsy and no resection. Because these are rare tumors, and there is no proof of the efficacy of a laparoscopic approach, quickly re-establish pneumoperitoneum after removing the specimen.

ILEOCOLECTOMY

Indications

An ileocolectomy is most frequently indicated in patients with benign disease, i.e. Crohn's disease, cecal diverticulitis, intestinal tuberculosis, enteric Behçet's disease, submucosal tumors (lipoma, gastrointestinal stromal tumor, lymphoma, carcinoid, etc.), giant villous adenoma and polyps, located in the ileocecal regions. Indications for performing a limited ileocecal resection for malignancies of the terminal ileum, the appendix, or the cecum are rare. This may be the procedure of choice in palliative resection for cecal cancer.

Before the surgery for Crohn's disease, patients should have a computed tomography scan, small bowel series, and a full colonoscopy to assess the localization and dimension of any phlegmon or abscess or the presence of small bowel stricture or fistula, respectively. The preoperative computed tomography scan is also useful to evaluate periureteral inflammation and to aid in the decision to use intraoperative ureteric catheters. Preoperative enteral or parenteral nutritional support should be considered in selected patients.

Most surgeons would agree that the laparoscopic approach is contraindicated in patients with nonlocalized intra-abdominal abscesses, multiple previous bowel operations with possible dense adhesions, fixed mass with multiple fistulas, acute intestinal obstruction, and perforation. Although the entire operation can be performed laparoscopically, most surgeons prefer a laparoscopic-assisted procedure by laparoscopic mobilization and extracorporeal resection and anastomosis.

Operative Technique

The patient is placed in the Trendelenburg position, and three or four ports are inserted according to base ball diamond concept. For establishment of pneumoperitoneum, CO_2 is channeled through the infraumbilical trocar until the intra-abdominal pressure reaches 12 mm Hg. Both the operating surgeon and

Section Three

camera holder stand on the patient's left side. After abdominal exploration, the operation table is rotated left side down so the small intestine falls toward the left upper quadrant.

The ascending colon is thoroughly mobilized from the base of the appendix up to the hepatic flexure by cutting the retroperitoneal attachments with electrosurgical scissors and laparoscopic coagulating shears, and bluntly dissecting the retroperitoneal fusion fascia and loose connective tissue. With this procedure, the duodenum, Gerota's fascia, and sometimes more inferiorly the right ureter and the gonadal vessels become visible beneath the retroperitoneal fusion fascia. During dissection, the direct grasping and handling of diseased bowel loops should be avoided, to prevent incidental myotomies and enterotomies.

In patients of Crohn's disease with ileovesical, ileorectal, and gastrocolic fistulas, division with an intracorporeal stapling device by one or two firings of the 45-or 60-mm stapler can be done. After mobilization of the entire ascending colon, meticulous hemostasis is made. Then, the patient is placed in a reversed Trendelenburg position temporarily and the abdomen is irrigated with warm sterile saline. The patient is placed in a flat supine position, and pneumoperitoneum is released.

To exteriorized the bowel loop a small laparotomy is performed through a 5-cm long skin incision made at the umbilical trocar site or through a Pfannenstiel incision. A wound protector is inserted and the segments of the colon are delivered through this incision. Mesenteric division, ileocolic resection, and anastomosis by Gambee's procedure using 4-0 absorbable sutures, or functional end-to-end anastomosis using linear staplers are performed extracorporeally. After closure of the mesenteric defect, the entire residual small bowel is examined through the incision, and drain tube is left in cul-de-sac through the right lateral trocar site if necessary, and every trocar site incision is closed with skin staplers.

Laparoscopic-assisted approach, with an extracorporeal anastomosis, rather than an entirely laparoscopic approach with an intracorporeal anastomosis is more popular. Laparoscopic-assisted approach provides the benefits of laparoscopic surgery while maintaining the advantages of open vascular division and anastomosis, i.e. speed, low risk of intra-

abdominal stool spillage. Laparoscopic colorectal surgery for benign conditions continues to evolve. When performed by surgeons with adequate experience, laparoscopic surgery seems to demonstrate advantages over conventional operations. We believe at this time that laparoscopic ileocolectomy should be considered the first-line surgical option for most primary resections for Crohn's disease localized to the ileocolic region.

BIBLIOGRAPHY

1. Altman DG. Practical Statistics for Medical Research. London, England: Chapman and Hall; 1991.
2. American Thoracic Society. Standardization of spirometry: 1987 update. Am Rev Respir Dis 1987;136:1285-98.
3. Azagra JS, Goergen M, Gilbert E, Jacobs D, Lejeune P, Carlier E. Anterior resection: The total laparoscopic approach. In: Monson JRT, Darzi A, eds. Laparoscopic Colorectal Surgery. Oxford, England: Isis Medical Media; 1995:38-55.
4. Bartlett RH, Brennan ML, Gazzaniga AL, Hanson EL. Studies on the pathogenesis and prevention of postoperative pulmonary complications. Surg Gynecol Obstet. 1973;137:925-33.
5. Beecher HK. The measured effect of laparotomy on the respiration. J Clin Invest 1933;12:639-50.
6. Benhamou D, Simonneau G, Poynard T, Goldman M, Chaput JC, Duroux P. Diaphragm function is not impaired by pneumoperitoneum after laparoscopy. Arch Surg 1993;128:430-32.
7. Berstein MA, Dawson JW, Reissman P, Weiss EG, Nogueras JJ, Wexner SD. Is complete laparoscopic colectomy superior to laparoscopic assisted colectomy? Am Surg 1996;62:507-11.
8. Bo¨hm B, Nouchirvani K, Hucke HP, Stock W. Morbidity and mortality after elective resections of colorectal cancers [in German]. Langenbecks Arch Chir 1991;376:93-101.
9. Bonnet F, Blery C, Zatan M, Simonet O, Brage D, Gaudy J. Effect of epidural morphine on post-operative pulmonary dysfunction. Acta Anaesthesiol Scand 1984;28:147-51.
10. Chen HH, Wexner SD, Weiss EG, et al. Laparoscopic colectomy for benign colorectal disease is associated with a significant reduction in disability as compared with laparotomy. Surg Endosc 1998;12:1397-1400.
11. Christensen EF, Schultz P, Jensen OV. Postoperative pulmonary complications and lung function in high-risk patients: a comparison of three physiotherapy regimens after upper abdominal surgery in general anesthesia. Acta Anaesthesiol Scand 1991;35:97-104.
12. Craig DB. Postoperative recovery of pulmonary function. Anesth Analg 1981;60:46-52.
13. Dean PA, Beart RW, Nelson H, Elftmann TD, Schlinkert RT. Laparoscopicassisted segmental colectomy: early Mayo Clinic experience. Mayo Clin Proc 1994;69:834-40.

14. Duepree HJ, Senagore AJ, Delaney CP, Brady KM, Fazio VW. Advantages of laparoscopic resection for ileocecal Crohn's disease. Dis Colon Rectum. 2002;45:605-10.

15. Dureuil B, Cantineau JP, Desmonts JM. Effects of upper or lower abdominal surgery on diaphragmatic function. Br J Anaesthiol 1987;59:1230-5.

16. Dureuil B, Viires N, Cantineau JP, Aubier M, Desmonts JM. Diaphragmatic contractility after upper abdominal surgery. J Appl Physiol 1986;61:1775-80.

17. Erice F, Fox GS, Salib YM, Romano E, Meakins JL, Magder SA. Diaphragmatic function before and after laparoscopic cholecystectomy. Anesthesiology 1993; 79:966-75.

18. Ford GT, Whitelaw WA, Rosenal TW, Cruse PJ, Guenter CA. Diaphragm function after upper abdominal surgery in humans. Am Rev Respir Dis 1983;127:431-6.

19. Franklin ME, Rosenthal D, Norem RF. Prospective evaluation of laparoscopic colon resection versus open colon resection for adenocarcinoma. Surg Endosc 1995;9:811-6.

20. Frazee RC, Roberts JW, Okeson GC, et al. Open versus laparoscopic cholecystectomy: a comparison of postoperative pulmonary function. Ann Surg 1991; 213:651-4.

21. Gunnarsson L, Tokics L, Gustavsson H, Hedenstierna G. Influence of age on atelectasis formation and gas exchange impairment during general anaesthesia. Br J Anaesth 1991;66:423-32.

22. Hansen G, Drablos PA, Steinert R. Pulmonary complications, ventilation and blood gases after upper abdominal surgery. Acta Anaesthesiol Scand 1977;21:211-5.

23. Hansen O, Schwenk W, Hucke HP, Stock W. Colorectal stapled anastomoses: experiences and results. Dis Colon Rectum 1996;39:30-6.

24. Hedenstierna G. Mechanisms of postoperative pulmonary dysfunction. Acta Chir Scand Suppl 1989;550:152-8.

25. Hendolin H, Lahtinen J, Lansimies E, Tuppurainen T, Partanen K. The effect of thoracic epidural analgesia on respiratory function after cholecystectomy. Acta Anaesthesiol Scand 1987;31:645-51.

26. Kanellos I, Zarogilidis K, Ziogas E, Dadoukis I. Prospektiv-vergleichende Studie der Lungenfunktion nach laparoskopischer, Mini-Lap oder konventioneller Cholezystektomie. Minim Invasive Chir 1995;4:169-71.

27. Kum CK, Eypasch E, Aljaziri A, Troidl H. Randomized comparison of pulmonary function after the "French" and "American" techniques of laparoscopic cholecystectomy. Br J Surg 1996;83:938-41.

28. Latimer RG, Dickmann M, Day EC. Ventilatory pattern and pulmonary complications after upper abdominal surgery determined by preoperative and postoperative computerized spirometry and blood gas analysis. Am J Surg 1971;122:622-32.

29. Lindberg P, Gunnarsson L, Tokics L, et al. Atelectasis and lung function in the postoperative period. Acta Anaesthesiol Scand 1992;36:546-53.

30. Ludwig KA, Milson JW, Church JM, Fazio VW. Preliminary experience with laparoscopic intestinal surgery for Crohn's disease. Am J Surg 1996;171:52-6.

31. Marshall BE, Wyche MQ Jr. Hypoxemia during and after anesthesia. Anesthesiology. 1972;37:178-209.

32. McMahon AJ, Baxter JN, Kenney G, O'Dwyer PJ. Ventilatory and blood gas changes during laparoscopic and open cholecystectomy. Br J Surg 1993;80:1252-4.

33. Milsom JW, Bo¨hm B. Laparoscopic Colorectal Surgery. New York, NY: Springer-Verlag NY Inc; 1996.

34. Milsom JW, Hammerhofer KA, Bohm B, Marcello P, Elson P, Fazio VW. Prospective, randomized trial comparing laparoscopic vs conventional surgery for refractory ileocolic Crohn's disease. Dis Colon Rectum 2001;44:1-9.

35. Milson JW, Lavery IC, Bohm B, Fazio VW. Laparoscopically assisted ileocolectomy in Crohn's disease. Surg Laparosc Endosc 1993;3:77-80.

36. Msika S, Iannelli A, Deroide G, et al. Can laparoscopy reduce hospital stay in the treatment of Crohn's disease? Dis Colon Rectum 2001;44:326-31.

37. Peters WR. Laparoscopic total proctocolectomy with creation of ileostomy for ulcerative colitis: report of two cases. J Laparoendosc Surg 1992;2:175-81.

38. Rademaker BM, Ringers J, Odoom JA, de Wit LT, Kalkman CJ, Oosting J. Pulmonary function and stress response after laparoscopic cholecystectomy: comparison with subcostal incision and influence of thoracic epidural analgesia. Anesth Analg 1992;75:381-5.

39. Rinnert-Gongora S, Tartter PI. Multivariate analysis of recurrence after anterior resection for colorectal carcinoma. Am J Surg 1989;157:573-6.

40. Sardinha TC, Wexner SD. Laparoscopy for inflammatory bowel disease: pros and cons. World J Surg 1998;22:370-4.

41. Schauer PR, Luna J, Ghiatas AA, Glen ME, Warren JM, Sirinek KR. Pulmonary function after laparoscopic cholecystectomy. Surgery 1993;114:389-99.

42. Schoetz DJ, Bockler M, Rosenblatt MS, et al. "Ideal" length of stay after colectomy: whose ideal? Dis Colon Rectum 1997;40:806-10.

43. Senagore AJ, Luchtefeld MA, Mackeigan JM, Mazier PW. Open colectomy versus laparoscopic colectomy: Are there differences? Am Surg 1993;59:549-53.

44. Senagore AJ, Lutchfeled MA, Mackeigan JM, Maizer WP. Open colectomy versus laparoscopic colectomy: Are there differences? Am Surg 1993;59:549-53.

45. Simonneau G, Vivien A, Sartene R, et al. Diaphragm dysfunction induced by upper abdominal surgery: role of postoperative pain. Am Rev Respir Dis 1983;128:899-903.

46. Sprung J, Cheng EY, Nimphius N, Hubmayr RD, Rodarte JR, Kampine JP. Diaphragm dysfunction and respiratory insufficiency after upper abdominal surgery. Plucne Bolesti 1991;43:5-12.

47. Stage JG, Schulze S, Moller P, et al. Prospective randomized study of laparoscopic versus open colonic resection for adenocarcinoma. Br J Surg 1997;84:391-6.

48. Stocchi L, Nelson H, Young-Fadok TM, Larson DR, Ilstrup DM. Safety and advantages of laparoscopic vs open colectomy in the elderly. Dis Colon Rectum 2000;43:326-32.

Section Three

49. Tabet J, Hong D, Kim CW, Wong J, Goodrace R, Anvari M. Laparoscopic versus open bowel resection for Crohn's disease. Can J Gastroenterol 2001;15:237-42.

50. Union Internationale Contre le Cancer. TNM Classification of Malignant Tumours. Berlin, Germany: Springer Publishing Co; 1987.

51. Wahba RWM. Perioperative functional residual capacity. Can J Anaesth 1991; 38:384-400.

52. Williams CD, Brenowitz JB. Ventilatory patterns after vertical and tranverse upper abdominal incisions. Am J Surg 1975;130:725-28.

53. Wu JS, Birbaum EH, Kodner IJ, Read TE, Fleshman JW. Laparoscopic-assisted ileocolic resections in patients with Crohn's disease: are abscess, phlegmons, or recurrent disease contraindications? Surgery 1997;122:682-9.

25

Laparoscopic Colorectal Surgery

INTRODUCTION

Laparoscopic colon resections are being performed with increasing frequency all over world, though the use of minimal access surgery in colorectal surgery has lagged behind its application in other surgical fields. Since the first laparoscopic colectomy was described in 1991, a great deal of controversy has surrounded its use, particularly in the management of colorectal cancer. After the successful introduction of laparoscopic colectomy by Jacobs, laparoscopic surgery for the treatment of colorectal cancer, especially laparoscopic rectal surgery, has been developed considerably. Several important new studies have demonstrated the benefits and safety of laparoscopic colorectal surgery, making it now the preferred approach in the surgical management of many colorectal diseases.

The technique of laparoscopic colectomy has a long learning curve because of the advanced laparoscopic skills it entails. Unlike other laparoscopic procedures, such as the Nissen fundoplication or cholecystectomy, colorectal procedures involve dissection and mobilization of intra-abdominal organs in multiple quadrants. *Tilting of the operating-room table in various positions during an operation uses gravity to allow intra-abdominal organs to fall away from the area of dissection*, providing necessary exposure that would normally be achieved through the use of retractors. Intestinal resection requires laparoscopic ligation of large vessels, mobilization and removal of a long floppy segment of colon, and restoration of intestinal continuity. Once the colon segment has been completely mobilized and its blood supply divided, a small skin incision is made to exteriorize the colon, a resection and anastomosis are performed extra-corporeally, and the rejoined colon is placed back into the abdomen.

The laparoscopic approach continues to gain popularity and has evolved to include not just "pure" laparoscopic techniques but also hand-assist devices. Hand-assisted surgery can be used as a bridge for surgeons who are not completely familiar or facile with laparoscopic techniques, and even for the most experienced laparoscopic surgeons, it is often the preferred technique for surgery involving left-sided pathology (Fig. 25.1). Use of a hand-assist device provides tactile feedback for the surgeon, and shortens operating-room time while still preserving many of the advantages of laparoscopic surgery. By combining laparoscopic surgery with the tactile feedback of a hand-assisted device, surgeons can reduce operating-room time and have a lower procedure conversion rate. The technique involves making an incision the width of a hand and placing a hand-assist device to facilitate laparoscopic dissection. New hand port devices make this technique possible without loss of pneumoperitoneum, which is essential for performing laparoscopic procedures. Because an incision (4-5 cm) is necessary to remove the colon specimen at the end of a laparoscopic operation, the difference between a pure laparoscopic procedure and a hand-assisted operation is generally a few additional centimeters (3-4 cm) of incision length. Several clinical trials have demonstrated that there is no difference in patient recovery or discharge for laparoscopic versus

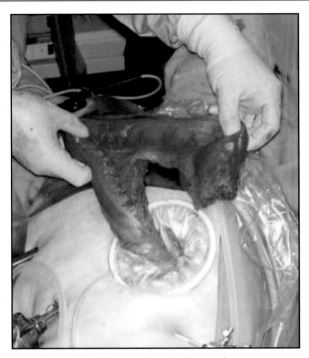

Fig. 25.1: Hand assisted colorectal surgery

hand-assisted techniques. Larger incisions are often needed and because of the increased risk of wound infections and pulmonary complications, this technique has particular advantages with overweight or obese patients.

Most patients are candidates for a laparoscopic approach. When the surgeon is experienced, even patients with a history of abdominal surgery are candidates. Though there are clear benefits, they have not been as compelling when compared to the clear advantages associated with other laparoscopic procedures. The main reason is that a colectomy, whether open or laparoscopic, results in a delayed return of bowel function. Though recovery of bowel function is quicker after laparoscopic surgery, the difference is on the order of one or two days, resulting in a similar reduction in length of hospital stay. Also, the laparoscopic approach is associated with longer operating-room times. Even if long-term benefits are equivalent between open and laparoscopic techniques, the short-term benefits are real advantages for patients. In practical terms, the laparoscopic approach is associated with less pain, a faster recovery, earlier return of bowel function, a shorter hospital stay, possible immune benefits, and smaller scars, making it the preferred method for intestinal resection.

The lack of tactile feedback during laparoscopic surgery can make tumor localization difficult, especially if the lesion location has not been tattooed on the colon wall before surgery. It is imperative that the exact location of the tumor is known prior to proceeding with colectomy. Even when the lesion location has been tattooed onto the colon, often the mark can be difficult to see, or there may be confusion regarding the location of the tattoo in relation to the tumor (proximal or distal), which can affect surgical margins. Intraoperative colonoscopy is a way of definitively localizing a lesion and should be available during all laparoscopic colectomies. Traditional colonoscopy uses room air as the insufflating gas, which leads to significant bowel distension and requires clamping of the proximal colon to minimize this effect. Clamping the bowel can lead to injury, and even when it is successfully performed, the degree of distension often makes simultaneous laparoscopic visualization difficult. These problems can be circumvented with the use of CO_2, rather than room air, as the insufflating gas. Because CO_2 is absorbed much more rapidly than room air, bowel distension is minimized and dissipates quickly, making proximal clamping unnecessary. Use of CO_2 allows for laparoscopic and endoscopic procedures to be performed simultaneously, and this technique has been shown to be safe and clinically useful. Besides tumor localization, CO_2 colonoscopy may have other potential applications.

Port Site Metastasis

In the early experience of laparoscopic colectomy for cancer, a few reports described immediate tumor recurrence at the laparoscopic incision sites, referred to as port site recurrences (Fig. 25.2). It was hypothesized such early cancer recurrence happened after laparoscopy due to tumor shedding and/or accelerated tumor growth, secondary to the presence of gas in the peritoneal cavity. However, multiple reviews have indicated that this is not the case. In one such study, which included over 2600 cases, the rate of port site recurrence was approximately 1 percent, which is similar to that noted in open colorectal surgery. It is not currently believed that laparoscopic colectomy is associated with early wound recurrences.

Section Three

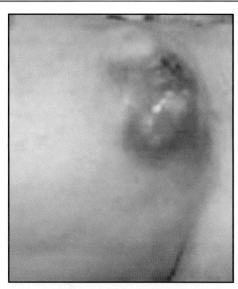

Fig. 25.2: Port side metastasis after laparoscopic surgery

Port site implantation was a concern in early period but it has been shown now that it can be prevented by:
1. Proper protection of port site while delivering the specimen. (Endobags ® and pouches).
2. Avoid squeezing of the specimen by taking a liberal incision.
3. Thorough wash to the wound, 5FU solution irrigation of all ports.
4. Slow release of pneumo-peritoneum.
5. Lap-lift technique

Cost can be brought down by either doing a hand sewn anastomosis through the specimen delivery site or use of conventional stapler for extra-corporeal stapled anastomosis. Minimal use of disposable ports and instruments can further cut down the cost. Use of ultrasonic energy source in form of harmonic shears (Ethicon ® and USSC ®) has added to the cost of lap surgery.

The two burning issues are port site metastasis in malignancies and cost factor due to use of endostaplers. As mentioned earlier for benign condition like rectal prolapse, adenomas, rectal polyposis and inflammatory condition like tuberculosis, ulcerative colitis, simple diverticulitis, and laparoscopic surgery offers a patient friendly technique. Crohn's though not very common in India, but laparoscopy can be offered for diagnosis, lymph node sampling and curative resection. Ileocecal tuberculosis is commonly seen in our country and it is a good option to offer the benefits of laparoscopy to these patients whenever surgery is

indicated. Incidental colonic resection is unlikely to help the laparoscopic surgeon team in mastering the techniques. Reduction of OT time due to better coordination and cost benefit to patients can only be offered by repetitive performances. A dedicated team effort will surely bring this speciality under the umbrella of minimal access surgery as has happened in western world.

Bowel Preparation in Colorectal Surgery

Though widely accepted as sensible and logical it has never been subjected to any really stringent scrutiny. The ideal method of mechanical preparation should be simple, inexpensive, without distress and side effects to the patient. However, such an ideal method does not exist. It must be chosen with respect to patient acceptability, efficiency and influence on fluid and electrolyte imbalance and on faecal micro flora. The conventional method involves a 3 day regimen consisting of low residue and clear liquid diet combined with purgation using laxatives and enemas. Although satisfactory in bowel cleansing in about 70 percent of patient, it is rather exhausting due to reduced calorie intake. It is time consuming and may result in dehydration if the patient drinks inadequate amount of fluids. These disadvantages stimulated the development of more reliable, efficient and quicker methods which includes:

Elemental Diets

Low residue liquid or elemental diets were used with the intention that nutrients could be absorbed in the small intestine. Although, these result in a low fecal bulk, satisfactory cleansing is obtained in only 17 percent of the patients. Nausea and vomiting can occur and evidence does not favor elemental diets as a sole means of bowel preparation.

Whole Gut Irrigation

Saline: Normal saline is instilled through a nasogastric tube at a constant rate of 50 to 70 ml per minute in 4 hours requiring a total of 10 to 14 liters of fluid. Cleansing effect is achieved in 90 percent of the patients however the concentration of colonic bacteria is not reduced unless antibiotics are added. Many patients complain of abdominal distension, nausea and vomiting. Other drawbacks of this method include the large volume of irrigant, need of nasogastric tube, risk of electrolyte disturbance and water retention and nursing care required to assist the patient. It is contradicted in patients with gastrointestinal obstruction, perforation, toxic colitis and has to be used with caution in patient with cardiac problems.

Castor Oil: (30-60 ml) orally achieves good cleansing but requires large volume of magnesium citrate purgative to achieve the desired results and requires to be given to days before surgery followed by anal washouts a day prior which entails preoperative admissions for 3 to 4 days. Unpalatibilty is another drawback.

Mannitol: Mannitol is a nonabsorbable oligosaccharide which acts as an osmotic agent by pulling fluid into the bowel and producing a purgative effect by irritating the colon. Being a sugar it is quite palatable and can be flavored by mixing with fruit juice. Usually 4 liters of 5 percent solution are consumed over 4 hours which can be difficult and can result in abdominal discomfort and nausea. To avoid these side effects, hypertonic solutions (10 to 20%) can be used but these predispose to dehydration and electrolyte losses. Overall, good cleansing is produced in about 80 percent of the patients a high wound infection rate probably by acting as a bacterial nutrient and production of explosive gases as a result of fermentation into methane and hydrogen by anaerobic bacteria is seen. The same can be overcome by using of an antibiotic.

Polyethylene Glycol: To overcome the drawbacks of mannitol, polyethylene glycol (PEGLAC) in a balanced electrolyte solution was introduced which also acts as an osmotic purgative (Fig. 25.3).

To achieve satisfactory cleansing in more than 90 percent of the patients, an average of 2 to 4 liter of PEGLAC solution must be ingested with tea and lemon. Studies using PEG have shown significantly lower incidence of fluid retention and lesser aerobic and anaerobic faecal bacterial counts compared to other agents. It is nowadays used as an agent of choice for preparations of the bowel before endoscopy and colonic surgery in a non obstructed patient.

Picolax: It (sodium picosulphate and magnesium citrate) is a stimulant purgative that acts mainly on the left colon after activation by colonic bacteria and on osmotic laxative that cleanses the proximal colon. Two sachets in 2 liters of water are administered with dietary restriction to improve effectiveness. Although acceptable cleansing is achieved in 85 percent of patients undergoing barium enema and colonoscopy, its efficacy for elective colorectal operations is poorly documented. Picolax is well tolerated but does produce fluid and electrolyte losses.

Antibiotic Bowel Preparations

Mechanical cleansing alone has failed to achieve a significant reduction in the total bacterial load of the colon and therefore the associated septic complications. Addition of antibiotics oral as well as parenteral to mechanical cleaning has resulted in significant reduction of the infection rate from 30 to 60 percent in an uncovered patient to 2-10 percent in otherwise patients covered with wide spectrum antibiotics.

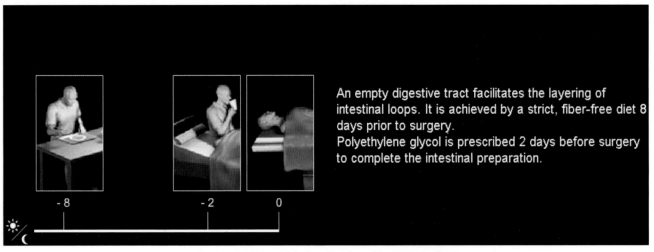

An empty digestive tract facilitates the layering of intestinal loops. It is achieved by a strict, fiber-free diet 8 days prior to surgery.
Polyethylene glycol is prescribed 2 days before surgery to complete the intestinal preparation.

Fig. 25.3: Bowel preparation in colorectal surgery

Oral Antibiotics

Because the aerobic Escherichia coli and the anaerobic bacteroides fragilis are frequently involved organisms in septic complications following colorectal operations, oral antibiotics active against both types of bacteria must be given. Oral administration of erythromycin, neomycin and metronidazole are popular. Several studies have documented the efficacy of oral antibiotics however antimicrobial used alone without mechanical cleansing has little impact on the postoperative infection rate.

Parenteral Antibiotics

Since parenteral antibiotics are effective only when adequate tissue levels are present at the time of contamination, systemic administration should start immediately before the surgery. A second or third generation cephalosporin with metronidazole is the most commonly preferred agents. Studies have shown conflicting results when parenteral antibiotics were compared with oral or both. Whether antibiotics bowel preparation should be oral, systemic or both are still a controversial issue. Majority of the surgeons would prefer parenteral antibiotics or with concomitant administration of oral antimicrobials together with oral PEGLAC electrolyte solution as the method of choice of preoperative bowel preparation.

Though observational data suggest that mechanical bowel preparation before colorectal surgery reduces fecal mass and bacterial count in the lumen, but the practice has been questioned because the bowel preparation liquefies feces, which could increase the risk for intraoperative spillage, and may be associated with bacterial translocation and electrolyte disturbance. Though commonly practiced without the benefit of evidence from randomized trials, and 2 of 3 meta-analyses suggest a higher rate of anastomotic leakage with mechanical bowel preparation thus calling for an end to the practice of mechanical bowel preparation in view of the possible disadvantages of this practice, patient discomfort, and the absence of clinical value. There are others who accept that though routine preoperative bowel cleansing is no longer justified prior to colorectal surgery in general, they call for further evaluation in cases such as total mesorectal resection with low anastomosis where it may still have a role and therefore to consider each case carefully, otherwise the chance of making an inappropriate decision exists with great consequences for patients.

Majority of surgeons believe that patients should have a standard bowel preparation 48 hours before the operation and should receive a single-dose antibiotic dose immediately preoperatively. For the bowel preparation, patients follow a strictly fibre-free diet 8 days before surgery, and take a sodium phosphate oral solution the day before surgery. This method is very effective because it ensures an empty digestive tract and a flat small bowel, which facilitates the layering of intestinal loops, a crucial point for achieving adequate exposure. Alternatively, polyethylene glycol can be used. In this case, administration 2 days before surgery is preferable to avoid distension of small bowel loops that may be difficult to handle during the surgery.

Right Colectomy

A right colectomy, or ileocolic resection is the removal of all or part of the right colon and part of the ileum (Fig. 25.4). These operations are performed for removal of cancers, certain non-cancerous growths as well as severe Crohn's disease. If performed by expert laparoscopic surgeon, laparoscopic right colectomy and ileocolic resection are as safe as "open" surgery in carefully selected cases.

Indications

The advanced laparoscopic skills required for laparoscopic resection of the colon and rectum has

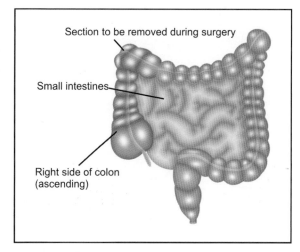

Fig. 25.4: Section to be removed in right colectomy

precluded wide dissemination of this procedure. By applying certain key principles, laparoscopic right hemicolectomy can be made simple, reproducible, easy to teach, easy to learn, and cost-effective. Although benign tumors not resectable by a colonoscopic procedure and stricturing inflammatory bowel disease may be good indications for laparoscopy, they are not so common. The most common disease for right colectomy is right-sided colon cancer. Colon cancer seems to be a good indication for laparoscopic surgery if performed using proper oncologic methods, i.e. early proximal ligation of the major mesenteric vessels and wide mesenteric and intestinal resection with complete lymphadenectomy. For right colectomy, laparoscopic mobilization of the bowel, mesenteric resection, or both is performed as for open colectomy, and bowel division and creation of the anastomosis are performed extracorporeally.

Contraindications

1. Patients with complete obstruction caused by the cancer
2. Cancer extensively invading adjacent organs
3. Bulky cancer larger than 10 cm in size should be excluded.

According to these concepts, a proper oncologic approach using laparoscopy for right colon cancer is described in this chapter.

Equipment and Instruments

One can use the same basic equipment, such as light source, insufflator, 30-degree angled laparoscope, and 5-mm graspers. To this basic equipment can be added reusable instruments such as Babcock and alligator clamps, which should be at least 38 to 40 cm in length to reach from the depths of the pelvis to the upper abdomen using limited port sites. In developing country these reusables can be used keeping disposable equipment to a minimum. Three 10-mm or 12-mm trocars with stability threads, plus reducers for 5-mm instruments should be used. Cannulas should allow instruments to move through smoothly while maintaining a good seal after multiple instrument passages. An energy source device of one's choice can also be added either bipolar, ligasure or harmonic scalpel can be used. Additional disposable equipment is kept readily available in the operating room and opened only as needed. These include a clip applier, linear vascular stapler, suction irrigator, and fan retractor.

Patient Positioning and Operating Room Setup

The patient is placed supine, and straps are used to secure the patient during steep table position changes. The patient is fixed in a moldable "bean bag" form with both arms tucked in, and placed in a modified lithotomy position using levitator stirrups (Figs 25.5 and 25.6). A urinary catheter is placed in the bladder, and the stomach is decompressed with a nasogastric tube. Identical operating room personnel are used for the laparoscopic case as for an open right hemicolectomy.

The nurse is on the patient's right. This is also where the assistant starts, with the surgeon on the patient's left side facing the right colon. Hasson (open) technique is preferred to safely insert the first port

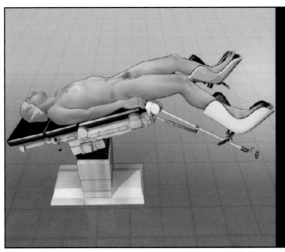

It is essential that the patient be appropriately positioned to avoid complications (nerve and vein compression, injuries to the brachial plexus) and to facilitate the procedure and anesthetic monitoring.
- Trendelenburg position with a 15° to 25° tilt and a 5° to 10° right tilt;
- lithotomy position;
- buttocks placed at the distal edge of the table;
- thighs and legs stretched apart with a slight flexure;
- right arm alongside the body;
- left arm at a right angle or alongside the body (surgeon's preference);
- gastric tube and urinary catheter;
- heating device.

Fig. 25.5: Position of patient for colorectal surgery

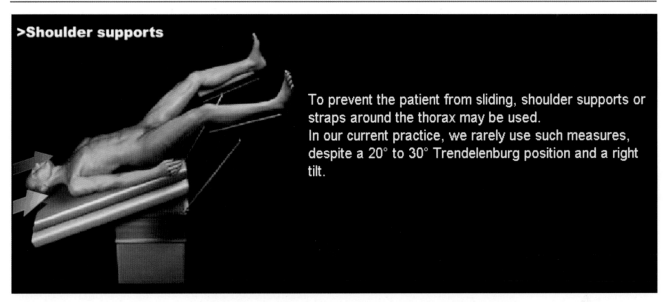

>Shoulder supports

To prevent the patient from sliding, shoulder supports or straps around the thorax may be used.
In our current practice, we rarely use such measures, despite a 20° to 30° Trendelenburg position and a right tilt.

Fig. 25.6: Shoulder support to prevent sliding during colorectal surgery

through the umbilicus. After establishing pneumo-peritoneum, the surgeon stands on the patient's left side to expose the right mesocolon and to mark the lower border of the ileocolic vessels.

After initial exploration ensures no prohibitive adhesions, two additional 10 to 12 mm ports are placed under direct visualization, one in the left upper quadrant (in or lateral to the rectus, avoiding the epigastric vessels, approximately a handbreadth from the supraumbilical port) and one in the suprapubic midline. Once all the trocars are in place, the assistant moves to the patient's left side to direct the camera.

To start the initial dissection the surgeon moves between the patient's legs, the assistants position themselves on the patient's left side and the nurse stands near the patient's right knee. The main monitor is placed near the patient's right shoulder to give the surgeon and the assistant's optimal viewing (Fig. 25.7).

The second monitor is placed on the left side close to the head, a location that gives the best view for the nurse. After completing the proximal vessel ligation with lymphadenectomy and mobilization of the terminal ileum and the cecum, the surgeon moves back to the patient's left side and the first assistant stands between the patient's legs for take-down of right flexure and whole mobilization of the right colon (Fig. 25.8).

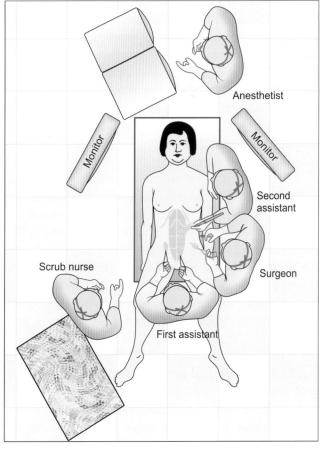

Fig. 25.7: Position of surgical team during colorectal surgery

Section Three

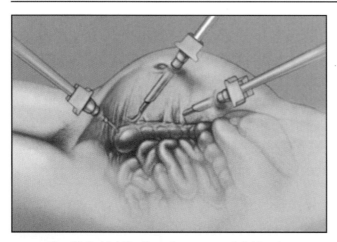

Fig. 25.8: Mobilization of cecum and right colon

Operative Technique

Right colectomy can be broadly divided in following steps:

1. Ligation of ileocolic vessels
2. Identification of right ureter
3. Dissection along superior mesenteric vein
4. Division of omentum
5. Division of right branch of middle colic vessels
6. Transection of transverse colon
7. Mobilization of right colon
8. Transection of terminal ileum
9. Ileocolic anastomosis
10. Delivery of specimen

The patient is positioned in Trendelenburg with the right side inclined upward. This allows the small bowel and omentum to fall toward the left upper quadrant, exposing the cecum and assisting in retraction. The omentum and transverse colon are moved toward the upper abdomen, the ventral side of the right mesocolon is well visualized, and the optimal operative field can be achieved. The small bowel is mobilized out of the pelvis by grasping the peritoneum, not bowel wall, near the base of the cecum and pulling cephalad and to the left. The appropriate plane along the base of the small bowel mesentery and around the cecum can be seen and the peritoneum overlying it carefully opened, exposing the correct retroperitoneal plane.

The ureter is identified either before opening the peritoneum in a thin patient or after, being visualized as it courses over the right iliac vessels. Dissection is then continued around the base of the cecum. Moving cephalad and laterally, the white line of Toldt is incised as the right colon is retracted medially and cephalad by grasping the cut edge of peritoneum, not the bowel.

Before starting the dissection, the ileocolic pedicle must be definitively identified by retracting the right mesocolon. Various approaches, such as lateral-to-medial (lateral approach), medial-to-lateral (medial approach), and retroperitoneal approach can be tried. The medial approach is quite effective for complete lymphadenectomy with early proximal ligation, minimal manipulation of the tumor-bearing segment, and ideal entry to proper retroperitoneal plane.

Various approaches to the right colon mobilization have been described.
A: Lateral to medial ("classic" open approach);
B: Medial to lateral approach);
C: Retroperitoneal approach.

It is believed that the medial approach is optimal in order to maintain conventional oncologic principles. First, the mesocolon near the ileocecal junction is lifted to confirm the ileocolic pedicle. The root of ileocolic pedicle is usually located at the lower border of duodenum. The independent right colic vessels, if present, are located at the upper border at duodenum. However, the majority of patients do not have the independent right colic vessels (vessels originating directly from the superior mesenteric artery and vein (Figs 25.9A and B). The surgeon should initially stand on the patient's left side to confidently know the ileocolic pedicle from the superior mesenteric vessels, and to mark the lower border of ileocolic pedicle.

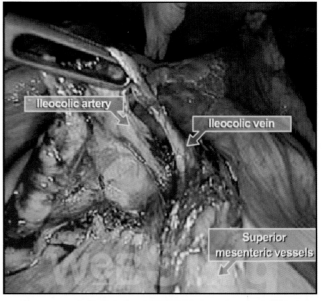

Fig. 25.9A: Position of major blood vessels at the time of surgery

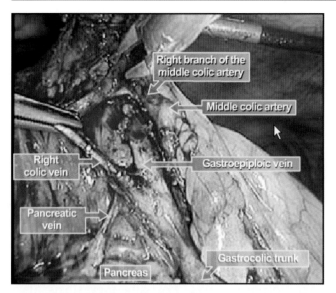

Fig. 25.9B: Important vessels supplying right side of colon

Once the iliocolic pedicle is identified, the surgeon moves between the patient's legs and the scope is inserted through the suprapubic port. The medial side of the right mesocolon is first incised starting from the previously marked region below the ileocolic pedicle, followed by the incision of the peritoneum over to the superior mesenteric vessels. This is done before mobilization of the right colon. With adequate traction of mesocolon toward the right upper quadrant, the ileocolic vessels are easily mobilized from the subperitoneal fascia leading onto the duodenum. Their origins are identified from the superior mesenteric vessels at the lower border of the duodenum and divided.

The surgeon's first step in the dissection is to mark the inferior border of the ileocolic pedicle. From between the legs, the surgeon dissects the peritoneum overlying the ileocolic vascular pedicle over to the superior mesenteric vessels.

After mobilization of the ileocolic pedicle from the duodenum, the dissection of the ventral side of the superior mesenteric vein leads to the dissection of the origin of ileocolic artery. In type B, the ileocolic artery is running behind the superior mesenteric vein. After mobilization and division of the ileocolic pedicle from the duodenum, the dissection of the ventral side of the superior mesenteric vein leads to a complete dissection of the root of the middle colic artery and vein.

Careful dissection onto the duodenum and the caudad portion of the pancreas must be exercised in the exposure of the middle colic vessels. Dissection around Henle's trunk (the truck of mesenteric veins consisting of the gastroepiploic vein fusing with the right branch of the middle colic vein or the main middle colic vein) may lead to the exposure of an accessory right colic vein. Accessory right colic vein and right branches of middle colic vessels are clipped and divided. However, if an accessory right colic vein is difficult to confirm in this situation, this vein may be easily detected later at the take-down of right flexure.

After securing the vessels, the operating table is tilted into the steep Trendelenburg position with the right side down to move the small intestine toward the right upper quadrant. After confirming the right ureter and gonadal vessels through the subperitoneal fascia at the right pelvic brim, the peritoneum is incised along the base of the ileal mesentery upward to the duodenum, and the ileocecal region is mobilized medial to lateral. After this mobilization, the surgeon moves back to the patient's left side and the scope is inserted through the umbilical port. The right mesocolon is mobilized from medial to lateral. Again, this approach allows dissection into the proper retroperitoneal plane. The right gonadal vessels and ureter are safe from injury in this plane, so exposing them is not necessary. This approach also allows the surgeon to work in a straight path from medial to lateral, without tissue to obstruct the vision that can occur working from lateral to medial. This plane connects the previous dissection plane from the caudad side.

The anatomy around the right flexure is very important to avoid inadvertent bleeding especially from around Henle's (gastrocolic) trunk. However, if the previous mesenteric dissection is fully performed from the caudad side and the accessory right colic vein is divided, the right flexure is easily taken down only by dividing the hepatocolic ligament. If the accessory right colic vein is difficult to detect at the previous dissection, it can be easily confirmed from Henle's trunk at this situation and should be divided before extracting the right colon to avoid its injury. Up to this point, the primary tumor has been minimally manipulated using medial to lateral approach. Finally, the right flexure and right colon including the tumor bearing segment are detached laterally, which completes the mobilization of the entire right colon (Fig. 25.10).

Section Three

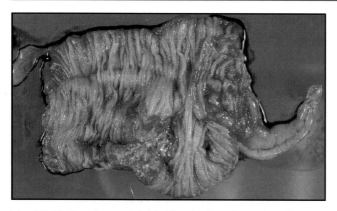

Fig. 25.10: Specimen of right side of colon after right colectomy

Once the entire right colon is freed, it is withdrawn through an enlargement of port site at the umbilicus. The wound must be covered with wound protector to prevent contamination or metastasis. The resection of ileum and transverse colon, and the anastomosis are accomplished extracorporeally by functional end to end anastomotic method using conventional staplers or by a hand-sewn method (Fig. 25.11). The anastomotic site is returned to the peritoneal cavity. Wounds and peritoneal cavity are copiously irrigated. All wounds are closed and operation is completed.

The identification of a small tumor in the colon may be difficult even in conventional open surgery. In laparoscopic surgery, where there is no tactile sensation, pre- or intraoperative marking of the tumor is frequently needed. Various kinds of marking methods, e.g. dye injection and mucosal clip placement by preoperative colonoscopy, have been reported for

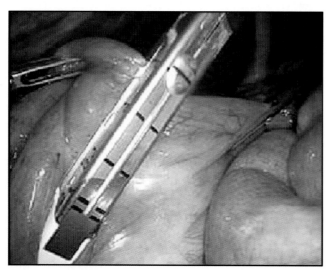

Fig. 25.11: Transaction of ileum by stapler

the tumor localization. Several reports demonstrated the usefulness of tattooing the colonic wall adjacent to the tumor with India ink in four quadrants using preoperative colonoscopy. However, effective injection in all four points of the bowel is sometimes difficult to achieve. In some cases, surgeon failed to achieve serosal staining visible at laparoscopy, which forced them to use intraoperative colonoscopy. This complicated the laparoscopic colon resection because of the distended bowel related to air insufflation during colonoscopy.

Conclusion

Right-sided colon cancer can be adequately treated by proper laparoscopic procedures adherent to the oncologic principles. Port-site metastasis after laparoscopic colon cancer surgery is unlikely to be a major risk factor when the procedure is performed according to oncologic principles. It is believed that laparoscopic right colectomy for cancer performed by expert surgeons is accepted as less invasive surgery without sacrificing the survival benefit compared with conventional open right colectomy.

SIGMOIDECTOMY

Laparoscopic sigmoid colon resection is indicated for both benign (diverticulitis, segmental Crohn's disease, polyp unresectable by colonoscopy) and malignant (primary colon cancer) etiologies, and is one of the most common operations done by laparoscopic methods. In chronic diverticular disease, the indications for laparoscopic sigmoid resection are the same as for open surgery. Sigmoid colectomy for diverticulitis can be technically challenging because of severe inflammation in the left-lower quadrant and pelvis.

Patient Positioning and Operating Room Setup

A proper patient position is key to both facilitating operative maneuvers and preventing complications such as nerve and vein compression, and traction injuries to the brachial plexus. The patient is placed supine, in the modified lithotomy position, with legs abducted and slightly flexed at the knees. The patient's right arm is alongside the body, whereas the left arm is usually placed at a 90° angle. Adequate padding is used to avoid compression on bone prominences.

A nasogastric or orogastric tube and a urinary catheter are placed. Adequate thromboembolism prophylaxis should be used, as preferred by the surgeon, and intermittent leg compression stockings can be used as well. The procedure is usually performed with two assistants and a scrub nurse (Fig. 25.12). The surgeon is on the right side of the patient and the second assistant is also on the right side. The first assistant stands between the patient's legs and the scrub nurse at the lower right side of the table. The team remains in the same position throughout the entire procedure. It is advisable to use a table that can be easily tilted laterally and placed into steep Trendelenburg and reverse Trendelenburg position, in order to facilitate exposure of the pelvic space and of the splenic flexure. The laparoscopic unit with the main monitor is located on the left side of the table. It is useful to use a second monitor placed above the patient's head.

Cannula Positioning

Standardize cannula placement are five or six cannulae for left-sided colectomies. This allows to achieve an excellent exposure which may be particularly valuable at the beginning of a surgeon's learning curve. Using six cannulae allows the use of more instruments in the abdominal cavity for retraction of bowel and structures especially in the presence of abundant intra-abdominal fat or of dilated small bowel, as well as during mobilization of the splenic flexure.

Cannula fixation to the abdominal wall is important, to avoid CO_2 leakage, and in cases of malignancy, to minimize the passage of tumor cells and help reduce the incidence of port-site metastases. This is mainly achieved by fitting the size of the incision to the cannula size or by fixing the cannula to the abdomen with a suture placed around the stopcock of the cannula. Use of screw-like cannulae, has drawback that it increases the parietal trauma. Generally it is better to perform an "open" technique for the insertion of the first cannula, which is placed at the midline, above the umbilicus, to reduce the risk of injury of abdominal organs. With some experience, the task becomes easy and very rapid. However, in the case of previous abdominal surgery, we usually inflate the abdominal cavity using the Veress needle in the left subcostal area, in order to insert the first cannula as far lateral as possible, in the right hypochondrium, to avoid potential areas of adhesions.

The first cannula (12 mm), which is used for the optical device, is positioned on the midline 3-4 cm above the umbilicus. The two operating cannulae are introduced, one at the junction between the umbilical line and the right midclavicular line, and the other 8-10 cm inferiorly, on the same line. The latter is a 12 mm operating cannula to allow the introduction of

Section Three

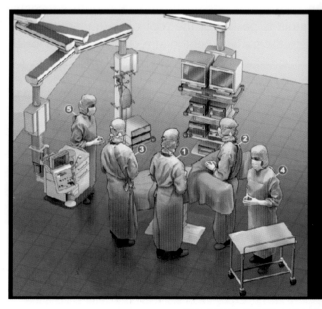

1. Surgeon
2. First assistant
3. Second assistant
4. Scrub nurse
5. Anesthesiologist
Although the procedure can be performed with a single assistant, it is preferable to have 2 assistants and a scrub nurse, especially when experience in performing the procedure is limited.
The team can remain in the same position throughout the entire procedure.

Fig. 25.12: Position of surgical team in colorectal surgery

a linear stapler at the time of bowel resection. This cannula accommodates the following: scissors (monopolar, high frequency hemostasis device, clip, staplers), a monopolar hook, surgical loops, a suction-irrigation device, and an atraumatic grasper. A fourth cannula is placed on the left midclavicular line, at the level of the umbilicus. This is a 5 mm cannula, which accommodates an atraumatic grasper used for retraction and exposure during the medial approach for the dissection of the left mesocolon. When performing mobilization of the splenic flexure, this cannula becomes an operating cannula. A fifth 5 mm cannula is placed 8-10 cm above the pubic bone, on the midline, and is used for retraction (Figs 25.13 and 25.14).

For most of the procedure, it accommodates a grasper used to expose the sigmoid and descending mesocolon. At the end of the procedure, the incision

at this cannula's site is lengthened to allow extraction of the specimen. Some surgeons sometimes use an additional cannula, which is a 5 mm cannula situated on the right midclavicular line in the subcostal area and accommodates an atraumatic grasper used to retract the terminal portion of the small intestine laterally at the beginning of the dissection, and to retract the transverse colon during the mobilization of the splenic flexure.

Operative Technique

Exposure

To complete exposure of the operative field, active positioning of the bowel is usually necessary in addition to the passive action of gravity, especially in the presence of obesity or bowel dilatation. The greater omentum and the transverse colon are placed in the left subphrenic region and maintained in this position by the Trendelenburg tilt. An atraumatic retractor, introduced through the cannula on the left side, may also be used. Subsequently, the proximal small bowel loops are placed in the right upper quadrant using gentle grasping (Fig. 25.15).

The distal small bowel loops are placed in the right lower quadrant with the cecum, and maintained there with gravity. If gravity is not sufficient, as occurs especially in the presence of abundant intraabdominal fat or dilated bowel, an additional maneuver is used. An instrument passed through the right subcostal cannula is passed at the root of the mesentery and grasps the parietal peritoneum of the right iliac fossa;

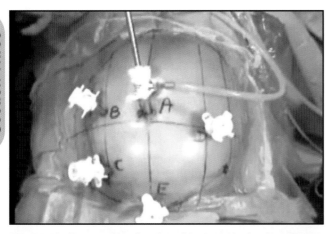

Fig. 25.13: Port position for sigmoidectomy for benign disease

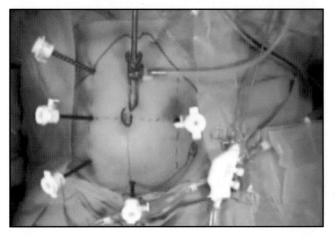

Fig. 25.14: Alternating post position for sigmoidectomy for malignant disease

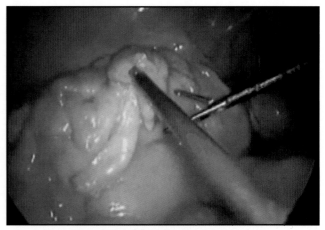

Fig. 25.15: Exposure of sigmoid colon after shifting the omentum upward

the shaft of the grasper thus provides an auto static retraction of the bowel loops, keeping them away from the midline and from the pelvic space. This technique of exposure provides an excellent view of the sacral promontory and of the aortoiliac axis. This particular view on the operative field is essential for the medial to lateral vascular approach.

The uterus may be an obstacle to adequate exposure in the pelvis. In postmenopausal women, the uterus can be suspended to the abdominal wall by a suture (Fig. 25.16). This suture is introduced halfway between the umbilicus and the pubis, and opens the rectovaginal space. In younger women, the uterus can be retracted using a similar suspension by a suture around the round ligaments or using a 5 mm retractor passed through the suprapubic cannula. Very often, conversion to open surgery is caused by difficulty in exposure, not only at the beginning, but also throughout the procedure.

To perform a medial approach, time is dedicated to the perfect achievement of this exposure, which will serve not only for the initial vascular approach, but also for about half of the remaining operative time. After adequate exposure has been achieved, the following steps of the technique include the vascular approach, the medial posterior mobilization of the sigmoid, the extraction of the specimen, and the anastomosis. Additional steps include the mobilization of the splenic flexure, performed when further

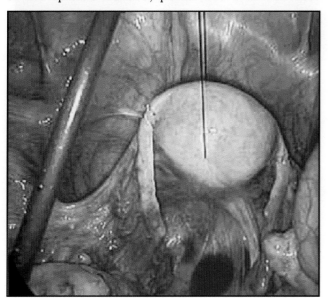

Fig. 25.16: Securing the uterus by suture for proper exposure of rectum

lengthening of the bowel is needed to perform a tension-free anastomosis.

The step of the exposure is preliminary, and it is done in a similar manner, regardless of the type of disease. The remainder of the procedure is different if the indication for surgery is a cancer or a benign disease.

Sigmoid Colon Resection for Cancer

In laparoscopic colorectal sigmoidectomy for cancer or for benign disease, the vascular approach is the first step of the dissection. It is believed that it allows us to avoid unnecessary manipulation of the colon and tumor, which may cause tumor cell exfoliation, and to perform a good lymphadenectomy following the vascular anatomy. The vessels are gradually exposed once the peritoneum at the base of the sigmoid mesocolon is incised (Figs 25.17A and B). The medial to lateral view allows us to see the sympathetic nerve plexus trunks, the left ureter, and gonadal vessels, avoiding ureteral injuries and possibly preserving genital function.

Primary Vascular Approach (Medial Approach)

Peritoneal Incision

The sigmoid mesocolon is retracted anteriorly, using a grasper introduced through the suprapubic cannula: This exposes the base of the sigmoid mesocolon. The visceral peritoneum is incised at the level of the sacral promontory (Figs 25.18A and B). The incision is continued upward along the right anterior border of the aorta up to the ligament of Treitz. The pressure of the pneumoperitoneum facilitates the dissection, as the diffusion of CO_2 opens the avascular planes.

Identification of the Inferior Mesenteric Artery

The dissection of the cellular adipose tissue is continued upward by gradually dividing the sigmoid branches of the right sympathetic trunk. The dissection behind the Inferior mesenteric artery involves preservation of the main hypogastric nerve trunks, but also division of the small branches travelling to the colon to expose the origin of the inferior mesenteric artery (Figs 25.19A and B). To ensure an adequate lymphadenectomy, the first 2 cm of the inferior mesenteric artery are dissected free and the artery is skeletonized before it is divided.

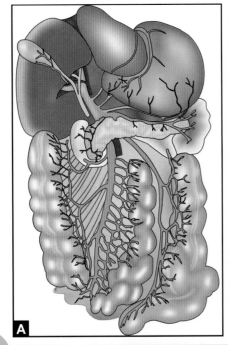

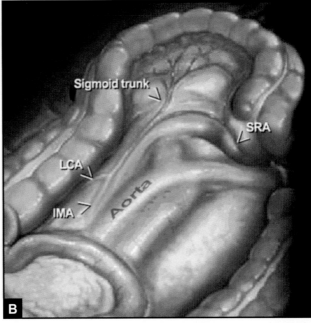

Figs 25.17A and B: Vascular supply of left side of colon

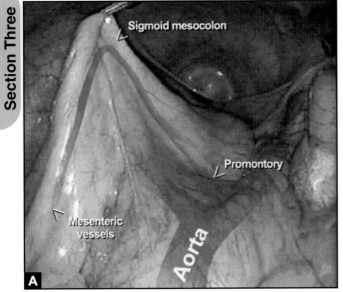

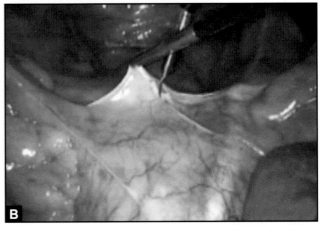

Figs 25.18A and B: Incision of peritoneum over sacral promontory

This dissection at the origin of the inferior mesenteric artery involves a risk of injury to the left sympathetic trunk situated on the left border of the inferior mesenteric artery. A meticulous dissection of the artery (skeletonization) helps to avoid this risk, because only the vessel will be divided, and not the surrounding tissues. Dissection performed close to the artery also minimizes the risk of ureteral injury during the ligation of the inferior mesenteric artery. The inferior mesenteric artery can then be divided between clips, or by using a linear stapler (vascular 2.5 or 2.0 mm cartridges. The artery is divided at 1-2 cm distal to its origin from the aorta ideally after the take off of the left colic artery (Figs 25.20A to D).

Identification of the Inferior Mesenteric Vein

The inferior mesenteric vein (IMV) terminates when reaching the splenic vein, which goes on to form the portal vein with the superior mesenteric vein (SMV). Anatomical variations include the IMV draining into the confluence of the SMV and splenic vein and the IMV draining in the SMV.

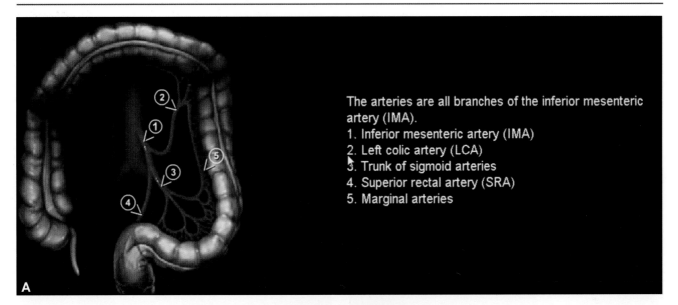

The arteries are all branches of the inferior mesenteric artery (IMA).
1. Inferior mesenteric artery (IMA)
2. Left colic artery (LCA)
3. Trunk of sigmoid arteries
4. Superior rectal artery (SRA)
5. Marginal arteries

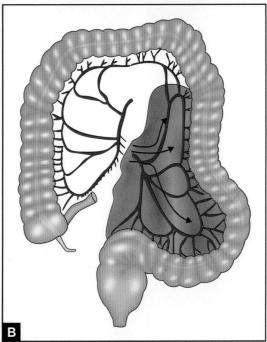

Figs 25.19A and B: Arterial supply of sigmoid colon

The inferior mesenteric vein (IMV) is identified to the left of the IMA or in case of difficulty, higher, just to the left of the ligament of Treitz junction (Fig. 25.21). The vein is divided below the inferior border of the pancreas or above the left colic vein. Once again, clips are sure options to ligate and divide this vessel (Figs 25.22 A and B).

Mobilization of the Sigmoid and Descending Colon

The mobilization of the sigmoid colon follows the division of the vessels. This step includes the freeing of posterior and lateral attachments of the sigmoid colon and mesocolon and the division of the rectal and sigmoid mesenteries. The approach is either

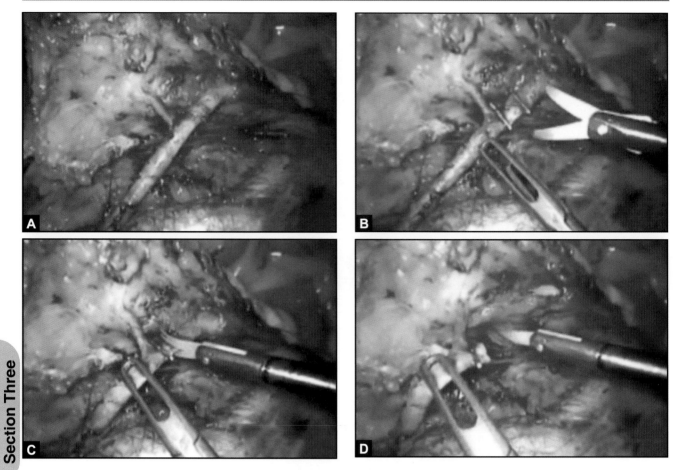

Figs 25.20A to D: Dissection of Inferior mesenteric artery

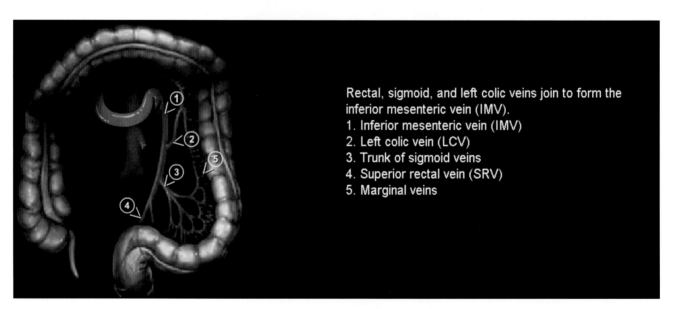

Rectal, sigmoid, and left colic veins join to form the inferior mesenteric vein (IMV).
1. Inferior mesenteric vein (IMV)
2. Left colic vein (LCV)
3. Trunk of sigmoid veins
4. Superior rectal vein (SRV)
5. Marginal veins

Fig. 25.21: Venous supply of sigmoid colon

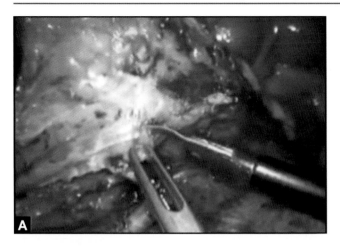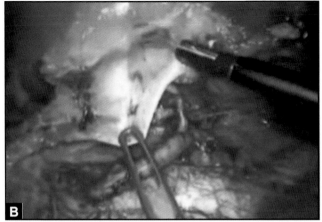

Figs 25.22A and B: Dissection of inferior mesenteric vein

medial or lateral. It is wise to routinely perform this medial-to-lateral laparoscopic dissection for all indications. The medial approach is well adapted for laparoscopy because it preserves the working space and demands the least handling of the sigmoid colon. In a randomized trial comparing the medial-to-lateral laparoscopic dissection with the classical lateral-to-medial approach for resection of rectosigmoid cancer, Liang et al showed that the medial approach reduces operative time and the postoperative proinflammatory response. Besides the potential oncologic advantages of early vessel division and "no-touch" dissection, it is believed that the longer the lateral abdominal wall attachments of the colon are preserved, the easier are the exposure and dissection.

Posterior Detachment

The sigmoid mesocolon is retracted anteriorly using the suprapubic cannula to expose the posterior space. The plane between Toldt's fascia and the sigmoid mesocolon can then be identified. This plane is avascular and easily divided. The dissection continues posterior to the sigmoid mesocolon going laterally toward Toldt's line. The sigmoid colon is then completely free, and the lateral attachments can then be divided using a lateral approach.

Lateral Mobilization

Extent of the dissection is superiorly for the inferior border of the pancreas, laterally following Gerota's fascia and inferiorly for the psoas muscle where the ureter crosses the iliac vessels. The sigmoid loop is

pulled toward the right upper quadrant (grasper in right subcostal cannula) to exert traction on the line of Toldt (Fig. 25.23). The peritoneal fold is opened cephalad and caudad, and the dissection joins the one previously performed medially. During this step, care must be taken to avoid the gonadal vessels and the left ureter because they can be attracted by the traction exerted on the mesentery. Ureteral stenting (infrared stents) can be useful in cases in which inflammation, tumoral tissue, or adhesions and endometriosis make planes difficult to recognize.

Dissection of the Upper Mesorectum

This area of dissection should be approached with caution, especially on the left side: The mesorectum there is closely attached to the parietal fascia where

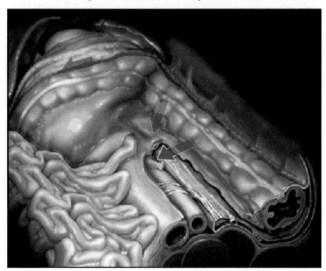

Fig. 25.23: Lateral approach

Section Three

the superior hypogastric nerve and the left ureter are situated. The upper portion of the rectum is mobilized posteriorly following the avascular plane described before, then laterally, until a sufficient distal margin is achieved (Figs 25.24A and B).

Resection of the Specimen

Division of the Rectum

Once the upper rectum is freed, the area of distal resection is chosen, allowing a distal margin of at least 5 cm. The fat surrounding this area is cleared, using monopolar cautery, ultrasonic dissection, or the LigaSure device. Doing so, the superior hemorrhoidal arteries are divided in the posterior upper mesorectum. The distal division is performed using a linear stapler.

The stapler is introduced through the right lower quadrant cannula. It is wise to use stapler loads 3.5 mm, 45 mm blue cartridges, which are applied perpendicular to the bowel (Figs 25.25A to C). Articulated staplers can also be useful, although they are usually unnecessary at the level of the upper rectum (Figs 25.26A and B).

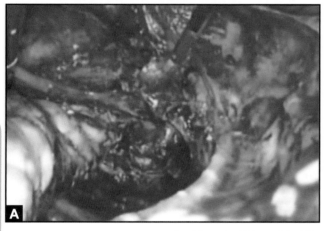
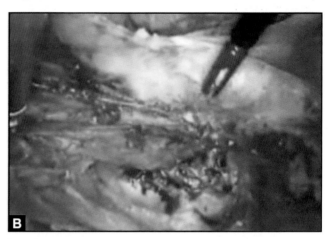

Figs 25.24A and B: Dissection of upper mesorectum

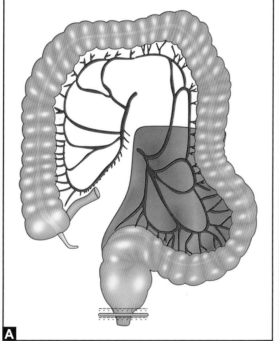
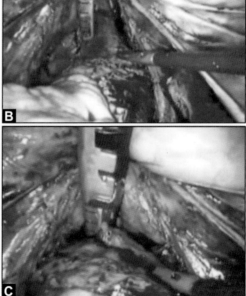

Figs 25.25A to C: Division of rectum using stapler

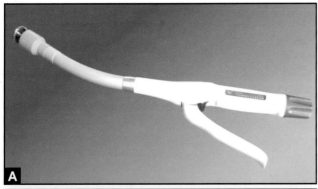

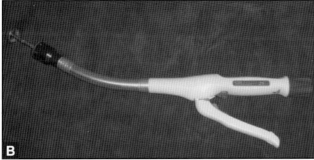

Figs 25.26A and B: Disposable circular staplers used in colorectal surgery

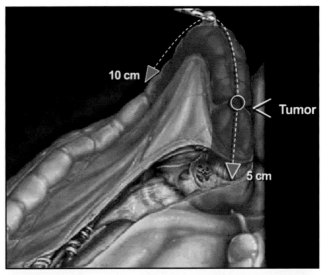

Fig. 25.27: Division 10 cm proximal and 5 cm distal to tumor

Proximal Division

The proximal division site should be located at least 10 cm proximal to the tumor. It is performed by first dividing the mesocolon and subsequently the bowel (Fig. 25.27). The division of the mesocolon is more easily performed with the harmonic scalpel, or the LigaSure, although linear staplers can also be used. The distal portion of the divided IMA is identified, and the division of the mesocolon starts right at this level and continues toward the chosen proximal section site at a 90° angle. A linear stapler is then fired across the bowel. The stapler (blue load) is introduced through the right lower quadrant cannula. The specimen is placed in a plastic retrieval sac introduced through the same cannula. This permits continuation of the procedure without manipulation of the bowel and tumor. If the resected specimen is large and obscures the operative fields, the extraction can be done before completing mobilization of the left colon.

Mobilization of the Splenic Flexure

In the frequent event that a long segment of sigmoid colon has been resected, mobilization of the splenic flexure is required. This can be achieved in different ways. It is important for the surgeon to be familiar with all approaches in order to select the most suitable approach. Sufficient mobilization of the splenic flexure may be achieved by simply freeing the posterior and lateral attachments of the descending colon. This is begun by a medial approach to free the posterior attachments of the descending and distal transverse colon, followed by the dissection of the lateral attachments, or by doing the same task in the reverse order. A lateral mobilization is sometimes sufficient in cases of sigmoid cancer, where the posterior mobilization can be omitted.

Lateral Mobilization of the Splenic Flexure

This approach is often used in open surgery and can also be used in simple laparoscopic colectomies. The first step is the section of the lateral attachments of the descending colon. An ascending incision is made along the line of Toldt using scissors introduced via the left-sided cannula. The phrenocolic ligament is then divided using scissors introduced through this cannula. Retraction of the descending colon and the splenic flexure toward the right lower quadrant using graspers introduced through the right lower and suprapubic cannulae helps to expose the correct plane (Figs 25.28A and B). The attachments between the transverse colon and the omentum are divided close to the colon until the lesser sac is opened. Division of these attachments is continued as needed, to facilitate the mobilization of the colon into the pelvis.

Section Three

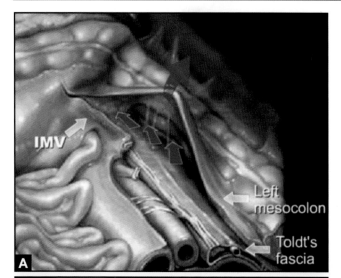

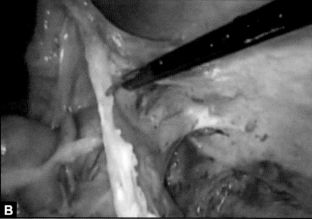

Figs 28A and B: Mobilization of splenic flexure of colon

Medial Mobilization

This approach dissects the posterior attachments of the transverse and descending colon first. The dissection plane naturally follows the plane of the previous sigmoid colon mobilization, cephalad and anterior to Toldt's fascia. The transverse colon is retracted anteriorly to expose the inferior border of the pancreas, and the root of the transverse mesocolon is divided anterior to the pancreas and at a distance from it; to enter the lesser sac. The dissection then follows toward the base of the descending colon and distal transverse colon, dividing the posterior attachments of these structures. The division of the lateral attachments, as described above, then follows the full mobilization of the splenic flexure. If the mobilized colon reaches the pelvis easily, it may be safely assumed the anastomosis will be tension free as well.

Extraction of Colon

The extraction of the specimen is performed using a double protection: A wound protector as well as a retrieval sac (Figs 25.29 and 25.30). The wound protector is also helpful to ensure that there is no CO_2 leak during the intracorporeal colorectal anastomosis, which follows the extraction. This allows reduction of the size of incision and potentially minimizes the risk of tumor cell seeding.

Incision to Extract the Specimen

The size of the incision, its location, and the extraction technique take into account the volume of the specimen, the patient's body habitus, cosmetic concerns, and the type of disease. The incision is generally performed in the suprapubic region. The proximal division is performed intracorporeally, as described above, and the specimen placed into a thick plastic bag before being extracted through the incision at the suprapubic area.

Anastomosis

For anastomosis a mechanical circular stapling device passed transanally to perform the anastomosis. Performing the anastomosis includes an extra-abdominal preparatory step and an intra-abdominal

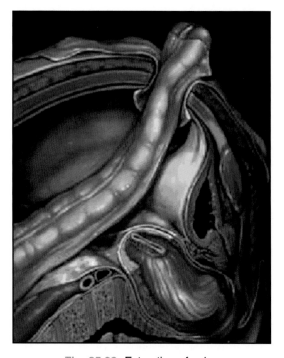

Fig. 25.29: Extraction of colon

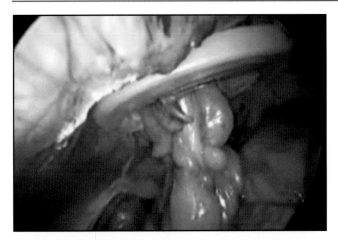

Fig. 25.30: Extraction of specimen through wound protector

step performed laparoscopically. The extra-abdominal step takes place after the extraction of the specimen.

The instrument holding the proximal bowel presents it at the incision where it can easily be grasped with a Babcock clamp and pulled out. If necessary, the colon

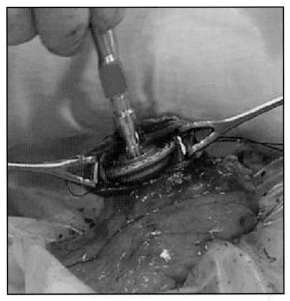

Fig. 25.32: Fixing the anvil on the proximal loop of colon

is divided again in a healthy and well-vascularized zone (Figs 25.31A and B).

The anvil (at least 28 mm in diameter) is then introduced into the bowel lumen and closed with a purse string; then the colon is reintroduced into the abdominal cavity (Fig. 25.32). The abdominal incision is closed to re-establish the pneumoperitoneum. For an air-tight closure, it is sufficient to twist the wound protector at the level of the incision using a large clamp (Fig. 25.33). The circular stapler is introduced into the rectum through the gently dilated anus. The rectal stump is then transfixed with the tip of the head of the circular stapler. In women, the posterior vaginal wall should be retracted anteriorly by the assistant passing the stapler (Fig. 25.34). Once the center rod and anvil

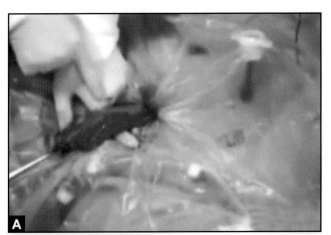

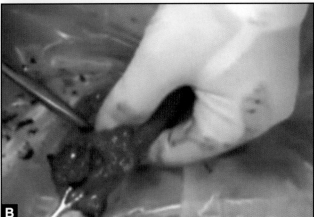

Fig. 25.31A and B: Preparation of the proximal loop of the colon for anastomosis

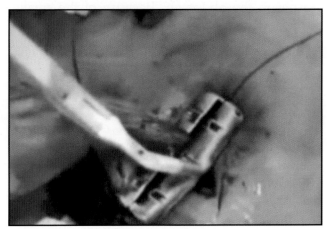

Fig. 25.33: Clamping and twisting of wound protector to prevent gas leak

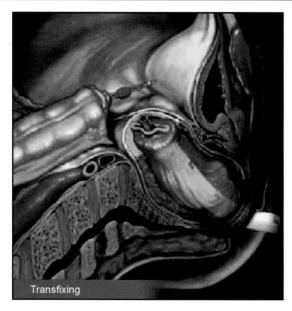

Fig. 25.34: Anvil and stapler ready for anastomosis

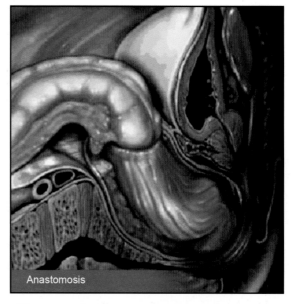

Fig. 25.35: End to end anastomosis done with the help of circular stapler

are clicked into the distal part of the circular stapler should be checked for twisting of the colon and the mesentery. The stapler is then fired after ensuring that the neighboring organs are away from the stapling line. The stapler is then twisted open and withdrawn. The anastomosis is checked for leaks by verifying the integrity of the proximal and distal rings, as well as performing an air test (Figs 25.35 and 25.36A to F).

Wound Closure

The cannula sites are checked internally for possible hemorrhage. To do so, a grasper is passed through the cannula and the cannula is removed leaving the grasper in the abdomen. Because of the smaller diameter of the grasper compared with the cannula, if a bleeding was so far concealed by the tamponade effect of the cannula, it would be revealed promptly. The cannula is then reintroduced to allow maintenance of the pneumoperitoneum while performing the same check at all cannula sites.

When the check is completed, the CO_2 is desufflated through the cannulae and cannulae are removed. No routine drainage of the anastomotic area is performed. The suprapubic incision is closed in layers using running absorbable sutures, and all fascial defects of 10 mm and more are closed. The skin is closed with a subcuticular absorbable suture.

Sigmoidectomy for Diverticular Disease

Outcomes after laparoscopic sigmoidectomy for diverticulitis are similar or even better to those seen in the open method, with faster recovery and decreased postoperative pain. Hand-assisted laparoscopic sigmoid resection for diverticulitis is also an attractive alternative to a "pure" laparoscopic method in complicated cases.

The vascular approach for patients with benign diseases of the sigmoid colon is performed with the following steps.

Peritoneal Incision

The peritoneal incision can be similar to the cancer technique particularly in difficult cases (obesity, inflammatory mesocolon). In most cases, surgeon should try to preserve the vascularization of the rectum and the left colic vessels. The opening of the peritoneum can be limited to the mesosigmoid parallel to colon at mid distance between the colon and the root of the mesosigmoid. An initial lateral mobilization of the sigmoid can be useful in this approach. The branches of the sigmoid arterial trunk can be divided separately anteriorly to inferior mesenteric vessels or together after creating windows in the mesentery to divide the various branches. A linear stapler or,

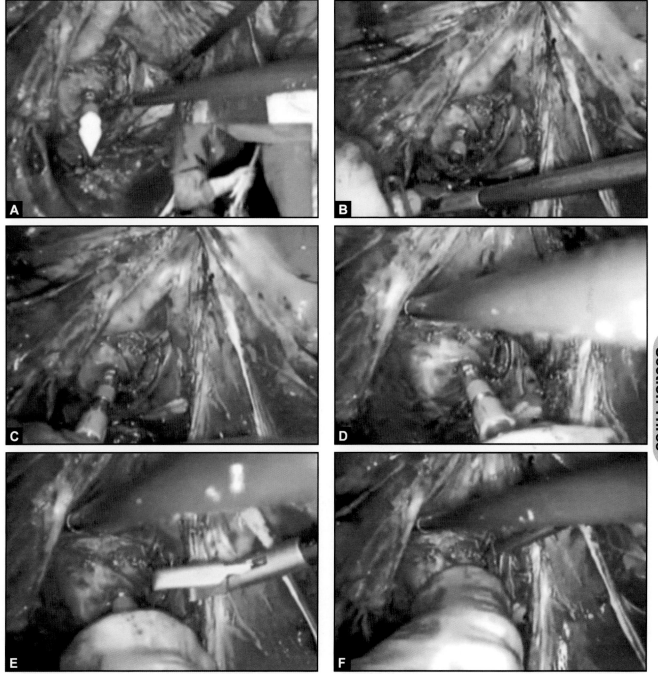

Figs 25.36A to F: Anastomosis by the help of circular stapler

better, the LigaSure Atlas 10 mm device can be used for this task.

Resection of the Specimen

In diverticular disease, one should perform the distal resection of the bowel below the rectosigmoid junction. The rectosigmoid junction is located just above the peritoneal reflexion, at the pouch of Douglas (Fig. 25.37). It is preferred to perform the mobilization of the splenic flexure at this moment, before resection at the proximal limit, using the same principles as described above.

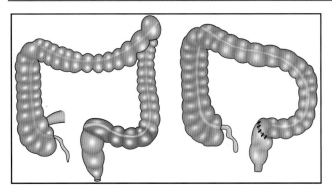

Fig. 25.37: Before and after sigmoidectomy

Extraction of the Specimen

Before extracting the colon, it is important to divide the mesocolon at the level of the proximal site of division. After adequate mobilization is achieved, the colon is extracted through a suprapubic incision, protected by the plastic drape described above, and proximal division performed externally on a compliant and well vascularized part of the colon. The anastomosis is performed as described above for cancer.

Special Considerations

Ureteral injuries are one of the most important complications, which can be avoided by a perfect exposure and the respect of the correct plane of dissection. Indeed, a dissection properly performed above the Toldt's fascia does not expose the ureter to accidental injury. Difficult cases, such as important inflammatory reaction, cancer invasion or adhesions, and, sometimes, endometriosis, may alter the anatomy of the region and render the identification of the ureter troublesome. In these special cases, prevention of ureteral injury may be facilitated by the use of infrared wires inserted in ureteral stents. The infrared light is cold and safe for use in close contact with the ureteral tissue, and, on the other side, makes it easy to recognize the structure under the light of an adequate laparoscope.

LOW ANTERIOR RESECTION

Two surgical procedures with curative intent are available to patients with rectal cancer:
1. Lower anterior resection and
2. Abdominoperineal resection

Lower anterior resection may improve quality of life and functional status. Lower anterior resection, formally known as anterior resection of the rectum and anterior excision of the rectum or simply anterior resection is a common surgery for rectal cancer. It is commonly abbreviated as LAR. LAR is generally the preferred treatment for rectal cancer insofar as this is surgically feasible. Laparoscopic low anterior resection for rectal cancer has gained wide acceptance among general surgeons. HALS LAR is also having equal acceptance mainly due to the technical difficulties encountered during pelvic dissection.

Patient Positioning

The patient is placed supine on the operating table (Fig. 25.38). After induction of general anesthesia and insertion of an orogastric tube and Foley catheter, the legs are placed in stirrups. The arms are tucked at the patient's side and the beanbag is aspirated. The abdomen is prepared with antiseptic solution and draped routinely.

Position of Surgical Team

The primary monitor is placed on the left side of the patient at approximately the level of the hip. Operating nurse is placed between the patient's legs. There should be sufficient space to allow the surgeon to move from either side of the patient to between the patient's legs, if necessary. The primary operating surgeon stands on the right side of the patient with the assistant

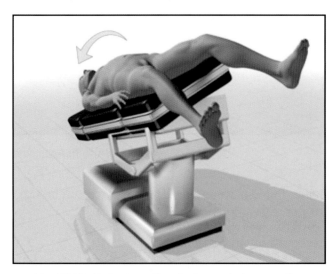

Fig. 25.38: Patient position for low anterior resection

standing on the patient's left, and moving to the right side, caudad to the surgeon, once ports have been inserted (Fig. 25.39). A 30 degree telescope is used.

Port Position

The primary optical port is introduced subumbilical using a modified Hasson approach. Having confirmed entry into the peritoneal cavity, a purse-string suture is placed around the subumbilical fascial defect. The abdomen to be insufflated with CO_2 to a pressure of 12 mm Hg.

The telescope is inserted into the abdomen and an initial diagnostic laparoscopy is performed, carefully evaluating the liver, small bowel, and peritoneal surfaces. A 12 mm port is inserted in the right lower quadrant approximately 2 to 3 cm medial and superior to the anterior superior iliac spine. It is carefully inserted lateral to the inferior epigastric vessels, paying attention to keep the tract of the port going as perpendicular as possible through the abdominal wall. A 5 mm port is then inserted in the right upper quadrant at least a hand's breadth superior to the lower quadrant port. A left lower quadrant 5 mm port is inserted. A 5 mm left upper quadrant port is also inserted to aid splenic flexure mobilization. Again, all of these remaining ports are kept lateral to the epigastric vessels. This may be ensured by diligence to anatomic port site selection and using the laparoscope to transilluminate the

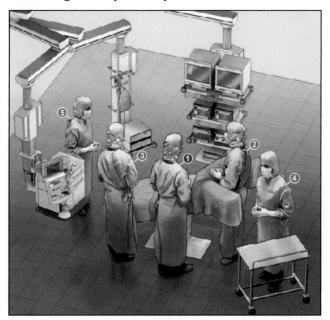

Fig. 25.39: Position of surgical team for LAR

abdominal wall before making the port site incision to identify any obvious superficial vessels.

The assistant now moves to the patient's left side, standing caudad to the surgeon. The patient is rotated with the left side up and right side down, to approximately 15 to 20 degrees tilt, and often as far as the table can go. This helps to move the small bowel over to the right side of the abdomen. The patient is then placed in the Trendelenburg position. This again helps gravitational migration of the small bowel away from the operative field. The surgeon then inserts two atraumatic bowel clamps through the two right-sided abdominal ports. The greater omentum is reflected over the transverse colon so that it comes to lie on the stomach. If there is no space in the upper part of the abdomen, one must confirm that the orogastric tube is adequately decompressing the stomach. The small bowel is moved to the patient's right side allowing visualization of the medial aspect of the rectosigmoid mesentery. This may necessitate the use of the assistant's 5 mm atraumatic bowel clamp through the left lower quadrant to tent the sigmoid mesentery cephalad.

Defining and Dividing the Inferior Mesenteric Pedicle

An atraumatic bowel clamp is placed on the rectosigmoid mesentery at the level of the sacral promontory, approximately half way between the bowel wall and the promontory itself. This area is then stretched up toward the left lower quadrant port, stretching the inferior mesenteric vessels away from the retroperitoneum. In most cases this demonstrates a groove between the right or medial side of the inferior mesenteric pedicle and the retroperitoneum. Electrosurgery or harmonic is used to open the peritoneum along this line, opening the plane cranially up to the origin of the inferior mesenteric artery, and caudally up to the sacral promontory. Blunt dissection is then used to lift the vessels away from the retroperitoneum and presacral autonomic nerves. The ureter is then looked for under the inferior mesenteric artery. If the ureter cannot be seen, and the dissection is in the correct plane, the ureter should be just deep to the parietal peritoneum, and just medial to the gonadal vessels. Care must be taken not to dissect too deep and injure the iliac vessels.

If the ureter cannot be found, it has usually been elevated on the back of the inferior mesenteric pedicle, and one needs to stay very close to the vessel not only to find the ureter but also to protect the autonomic nerves. If the ureter still cannot be found, the dissection needs to come in a cranial direction, which is usually into clean tissue allowing it to be found. If this fails, a lateral approach can be performed. This usually gives a fresh perspective to the tissues, and the ureter can often be found quite easily. In very rare cases, the ureter still may not be found. Ureteric stent should be used and it helps in easy identification of ureter and prevents it to get injured. It is good not to proceed if the ureter cannot be defined. The dissection is continued up to the origin of the inferior mesenteric artery, which is carefully defined and divided using a high ligation, above the left colic artery. A clamp is placed on the origin of the vessel to control it if clips or other energy sources do not adequately control the vessel. Endogia stapler can also be used for easy division of the vessel.

Having divided the vessels at the origin of the artery, the plane between the descending colon mesentery and the retroperitoneum is developed laterally, out toward the lateral attachment of the colon, and superiorly, dissecting the bowel off the anterior surface of the Gerota's fascia up toward the splenic flexure. This makes the inferior vein quite obvious and this vessel can also be divided just inferior to the pancreas. This allows increased reach for a coloanal anastomosis with or without neorectal reservoir.

Mobilization of the Lateral Attachments of the Rectosigmoid and Descending Colon

The surgeon now grasps the rectosigmoid junction with his left-hand instrument and draws it to the patient's right side. This allows the lateral attachments of the sigmoid colon to be seen and divided using electrosurgery or harmonic. Bruising from the prior retroperitoneal mobilization of the colon can usually be seen in this area. Once this layer of peritoneum has been opened, one immediately enters into the space opened by the retroperitoneal dissection. Dissection now continues up along the white line of Toldt, toward the splenic flexure. As the dissection continues, the surgeon's left-hand instrument needs to be gradually moved up along the descending colon to keep the lateral

attachments under tension. In this way, the lateral and any remaining posterior attachments are freed, making the left colon and sigmoid a midline structure. Elevating the descending colon and drawing it medially is useful, as this keeps small bowel loops out of the way of the dissecting instrument and facilitates the dissection. In some patients, particularly very obese or otherwise large patients, it is difficult to reach high enough through the right lower quadrant port. For this reason, the surgeon's right-hand instrument is moved to the left lower quadrant port site. This permits greater reach along the descending colon.

Mobilization of the Splenic Flexure

Complete lateral mobilization of the left colon up to the splenic flexure is performed as an initial step. The descending colon is pulled medially using an atraumatic bowel clamp in the right lower quadrant port and the scissors are placed in the left iliac fossa port. A 5-mm left upper quadrant port may be necessary, particularly in those with a very high splenic flexure, or in very tall or obese individuals. The lateral attachments of the left colon are divided and the colon is dissected off the Gerota's fascia over the left kidney.

Once the lateral attachments of the colon have been freed, it is necessary to move medially and enter the lesser sac. Some surgeons prefer to perform this as an initial step before lateral mobilization. To enter the lesser sac, the patient is tilted to a slight reverse Trendelenburg position. An atraumatic bowel clamp is inserted through the right upper quadrant port. If the left upper quadrant port is available this is also used. The assistant holds up the greater omentum, toward its left side, like a cape. The surgeon grasps the transverse colon toward the left side using a grasper in the right lower quadrant port to aid identification of the avascular plane between the greater omentum and the transverse mesocolon. Harmonic scalpel or monopolar scissors can be used through the left lower quadrant port to dissect this plane and enter the lesser sac. The surgeon usually moves to stand between the patient's legs for this part of the procedure. This dissection is continued toward the splenic flexure.

Following separation of the omentum off the left side of the transverse colon, connection to the lateral dissection allows the splenic flexure to be fully mobilized. The colon at the flexure is retracted caudally and medially, and any remaining restraining attachments are divided.

Rectal Mobilization

The patient is returned to the Trendelenburg position, and the small bowel is reflected cranially. Atraumatic bowel clamps inserted through the left-sided ports are used to elevate the rectosigmoid colon out of the pelvis and away from the retroperitoneum and sacral promontory, to enable entry into the presacral space. The posterior aspect of the mesorectum can be identified and the mesorectal plane dissected with diathermy, preserving the hypogastric nerves as they pass down into the pelvis, anterior to the sacrum. Dissection continues down the presacral space in this avascular plane toward the pelvic floor.

Attention is now switched to the peritoneum on the right side of the rectum. This is divided to the level of the seminal vesicles or rectovaginal septum. This is repeated on the peritoneum on the left side of the rectum. This facilitates further posterior dissection along the back of the mesorectum to the pelvic floor, to a level inferior to the lower edge of the mesorectum, just posterior to the anal canal. For a low anterior resection, it is necessary to perform a total mesorectal excision and hence the rectum must be dissected down to the muscle tube of the rectum below the inferior extent of the mesorectum. In many cases, particularly in those who are obese or men with a narrow pelvis, some or all of the anterior and lateral dissection must be completed to get adequate visualization, to complete the posterior dissection.

An atraumatic bowel clamp through the left iliac fossa port is used to retract the peritoneum anterior to the rectum forward. The peritoneal dissection is continued from the free edge of the lateral peritoneal dissection, anteriorly. Lateral dissection is continued on both sides of the rectum and is extended anterior to the rectum, posterior to Denonvillier's fascia, separating the posterior vaginal wall from the anterior wall of the rectum or down to the level of the prostate in men. The difficulty of dissection will vary depending on the body habitus of the patient, the diameter of the pelvis, and the size of the tumor. Occasionally, rectal mobilization can be very difficult to perform laparoscopically. In some cases, it may need to be completed in an open manner through a small Pfannenstiel incision.

Division of Rectum

The lower rectum may be divided with a stapler either laparoscopically or by open surgery, depending on the ease of access related to the size of the pelvis (Fig. 25.40). A rotaculator laparoscopic stapler may be used to divide the muscle tube of the rectum below the level of the mesorectum. The stapler is inserted through the right lower quadrant incision, and two firings of the stapler are usually required to divide the rectum. There is no residual mesorectum to divide at this level. Digital examination is performed to confirm the location of the distal staple line, and if there is any doubt about adequacy of the distal margin, a rigid proctoscopy is performed.

It is sometimes impossible to divide the rectum laparoscopically as the angulation of the endovascular stapler is limited to 45 degrees, necessitating open division of the rectum. In some patients, getting an assistant to push up on the perineum with their hand may lift the pelvic floor enough to get the first cartridge of the stapler low enough. In some cases, placing a suprapubic port allows easier access with the stapler to allow division of the rectum.

Some patients are either too obese or have a very narrow pelvis or a long anal canal, and the stapler cannot be passed low enough. Two options exist. One is to perform a transanal intersphincteric dissection, remove the specimen, and then perform a hand-sewn coloanal anastomosis. The second is to perform a short Pfannenstiel incision, which allows a linear 30 mm stapler to be positioned and the rectum divided.

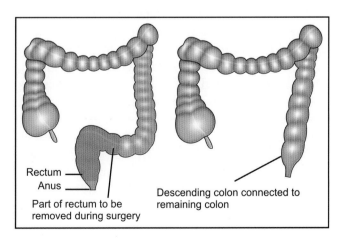

Rectum
Anus

Part of rectum to be removed during surgery

Descending colon connected to remaining colon

Fig. 25.40: Low anterior resection

Extraction and Anastomosis

The specimen can be extracted either through a Pfannenstiel incision or a left iliac fossa incision; in both incisions, a wound protector is used in cases with a polyp or cancer to reduce the risk of tumor implantation in the wound. The left colon mesentery is divided with cautery. The left colon is divided and the specimen is removed. Pulsatile mesenteric bleeding is confirmed and the vessels ligated with 0 polyglycolate suture ties. Depending on the preference of the operating surgeon, a colonic pouch or coloplasty may be performed. A 2/0 Prolene purse-string suture is inserted into the distal end of the left colon or pouch, the anvil of a circular stapling gun inserted, and the purse-string suture is tied tightly. If a Pfannenstiel incision has been made, the coloanal anastomosis can be performed under direct vision and open manipulation following insertion of a circular stapling gun into the rectal stump. If a left iliac fossa incision has been used, the colon is returned to the abdomen and the incision closed, the pneumoperitoneum recreated, and the anastomosis is formed laparoscopically. The anastomosis can be leak-tested by filling the pelvis with saline and inflating the neorectum using a proctoscope or bulb syringe.

ABDOMINOPERINEAL RESECTION

A laparoscopic abdominoperineal resection is an operation in which the anus, rectum, and sigmoid colon are removed (Fig. 25.41). It is used to treat cancer located very low in the rectum or in the anus, close to the sphincter muscles. Laparoscopic surgery for anorectal carcinoma is steadily gaining acceptance. The advantage offered by laparoscopy has always centered on improved vision. This advantage seems to be put to best use in the case of rectal cancer surgery, where logistic impediments, viz. narrow pelvis and impaired visibility as the dissection proceeds caudad, have proved to be obstacles to colorectal surgeons during open surgery. The recent studies have shown that the size of the tumor does not hamper the feasibility of performing laparoscopic abdomino-perineal resection. We need to consider the possibility of an increased circumferential margin rate for large-size tumors. This may be addressed by preoperative radiotherapy and chemotherapy before undertaking surgery on these large tumors. It is important to note,

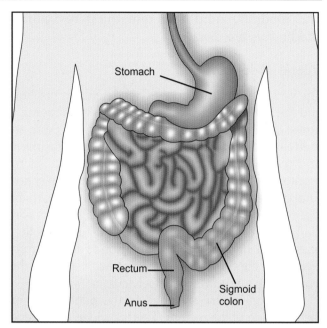

Fig. 25.41: Anus, rectum, and sigmoid colon removed in APR

though, that the oncological safety is not only dependant on the abdominal procedure but also on the adequacy of the perineal part of the operation. Besides, should tumor injury be detected intraoperatively, it is advisable to convert to open surgery to control the amount of contamination and complete the rest of the procedure.

Patient Position

The patient is placed supine on the operating table on a beanbag. After induction of general anesthesia and insertion of an orogastric tube and Foley catheter, the legs are placed stirrups. The arms are tucked at the patient's side. The abdomen is prepared with antiseptic solution and draped routinely.

Position of Surgical Team

The primary monitor is placed on the left side of the patient up toward the patient's feet. The secondary monitor is placed on the right side of the patient at the same level, and is primarily for the assistant during the early phase of the surgery and port insertion. The operating nurse's instrument table is placed between the patient's legs. There should be sufficient space to allow the surgeon to move from either side of the patient to between the patient's legs, if necessary. The primary operating surgeon stands on the right side of the patient with the assistant standing on the patient's left, and moving to the right side, caudad to the surgeon, once ports have been inserted.

Port Position

This is performed using a Hasson approach. A 10 mm smiling subumbilical incision is made. This is deepened down to the linea alba, which is then grasped on each side of the midline using Kocher clamps. A scalpel (No. 15 blade) is used to open the fascia between the Kocher clamps and a Kelly forceps is used to open the peritoneum bluntly. Having confirmed entry into the peritoneal cavity, a purse-string suture of 0 polyglycolic acid is placed around the subumbilical fascial defect. A 10 mm reusable port is inserted through this port wound allowing the abdomen to be insufflated with CO_2 to a pressure of 12 mm Hg. The laparoscope is inserted into the abdomen and an initial laparoscopy is performed, carefully evaluating the liver, small bowel, and peritoneal surfaces. A 12 mm port is inserted in the right lower quadrant approximately 2 to 3 cm medial and superior to the anterior superior iliac spine. This is carefully inserted lateral to the inferior epigastric vessels, paying attention to keep the tract of the port going as perpendicular as possible through the abdominal wall. A 5 mm port is then inserted in the right upper quadrant at least a hand's breadth superior to the lower quadrant port. A left lower quadrant 5 mm port is also inserted.

Exposure and Dissection of Retroperitoneum

The assistant now moves to the patient's left side, standing caudad to the surgeon. The patient is rotated with the left side up and right side down, to approximately 15 to 20 degrees tilt, and often as far as the table can go. This helps to move the small bowel over to the right side of the abdomen. The patient is then placed in the Trendelenburg position. This again helps gravitational migration of the small bowel away from the operative field. The surgeon then inserts two atraumatic bowel clamps through the two right-sided abdominal ports. The greater omentum is reflected over the transverse colon so that it comes to lie on the stomach. If there is no space in the upper part of the abdomen, one must confirm that the orogastric tube is adequately decompressing the stomach. The small bowel is moved to the patient's right side allowing visualization of the medial aspect of the rectosigmoid

mesentery pedicle. This may necessitate the use of the assistant's 5 mm atraumatic bowel clamp through the left lower quadrant to tent the sigmoid mesentery cephalad. Complete mobilization of the left colon is not required. Adequate mobilization must allow formation of a left iliac fossa colostomy without tension. Following division of the inferior mesenteric artery, the left mesocolon is separated from the retroperitoneum in a medial-to-lateral direction using a spreading movement. An atraumatic bowel clamp inserted through a right-sided port is placed under the left colonic mesentery, which is elevated away from the retroperitoneum, and using a scissors inserted through the other right-sided port, the attachments to the retroperitoneum are swept down, until the lateral abdominal wall is reached.

Division of the Left Colon

The mesentery of the left colon is divided from the free edge, cranial to the previously divided inferior mesenteric artery, toward the left sigmoid colon. The mesentery can be divided with diathermy and the marginal artery can be clipped and then divided. Alternatively, an energy source such as a LigaSure may be used to divide the mesentery up to the edge of the bowel. This may be done before freeing the lateral attachments of the sigmoid and left colon as it aids in retraction.

After division of the mesentery, the lateral attachments of the sigmoid to the abdominal wall are divided along the white line. Care is taken to avoid damage to the retroperitoneal structures. The colon is then divided using a linear endoscopic stapler at the site where the colonic mesentery has been divided.

Rectal Mobilization

In women, the uterus may be hitched out of the area of dissection with a suture. Atraumatic bowel clamps that are inserted through the left-sided ports are used to elevate the rectosigmoid colon out of the pelvis and away from the retroperitoneum and sacral promontory, to enable entry into the presacral space. The posterior aspect of the mesorectum can be identified and the mesorectal plane dissected with diathermy, preserving the hypogastric nerves passing down into the pelvis anterior to the sacrum. Dissection continues down the presacral space in this avascular plane toward the pelvic floor. Attention is now switched to the peritoneum on the right side of the rectum. This is divided to the level of the seminal vesicles or rectovaginal septum. This is repeated on the peritoneum on the left side of the rectum. This facilitates further posterior dissection along the back of the mesorectum to the pelvic floor, to a level inferior to the lower edge of the mesorectum. Usually, when the approach is low on the posterior surface of the mesorectum, it becomes necessary to perform a lateral and anterior dissection.

A bowel grasper inserted through the left iliac fossa port is used to retract the peritoneum anterior to the rectum forward. The peritoneal dissection is continued from the free edge of the lateral peritoneal dissection, anteriorly. Lateral dissection is continued on both sides of the rectum and is extended anterior to the rectum in front of Denonvillier's fascia, separating the posterior vaginal wall from the anterior wall of the rectum or down past the level of the prostate in men. The most inferior rectal dissection can be completed from the perineal approach. For anterior tumors, the dissection may be performed anterior to Denonvillier's fascia, or by taking one side of the fascia to protect the anterolateral nerve bundle.

It is necessary to perform a total mesorectal excision and hence the rectum must be dissected down close to the muscle tube of the rectum below the level of the mesorectum. The levators may then be divided from above, staying well wide of any potential tumor, or the division may be performed from below after making the perineal incision.

Formation of Trephine Left Iliac Fossa Colostomy

The divided distal end of the left sigmoid colon is grasped with atraumatic bowel clamps, which are locked. A trephine colostomy is made in the left iliac fossa at a site that has been marked by an enterostomal therapist before surgery. A skin disk is excised, and a longitudinal incision is made in the anterior rectus sheath and the left rectus muscle is split. The peritoneum is held with two hemostats and incised. The stapled colon is delivered to the trephine and grasped with Babcock forceps and delivered through the trephine. The staple line is excised and the end colostomy is matured using 3/0 chromic catgut sutures.

Perineal Dissection

The perineal dissection is performed with a conventional open approach (Fig. 25.42). The anus is sutured closed with 0 nylon and an elliptical skin incision is made. The incision is deepened using diathermy and the ischiorectal fossae are entered on either side, well lateral to the external sphincter muscle. The dissection continues laterally and posteriorly to expose the levator ani muscles (Fig. 25.43). The tip of the coccyx is used as the posterior landmark and the pelvic cavity is entered by dividing the levator ani muscle just anterior to the tip of the coccyx. A finger can be placed into the pelvis onto the upper border of levator ani, which is divided with diathermy onto the underlying finger. Care is taken anteriorly to divide the remaining levator ani while protecting the posterior surface of the vagina or prostate/urethra. The specimen may then be delivered out of the pelvis, which facilitates division of the remaining anterior attachments of the rectum, reducing the risk of damage to the prostate or posterior wall of the vagina. The specimen is removed, the pelvic cavity irrigated of blood or debris, and the perineal tissue closed in layers using polydioxanone sutures.

HARTMANN REVERSAL

The Hartmann procedure is a standard life-saving operation for acute left colonic complications. It is

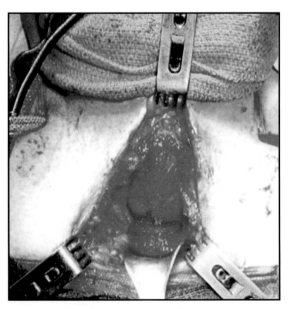

Fig. 25.42: Perineal dissection

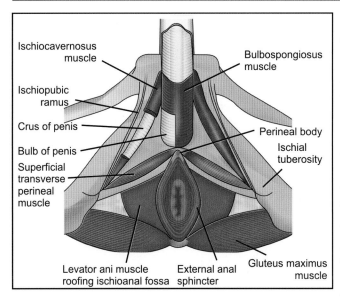

Fig. 25.43: Perineal anatomy

usually performed as a temporary procedure with the intent to reverse it later on. This reversal is associated with considerable morbidity and mortality by open method. The laparoscopic reestablishment of intestinal continuity after Hartmann procedure has shown better results in terms of decrease in morbidity and mortality.

There are several laparoscopic techniques of reversal of Hartmann procedure. The principle common to all techniques is a tension-free intracorporeal stapler anastomosis. The introduction of circular stapler in the rectal stump helps in identification and mobilization of the rectal stump. Others have mobilized the colostomy first and have used the colostomy site as a first port or used a standard umbilical port.

It is technically challenging and requires an experienced laparoscopic surgeon but offers clear advantages to patients. Main reasons reported for conversion to open were dense abdominal-pelvic adhesions secondary to diffuse peritonitis at the primary operation, short delay before the reconstruction, difficulty in finding the rectal stump and rectal scarring. Leaving long nonabsorbable suture ends at the rectal stump or suturing it to the anterior abdominal wall helps in its localization. Other relative limitation factors could be a large incisional hernia from the previous laparotomy and contraindications to general anesthesia and laparoscopy.

Patient Position

The patient is placed supine on the operating table, on a beanbag. After induction of general anesthesia and insertion of an orogastric tube and Foley catheter, the legs are placed in lithotomy stirrup position. The arms are tucked at the patient's side and the beanbag is aspirated. The abdomen is prepared with antiseptic solution and draped routinely.

Position of Surgical Team

The primary monitor is placed on the left side of the patient at approximately the level of the hip. The secondary monitor is placed on the right side of the patient at the same level, and is primarily for the assistant during the early phase of the surgery and port insertion. The operating nurse's instrument table is placed between the patient's legs. There should be sufficient space to allow the surgeon to move from either side of the patient to between the patient's legs, if necessary. The primary operating surgeon stands on the right side of the patient with the assistant standing on the patient's left, and moving to the right side, caudad to the surgeon once ports have been inserted. A 30 degree camera lens is better to be used.

The colostomy is mobilized and all adhesions dissected through the fascial opening until an adequate segment of bowel has been freed from the surrounding tissues. The bowel is trimmed as necessary and a purse-string suture is positioned before insertion of the anvil of a curved EEA stapling device. The bowel is returned to the abdomen, the fascia is closed with a monofilament suture, but before tying the suture a 12 mm port is inserted at this site, and the abdomen is insufflated.

The laparoscope is inserted into the abdomen through the stoma port to assess adhesions and allow direct visualization for subsequent port insertion and an initial laparoscopy is performed, carefully evaluating the liver, small bowel, and peritoneal surfaces. A 10 mm port is inserted in the umbilicus for camera location. A 5 mm right lower quadrant trocar is placed approximately 2 to 3 cm medial to the anterior superior iliac spine. This is carefully inserted lateral to the inferior epigastric vessels, paying attention to keep the tract of the port going as perpendicular as possible through the abdominal wall. A 5 mm port is then inserted in the right upper quadrant at least a hand's breadth superior to the lower quadrant port. A left upper quadrant 5 mm port is inserted. Again all of these remaining ports are kept lateral to the epigastric vessels. This may be ensured by diligence to anatomic port site selection and using the laparoscope to transilluminate the abdominal wall before making the port site incision to identify any obvious superficial vessels.

The assistant now moves to the patient's right side, standing caudad to the surgeon. The patient is rotated with the left side up and right side down, to approximately 15 to 20 degrees tilt, and often as far as the table can go. This helps to move the small bowel over to the right side of the abdomen. The patient is then placed in the Trendelenburg position. This again helps gravitational migration of the small bowel away from the operative field. The surgeon then inserts two atraumatic bowel clamps through the two right-sided abdominal ports. The greater omentum is reflected over the transverse colon so that it comes to lie on the stomach. If there is no space in the upper part of the abdomen, one must confirm that the orogastric tube is adequately decompressing the stomach. The small bowel is moved to the patient's right side allowing visualization of the proximal rectum. Variable degrees of adhesiolysis may be required. This may necessitate the use of the assistant's 5 mm atraumatic bowel clamp through the stoma trocar or left upper quadrant.

Left Colon Mobilization

An atraumatic bowel clamp is placed on the descending colon to take down the inflammatory and native attachments to free it laterally. The omentum is dissected off the transverse colon and the lesser sac is entered. The splenic flexure is released to allow a tension-free reach to the proximal rectum. The colonic mesentery should be mobilized off the Gerota's fascia. The left ureter is identified at the pelvic brim and freed from the proximal rectum to avoid injury. The ureter should be just deep to the parietal peritoneum, and just medial and posterior to the gonadal vessels. Care must be taken not to dissect too deep or caudad, leading to injury of the iliac vessels.

Mobilization of Rectum

An atraumatic bowel clamp inserted through the left lower quadrant port is used to elevate the proximal rectum out of the pelvis and away from the

retroperitoneum and sacral promontory, to enable entry into the presacral space. The posterior aspect of the mesorectum can be identified and the mesorectal plane dissected with diathermy, preserving the hypogastric nerves as they pass down into the pelvis anterior to the sacrum. Dissection needs to progress only to allow advancement of the circular stapler to the end of the rectum and assure that all the sigmoid has been resected. If residual sigmoid is present, the linear endoscopic stapler should be used to divide the bowel at the level of the proximal rectum. A site for rectal division should be chosen in proximal, peritonealized rectum, which assures that the anastomosis will be distal to the sacral promontory. The rectum is divided laparoscopically with a linear endoscopic stapler through the right lower quadrant trocar. One or two firings of the stapler may be required to divide the rectum. The mesorectum is divided using monopolar and bipolar cautery at this level.

Specimen Extraction and Anastomosis

If residual sigmoid is required, the specimen is extracted through the stoma site port. Pneumoperitoneum is recreated, and the circular stapled anastomosis is formed under laparoscopic guidance. The anastomosis can be leak-tested by filling the pelvis with saline and inflating the neorectum using a proctoscope or bulb syringe and the orientation and lack of tension confirmed. Fascia of all the 10 mm or above port is closed and skin dressing is applied by usual manner.

Conclusion

The reversal of Hartmann procedure can be difficult due tendency of Hartmann segment to become densely adherent deep in the pelvis. The laparoscopic reversal has made this major operation easier, safe and practical. As a majority of these patients is in the elderly age group, it has the advantage of early mobilization, less pain, short hospital stay and return to normal life.

RESECTION RECTOPEXY

Total rectal prolapse with chronic constipation and anal incontinence is a devastating disorder. It is more common in the elderly, especially women, although why it happens is unclear. Rectal prolapse can cause complications (such as pain, ulcers and bleeding), and cause fecal incontinence (Figs 25.44A and B).

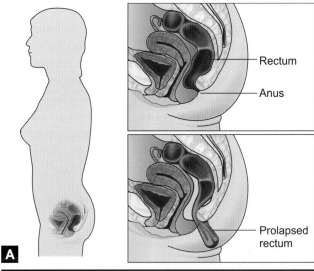

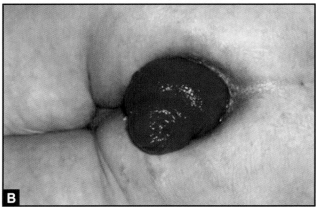

Figs 25.44A and B: Rectal prolapse

Surgery is commonly used to repair the prolapse. Rectopexy with or without bowel resection is the most frequent surgical procedure, with 0 to 9 percent recurrence rates in many years. Laparoscopic resection rectopexy is safely feasible as a minimally-invasive treatment option for rectal prolapse.

Patient Position

The patient is placed supine on the operating table, on a beanbag. After induction of general anesthesia and insertion of an orogastric tube and Foley catheter, the legs are placed in Dan Allen stirrups. The arms are tucked at the patient's side. The abdomen is prepared with antiseptic solution and draped routinely.

Position of Surgical Team

The primary monitor is placed on the left side of the patient at approximately the level of the hip. The secondary monitor is placed on the right side of the patient at the same level, and is primarily for the assistant during the early phase of the surgery and port insertion. The operating nurse's instrument table is placed between the patient's legs. There should be sufficient space to allow the surgeon to move from either side of the patient to between the patient's legs, if necessary. The primary operating surgeon stands on the right side of the patient with the assistant standing on the patient's left, and moving to the right side, caudad to the surgeon once ports have been inserted. A 0 degree camera lens is used.

Port Position

This is performed using a Hasson approach. A smiling 10 mm subumbilical incision is made. This is deepened down to the linea alba, which is then grasped on each side of the midline using Kocher clamps. A scalpel (No. 15 blade) is used to open the fascia between the Kocher clamps and a Kelly forceps is used to open the peritoneum bluntly. The telescope is inserted into the abdomen and an initial laparoscopy is performed, carefully evaluating the liver, small bowel, and peritoneal surfaces. A 12 mm port is inserted in the right lower quadrant approximately 2 to 3 cm medial and superior to the anterior superior iliac spine. This is carefully inserted lateral to the inferior epigastric vessels, paying attention to keep the tract of the port going as perpendicular as possible through the abdominal wall. A 5 mm port is then inserted in the right upper quadrant at least a hand's breadth superior to the lower quadrant port. A left lower quadrant 5 mm port is inserted. All the ports are more or less obeying the baseball diamond concept.

Dissection

The patient is rotated with the left side up and right side down, to approximately 15 to 20 degrees tilt, and often as far as the table can go. This helps to move the small bowel over to the right side of the abdomen. The patient is then placed in the Trendelenburg position. This again helps gravitational migration of the small bowel away from the operative field. The surgeon then inserts two atraumatic bowel clamps through the two right-sided abdominal ports. The greater omentum is reflected over the transverse colon so that it comes to lie on the stomach. If there is no space in the upper

Section Three

part of the abdomen one must confirm that the orogastric tube is adequately decompressing the stomach. The small bowel is moved to the patient's right side allowing visualization of the medial aspect of the rectosigmoid mesentery. This may necessitate the use of the assistant's 5 mm atraumatic bowel clamp through the left lower quadrant to tent the sigmoid mesentery cephalad.

Division of Inferior Mesenteric Vessel

An atraumatic bowel clamp is placed on the rectosigmoid mesentery at the level of the sacral promontory, approximately half way between the bowel wall and the promontory itself. This area is then stretched up towards the left lower quadrant port, stretching the inferior mesenteric vessels away from the retroperitoneum. In most cases, this demonstrates a groove between the right or medial side of the inferior mesenteric pedicle and the retroperitoneum. Cautery is used to open the peritoneum along this line, opening the plane cranially up to the origin of the inferior mesenteric artery, and caudally past the sacral promontory. Blunt dissection is then used to lift the vessels away from the retroperitoneum and presacral autonomic nerves. The ureter is then looked for under the inferior mesenteric artery. If the ureter cannot be seen, and the dissection is in the correct plane, the ureter should be just deep to the parietal peritoneum, and just medial to the gonadal vessels. Care must be taken not to dissect too deep or caudad leading to injury of the iliac vessels.

If the ureter cannot be found, it has usually been elevated on the back of the inferior mesenteric pedicle, and one needs to stay very close to the vessel not only to find the ureter but also to protect the autonomic nerves. If the ureter still cannot be found, the dissection needs to come in a cranial dissection, which is usually into clean tissue allowing it to be found. If this fails, a lateral approach can be performed. This usually gives a fresh perspective to the tissues, and the ureter can often be found quite easily. In very rare cases the ureter still may not be found.

The dissection should allow sufficient mobilization of the inferior mesenteric artery so that the origin of the left colic artery is seen. The vessel is carefully defined and divided just distal to the left colic artery. A clamp is placed on the origin of the vessel to control it if clips or other energy sources do not adequately control the vessel. In general, a cartridge of the endoscopic linear stapler is used to divide the vessel. Having divided the pedicle, the plane between the sigmoid colon mesentery and the retroperitoneum is developed laterally, out towards the lateral attachment of the colon. Limited mobilization of the mesentery off the anterior surface of Gerota's fascia and of the left colon should be performed to enhance fixation of the rectum.

Mobilization of the Lateral Attachments of the Rectosigmoid

The surgeon now grasps the rectosigmoid junction with his left-hand instrument and draws it to the patient's right side. This allows the lateral attachments of the sigmoid colon to be seen and divided using cautery. Bruising from the prior retroperitoneal mobilization of the colon can usually be seen in this area. Once this layer of peritoneum has been opened, one immediately enters into the space opened by the retroperitoneal dissection. No dissection should be performed more proximally along the white line of Toldt, toward the splenic flexure.

Mobilization of Rectum

An atraumatic bowel clamp inserted through the left lower quadrant port is used to elevate the rectosigmoid colon out of the pelvis and away from the retroperitoneum and sacral promontory, to enable entry into the presacral space. The posterior aspect of the mesorectum can be identified and the mesorectal plane dissected with diathermy, preserving the hypogastric nerves as they pass down into the pelvis anterior to the sacrum. Dissection continues down the presacral space in this avascular plane toward the pelvic floor. Only the posterior 60 percent of the rectum needs to be mobilized; however, dissection should be continued all the way to the levator ani muscles. A transanal examining finger should be used to confirm the distal extent of the dissection. The lateral stalks should be preserved. The peritoneum on either side of the rectum should be incised to the level of the lateral stalks. The lateral stalks should generally be preserved, the exception being when further dissection must completely reduce a very distal prolapsing segment.

Rectal Division

The fully mobilized rectum should be elevated out of the pelvis and a site selected for optimal rectal tension to maintain full reduction of the prolapse. A site for rectal division should be chosen in proximal, peritonealized rectum, which assures that the anastomosis will be rostral to the sacral promontory. The rectum is divided laparoscopically with a linear endoscopic stapler through the right lower quadrant trocar. One or two firings of the stapler may be required to divide the rectum. The mesorectum is divided using monopolar and bipolar cautery at this level.

Specimen Extraction and Anastomosis

The specimen is extracted through a left iliac fossa incision. Before making the incision, the proximal colonic transaction point should be grasped with a locking atraumatic bowel grasper. This site should allow a colorectal anastomosis that will provide a safe amount of tension on the rectum to maintain prolapse reduction. After extracorporeal bowel transaction, adequate vascularity of the colon should be assured. A 2/0 Prolene purse-string suture is inserted into the distal end of the left colon, the anvil of a circular stapling gun is inserted and the purse-string suture is tied tightly. The colon is returned to the abdomen and the left iliac fossa incision is closed in layers with 0 polyglycolic acid suture. Pneumoperitoneum is recreated, and the circular stapled anastomosis is formed under laparoscopic guidance. The anastomosis can be leak-tested by filling the pelvis with saline and inflating the neorectum using a proctoscope or bulb syringe.

Rectopexy (Figs 25.45A and B)

The rectum is retracted rostrally to the desired tension to allow complete reduction of the prolapse. The rectopexy is then performed from the right side using the two remaining ports. Two or three nonabsorbable sutures are used to attach the mesorectum distal to the anastomosis to the sacral promontory. Alternatively, nitinol or titanium tackers may be employed using one of the mechanical fixation devices used for mesh hernia repairs.

WELLS OR MARLEX RECTOPEXY

Rectal prolapse is a distressing condition especially when associated with fecal incontinence and

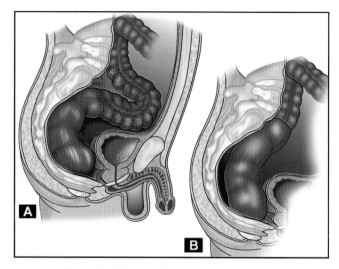

Figs 25.45A and B: Resection rectopexy

constipation. It usually occurs in children or elderly. Presently laparoscopic approach is favored as it has better results especially in terms of less postoperative pain, shorter hospital stay and lower cost. The pelvic sympathetic and parasympathetic nerves run along the rectum; if dissection is not carried out in the proper plane, injury can occur, leading to bladder dysfunction, impotence, and/or retrograde ejaculation. This is an important consideration when trying to decide which procedure to perform, especially in men, although the risk of injury should be less than 1-2 percent. Perineal procedures and anterior resection have a low risk of outlet obstruction. Abdominal procedures of rectopexy that tack the rectum to the sacrum can cause outlet obstruction if the rectum is wrapped circumferentially, often requiring release of the fixation to treat the problem.

In a Marlex rectopexy (Ripstein procedure), the entire rectum is mobilized down to the coccyx posteriorly, the lateral ligaments laterally, and the anterior cul-de-sac anteriorly. A nonabsorbable material, such as Marlex mesh or an Ivalon sponge, is then fixed to the presacral fascia. The rectum is then placed on tension, and the material is partially wrapped around the rectum to keep it in position. The anterior wall of the rectum is not covered with the sponge or mesh in order to prevent a circumferential obstruction. The peritoneal reflections are then closed to cover the foreign body. The Marlex mesh or sponge causes an inflammatory reaction that scars and fixes the rectum into place.

The Wells procedure was followed by rectal dysfunction accompanied by increased constipation and evacuation problems. The Ripstein procedure, preserving the lateral ligaments, appears not to affect such symptoms adversely. Modified mesh rectopexy aligns the rectum, avoids excessive mobilization and division of lateral ligaments thus preventing constipation and preserving potency. We recommend this technique for patients with complete rectal prolapse with up to grade 1, 2 and 3 incontinence based on Browning and Parks classification.

During wells rectopexy the dissection should allow sufficient mobilization of the inferior mesenteric artery so that the origin of the left colic artery is seen. The pedicle is not divided.

The plane between the sigmoid colon mesentery and the retroperitoneum is developed laterally, out toward the lateral attachment of the colon. Limited mobilization of the mesentery off the anterior surface of Gerota's fascia and of the left colon should be performed to enhance fixation of the rectum.

Ripstein's operation often improved anal continence in patients with rectal prolapse and rectal intussusception. This improvement was accompanied by increased Maximum resting pressure in patients with rectal prolapse, indicating recovery of internal anal sphincter function. In one of the study at Department of Surgery, Karolinska Institute at Danderyd Hospital, Stockholm, Sweden maximum resting pressure (52+/- 23 mmHg) was found in Ripstein operation than patients with rectal prolapse. No postoperative increase in MRP was found in patients with rectal intussusception. This suggests an alternate mechanism of improvement in patients with rectal intussusception.

Mobilization of the Lateral Attachments of the Rectosigmoid

For rectal prolapse surgery lateral mobilization the surgeon grasps the rectosigmoid junction with his left-hand instrument and draws it to the patient's right side. This allows the lateral attachments of the sigmoid colon to be seen and divided using cautery. Bruising from the prior retroperitoneal mobilization of the colon can usually be seen in this area. Once this layer of peritoneum has been opened, one immediately enters into the space opened by the retroperitoneal dissection.

No dissection should be performed more proximally along the white line of Toldt, toward the splenic flexure.

Rectal Mobilization

An atraumatic bowel clamp inserted through the left lower quadrant port is used to elevate the rectosigmoid colon out of the pelvis and away from the retroperitoneum and sacral promontory, to enable entry into the presacral space. The posterior aspect of the mesorectum can be identified and the mesorectal plane dissected with diathermy, preserving the hypogastric nerves as they pass down into the pelvis anterior to the sacrum. Dissection continues down the presacral space in this avascular plane toward the pelvic floor. Only the posterior 60 percent of the rectum needs be mobilized; however, dissection should be continued all the way to the levator ani muscles. A transanal examining finger should be used to confirm the distal extent of the dissection. The peritoneum on either side of the rectum should be incised to the level of the lateral stalks. The lateral stalks should generally be preserved, the exception being when further dissection must completely reduce a very distal prolapsing segment. The rectum is not divided in case of wells rectopexy.

Rectopexy

A 2 to 4 cm portion of polypropylene mesh is rolled and inserted through the umbilical trocar. The camera is reinserted and the mesh is positioned at the sacral promontory. A mechanical device used for hernia mesh fixation is used to fix the mesh to the promontory. This may be inserted through the right lower quadrant port, but if adequate access cannot be obtained, a 5 mm suprapubic port may be inserted. Great care must be taken not to tear or strip off the presacral fascia when stapling the mesh in place.

The rectum is retracted rostrally to the desired tension to allow complete reduction of the prolapse, which is confirmed by digital rectal examination. The rectopexy is then performed from the right side using the two right-sided trocars. Two or three nonabsorbable sutures are used to attach the distal mesorectum to the mesh at the promontory, sufficient to maintain adequate tension. Alternatively, the mechanical fixation device used for mesh fixation may be employed.

Complication of Colorectal Surgery

The exact frequency and severity of complications are difficult to determine due to heterogeneous definitions, patient populations, procedures, comobidities, and intensity of follow up. One perspective of the incidence of complications can be gleaned from four recent randomized controlled trials comparing laparoscopic to open colon resections for cancer (Table 25.1).

Wound Infection

Superficial wound infections are the most common complication of colorectal surgery. The previously held belief that preoperative cathartic and oral antibiotic bowel preparation was mandatory to prevent postoperative infections has recently been debunked by multiple randomized controlled trials. Superficial wound infections are recognized by any combination of erythema, induration, tenderness, or drainage at the wound site. Systemic signs of fever and tachycardia may also be present. The infection may manifest as an abscess, cellulitis, or a combination of the two. When suspected, the wound should be carefully inspected and when a collection is detected, it is drained by reopening the wound. Gram stain can assist in management and antibiotic selection.

Anastomotic Leak

During laparoscopic colorectal surgery anastomotic leak is a common, potentially life threatening complication associated with significant morbidity, increased risk of local recurrence of cancer, decreased functional outcomes, increased length of stay, high risk of (permanent) ostomy, and death. Leaks are variably defined in the literature, but in general regarded as perianastomotic stool, gas, or abscess, peritonitis, or a fecal fistula. The incidence of anastomotic leak following colectomy is generally reported between 2 and 6 percent. Anastomotic leaks present in one of three ways.

1. Asymptomatic leak
2. Subtle insidious leak
3. Dramatic early leak

After surgery the asymptomatic leak is incidentally found during endoscopic or radiographic studies. The incidence of radiographically detected leaks is 4-6 times higher than clinically detected leaks. These leaks, which often present weeks or months later, are typically walled off sinuses, and are, as a general rule, harmless. Treatment is rarely necessary. The subtle insidious leak can present perioperatively with nonspecific signs and symptoms common in the postoperative period. Such signs include low grade fevers, mild leukocytosis, protracted ileus, and failure to thrive and occur 5-14 days following surgery. Management of the stable patient without signs of peritonitis usually begins with imaging to identify and localize the process. Traditionally, water-soluble contrast enema has been the primary study to identify leaks. Drawbacks include lower sensitivity for right-sided anastomosis as the contrast dilutes out before reaching the proximal bowel. It also provides little information on extracolonic conditions such as ileus and collections. Abdominopelvic CT scan with triple contrast (oral,

Table 25.1: Complication rates following laparoscopic and open colon resections

	Barcelona Trial	Cost Trial	Classic Trial	Color Trial
Wound infection	11.9 percent	2.5 percent	8.7 percent	3.3 percent
Persistent ileus	5.5 percent	2.8 percent		
Evisceration	0.9 percent			0.8 percent
Bleeding	0.5 percent	1.2 percent	4.8 percent	1.9 percent
Anastomotic leak	0.9 percent		6.0 percent	2.3 percent
Pneumonia	0 percent		6.5 percent	1.9 percent
UTI	0.5 percent	1.2 percent		2.3 percent
ARF	1.4 percent			
DVT			1 percent	
Cardiac		2.6 percent		1.2 percent

URI = urinary tract infection, ARF = acute renal failure, DVT = deep venous thrombosis

Section Three

intravenous, and rectal) has become the imaging modality of choice to evaluate suspected postoperative intra-abdominal infection. Specificity during the first five days postoperative, however, is reduced. During this period, infectious processes may be difficult to differentiate from acute postoperative inflammation and fluid collections. Sensitivity is much improved beyond 5-7 days. CT scan and contrast enema can also be used as complimentary studies.

If there is large collections, it can often amenable to percutaneous, transgluteal, or transanal image guided catheter drainage. The images should be reviewed with an interventional radiologist to identify a safe window of access that avoids vascular structures and other organs. Abscesses less than 3-4 cm are too small for most pigtail catheters and will often resolve with a course of antibiotics. In the era of modern CT scanning and interventional radiology, the routine practice of repeat laparotomy, abdominal washouts, large sump drains, and open abdominal wound management is rarely necessary and can be reserved for patients who fail to respond to, deteriorate following, or are not candidates for percutaneous drainage.

Sometime management of the patient with progressive generalized peritonitis with or without septic shock requires resuscitation in ICU with broad spectrum antibiotics and urgent laparotomy. Laparoscopic management may be considered if the surgeon has sufficient laparoscopic skills and reoperative experience. At the time of surgery, the anastomosis should be scrutinized for signs which led to its failure. This can guide the appropriate method of repair.

After laparoscopic colorectal surgery if the findings at operation show ischemia and necrosis of greater than one third of the anastomosis, the anastomosis should be resected with creation of a stoma. If the mucous fistula can be brought up to the skin, it should ideally be fashioned through the same site as the proximal ostomy. When performed in this fashion, subsequent ostomy reversal can be done via a circumstomal incision, obviating the need for formal laparotomy and its associated morbidity. If the findings at operation identify a smaller leak with healthy bowel, the anastomosis can usually be salvaged with suture repair, proximal diversion, and washout of the distal segment. Our preferred diversion is a loop ileostomy.

Early Postoperative Small Bowel Obstruction

After colorectal laparoscopic surgery early postoperative bowel obstruction is rare, occurring in 1 percent of patients. This time period accounts for 5-29 percent of all small bowel obstructions. Most obstructions are caused by adhesions which form within 72 hours of surgery then become very dense and vascular after two to three weeks. Obstructions are more common following colorectal and gynecological procedures than following appendectomy or procedures located above the transverse colon. Signs and symptoms of early postoperative small bowel obstruction are similar to and hard to differentiate from the more common paralytic ileus. Patients typically develop abdominal distention, nausea, and vomiting, but cannot tolerate nasogastric tube clamping or removal. Most patients have a slow, smoldering course with emergencies being the exception.

Surgeon should try to manage obstruction conservatively initially. There is a fine balance between waiting for the obstruction to resolve and rushing a patient to the operating room. In the first week following surgery, obstruction is hard to differentiate from ileus. Between 2 weeks and 2 months postoperative adhesions become thick, vascular and obliterate natural planes making surgery much more difficult and prone to complications. The decision to operate should, therefore, occur between 7-14 days.

If patient has symptoms of obstruction, plain films readily diagnose most small bowel obstructions. Oral administration of water soluble contrast followed by an abdominal plain film or CT scan 4 hours later is good predictor of resolution of a small bowel obstruction. Contrast in the colon indicates the obstruction is likely to resolve with non-operative means. CT scan may be useful in identifying signs of ischemia, other intraabdominal processes and in localizing the site of obstruction for operative planning.

Initial management of the stable patient involves fluid and electrolyte replacement, bowel rest, nasogastric tube drainage, and a nutritional evaluation. Total parenteral nutrition should be started after 7 days. Operation is advised for high grade or complete bowel obstruction, concern for strangulated bowel, or unresolved small bowel obstruction despite prolonged NGT decompression.

If proper care is insured most patients resolve with non-operative management. If surgery becomes necessary, it should occur prior to the two week mark after which the acute adhesions become dense, vascular, and problematic. Surgery involves careful re-exploration and lysis of adhesions. Operative findings usually reveal either a single adhesive band or multiple matted adhesions, each occurring with similar frequency.

After colorectal surgery if obstruction develops, laparoscopic exploration and adhesiolysis is being increasingly utilized for small bowel obstructions. Advanced laparoscopic skills and experience are a prerequisite because access is difficult in these patients. Poor candidates for laparoscopic management include patients with signs of peritonitis, multiple previous operations for small bowel obstruction, small bowel diameter greater than 4 cm, or other medical contraindication to laparoscopy. Pneumoperitoneum should be established with an open technique at a site remote from the previous incision. Atraumatic graspers are used to explore the bowel in a retrograde fashion beginning with decompressed bowel at the ileocecal valve. Distended bowel is fragile and should not be graped: grasping the adjacent mesentery reduces the risk of inadvertent bowel perforation. Adhesiolysis is best performed with scissors or bipolar cautery devices to reduce the risk of adjacent bowel injury. Conversion rates range from 7-43 percent. Proactive reasons to convert include poor visualization, non-viable intestine, multiple dense adhesions, deep pelvic adhesions, and failure to progress in a reasonable time.

TIPS AND TRICKS

To avoid intraoperative complications:
- Create adequate exposure
- Use proper traction and counter traction
- Develop the right planes
- Standardize the assistant's role
- Beware of the variations of vasculature and anatomy
- Should visualization be compromised during the procedure it is easy to switch to a 30° laparoscope for a more topographical view? Applying the angled 30° laparoscope can also be helpful to manage external arm collisions during tight set-up situations, as the camera arm angle changes depending on the endoscopy used. Additionally, with angled 30° laparoscope the surgeon has the ability to rotate the viewing angle of the scope (out of the horizontal image plane) and minimize collisions as well.
- Leave 1 to 1.5 cm on either side of the transacted IMA and IMV so that if any bleeding occurs grasping of the vessel is still possible to allow application of the hemostatic technique (clips, LigaSure™ or suture).
- Distance the ports as much as possible from each other during initial port placement (minimum of 7.5 cm). Placing the patient in a steeper Trendelenburg position can increase the vertical spacing between the arms and potentially eliminate or minimize arising collisions.
- Before dividing any tissues, identify the ureter and gonadal vessels one more time.
- During all procedure steps clear communication with the patient-side assistant is essential.

CONCLUSION

The laparoscopic technique reduces the parietal aggression and achieves the same results as traditional surgery. Patients recover faster and experience less pain, with fewer wound infections, postoperative hernias, less time in hospital and reduced costs. But laparoscopic colonic surgery requires extensive and highly specialized training, with few surgeons qualified to perform these procedures. The recent conclusion of the oncologic debate together with the rapid development of technological means and the increase in public awareness will probably result in a substantial increase in the number of surgeons performing laparoscopic colorectal surgery. Laparoscopic technique is an excellent approach though not yet the gold standard. A smooth performance of this technique depends on: the quality of the equipment; perfect knowledge of the operative steps; exposure of operative field; the experience of the surgical team. Operative times are somewhat longer than open procedures but become shorter along the learning curve. Right colectomies are shorter and easier to perform than left-sided and rectal resections and should be employed for teaching residents. The conversion rate would not necessarily drop after the first 50 cases and should reflect good surgical judgment rather than a surgical failure.

BIBLIOGRAPHY

1. Anderson J, Luchtefeld M, Dujovny N, et al. A comparison of laparoscopic, hand-assist and open sigmoid resection in the treatment of diverticular disease. Am J Surg 2007 Mar;193(3):400-3.
2. Belizon A, Balik E, Feingold DL, et al. Major abdominal surgery increases plasma levels of vascular endothelial growth factor: open more so than minimally invasive methods. Ann Surg 2006 Nov;244(5):792-8.
3. Bender JS, Magnuson TH, Zenilman ME, et al. Outcome following colon surgery in the octogenarian. Am Surg 1996;62:276-9.
4. Berends FJ, Kazemier G, Bonjer HJ, Lange JF. Subcutaneous metastases after laparoscopic colectomy. Lancet 1994 Jul 2;344(8914):58.
5. Chang YJ, Marcello PW, Rusin C, Roberts PL, Schoetz DJ. Hand-assisted laparoscopic sigmoid colectomy: helping hand or hindrance? Surg Endosc 2005 May;19(5):656-61.
6. Dean PA, Beart RWJr, Nelson H, Elftmann TD, Schlinkert RT. Laparoscopic-assisted segmental colectomy: early Mayo Clinic experience. Mayo Clin Proc 1994;69:834-40.
7. Djokovic JL, Hedley-Whyte J. Prediction of outcome of surgery and anaesthesia in patients over 80. JAMA 1979; 242:2301-6.
8. Döbrönte Z, Wittmann T, Karácsony G. Rapid development of malignant metastases in the abdominal wall after laparoscopy. Endoscopy 1978 May;10(2):127-30.
9. Falk PM, Beart RW Jr, Wexner SD, et al. Laparoscopic colectomy: a critical appraisal. Dis Colon Rectum 1993; 36:28-34.
10. Fallahzadeh H, Mays ET. Preexisting disease as a predictor of the outcome of colectomy. Am J Surg 1991; 162:497-8.
11. Fleshman JW, Fry RD, Birnbaum EH, Kodner IJ. Laparoscopic-assisted and minilaparotomy approaches to =colorectal diseases are similar in early outcome. DisColon Rectum 1996;39:15-22.
12. Franklin ME Jr, Rosenthal D, Abrego-Medina D, et al. Prospective comparison of open vs. laparoscopic colon surgery for carcinoma: five-year results. Dis Colon Rectum 1996;39(Suppl):S35-46.
13. Franklin ME, Rosenthal D, Abrego-Medina D, et al. Prospective comparison of open vs laparoscopic colon surgery for carcinoma. Five-year results. Dis Colon Rectum 1996 Oct;39(10 Suppl):S35-46.
14. Frazee RC, Roberts JW, Okeson GC, et al. Open versus laparoscopic cholecystectomy. A comparison of postoperative pulmonary function. Ann Surg 1991;213:651-3.
15. Gellman L, Salky B, Edye M. Laparoscopic assisted colectomy. Surg Endosc 1996;10:1041-4.
16. Goh YC, Eu KW, Seow-Choen F. Early postoperative results of a prospective series of laparoscopic vs. open anterior resections for rectosigmoid cancers. Dis Colon Rectum 1997;40:776-80.
17. Hasegawa H, Kabeshima Y, Watanabe M, Yamamoto S, Kitajima M. Randomized controlled trial of laparoscopic versus open colectomy for advanced colorectal cancer. Surg Endosc 2003 Apr;17(4):636-40.
18. Hoffman GC, Baker JW, Fitchett CW, Vansant JH. Laparoscopic-assisted colectomy. Initial experience. Ann Surg 1994;219:732-40.
19. Hughes ESR, McDermott FT, Polglase AL, Johnson WR. Tumor recurrence in the abdominal wall scar after large-bowel cancer surgery. Dis Colon Rectum 1983 Sep;26(9):571-2.
20. Keats AS. The ASA classification of physical status-a recapitulation. Anesthesiology 1978;49:233-6.
21. Khalili TM, Fleshner PR, Hiatt JR, et al. Colorectal cancer: comparison of laparoscopic with open approaches. Dis Colon Rectum 1998;41:832-8.
22. Kirman I, Cekic V, Poltoratskaia N, et al. Open surgery induces a dramatic decrease in circulating intact IGFBP-3 in patients with colorectal cancer not seen with laparoscopic surgery. Surg Endosc 2005 Jan;19(1):55-9.
23. Kranczer S. Banner year for US longevity. Star Bull Metrop Insur Co 1998;79:8-14.
24. Lacy AM, García-Valdecasas JC, Delgado S, et al. Laparoscopy-assisted colectomy versus open colectomy for treatment of non-metastatic colon cancer: a randomised trial. Lancet 2002 Jun 29;359(9325):2224-9.
25. Lacy AM, Garcia-Valdecasas JC, Pique JM, et al. Shortterm outcome analysis of a randomized study comparing laparoscopic vs open colectomy for colon cancer. Surg Endosc 1995;9:1101-5.
26. Lechaux D, Trebuchet G, Le Calve JL. Five-year results of 206 laparoscopic left colectomies for cancer. Surg Endosc 2002 Oct;16(10):1409-12.
27. Liberman MA, Phillips EH, Carroll BJ, Fallas M, Rosenthal R. Laparoscopic colectomy vs traditional colectomy for diverticulitis. Outcome and costs. Surg Endosc 1996;10:15-8.
28. Lord SA, Larach SW, Ferrara A, Williamson PR, Lago CP, Lube MW. Laparoscopic resections for colorectal carcinoma: a three-year experience. Dis Colon Rectum 1996; 39:148-54.
29. Loungnarath R, Fleshman JW. Hand-assisted laparoscopic colectomy techniques. Semin Laparosc Surg 2003 Dec;10(4):219-30.
30. Lumley JW, Fielding GA, Rhodes M, Nathanson LK, Siu S, Stitz RW. Laparoscopic-assisted colorectal surgery: lessons learned from 240 consecutive patients. Dis Colon Rectum 1996;39:155-9.

31. Milsom JW, Böhm B, Hammerhofer KA, et al. A prospective, randomized trial comparing laparoscopic versus conventional techniques in colorectal cancer surgery: a preliminary report. J Am Coll Surg 1998 Jul;187(1):46-54.

32. MilsomJW, Bohm B, Hammerhofer KA, Fazio V, Steiger E, Elson P. A prospective, randomized trial comparing laparoscopic versus conventional techniques in colorectal cancer surgery: a preliminary report. J Am Coil Surg 1998;187:46-54.

33. Nakajima K, Lee SW, Sonoda T, Milsom JW. Intraoperative carbon dioxide colonoscopy: a safe insufflation alternative for locating colonic lesions during laparoscopic surgery. Surg Endosc 2005 Mar;19(3):321-5.

34. Ng CSH, Whelan RL, Lacy AM, Yim AP. Is minimal access surgery for cancer associated with immunologic benefits? World J Surg 2005 Aug;29(8):975-81.

35. Ortega AE, Beart RW Jr, Steele GD Jr, Winchester DP, Greene FL. Laparoscopic bowel surgery registry: preliminary results. Dis Colon Rectum 1995;38:681-5.

36. Peters WR, Barrels TL. Minimally invasive colectomy: are the potential benefits realized? Dis Colon Rectum 1993; 36:751-6.

37. Peters WR, Fleshman JW. Minimally invasive colectomy in elderly patients. Surg Laparosc Endosc 1995;5:477-9.

38. Reilly WT, Nelson H, Schroeder G, et al. Wound recurrence following conventional treatment of colorectal cancer. Dis Colon Rectum 1996 Feb;39(2):200-7.

39. Reissman P, Agachan F, Wexner SD. Outcome of laparoscopic colorectal surgery in older patients. Am Surg 1996;62:1060-3.

40. Senagore AJ, Luchtefeld MA, Mackeigan JM, Mazier WP. Open colectomy versus laparoscopic colectomy: are there differences? Am Surg 1993;59:549-53.

41. Spivak H, Maele DV, Friedman I, Nussbaum M. Colorectal surgery in octogenarians. J Am Coil Surg 1996; 183:46-50.

42. Stocchi L, Nelson H. Laparoscopic colectomy for colon cancer: trial update. J Surg Oncol 1998;68:255-67.

43. Veldkamp R, Kuhry E, Hop WC; Colon cancer Laparoscopic or Open Resection Study Group (COLOR). Laparoscopic surgery versus open surgery for colon cancer: short-term outcomes of a randomized trial. Lancet Oncol 2005 Jul;6(7):477-84.

44. Vukasin P, Ortega AE, Greene FL, et al. Wound recurrence following laparoscopic colon cancer resection. Results of the American Society of Colon and Rectal Surgeons Laparoscopic Registry. Dis Colon Rectum 1996 Oct;39(10 Suppl):S20-3.

45. Walsh TH. Audit of outcome of major surgery in the elderly. Br J Surg 1996;83:92-7.

46. Weeks JC, Nelson H, Gelber S; Clinical Outcomes of Surgical Therapy (COST) Study Group. Short-term quality of life outcomes following laparoscopic-assisted colectomy vs open colectomy for colon cancer: a randomized trial. JAMA 2002 Jan 16;287(3):321-8.

47. Whittle J, Steinberg EP, Anderson GF, Herbert R. Results of colectomy in elderly patients with colon cancer, based on Medicare claims data. Am J Surg 1992;163: 57245.

48. Wise WE Jr, Padmanabhan A, Meesig DM, Arnold MW, Aguilar PS, Stewart WR. Abdominal colon and rectal operations in the elderly. Dis Colon Rectum 1991;34: 959-63.

49. Young-Fadok T, Radice E, Nelson H. Benefits of laparoscopic-assisted colectomy for colon polyps: a casematched series. [meeting abstract] Dis Colon Rectum 1998;41:A47.

Section Three

26 Laparoscopic Adhesiolysis

Peritoneal adhesion is a common cause of bowel obstruction, pelvic pain and infertility. Proper technique of adhesiolysis is important and operating surgeons should have clear concept of mechanism of adhesion formation.

Normal fibrinolytic activity prevents fibrinous attachments for 72 to 96 hours after surgery and mesothelial repair occurs within 5 days of trauma. Within these 5 days a single cell layer of new peritoneum covers the injured raw area, replacing fibrinous exudates. However, if fibrinous activity of the peritoneum is suppressed, fibroblast will migrate, proliferate and form fibrous adhesion. Collagen is deposited and neovascular formation starts.

The most important factors which suppress fibrinolytic activity and promote adhesion formation are:

- Port wound just above the target of dissection
- Tissue ischemia
- Drying of serosal surfaces
- Excessive suturing omental patches
- Traction of peritoneum
- Blood clots, stones or dead tissue retained inside
- Prolonged operation
- Visceral injury
- Infection
- Delayed postoperative mobilization of patient
- Postoperative pain due to inadequate analgesia.

Contraindications

- Hemodynamic instability
- Uncorrected coagulopathy
- Severe cardiopulmonary disease
- Abdominal wall infection
- Multiple previous upper abdominal procedures
- Late pregnancy.

Patient Position

The anesthetized patient is placed on the operating table with the legs straight or lithotomy position if female. The lithotomy position will allow the gynecologists and assistant to work simultaneously and uterine manipulation would be possible. The thighs must not be flexed onto the abdominal wall as they would be in the full lithotomy position used for other open surgical gynecological procedures. The operating table is tilted head up or down by approximately 15° depending on the main area of examination. Compression bandage may be used on leg during the operation to prevent thromboembolism especially if patient is in lithotomy position.

Position of the Surgical Team

Before starting diagnostic laparoscopy a best guess is made about the quadrant in which adhesion is more likely to be found. The surgeon should stand opposite to this quadrant to allow direct view into this quadrant. If the pathology is more likely in pelvic cavity the surgeon stands on left side of the patient. The first assistant, whose main task is to position the video camera, is also on the patient's left side. The instrument trolley is placed on the patient's left, allowing the scrub nurse to assist with placing the appropriate instruments in the operating ports. Television monitors are positioned on either side of the top end of the

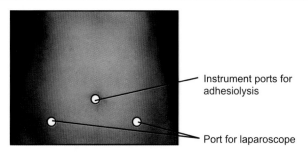

Fig. 26.1: Three ports for pelvic adhesiolysis

Instrument ports for adhesiolysis

Port for laparoscope

operating table at a suitable height for surgeon, anesthetists, as well as assistant to see the procedure.

Port Position

For adhesiolysis of gynecological purposes, generally one optical port in umbilicus and two 5 mm port in left and right iliac fossa should be introduced according to base ball diamond concept after visualizing the target of dissection. Port should be in a position to provide elevation angle of 30° and manipulation angle of 60°, which is ergonomically better. Some gynecologist use suprapubic port, with suprapubic port, elevation angle of instrument and tubal structure is 90° and hence lifting up of ovary and tube may be difficult without grasping it.

A three-port approach should be used if there is any difficulty in manipulation with two ports especially in case of extensive adhesion (Fig. 26.1).
• 10 mm umbilical (optical)
• 5 mm suprapubic
• 5 mm right hypochondrium.

A 30° telescope is employed in most instances, as this facilitates easier inspection of the deeper peritoneal cavity and abdominal organs. The secondary ports are inserted under laparoscopic vision. The selected site on the abdominal wall is identified by finger indentation of the parietal peritoneum.

The open technique for trocar insertion is recommended if extensive adhesion is suspected. At the time of laparoscopic adhesiolysis, surgeon should try to be very gentle with the tubal structure and bowel so that re-adhesion will not form and stricture of tube will not occur.

Viewing of lateral pelvic organs is helped by the manipulation of mobile structure with a solid port introduced through the left iliac fossa port.

LAPAROSCOPIC ADHESIOLYSIS

Animal studies have proved that laparoscopy leads to less adhesion formation compared to open surgery. The less adhesion formation after laparoscopic surgery is because retraction is not used much, packing of the abdominal cavity is not required that can damage peritoneum. In laparoscopic surgery, there is less chance of drying of tissue because inside environment is cut off from outside. Also, the excellent visualization and magnification result into less tissue injury and adhesion. In laparoscopy, port wound and wound at the target of dissection is far away from each other so the chances of adhesion are less to the peritoneum because, for adhesion both the layer which tends to

Section Three

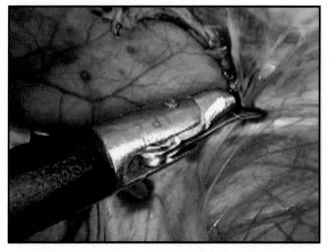

Fig. 26.2: Sharp dissection with scissors for bowel adhesion

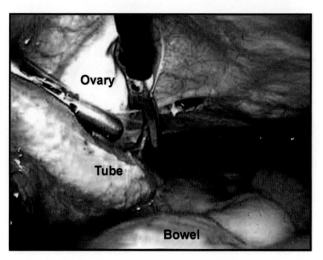

Ovary

Tube

Bowel

Fig. 26.3: Sharp dissection with scissors if bowel is involved

adhere should be in contact. At least three ports should be used to perform laparoscopic adhesiolysis. After access and introduction of telescope two other ports should be introduced according to baseball diamond concept keeping in mind, the center of adhesion as target of dissection.

If the adhesion is thin and avascular, it is easily lysed and the chances of recurrence are not much. In contrast if adhesion is thick and highly vascular it is difficult to separate. Theses adhesion requires use of energy (Ultrasonic dissector, Unipolar or Bipolar). After achieving hemostasis sharp dissection with scissors are necessary (Fig. 26.3).

An atraumatic grasper is introduced to hold the adhesion or involved organ. It should be stretched gently and boundaries of adhesion are identified. The avascular area is choosen with the close-up magnified view of telescope. The opposite trocar on the side of

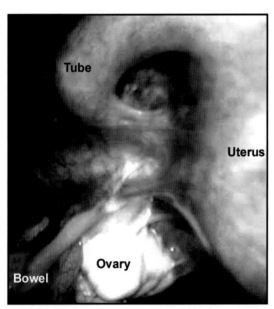

Fig. 26.4: Tubo-ovarian mass with bowel involvement

the surgeon is used for scissors and adhesion should be cut close to the affected organ. Vascular adhesions should be coagulated using electrosurgical instrument preferably, bipolar. Scissors should be used only if flimsy avascular adhesion is found (Fig. 26.2). Thick vascular adhesion first should be tried with blunt dissection, otherwise must be coagulated before being cut. Suction irrigation instrument is good if blunt dissection is thought.

Bowel injury is common during enterolysis and patient who have a history of previous laparotomy should undergo a bowel preparation (Fig. 26.4). If injury, results enterorrhaphy can be accomplished with one layer closure using vicryl. Details of intracorporeal suturing can be found in chapter of laparoscopic suturing and knotting.

After adhesiolysis some fluid can be left inside to prevent recurrence. Steroids and antihistamines were tried but are used infrequently because of adverse effect delayed wound healing and high-risk of dehiscence.

High molecular weight dextran was tried to prevent re-adhesion because it is absorbed over a period of 7 to 10 day. Its osmotic effect draws the fluid into the peritoneal cavity and so the mobile peritoneal organ floats reducing adherence between intraperitoneal organs. Although study in animals has demonstrated reduced postoperative adhesion, it is not fully confirmed for its efficacy.

Adhesion barrier membrane was also tried. These absorbable membrane separate peritoneal membrane from adhered organ and thus prevent fibrous bands from binding different structure. Two such materials are Interceed and Gore-Tex. Interceed is an absorbable fabric of oxidized regenerated cellulose, and Gore-Tex is nonabsorbable, nonreactive surgical membrane. Animal studies have demonstrated good results using these membranes.

BIBLIOGRAPHY

1. De Wilde RL. Goodbye to late bowel obstruction after appendicectomy. Lancet 1991;338:1012.
2. Diamond MP, Daniell JF, Feste J, Surrey MW, McLaughlin DS, Friedman S, Vaughn WK, Martin DC. Adhesion reformation and de novo adhesion formation after reproductive pelvic surgery. Fertil Steril 1987;47(5):864-6.
3. Easter DW, Cushieri A, Nathanson LK, Lavelle-Jones M. The utility of diagnostic laparoscopy for abdominal disorders. Audit of 120 patients. Arch Surg 1992;127(4):379-83.
4. Eypasch E, Spangenberger W, Williams JI, Ure B, Neugebauer W, Wood-Dauphinee S, Troidl H. Frfihe postoperative Verbesserung der Lebensqualitfit nach laparoskopischer Cholecystektomie. In: Hfiring R (ed) iagnostik und Therapie des Gallensteinleidens im Wandel der Zeit. Blackwell, Berlin, 1992;481-91.
5. Fervers C. Die Laparoskopie mit dem Cystoskop. Ein Beitrag zur Vereinfachung der Technik und zur endoskopischen Strangdurchtrennung in der Bauchh6hle. Med Klin Chir 1933;178:288.
6. Fuchs KH, Freys SM, Heimbucher J, Thiede A. Laparoskopische Cholecystektomie—lohnt sich die

laparoskopische Technik in "schwierigen" Ffillen? Chirurg 1992;63:296-304.

7. Klaiber C, Metzger A. Manual der laparoskopischen Chirurgie. Verlag Hans Huber, Bern, 1992;185-206.

8. Kolmorgen K, Schulz AM. Results of laparoscopic lysis of adhesions in patients with chronic pelvic pain. Zentralbl Gynakol 1991;113(6):291-5.

9. Kresch AJ, Seifer DB, Sachs LB, Banner I .Laparoscopy in 100 women with chronic pelvic pain. Obstet Gynecol 1984;64(5):672-4.

10. Luciano AA, Maier DB, Koch EI, Nulsen JC, Whitman GF. A comparative study of postoperative adhesions following laser surgery by laparoscopy versus laparotomy in the rabbit model. Obstet Gynecol 1989;74(2): 220-4.

11. Mecke H, Semm K. Pelviscopic adhesiolysis. Successes in the treatment of chronic abdominal pain caused by adhesions in the lower and middle abdomen. Geburtshilfe Frauenheilkd 1988;48(3):55-9.

12. Meiser G, Waclawiczek HW, Heinerman M, Boeckl O. Der intermittierende inkomplette Dtinndarmileus— sonographische Diagnostik und Trendbeobachtung. Chirurg 1990;61:651-6.

13. Nezhat CR, Nezhat FR, Metzger DA, Luicano A. Adhesion reformation after reproductive surgery by video-laseroscopy. Fertil Steril 1990;53(6):1008-11.

14. Peters AA, Trimbos-Kemper GC, Admiraal C, Trimbos JB, Hermans J. A randomized clinical trial on the benefit of adhesiolysis in patients with intraperitoneal adhesions and chronic pelvic pain. Br J Obstet Gynaecol 1992;99(1): 59-62.

15. R, LE. Causes of abdominal adhesions in cases of intestinal obstruction. Acta Chir Scand 1969;135:73-6.

16. Rapkin AJ (1986) Adhesions and pelvic pain: a retrospective study. Obstet Gynecol 68(1):13-15.

17. Riedel HH, Haag GM (1989) Late sequelae of appendectomy with special reference to adhesions in the lower abdomen, chronic abdominal pain and sterility. Zentralbl Gynakol 111 (16):1101-12.

5. Riedel HH, Lehmann-Willenbrock E, Mecke H, Serum K. The frequency distribution of various pelviscopic (laparoscopic) operations, including complications rates—statistics of the Federal Republic of Germany in the years 1983-1985. Zentralbl Gynakol 1989;111:78-91.

18. Serum K. Operationslehre ftir endoskopische Abdominal-chirurgie. Schattauer, Stuttgart 1984.

19. Serum K. Sichtkontrollierte Peritoneumperforation zur operativen Pelviskopie. Geburtshilfe Frauenheilkd 1988;48:436-39.

20. Tavmergen EN, Mecke H, Serum K. Hfiufigkeit intra-abdomineller Adhfisionen nach Pelviskopie und Laparotomie. Zentralb Gynakol 1990;112:1163-9.

21. Troidl H, Spangenberger W, Dietrich A, Neugebauer F. Laparoskopische Cholecystektomie. Erste Erfahrungen und Ergebnisse bei 300 Operationen: eine prospektive Beobachtungsstudie. Chirurg 1991;62:257-265.

Laparoscopic Sterilization

Laparoscopic sterilization was the first popular minimal access surgical procedure ever performed. Laparoscopic sterilization is straightforward procedure. Worldwide laparoscopic sterilization is now the most commonly method used for family planning (Fig. 27.1).

Laparoscopic sterilization has evolved by Palmer and Steptoe in USA by monopolar technique. Rioux and Kleppinger developed bipolar technique for sterilization because of more cases of bowel injury were reported with the use of monopolar. Later silastic band and spring clips were invented for occlusive method of sterilization.

LAPAROSCOPIC ANATOMY

From anterior to posterior, following important tubular structures are found crossing the brim of true pelvis: The round ligament of the uterus, the infundibulopelvic ligament, which contains the gonadal vessels and the ureter. The ovaries and fallopian tube is found between the round ligament and the infundibulopelvic ligament.

The main problem in laparoscopic sterilization surgery is mistaking the round ligament for fallopian tube. This mistake was more common when single puncture sterilization was used with laparocator.

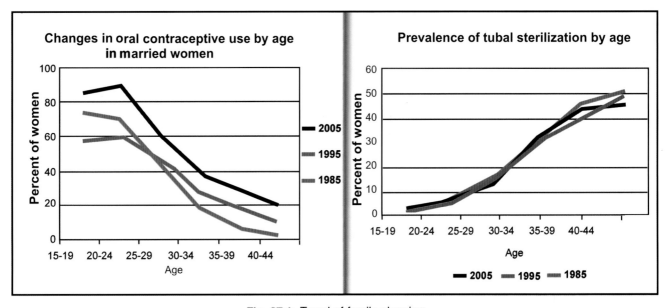

Fig. 27.1: Trend of family planning

In laprocator the image of the target organ and instrument were in the same axis and this was the cause of more incidence of failure. The next most common mistake is injury of the ureter during dissection of the infundibulopelvic ligament. If the uterus is deviated to the contralateral side with the help of uterine manipulator infundibulopelvic ligament is spread out and a pelvic side wall triangle is created. The base of this triangle is the round ligament, the medial side is the infundibulopelvic ligament, and the lateral side is the external iliac artery. The apex of this triangle is the point at which the infundibulopelvic ligament crosses the external iliac artery.

CONTRAINDICATIONS

- Hemodynamic instability
- Uncorrected coagulopathy
- Severe cardiopulmonary disease
- Abdominal wall infection
- Multiple previous upper abdominal procedures
- Late pregnancy.

Patient Position

Patient should be in steep Trendelenburg's and lithotomy position. One assistant should remain between the legs of patient to do uterine manipulation whenever required.

Port Position

Generally laparoscopic sterilization is possible with two ports only. Many gynecologists like to perform tube ligation with one port in umbilicus and other in suprapubic region. In our practice we like to put port in left iliac fossa. The left iliac fossa port will allow elevation angle of instrument at 30° and this angle is better for manipulation of fallopian tube and good ergonomics. If the cyst is on left side, one port should be in right iliac fossa and another below left hypochondrium (Fig. 27.2).

Operative Procedure

Methods of Tubal Sterilization (Fig. 27.3)

- *Destructive*
  1. Unipolar
  2. Bipolar

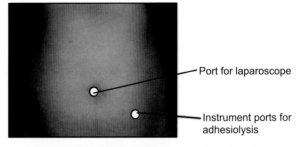

Fig. 27.2: Port position for tubal sterilization

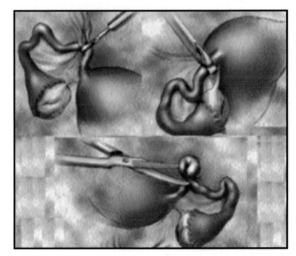

Fig. 27.3: Methods of sterilization

  3. Coagulation using thermal cautery
  4. Ligation and cutting by scissors (Pomeroy technique)
- *Occlusive (Figs 27.4 and 27.5)*
  1. Filshie clip
  2. Fallop ring
  3. Hulka clip.

Laparoscopic sterilization by occlusive method is most popular method of interval sterilization in USA. Use of laparoscopic sterilization in immediate postpartum period is not wise and usually planned 4 to 6 weeks after delivery. At the time of postpartum laparoscopic tubal sterilization there are chances of some complications if performed laparoscopically. At the time of immediate postpartum, the uterus is approximately 20 weeks in size and fills the entire pelvis, rendering insertion of the Veress needle and laparoscopic trocar difficult. Making the sub-umbilical mini-laparotomy incision is fast and easy; often it can be performed under regional anesthesia. There is no advantage to performing postpartum tubal sterilization laparoscopically.

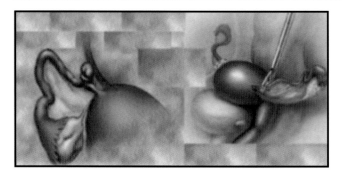

Fig. 27.4: Fallop ring and Filshie clip

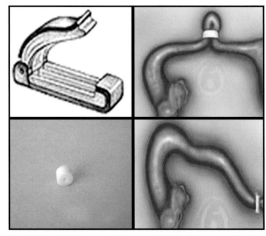

Fig. 27.5: Various occlusive devices for sterilization

Laparoscopic sterilization can be planned together with first trimester MTP but in second trimester again interval of 6 weeks is essential. The main risk of laparoscopic sterilization just after delivery or after second trimester MTP is because uterus is large and may be injured by trocar.

The occlusion of tube in the luteal phase may lead to pregnancy just after sterilization. This creates a medicolegal problem for gynecologist. To avoid this problem, a urine pregnancy test should be obtained on the morning of surgery and patient should be advised to return for MTP if sign of intrauterine or ectopic pregnancy develops.

BIPOLAR COAGULATION

Two port techniques are used for sterilization by electrosurgery. One in umbilicus and one in left iliac fossa. Gynecologist stands left to the patient and camera assistant right to the gynecologist. Uterine manipulator is helpful to bring both the tube under vision.

Fallopian tube is grasped 2 cm lateral to the uterine end and bipolar is activated. If tube is coagulated very close to uterus, there is chance of development of uteroperitoneal fistula containing endometrial tissue due to continuous contractility of uterus. Activation of bipolar should be intermittent and after each activation jaw of bipolar should be slightly opened to avoid sticking of jaw of bipolar with tube. The procedure should be repeated at three adjacent areas.

If the jaw of bipolar adhered with tube forceps should be gently twisted clockwise and counter-clockwise and at the same time the pressure from the handle of grasper is decreased.

Some gynecologist prefer coagulation and division of tube between coagulated area but study has shown that coagulation of 2 to 3 cm of tube without division is better because division lead to significant incidence of bleeding from underlying vessels. Bipolar should be applied always at three places. If only one place bipolar coagulation per tube is performed, there is always a risk of spontaneous re-canalization in about three months.

FALLOP RING APPLICATION

Yoon in 1974, described silastic band technique for occlusive tubal sterilization. The Fallop ring is applied with the help of Fallop ring applicator (Fig. 27.8).

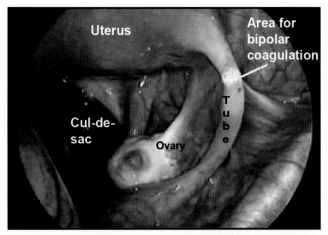

Fig. 27.6: Preferred area of sterilization is isthmus

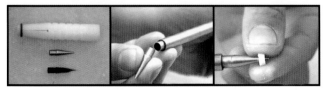

Fig. 27.7: Ring loading

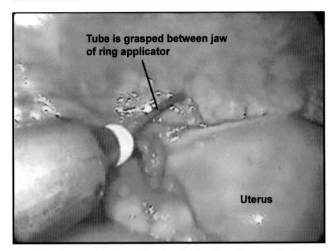

Fig. 27.8: Tubal sterilization by Fallop ring applicator

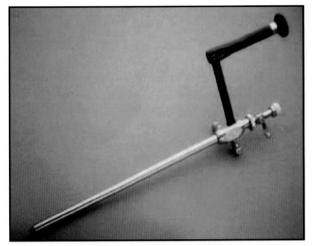

Fig. 27.9: Laprocator for single puncture tubal ligation

Operative Technique

Sterilization using Fallop ring application gained popularity in the 1970s. Initially failure rate was high with single puncture technique using laprocator (Fig. 27.9).

These days double puncture technique is preferred and has less failure rate compared to single puncture technique. Pneumoperitoneum is created in usual manner. First of all diagnostic laparoscopy should be performed to exclude any other abnormality. The Filshie clip or Fallop ring is loaded into the receiving edge of the applicator (Fig. 27.7). The clip or ring should be applied across the narrow isthemic area about 2 cm from the cornua (Fig. 27.6). This area is very mobile and easy to see. In case of desired re-anastomosis, this area is easy to do anastomosis.

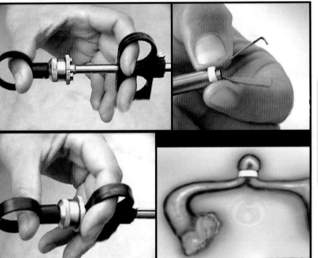

Fig. 27.10: Loading of Fallop ring

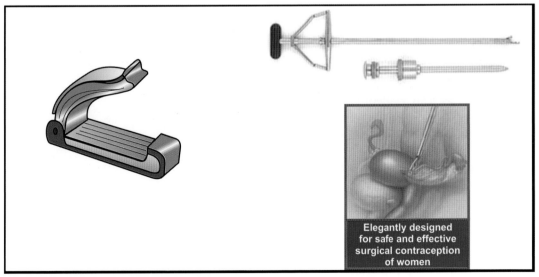

Fig. 27.11: Filshie clip

Section Three

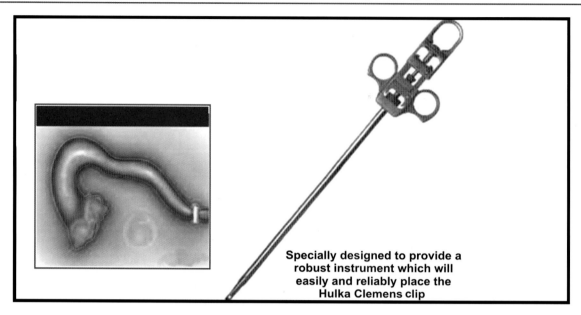

Specially designed to provide a robust instrument which will easily and reliably place the Hulka Clemens clip

Fig. 27.12: Hulka clip

Section Three

Once the fallopian tube is found the atraumatic grasping forceps is used to pick up one of the tubes, one to two cm lateral to the corneal end of uterus. The jaw of Fallop ring applicator is pushed out and tube is then drawn into the inner cylinder of Fallop ring applicator (Fig. 27.8). Once the Fallop ring applicator is fully fired either one or two silicon rubber bands are applied to the grasped segment of the fallopian tube. After application of Fallop ring the grasping forceps is moved forward out of the inner cylinder to release the occluded segment of tube (Fig. 27.10). In the similar manner the contralateral tube is grasped and the ring is applied. After both the tube is occluded some gynecologists inject indigo-caramine dye through uterus to confirm tubal lumen occlusion. The blenching of the tube after clip application can also be seen after successful application of ring. Blench is due to ischemia and this means that the sterilization is perfect.

If everything goes well, patient can be discharged on the same day. The snapshot pictures and video recording of all the procedure is good practice for future references.

Filshie and Hulka clip is also applied with same manner, only difference is that clips does not form loop. Hence, the chances of reversal of sterilization are better compared to Fallop rings (Figs 27.11 and 27.12).

BIBLIOGRAPHY

1. Benhamou, D, Narchi, P, Mazoit, JX and Fernandez, H. Postoperative pain after local anesthetics for laparoscopic sterilization. Obstet. Gynecol, 1994;84, 877-80.
2. Bordahl, PE, Raeder, JC, Nordentoft, J, Kirste, U and Refsdal, A. Laparoscopic sterilization under local or general anesthesia? A randomized study. Obstet. Gynecol, 1993;81: 137-41.
3. Cooper, JM. Hysteroscopic sterilization. Clin Obstet Gynecol, 1992;35:282-98.
4. Davis, A and Millar, JM. Postoperative pain: a comparison of laparoscopic sterilisation and diagnostic laparoscopy. Anaesthesia, 1988;43:796-7.
5. De Wilde RL. Goodbye to late bowel obstruction after appendicectomy. Lancet 1991;338:1012.
6. Diamond MP, Daniell JF, Feste J, Surrey MW, McLaughlin DS, Friedman S, Vaughn WK, Martin DC. Adhesion reformation and de novo adhesion formation after reproductive pelvic surgery. Fertil Steril 1987;47(5): 864-6.
7. Easter DW, Cushieri A, Nathanson LK, Lavelle-Jones M. The utility of diagnostic laparoscopy for abdominal disorders. Audit of 120 patients. Arch Surg 1992;127(4): 379-383.
8. Fraser, R.A, Hotz, SB, Hurtig, JB, Hodges, SN and Moher, D. The prevalence and impact of pain after day-care tubal ligation surgery Pain, 1989;39:189-201.
9. JF Kerin et al. Submitted on October 11, 2002; resubmitted on December 31, 2002; accepted on February 28, 2003,1230.
10. Kerin, JF, Carignan, CS and Cher, D. The safety and effectiveness of a new hysteroscopic method for permanent

birth control: results of the first Essure pbc clinical study. Aust. N Z J Obstet. Gynecol, 2001;41:364-70.

11. Kerin, JF, Williams, DB, San Roman, GA, Pearlstone, AC, Grundfest, W.S. and Surrey, E.S. Falloposcopic classification and treatment of fallopian tube lumen disease. Fertil. Steril., 1992;57:731-741.

12. Kerin, JF. New methods for transcervical cannulation of the fallopian tube. Int. J Gynaecol Obstet, 1995;51 (1): S29-S39.

13. Klaiber C, Metzger A. Manual der laparoskopischen Chirurgie. Verlag Hans Huber, Bern, 1992;185-206.

14. Kolmorgen K, Schulz AM. Results of laparoscopic lysis of adhesions in patients with chronic pelvic pain. Zentralbl Gynakol 1991;113(6): 291-5.

15. Kresch AJ, Seifer DB, Sachs LB, Banner I. Laparoscopy in 100 women with chronic pelvic pain. Obstet Gynecol 1984;64(5):672-4.

16. Ligt-Veneman, NG, Tinga, DJ, Kragt, H, Brandsma, G and van der Leij, G. The efficacy of intratubal silicone in the Ovabloc hysteroscopic method of sterilization. Acta Obstet. Gynecol. Scand., 1999;78:824-5.

17. Lindblom, B and Norstrom, A. The smooth-muscle architecture of the human Fallopian tube. In Siegler, AM and Ansari, AH (eds), The Fallopian Tube. Futura Publishing Company, Inc., Mount Kisco, New York, USA, 1986;13-20.

18. Luciano AA, Maier DB, Koch EI, Nulsen JC, Whitman GF. A comparative study of postoperative adhesions following laser surgery by laparoscopy versus laparotomy in the rabbit model. Obstet Gynecol 1989;74(2): 220-4.

19. MacKay, AP, Kieke, BA, Jr, Koonin, LM and Beattie, K. Tubal sterilization in the United States, 1994-1996. Fam. Plann. Perspect., 2001;33:161-5.

20. Mecke H, Semm K. Pelviscopic adhesiolysis. Successes in the treatment of chronic abdominal pain caused by adhesions in the lower and middle abdomen. Geburtshilfe Frauenheilkd 1988;48(3): 155-9.

21. Nezhat CR, Nezhat FR, Metzger DA, Luicano A. Adhesion reformation after reproductive surgery by video-laseroscopy. Fertil Steril 1990;53(6): 1008-1011.

22. Peters AA, Trimbos-Kemper GC, Admiraal C, Trimbos JB, Hermans J. A randomized clinical trial on the benefit of adhesiolysis in patients with intraperitoneal adhesions and chronic pelvic pain. Br J Obstet Gynaecol 1992;99(1):59-62.

23. Peterson, HB, Xia, Z, Hughes, JM, Wilcox, LS, Tylor, LR and Trussell, J. The risk of pregnancy after tubal sterilization: findings from the US Collaborative Review of Sterilization. Am J Obstet Gynecol, 1996;174, 1161-70.

24. R LE. Causes of abdominal adhesions in cases of intestinal obstruction. Acta Chir Scand 1969;135:73-6.

25. Rapkin AJ. Adhesions and pelvic pain: a retrospective study. Obstet Gynecol 1986;68(1): 13-5.

26. Riedel HH, Haag GM. Late sequelae of appendectomy with special reference to adhesions in the lower abdomen, chronic abdominal pain and sterility. Zentralbl Gynakol 1989;111 (16): 1101-12.

27. Ryder, RM and Vaughan, MC. Laparoscopic tubal sterilization. Methods, effectiveness, and sequelae Obstet Gynecol Clin North Am, 1999;26, 83-97.

28. Sciarra, JJ and Keith, L. Hysteroscopic sterilization. Obstet Gynecol Clin North Am., 1995;22:581-9.

29. Tool, AL, Kammerer-Doak, DN, Nguyen, CM, Cousin, MO and Charsley, M. Postoperative pain relief following laparoscopic tubal sterilization with silastic bands. Obstet. Gynecol., 1997;90:731-4.

30. Valle, RF, Carignan, CS and Wright, TC. Tissue response to the STOP microcoil transcervical permanent contraceptive device: results from a prehysterectomy study. Fertil Steril, 2001;76:974-80.

Laparoscopic Ovarian Surgery

Most ovarian abnormalities can be managed laparoscopically. First laparoscopic salpingo-oophorectomy was performed by Semm in 1984. He reported his experience with a laparoscopic approach to oophorectomy and salpingo-oophorectomy.

Laparoscopy may be an alternative of hysterectomy and more conservative management of pain caused by adnexal disease can be performed. If necessary, oophorectomy can be performed laparoscopically with a short hospital stay and recovery period at a later date.

LAPAROSCOPIC ANATOMY

The ovaries are seen clearly by laparoscope because of their whiteness and knobby texture (Fig. 28.1). It is seen more clearly if uterine manipulator is used and uterus is pushed towards anterior abdominal wall. Ovaries hang down in the laparoscopic field. A normal ovary is almond shaped, and approximately 3 cm in diameter (Fig. 28.2).

The ovarian ligaments run from the ovaries to the lateral border of the uterus. Ovary is attached to the pelvic side wall with infundibulopelvic ligament, which carries ovarian artery (Fig. 28.3). One of the common mistakes is injury of the ureter during dissection of the infundibulopelvic ligament. If the uterus is deviated to the contralateral side with the help of uterine manipulator infundibulopelvic ligament is spread out and a pelvic side wall triangle is created. The base of this triangle is the round ligament, the medial side is the infundibulopelvic ligament, and the lateral side is the external iliac artery. The apex of this triangle is the point at which the infundibulopelvic ligament crosses the external iliac artery.

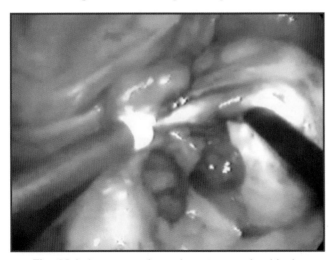

Fig. 28.1: Laparoscopic oophorectomy using bipolar

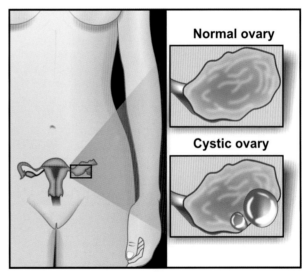

Fig. 28.2: Anatomy of ovary

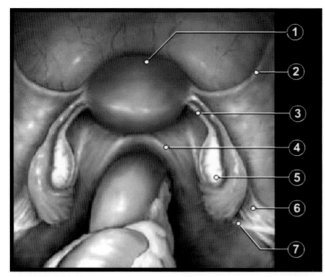

Fig. 28.3: Position of ovary, 1-Uterus, 2-Round ligament, 3-Utero-ovarian ligament (proper ovarian ligament), 4-Uterosacral ligament, 5-Ovary, 6-Suspensory ligament of the ovary, 7-Ureter

The ovarian arteries arise from the aorta to descend lateral to the ureter and genitofemoral nerve. The artery and accompanying vein cross over the external and internal iliac vessels to enter the pelvis. The left ovarian vein joins the left renal vein and right ovarian vein joins the inferior vena cava.

LAPAROSCOPIC MANAGEMENT OF OVARIAN CYST

Ovarian cysts are sacs filled with fluid or a semisolid material that develops on or within the ovary. Surgery is indicated if the growth is larger than 4 inch (10 cm), complex, growing, persistent, solid and irregularly shaped, on both ovaries, or causes pain or other symptoms.

Laparoscopic management of ovarian cyst depends on the patient's age, pelvic examination, sonographic images, and serum markers. A large, solid, fixed, or irregular adnexal mass accompanied by ascites is suspicious for malignancy. Cul-de-sac modularity, ascites, cystic adnexal structures, and fixed adnexae occur with endometriosis and ovarian malignancy. Before selecting any case for laparoscopy, Ca-125, an ovarian cancer marker, should be estimated, that may help to identify cancerous cysts in older women. Although ovarian neoplasms can occur at any age, the risk of malignancy is highest during prepuberty and

menopause. Malignancy is not the only concern in managing an ovarian cyst. Patients who wish to preserve their reproductive organ should have the least aggressive therapy. In a postmenopausal patient whose family has a history of ovarian cancer, Ca-125 levels may help to detect it in the early stages. However, surgeon should keep in mind that many benign gynecologic disorders are also associated with elevated Ca-125 levels, including fibroid uterus, endometriosis, and salpingitis that could lead to unnecessary concern and intervention.

Because the risk of malignancy is relatively low in young women, preoperative evaluation should include a history and physical examination. Pelvic ultrasound should be performed to evaluate both ovaries to rule out bilateral endometriomas or teratoma.

Hormone levels (such as LH, FSH, estradiol, and testosterone) may be checked to evaluate for associated hormonal conditions. The persistent ovarian cysts must be treated surgically, and evolving laparoscopic technology has enabled endoscopic management of most of them. Although most are benign, the possibility of malignancy usually requires a laparotomy using a midline incision.

Oral contraceptives have been prescribed for some small cystic adnexal masses in reproductive-aged women on the assumption that decreasing gonadotropin stimulation to a functional cyst will hasten its resolution. Either danazol (800 mg/d) or oral contraceptive pills with 50 pg estrogen are advised for any cyst suspected of being functional.

LAPAROSCOPIC ANATOMY

Crossing the true brim of pelvis following important tubular structures are found. The round ligament of the uterus, the infundibulopelvic ligament, which contains the gonadal vessels and the ureter. The ovaries and fallopian tube is found between the round ligament and the infundibulopelvic ligament.

The ovaries are seen clearly by laparoscope because of their whiteness and knobby texture. It is seen more clearly if uterine manipulator is used and uterus is pushed towards anterior abdominal wall. Ovaries hang own in the laparoscopic field. A normal ovary is almond shaped, and approximately 3 cm in its greatest diameter.

Section Three

The ovarian ligaments run from the ovaries to the lateral border of the uterus. Ovary is attached to the pelvic side wall with infundibulopelvic ligament, which carries ovarian artery. One of the common mistakes is injury of the ureter during dissection of the infundibulopelvic ligament. If the uterus is deviated to the contralateral side with the help of uterine manipulator infundibulopelvic ligament is spread out and a pelvic side wall triangle is created. The base of this triangle is the round ligament, the medial side is the infundibulopelvic ligament, and the lateral side is the external iliac artery. The apex of this triangle is the point at which the infundibulopelvic ligament crosses the external iliac artery.

Patient Position

Patient should be in steep Trendelenburg's and lithotomy position. One assistant should remain between the legs of patient to do uterine manipulation whenever required.

Port Position

Port position should be in accordance with baseball diamond concept. If the cyst is of right side, one port should be in left iliac fossa and another in right hypochondrium (Fig. 28.4).

Operative Procedure

After access, the pelvis and upper abdomen have been examined, the cyst contents should be aspirated. Once the capsule is opened, the interior of the capsule is examined and suspicious areas should be sent for biopsy. The entire cyst capsule must be removed to search for an early carcinoma. Whether to perform oophorectomy or cystectomy depends on the patient's age and characteristics of the mass.

Ovarian Cystectomy

Medical management of endometriomas has proven ineffective, either laparotomy or operative laparoscopy is necessary. Laparoscopic ovarian cystectomy removes the cyst with minimal trauma to the residual ovarian tissue. Laparotomy for ovarian cystectomy is not a good procedure because of increased risk of ovarian adhesion formation. Three methods to

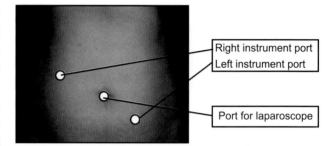
Fig. 28.4: Port position for right sided ovarian surgery

manage such cysts are drainage, excision and thermal coagulation. By excising the unruptured cyst, histopathologic examination is more complete and the risk of recurrence is minimized, but laparoscopic removal of intact cyst is very difficult and aspiration is recommended for functional cysts, which are diagnosed laparoscopically. Many cysts are ruptured during their manipulation despite a delicate technique.

Thermal ablation does not destroy the entire cyst wall, and the underlying ovarian cortex can be damaged by the heat. Therefore, excision of entire cyst wall with the help of blunt stripping and sharp dissection by scissors are recommended.

The removal of a cyst 10 cm or larger is difficult laparoscopically. Aspiration before removal of large cysts is practical and can be accomplished using an 18 gauge needle passed through the separate puncture of abdominal wall while stabilizing the cyst. The suction irrigation instrument can also be used to aspirate the content of the cyst (Fig. 28.5).

If gross characteristics of ovary look suspicious for malignancy. Some gynecologists recommend peritoneal washing before puncturing an ovarian cyst, because any cyst may be malignant. The peritoneal fluid or washings should be sent for cytological examination.

After aspiration capsule of cyst is stripped from the ovarian stroma using two grasping forceps and the suction-irrigator probe for traction and counter traction (Fig. 28.6). The electrosurgery can be used at low power to seal blood vessels at the base of the capsule and at higher powers to vaporize small remnants of capsule. Bipolar forceps also can be used to control bleeding. The open jaw of bipolar can touch the oozing are and hemostasis can be achieved.

Sometimes it is difficult to remove the capsule from the ovarian cortex so that injecting dilute vasopressin

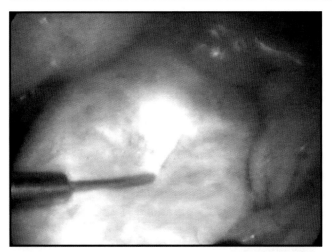
Fig. 28.5: Ovarian cyst is aspirated for ovarian cystectomy

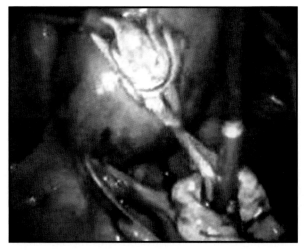
Fig. 28.7: Cyst is being separated from ovary

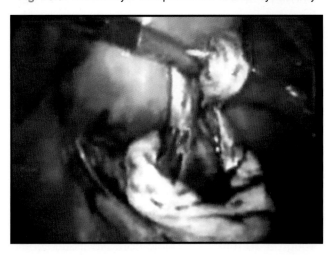
Fig. 28.6: Cystic wall is stripped out from ovarian cortex

forceps can be used to minimize thermal damage. Large cysts sometime need partial oophorectomy, to remove the distorted portion of the ovary, and the remaining cyst wall can be stripped from the ovarian stroma.

Teratoma often can be excised intact but often the cyst rupture. After extraction, if the ovarian edges overlap it self, the defect is left to heal without suturing because adhesions are more likely, following the use of suture. In rare instances one or two fine, absorbable monofilament sutures may be needed to approximate the ovarian edges. The sutures are placed inside the ovary to decrease formation of adhesions.

between the capsule and cortex facilitates the stripping procedure (Fig. 28.7). If the cyst wall cannot be identified clearly, the edge of the ovarian incision can be "freshened" with scissors and the resulting clean edge reveals the two layer, outer layer will be ovarian and inner cystic. If this does not free the capsule, the base of the cyst is grasped, and traction applied to the cyst with counter traction to the ovary. Sometime the complete cyst or portions of the wall may be densely adherent to the ovary, requiring sharp or electrosurgical dissection to completely free the cyst wall. Generally, when the cyst capsule is removed from the ovary, the contraction of the ovarian capsule provides significant hemostasis. Bleeding can occur at the base, particularly if the cyst was close to the hilum. Under these circumstances, a needle electrode or a fine bipolar

Endometriomas

Ovarian endometriosis causes the adhesions between the ovarian surface and the broad ligament. As the ovary enlarges, endometriomas form. Sometime surface endometrial implants penetrate more deeply into the cyst wall, making excision more difficult. The degree of endometrial invasion of the cyst wall forms the basis for differentiating between these two subtypes and is characterized by the progressive difficulty in removing the cyst wall.

The least invasive and the technically simplest approach to endometriomas involve laparoscopic fenestration and removal of "chocolate" fluid without cystectomy or ablation of the cyst wall. However, fenestration and irrigation are associated with a 50 percent recurrence rate compared to 8 percent in the group with the capsule removed. Postoperatively, either

Section Three

danazol 800 mg/d or a GnRH analog is used for 6 to 8 weeks. Large hematomas are associated with periovarian adhesions attaching them to the pelvic sidewall and the back of the uterus, and tend to rupture during separation. After mobilizing the ovary, the contents of the cyst are removed with the suction-irrigator probe and the cavity is irrigated. The inside of the cyst is evaluated and the portion of ovarian cortex involved with endometriosis is removed. Using the grasping forceps and the suction-irrigator probe, the cyst wall is grasped and separated from the ovarian stroma by traction and counter traction. Small blood vessels from the ovarian bed and bleeding from the ovarian hilum can be controlled with bipolar electro-coagulation. The remaining ovarian tissue is approximated with low-power laser or electrosurgery to avoid adhesions. Low-power, continuous laser or bipolar coagulation applied to the inside wall of the redundant ovarian capsule causes it to invert, but excessive coagulation of the adjacent ovarian stroma must be avoided. Sutures, if needed, are placed inside the capsule and 4-0 polydioxanone sutures used. Fewer sutures result in fewer adhesions.

The ability to diagnose and treat endometriosis at earlier stages may prevent its progression and invasion, reducing its adverse impact on health, quality of life, and fertility potential.

Benign Cystic Teratoma

These germ cell tumors occur predominantly in young women. A cystic teratoma contains sebaceous material that is irritating to peritoneal surfaces and can cause chemical peritonitis and possible adhesions. The surgeon should avoid rupturing the cyst. If the cyst is ruptured during excision, it is important to clean the body cavity of all sebaceous material and hair. If it ruptures at the time of excision, without spending much time, the suction-irrigator is placed in the cyst, the contents aspirated, and the cavity copiously irrigated. The interior of the cyst is inspected and its lining is grasped and removed from the ovary. The lining is removed from the pelvis through a 10 mm port, In case of intact cyst an Endobag may be necessary (Fig. 28.8). A colpotomy can be made through which the cyst is incised and drained and its capsule removed. These same procedures can be performed through a mini-laparotomy incision. The cyst wall is punctured

and the contents rapidly aspirated. The wall is removed, placed in an Endobag, and removed through the cul-de-sac or through one of the port wound. Following removal, it is critical to irrigate the pelvis copiously with 5 to 10 L of warm Ringer's lactate. The sebaceous material is less dense than water and will float, facilitating removal. Occasionally, when the cyst is mainly solid, it can be removed intact without rupturing. The cyst wall should be sent for histopathological examination. The pelvis is irrigated with lactated Ringer's solution until all evidence of sebaceous material is removed because incomplete removal of this material can cause peritonitis. During irrigation, the ovarian stroma is inspected to verify hemostasis. If bleeding is present, bleeder points are controlled with a monopolar fulguration or bipolar forceps.

If the teratomas are greater than 8 cm, the ovary can be placed in the cul-de-sac adjacent to a colpotomy incision. Cyst is removed transvaginally which minimizes the risk of contamination of upper abdomen and port wound and maintains a minimally invasive approach. The vagina should be cleaned thoroughly and prepared with betadine before colpotomy. In elderly women or for those patients in whom the ovary and tube cannot be conserved, salpingo-oophorectomy should be considered. When the cyst wall is benign and the tissue is fragmented, it can be removed through a 10 mm suprapubic port. No tissue should be left in the pelvic cavity or on the abdominal wall. Contamination of the anterior abdominal wall should be avoided and if this happens, all tissue must be

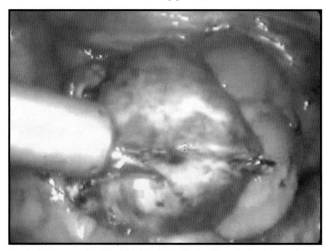

Fig. 28.8: Extraction of ovary

removed and the incision copiously irrigated and washed. Abdominal wall metastasis has been reported following contamination of the wall during laparoscopy for ovarian cancer.

LAPAROSCOPIC OOPHORECTOMY

Indications of Oophorectomy

The most common indications for oophorectomy are:
- Persistent localized pain despite previous lysis of adhesions or ablation of endometriosis
- Residual ovary syndrome
- Dysgenetic gonads
- Ovarian cysts greater than 5 cm
- Tubo-ovarian abscess
- Prophylactic therapy for advanced breast cancer
- Early ovarian cancer in young women.

CONTRAINDICATIONS

- Hemodynamic instability
- Uncorrected coagulopathy
- Severe cardiopulmonary disease
- Abdominal wall infection
- Multiple previous upper abdominal procedures
- Late pregnancy.

Operative Procedure

The port position is shown in Figure 28.9. Properly placed uterine manipulator is important to get a good exposure of ovary and tube. It is sometime difficult to immobilize the ovary because of its smooth surface and finer texture. In case of difficulty in immobilizing the uterus the uterine-ovarian ligament can be grasped by one of the atraumatic grasper to lift and isolate the ovary or the ovary can be wedged against the pelvic sidewall using the flattened edges of the opened or closed forceps. It is important to remember that overly aggressive manipulation can cause lacerations in the capsule, follicles, or cysts and result in bleeding. Before starting the procedure, it is important to observe the course of the ureter as it crosses the external iliac artery near the bifurcation of the common iliac artery at the pelvic brim. The left ureter can be more difficult to find because it is often covered by the base of the sigmoid mesocolon. If the ureter is difficult to identify transperitoneally it must be identified by retroperitoneal

approach. If previous hysterectomy is done it is better to insert a vaginal probe or sponge stick through the vagina so that the surgeon can maintain orientation, particularly with procedures involving extensive adhesions. Many time anatomic landmarks are distorted by adhesions, endometriosis, or prior surgical extirpation. In those cases dissection should be started from the most normal area and then it should proceed toward the more distorted parts of the operative field. Attention should be given that complete ovary must be removed to prevent ovarian remnant syndrome or tumor development in a dysgenetic gonad. At the end of the procedure, the operative field is inspected and any clots are removed with a suction-irrigator or grasping forceps. Pedicles are inspected under water and with decreased pneumoperitoneum and any bleeding if present can be controlled with bipolar electrocoagulation.

Dissection of the Infundibulopelvic Ligament

Three techniques have been described for managing the infundibulopelvic ligament:
- Bipolar electrodesiccation
- Suture ligation with pretied loop
- Stapling.

Patient cost for the linear stapler is approximately Rs. 4500 and Rs. 250 for each pretied ligature. Considering these expenses bipolar electrosurgery is most economical way of dissection and it is preferable for hemostasis of the infundibulopelvic ligament.

Endoloop cannot be applied in the presence of adhesions and distorted anatomy. Sometime it is difficult to place endoloop sutures on large bunch of pedicles such as the mesovarium and infundibulopelvic ligament. If extracorporeal slip knot is applied over wide pedicle, the slipknot can loosen under the tension of the large pedicle. It may increase the risk of intraoperative hemorrhage. If the stump is large a piece of the ovary may be left in the pedicle, predisposing the patient to ovarian remnant syndrome.

Aside from cost, the linear stapling device has several other drawbacks. It should be introduced though a 12 mm trocar. Insertion of bigger trocar can lead to injury of the inferior epigastric artery and predispose the patient to a postoperative hernia. The

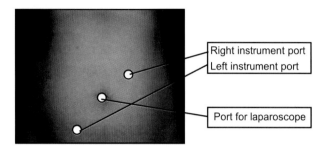

Fig. 28.9: Port position for laparoscopic oophorectomy

linear stapler instrument is bulky and the operator must be careful to its proximity to the ureter, bowel, and bladder. If correct size staple is not selected the staples may dislodge and bleeding may start.

Salpingo-oophorectomy

If complete salpingo-oophorectomy is planned, the ovary and tube can be approached either from the infundibulopelvic or utero-ovarian ligament. Filmy adhesion limiting the mobilization of ovary should be dissected first. If ovarian cyst is found it should be aspirated and deflated, making removal of the ovary easier. The preferred approach is dissection should begin with the infundibulo ligament because it is easier and this approach is essential if prior hysterectomy is performed. The lateral approach is essential if the hemostasis from ovarian vessel is thought. The ovary is held with a grasping forceps and infundibulopelvic ligament is put under traction by pulling it up and medially (Fig. 28.10).

The infundibulopelvic ligament is desiccated with bipolar forceps and cut with scissors from lateral to medial.

It is important to use appropriate traction away from lateral pelvic wall to prevent excessive coagulation and damage to the lateral pelvic structures like ureter or vessels in triangle of doom.

Laparoscopic linear stapling and cutting device can also be used for salpingo-oophorectomy in selected cases. Laparoscopic extra-corporeal Roeader's or Meltzer's knot can also be applied. Pretied loop are easy to use but pedicle should not be wide. In cases of wide pedicel window can be created in mid point of infundibulopelvic ligament and extra-corporeal knot for continuous structure should be applied.

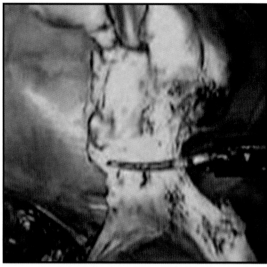

Fig. 28.10: Dissection at the level of infundibulopelvic ligament

Dysgenic Gonads

Sometime dysgenic gonads can be found at the time of laparoscopy and require gonadotomy to prevent gonadoblastoma. The laparoscopic removal technique of dysgenic gonad is same as removing an ovary with adhesion to lateral pelvic wall. In these difficult cases hydrodissection is of utmost importance.

Ovarian Wedge Resection and Ovarian Drilling

Drilling of polycystic ovary is a common procedure performed laparoscopically. Polycystic disease of ovary has various manifestations but its hallmark is chronic anovulation. Ovarian wedge resection is advocated for these enlarged ovaries. However, there is chance of returning to previous inoculators state is quite high after several month. There is also increased risk of adhesion formation after laparoscopic ovarian wedge resection. Availability of ovulation inducing medicines clomiphene citrate around 1970s has offered a non-surgical management of this disease. Initially wedge resection of polycystic ovary was tried but later laparoscopic ovarian drilling appears to be associated with comparable rates of ovulation and conception.

Theoretically wedge resection of ovary and ovarian drilling work by reducing androgen production by ovarian stroma. Ideal patient of ovarian wedge resection or ovarian drilling are woman who fail to ovulate after 3 to 4 months treatment with clomiphene citrate.

The laparoscopic technique uses a 5 mm or 10 mm umbilical port for telescope and 5 mm port in left iliac fossa or suprapubic region. With the help of one atraumatic grasper one ovary is kept held by tubo-ovarian ligament. At laparoscopy, multiple symmetrically placed holes are made over sub-capsular follicular cystic stroma. Polycystic drilling generally does not bleed like physiological follicular cyst following incision. Each ovary is treated symmetrically and cysts are vaporized. The ovaries are irrigated and hemostasis is obtained by the help of bipolar forceps. If aspiration needle is used for monopolar drilling 30 to 40 W current is used in a cutting mode. The power is activated just before touching the ovary and it should be penetrated at 4 to 8 sites at a depth of 4 mm.

Ovarian Torsion

Adnexal torsion is a surgical emergency and if diagnosed early the adnexae can be unwound. It occurs most frequently if there is an adnexal lesion. It occurs generally in young women in whom preservation of ovary may be necessary. If diagnosis is delayed the adnexae may become gangrenous (Fig. 28.11).

If conservative treatment is planned the torted structure is straightened to assess the viability and even ovary that appears infarcted at laparotomy regain normal color after untwisting. Causes of ovarian torsion include par ovarian cyst, functional and pathologic ovarian cyst. Ovarian hyperstimulation, ectopic pregnancy, adhesions, congenital malformation, ischemic structure straightened gently with the atraumatic forceps to avoid additional adnexal damage. In women with ovarian hyperstimulation, the functional cyst should be drained before untwisting. The abnormalities contributing to torsion should be treated. It may be necessary to shorten the utero-ovarian ligament, if its length has contributed to ovarian torsion. A running suture of monofilament material is placed along the utero-ovarian ligament and tied to shorten it, limiting ovarian mobility.

Ovarian Remnant Syndrome

In premenopausal women who had undergone bilateral oophorectomy, small piece of functional ovarian tissue can respond to hormonal stimulation with growth, cystic degeneration or hemorrhage and produce pain. Ovarian remnant remains because of dense adhesion and distorted anatomic relationship, which invariably worsen with subsequent operation. It is not unusual for these patients to have had previous attempt to excise an ovarian remnant. Removal of the ovarian tissue is preferred. Diagnosis is based on history and localization of pelvic pain. Although some patients have cystic adnexal structure or ill defined fixed masses, others have normal pelvic findings. Vaginal ultrasound helps to locate the ovarian remnants. Low or borderline FSH levels in patients with documented bilateral oophorectomy are consistent with the presence of active ovarian tissue. Hormonal suppression, with oral contraceptives or gonadotropin releasing hormone agonist provide no relieve in most patients. Clomiphene citrate or hMG may be used to increase the ovarian remnant size to confirm the diagnosis, preoperatively or to aid in locating the tissue intraoperatively.

The anatomy of the retroperitoneal space should be identified when the ovarian remnant is adherent to the lateral pelvic wall. Space beneath the peritoneum is injected with Ringer's lactate solution and the peritoneum is opened to the infundibulopelvic ligament

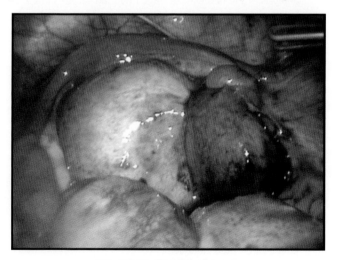

Fig. 28.11: Torsion of ovary

or its remnant. Adhesions are lysed until the course of the major pelvic blood vessels and ureter can be tressed and if necessary dissected. The ovarian blood supply is desiccated with bipolar forceps and ovarian tissue is excised and submitted for histological examination.

Par Ovarian Cysts

These cysts are most commonly found over the serosa surrounding the tubal fimbriae. Usually puncture with fine electrode is sufficient for these patients. Only 40 to 50 watt of cutting current is required for a fraction of second and cyst will burst. Sometime if these par ovarian cysts are large and intermingled with the serosa surrounding the fimbriae and may be attached with lateral pelvic wall. In these cases, opening of peritoneum is necessary for hydrodissection. Once the cyst will leave the pelvic wall; using scissors, laser or electrode it can be dissected nicely.

BIBLIOGRAPHY

1. Acs G. Serous and mucinous borderline (low malignant potential) tumors of the ovary. Am J Clin Pathol 2005;123:S13–S57.
2. Arnhill DR, Kurman RJ, Brady MF, Omura GA, Yordan E, Given FT, Kucera PR and Roman LD. Preliminary analysis of the behaviour of stage I ovarian serous tumors of low malignant potential: a Gynecologic Oncology Group study. J Clin Oncol 1995;13:2752–6. Borderline ovarian tumours and fertility 585.
3. Barnhill DR, Kurman RJ, Brady MF, et al. Preliminary analysis of the behavior of stage I ovarian serous tumors of low malignant potential: a Gynecologic Oncology Group study. J Clin Oncol 1995;13:2752–6.
4. Blanc B, D'Ercole C, Nicoloso E and Boubli L. Laparoscopic management of malignant ovarian cysts: a 78-case national survey. Part 2: Followup and final treatment. Eur J Obstet Gynecol Reprod Biol 1995;61,147–50.
5. Boran N, Cil AP, Tulunay G, Ozturkoglu E, Koc S, Bulbul D and Kose MF. Fertility and recurrence results of conservative surgery for borderline ovarian tumors. Gynecol Oncol 2005;97;845–51.
6. Bostwick DG, Tazelaar HD, Ballon SC, Hendrickson MR, Kempson RL. Ovarian epithelial tumors of borderline malignancy. A clinical and pathologic study of 109 cases. Cancer 1986; 58:2052–65.
7. Camatte S, Morice P, Atallah D, Thoury A, Pautier P, Lhomme C, Duvillard P and Castaigne D. Clinical outcome after laparoscopic pure management of borderline ovarian tumors: results of a series of 34 patients. Ann Oncol 2004;15: 605–9.
8. Camatte S, Morice P, Pautier P, Atallah D, Duvillard P and Castaigne D. Fertility results after conservative treatment of advanced stage serous borderline tumour of the ovary. BJOG 109,376–380.
9. Camatte S, Morice P, Pautier P, Atallah D, Duvillard P, Castaigne D. Fertility results after conservative treatment of advanced stage serous borderline tumour of the ovary. BJOG 2002; 109:376–80.
10. Candiani M, Vasile C, Sgherzi MR, Nozza A, Maggi F, Maggi R. Borderline ovarian tumors: laparoscopic treatment. Clin Exp Obstet Gynecol 1999; 26:39–43.
11. Chan JK, Lin YG, Loizzi V, Ghobriel M, DiSaia PJ and Berman ML. Borderline ovarian tumors in reproductive-age women. Fertility-sparing surgery and outcome. J Reprod Med 2003;48: 756–60.
12. Crispens MA. Borderline ovarian tumours: a review of the recent literature. Curr Opin Obstet Gynecol 2003; 15:39–43.
13. Darai E, Teboul J, Fauconnier A, Scoazec JY, Benifla JL and Madelenat P. Management and outcome of borderline ovarian tumors incidentally discovered at or after laparoscopy. Acta Obstet Gynecol Scand 1998;77:451–7.
14. Darai E, Teboul J, Fauconnier A, Scoazec JY, Benifla JL, Madelenat P. Management and outcome of borderline ovarian tumors incidentally discovered at or after laparoscopy. Acta Obstet Gynecol Scand 1998; 77:451–7.
15. Darai E, Teboul J, Walker F, et al. Epithelial ovarian carcinoma of low malignant potential. Eur J Obstet Gynecol Reprod Biol 1996; 66:141–5.
16. Deffieux X, Morice P, Camatte S, Fourchotte V, Duvillard P and Castaigne D. Results after laparoscopic management of serous borderline tumor of the ovary with peritoneal implants. Gynecol Oncol 2005;97:84–9.
17. Desfeux P, Camatte S, Chatellier G, Blanc B, Querleu D and Lecuru F. Impact of surgical approach on the management of macroscopic early ovarian borderline tumors. Gynecol Oncol 2005;98:390–5.
18. Donnez J, Bassil S. Indications for cryopreservation of ovarian tissue. Hum Reprod Update 1998; 4:248–59.
19. Donnez J, Munschke A, Berliere M, et al. Safety of conservative management and fertility outcome in women with borderline tumors of the ovary. Fertil Steril 2003; 79:1216–21.
20. Donnez J, Munschke A, Berliere M, Pirard C, Jadoul P, Smets M and Squifflet J. Safety of conservative management and fertility outcome in women with borderline tumors of the ovary. Fertil Steril 2003;79,1216–1221.
21. Fauvet R, Boccara J, Dufournet C, David-Montefiore E, Poncelet C, Darai E. Restaging surgery for women with borderline ovarian tumors: results of a French multicenter study. Cancer 2004; 100:1145–51.
22. Fauvet R, Poncelet C, Boccara J, Descamps P, Fondrinier E and Darai E. Fertility after conservative management for borderline ovarian tumors: a French multicenter study. Fertil Steril 2005;83:284–90.
23. Fauvet R, Poncelet C, Boccara J, Descamps P, Fondrinier E, Darai E. Fertility after conservative treatment for borderline ovarian tumors: a French multicenter study. Fertil Steril 2005; 83:284–90.

24. Gershenson DM. Contemporary treatment of borderline ovarian tumors. Cancer Invest 1999; 17:206–10.

25. Gotlieb WH, Flikker S, Davidson B, Korach Y, Kopolovic J and Ben-Baruch G. Borderline tumors of the ovary: fertility treatment, conservative management, and pregnancy outcome. Cancer 1998;82:141–6.

26. Gotlieb WH, Flikker S, Davidson B, Korach Y, Kopolovic J, Ben-Baruch G. Borderline tumors of the ovary: fertility treatment, conservative management, and pregnancy outcome. Cancer 1998;82:141–6.

27. Havrilesky LJ, Peterson BL, Dryden DK, Soper JT. Clarke-Pearson DL, Berchuck A. Predictors of clinical outcomes in the laparoscopic management of adnexal masses. Obstet Gynecol 2003; 102:243–51.

28. International Federation of Gynaecoloy and Obstetrics. Annual report and results of treatment in gynaecologic cancer. Int J Gynaecol Obstet 1989; 28:189–90.

29. International Federation of Gynecology and Obstetrics. Changes in definitions of clinical staging for carcinoma of the cervix and ovary. Am J Obstet Gynecol 1987;156: 263–4.

30. International Federation of Gynecology and Obstetrics. Classification and staging of malignant tumors in the female pelvis. Acta Obstet Gynecol Scand 1971; 50:1–7.

31. Kaern J, Trope CG, Abeler VM. A retrospective study of 370 borderline tumors of the ovary treated at the Norwegian Radium Hospital from 1970 to 1982. A review of clinicopathologic features and treatment modalities. Cancer 1993; 71:1810–20.

32. Lim-Tan SK, Cajigas HE, Scully RE. Ovarian cystectomy for serous borderline tumors: a follow-up study of 35 cases. Obstet Gynecol 1988; 72:775–81.

33. Lin PS, Gershenson DM, Bevers MW, Lucas KR, Burke TW, Silva EG. The current status of surgical staging of surgical staging of ovarian serous borderline tumors. Cancer 1999; 85:905–11.

34. Maneo A, Vignali M, Chiari S, Colombo A, Mangioni C and Landoni F. Are borderline tumors of the ovary safely treated by laparoscopy? Gynecol Oncol 2004;94,387–92.

35. Morice P, Camatte S, El Hassan J, Pautier P, Duvillard P, Castaigne D. Clinical outcomes and fertility after conservative treatment of ovarian borderline tumors. Fertil Steril 2001; 75:92–6.

36. Morice P, Camatte S, Wicart-Poque F, Atallah D, Rouzier R, Pautier P, Pomel C, Lhomme C, Duvillard P and Castaigne D. Results of conservative management of epithelial malignant and borderline ovarian tumours. Hum Reprod Update 2003;9:185–112.

37. Morice P, Camatte S, Wicart-Poque F, et al. Results of conservative management of epithelial malignant and borderline ovarian tumours. Hum Reprod Update 2003; 9:185–92.

38. Nezhat F, Nezhat C, Welander CE and Benigno B. Four ovarian cancers diagnosed during laparoscopic management of 1011 women with adnexal masses. Am J Obstet Gynecol 1992;167:790–6.

39. Pejovic T and Nezhat F. Laparoscopic management of adnexal masses the opportunities and the risks. Ann N Y Acad Sci 2001;943:255–68.

40. Querleu D, Papageorgiou T, Lambaudie E, Sonoda Y, Narducci F and LeBlanc E. Laparoscopic restaging of borderline ovarian tumours: results of 30 cases initially presumed as stage IA borderline ovarian tumours. BJOG 2003;110:201–4.

41. Querleu D, Papageorgiou T, Lambaudie E, Sonoda Y, Narducci F, LeBlanc E. Laparoscopic restaging of borderline ovarian tumours: results of 30 cases initially presumed as stage IA borderline ovarian tumours. BJOG 2003; 110: 201–4.

42. Rao GG, Skinner EN, Gehrig PA, Duska LR, Miller DS, Schorge J and Ottg. Fertility-sparing surgery for ovarian low malignant potential tumors. Gynecol Oncol 2005;98: 263–6.

43. Romagnolo C, Gadducci A, Sartori E, Zola P and Maggino T. Management of borderline ovarian tumors: Results of an Italian multicenter study. Gynecol Oncol 2006;101(2):255–60.

44. Rota SM, Zanetta G, Ieda N, et al. Clinical relevance of retroperitoneal involvement from epithelial ovarian tumors of borderline malignancy. Int J Gynecol Cancer 1999; 9: 477–80.

45. Salomon LJ, Lhommé C, Pautier P, Duvillard P and Morice P. Safety of simple cystectomy in patients with unilateral mucinous borderline tumors. Fertil Steril 2006;85:1510. e1–4.

46. Scully RE. World Health Organization classification and nomenclature of ovarian cancer. Natl Cancer Inst Monogr 1975;42:5–7.

47. Seidman JD, Kurman RJ. Ovarian serous borderline tumors: a critical review of the literature with emphasis on prognostic indicators. Hum Pathol 2000; 31:539–57.

48. Seracchioli R, Venturoli S, Colombo FM, Govoni F, Missiroli S and Bagnoli A. Fertility and tumor recurrence rate after conservative laparoscopic management of young women with early-stage borderline ovarian tumors. Fertil Steril 2001;76:999–1004.

49. Seracchioli R, Venturoli S, Colombo FM, Govoni F, Missiroli S, Bagnoli A. Fertility and tumor recurrence rate after conservative laparoscopic management of young women with early-stage borderline ovarian tumors. Fertil Steril 2001; 76:999–1004.

50. Steinberg M. Cox regression examples. In SPSS Advanced Models 9.0. SPSS Inc., 1999;258.

51. Tazelaar HD, Bostwick DG, Ballon SC, Hendrickson MR, Kempson RL. Conservative treatment of borderline ovarian tumors. Obstet Gynecol 1985; 66:417–22. C. 570 PONCELET ET AL.

52. Tinelli R, Tinelli A, Tinelli FG, Cicinelli E and Malvasi A. Conservative surgery for borderline ovarian tumours: a review. Gynecol Oncol 2006;100:185–91.

53. Trimble EL, Trimble LC. Epithelial ovarian tumors of low malignant potential. In: Markman M, Hoskins WJ (eds). Cancer of the Ovary, New York: Raven Press 1993:415–29.

Section Three

54. Trope CG, Kristensen G, Makar A. Surgery for borderline tumor of the ovary. Semin Surg Oncol 2000; 19:69–75.
55. Vergote I, De Brabanter J, Fyles A, et al. Prognostic importance of degree of differentiation and cyst rupture in stage I invasive epithelial ovarian carcinoma. Lancet 2001; 357:176–82. Cystectomy for borderline ovarian tumor 571
56. Winter WE III, Kucera PR, Rodgers W, McBroom JW, Olsen C, Maxwell GL. Surgical staging in patients with ovarian tumors of low malignant potential. Obstet Gynecol 2002; 100:671–6.
57. Zanetta G, Chiari S, Rota S, Bratina G, Maneo A, Torri V and Mangioni C (1997) Conservative surgery for stage I ovarian carcinoma in women of childbearing age. BJOG 104,1030–1035. Submitted on May 7, 2006; resubmitted on July 20, 2006; accepted on August 31,2006.
58. Zanetta G, Chiari S, Rota S, et al. Conservative surgery for stage I ovarian carcinoma in women of childbearing age. BJOG 1997;104:1030–5.
59. Zanetta G, Rota S, Chiari S, Bonazzi C, Bratina G, Mangioni C. Behavior of borderline tumors with particular interest to persistence, recurrence, and progression to invasive carcinoma: a prospective study. J Clin Oncol 2001; 19: 2658–64.

29

Laparoscopic Tubal Surgery

Tubal diseases are one of the frequent causes of infertility. The most common predisposing factor is pelvic inflammatory disease. Distal tubal obstruction has been managed previously by open surgery using microsurgical technique. The pregnancy rate after reconstructive surgery is 20 to 30 percent two years postoperatively. Laparoscopy for tubal infertility has been a significant factor in reducing- costs, hospitalization, and recuperation. Recently, in women with severe tubal damage, *in vitro* fertilization (IVF) offers a better chance for term pregnancy (72.3%) compared to reconstructive surgery (27.3%). Fimbrioplasty and lysis of peritubal and periovarian adhesions have been associated with good pregnancy rates. In these patients, IVF is appropriate when pregnancy is not achieved postoperatively after a few years.

LAPAROSCOPIC ANATOMY

The fallopian tubes arise from the superior portion of the uterus just above the attachment points of the round ligament. Laparoscopically, the round ligaments overhang the fallopian tube because of uterine manipulation and can be easily mistaken for them. The fallopian tubes towards its lateral end encircle the ovaries partially with their fimbriated ends (Fig. 29.1).

From anterior to posterior, following important tubular structures are found crossing the brim of true pelvis; the round ligament of the uterus, the infundibulopelvic ligament, which contains the gonadal vessels and the ureter. The ovaries and fallopian tube is found between the round ligament and the infundibulopelvic ligament.

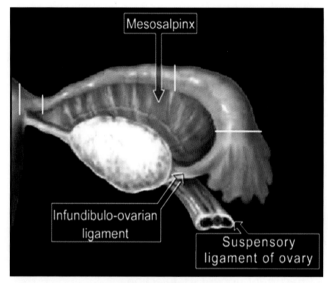

Fig. 29.1: Tubal anatomy

The ovarian ligaments run from the ovaries to the lateral border of the uterus. Ovary is attached to the pelvic side wall with infundibulopelvic ligament, which carries ovarian artery. One of the common mistakes is injury of the ureter during dissection of the infundibulopelvic ligament. If the uterus is deviated to the contralateral side with the help of uterine manipulator infundibulopelvic ligament is spread out and a pelvic side wall triangle is created. The base of this triangle is the round ligament, the medial side is the infundibulopelvic ligament, and the lateral side is the external iliac artery. The apex of this triangle is the point at which the infundibulopelvic ligament crosses the external iliac artery.

The ureters enter the pelvis in close proximity to the female pelvic organ and are at risk for injury during laparoscopic surgery of these organs. As the ureter course medially over the bifurcation of the iliac vessels, they pass obliquely under the ovarian vessels and then run in close proximity to the uterine artery.

Patient Position

Patient should be in steep Trendelenburg's and lithotomy position. One assistant should remain between the legs of patient to do uterine manipulation whenever required.

Port Position

Port position should be in accordance with baseball diamond concept. If the left side of tube has to be operated, one port should be in right iliac fossa and another below left hypochondrium (Fig. 29.2).

OPERATIVE PROCEDURE

Management of Acute PID

Pelvic inflammatory disease usually results from sexually transmitted diseases caused by Chlamydia or gonococcus infection, an intrauterine device (IUD), postpartum endometritis, or hysteroscopy at the time of endometrial infection.

Pelvic inflammatory disease has four primary sequelae:
1. Infertility
2. Ectopic pregnancy
3. Chronic pelvic pain
4. Recurrent upper GIT infection.

One of the worst outcomes of PID is adhesions of reproductive organ leading to infertility and pain. The degree of tubal damage and pelvic adhesions often depends on the severity of the infection, the number of PID episodes, and etiology. Severe peritonitis is associated with a 17 percent risk of infertility compared to 3 percent for mild infection. With each successive episode of PID, the risk of infertility doubles. Despite its typically mild presentation, chlamydial PID results in a three-fold increase in infertility compared to gono-coccal PID. The risk of ectopic pregnancy is 6 to 10 times higher in women who have had PID. In addition, chronic pelvic pain has been shown to occur in 15 to 18 percent of patients after PID, usually because of adhesions. Up to 20 to 25 percent of patients will have at least one recurrent infection because damaged fallopian tubes are more susceptible to infection.

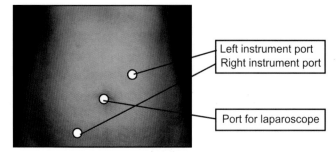

Left instrument port
Right instrument port

Port for laparoscope

Fig. 29.2: Port position tubal surgery

Laparoscopy is being used increasingly in patients suspected of having PID to make a precise diagnosis and thereby avoid the potential sequelae. Prompt surgical confirmation of the diagnosis is possible with laparoscopy. A tubo-ovarian abscess (TOA) can be drained, reducing the risk of serious morbidity associated with rupture. The clinical diagnosis of PID is difficult because of the wide variation in symptoms and signs. Many women with PID report subtle, vague, or mild symptoms that are not specific, such as dyspareunia, post-coital spotting, or abnormal uterine bleeding. In these situations, a bimanual examination may demonstrate cervical motion or adnexal tenderness.

Tubo-ovarian abscess is severe sequelae and occurs in as many as 34 percent of patients hospitalized with PID. Symptomatic or sub-clinical infections can progress rapidly into a TOA. These abscesses can rupture, resulting in severe peritonitis.

At present, surgical intervention is used only to treat a tubo-ovarian mass when medical management is ineffective. The laparoscopic procedure for managing pelvic abscesses has been described by several authors. Once TOA is diagnosed laparoscopically, two 5 mm trocars are placed in both the flanks according to baseball diamond concept through which a suction-irrigator probe and grasping forceps are inserted. The pelvis, upper abdomen, and pelvic gutters should be examined for free or loculated purulent material and the course of both ureters should be identified. Purulent fluid is aspirated from the pelvis, and cultures are taken from the aspirated fluid and the inflammatory exudates. If necessary, the suction-irrigator is used to mobilize the omentum, small bowel, rectosigmoid. Tubo-ovarian adhesions should be recognized until the abscess cavity is localized. After the abscess cavity is drained, the suction-irrigator is used to separate the bowel and omentum completely from the reproductive organs. Chromotubation is not indicated in case of PID because edema in the interstitial tissue of the tube occludes the lumen.

At the end of the procedure, whole peritoneal cavity is irrigated with normal saline until the effluent is clear. Between 300 and 400 ml of irrigation fluid are left in the pelvis to separate these organs during the early healing phase.

Adhesiolysis is technically difficult and associated with a high-risk of complications. Hydrodissection decreases the potential for intestinal or ureteral injury; the laser and electrosurgery should be used sparingly.

Laparoscopy for Adnexal Torsion

Adnexal torsion is a rare gynecologic emergency of women who are mostly at reproductive ages. So there is an increasing trend towards conservative approach for preservation of fertility in young women. Literature has all come to a point of agreement that as minimal surgery as possible and sparing of adnexa for these women of reproductive age since torted adnexa has a benign histopathology mostly. Operative laparoscopic procedures are being performed increasingly in gynecology in recent years. It presents some main advantages over laparotomy. Smaller surgical scars which have better healing process than a single big scar reduced postoperative pain and morbidity; and shorter hospital stays, recovery periods with a lower cost are the major advantages of laparoscopy. For a number of gynecologic conditions (ectopic pregnancy, benign ovarian cysts, tuba peritoneal infertility, etc. The results of laparoscopic treatment are comparable with those of laparotomy. For these reasons operative laparoscopy has become the surgical treatment of choice for the conditions listed above. Like all surgery, operative laparoscopy does bring with it a risk of complications which need to be assessed.

Since mostly the lesions are benign in nature simply detorsion of the torted adnexa and if necessary the cyst excision is the preferred procedure. But what is very important is the time period between the diagnosis and treatment of the pathology. Since the torsion of adnexa causes a relative ischemia of the ovarian tissue, it may result in failure and loss of ovarian function.

In older studies it was advised to remove the necrotic adnexa since they thought that it would cause pulmonary emboly. But in recent literature it is not advised to remove the adnexa even if the adnexa looks necrotic because even severely necrotic looking adnexa may save its function after surgery.

Some literature suggest that only simple detorsion procedure may cause retorsion and the rate of retortion is higher patients with normal looking adnexa and is lower in the patients who have pathologic adnexa and some other procedure also applied with detorsion. Ovariopexy may be applied additionally if especially there is a long ovarian pedicle, more studies are needed to evaluate its value.

In the literature it is shown in retrospective studies that in the patient selection for laparoscopic surgery, size of the adnexal cystic pathology are important criteria that are the mean size of the cyst is smaller in laparoscopic surgeries compared to laparotomy.

Risk factors for conversion to laparotomy are studied in some articles and it is found that the most important risk factor for conversion to laparotomy is previous pelvic surgery and especially hysterectomy. In cases where laparoscopic access cannot be performed, mini-laparotomy is an alternative method and the results are comparable to laparoscopic surgery.

Adnexal torsion in pregnant patients may occur due to drugs used for ovarian hyperstimulation at infertility therapy that increases the size of ovary or due to persistence of corpus luteum or other pathologic procedures of the adnexa. Laparoscopic detorsion and cyst excision procedures were safely applied in pregnant patients even in third trimester of pregnancy. The maternal and fetal outcomes after procedure were satisfactory and comparable to laparotomy. Open laparoscopy technique is advised in literature for the safety of the procedure in advanced pregnancy.

In case of premenarchal and adolescence period, although very rare, adnexal torsion may occur and sometimes an additional congenital malformation accompany. With the advent of new and smaller instrumentation, laparoscopic surgery has extended to include the neonate as well as the pediatric patient. Laparoscopic detorsion and the sparing of the adnexa is the type of treatment encouraged in the literature in case of benign neoplasm, although the patient's numbers are very limited. Some authors suggest contralateral oophoropexy in case of normal appearing adnexa.

In post-menopausal women due to increase in rate of malignant formations, preoperative investigations for predicting malignant and benign lesions is very important. Literature supports that in case of good analyses of the patient preoperatively and the criteria for the lesion to be benign are fulfilling, laparoscopic surgery is safe and if the intraoperative histopathological diagnosis is also benign, bilateral salphyngo-oophorectomy is the treatment of choice. But in advanced centers with a skilled surgeon at malignant procedures, laparoscopic surgery and laparoscopic staging may be performed in case suspicion of malignancy.

Laparoscopic Tubal Reconstruction and Anastomosis

Prior to laparoscopy, most tubal recanalization operations were performed by an operating microscope or with magnifying loupes (Figs 29.3 and 29.4). These reduced tissue trauma and increased the detection of abnormalities. Magnification, which enabled the use of microsurgical instruments and fine, nonreactive sutures, was an improvement over macrosurgical techniques. The combination of the laparoscope and the video monitor make it possible to perform tubal microsurgery using laparoscopic instruments due to magnification.

The serosa of the fallopian tube is delicate and easily traumatized, especially when graspers are used to apply traction. Although laparoscopic Babcock clamps allow atraumatic manipulation of the tube, it is still possible to tear the mesosalpinx and lacerate vessels. It is preferable to use a manipulating probe, a closed grasper, or the suction-irrigator to position the tube and apply traction. If necessary, the tubal serosa should be held behind the fimbria on the antimesenteric aspect using atraumatic grasping forceps.

The fimbria is very vascular and bleeds with little provocation. The bleeding is difficult to localize precisely and frequent attempts to achieve hemostasis may damage tubes. An injection of 3 to 5 ml of dilute Pitressin in the mesosalpinx can be used to decrease bleeding. The removal of any large clots is vital to prevent adhesion formation.

Outcome of tuboplasty depends on the extent of adnexal disease and the degree of postoperative adhesion formation. The adhesions can be filmy,

dense, and vascular and involve the tubes and ovaries. Tubal abnormality and other pelvic disease (i.e. endometriosis, fibroids) also affect the outcome.

Judicious use of suture can improve the operative outcome. A monofilament suture is recommended (i.e. 4 -0 PDS or similar type) (Fig. 29.3).

Desire to perform minimally invasive surgery resulted in the continued performance of anastomosis by laparoscopy. However, the reproductive outcome after tubal anastomosis by laparoscopy has been slightly poor than open procedure. Patients who want reversal of sterilization should show the documentation of the sterilization procedure previously. If previous sterilization is performed near fimbria, the reversal is seldom successful and in these patients, IVF is recommended. If the mechanical occlusion was used for previous sterilization, the tube is not much destroyed and reversal is more successful. The ability to perform laparoscopic tubal reversal is limited by the fine suture and needles required for anastomosis (Figs 29.5A and B). Gynecologists who want to perform recanalization surgery should have good practice of intracorporeal suturing. However, it is possible to prepare the tubes through the laparoscope and either bring the ends through a mini-laparotomy incision or bring the entire uterus out to perform the anastomosis under the operating microscope, using 8-0 polydioxanone suture.

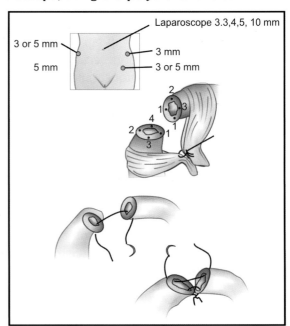

Fig. 29.3: Tubal recanalization surgery

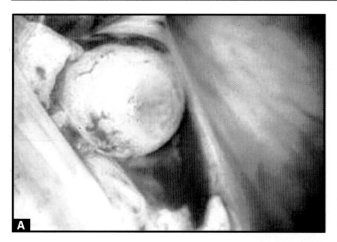
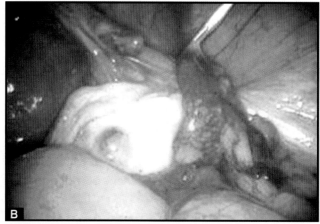

Figs 29.4A and B: Tubal recanalization

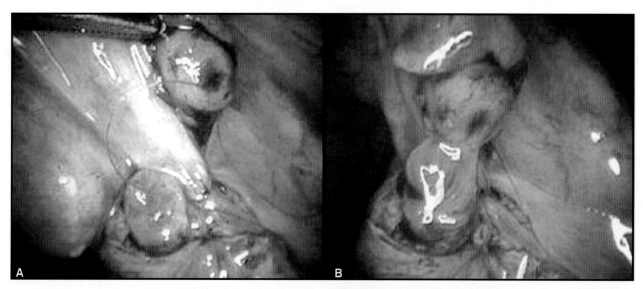

Figs 29.5A and B: 6-0 vicryl is used for tubal recanalization surgery

Successful tubal anastomosis depends on precise apposition of tissues to ensure and restore anatomic integrity (Fig. 29.6).

Fine suture material can minimize tissue reaction and excessive scar formation. Several obstacles have limited the performance of tubal anastomosis at laparoscopy. One of the limiting factors of less success rate of laparoscopic anastomosis is inappropriate intracorporeal suturing skill.

In Europe, the availability of fibrin glue has increased the options for joining tissues without suture. Recently performed randomized prospective study has compared microsurgical tubal anastomosis with anastomosis using fibrin glue. Postoperative

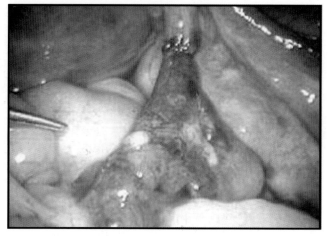

Fig. 29.6: Chromotubation after recanalization

Section Three

adhesions and pregnancy rates did not differ between the two groups.

If surgeon does not have sufficient laparoscopic intracorporeal suturing skill, the ends of the tube are exteriorized through a mini-laparotomy incision and the lumen is approximated with 8-0 or finer vicryl. Exteriorization is aided by using traction on the uterine manipulator to properly position the uterus. Patients are discharged the same day or the following morning.

The anastomosis has been completed after four 6/0 sutures have been tied. Methylene blue dye injected into the uterine cavity emerges from the end of the tube with no leakage at the joint.

With continuous progress in laparoscopic micro-instruments, with refinement of videocameras, and with further improvement of endoscopic surgical suturing skills, it is now possible to perform tubal anastomosis entirely by laparoscopy. However, the success of the anastomosis should never be sacrificed for the sake of performing the procedure by laparoscopy and increasing skill on human patients.

Laparoscopic Management of Distal Tubal Occlusion

A hydrosalpinx is caused by distal tubal occlusion and is characterized by a dilated tube filled with clear fluid. It is usually a consequence of infectious salpingitis and is associated with intrinsic tubal disease. Distal tubal obstruction also can be caused by ruptured appendix, adhesions from previous pelvic surgery, or endometriosis, all of which result in extrinsic disease and do not significantly affect the delicate tubal mucosa.

The pregnancy outcome following tuboplasty is related to many variables that reflect the severity of pre-existing disease. Only a small percentage of patients achieve intrauterine pregnancy.

In contrast, pregnancy rates approached zero when there were numerous dense adhesions. No clear pattern was associated with the risk for ectopic pregnancy. Several scoring systems have been proposed to predict the probability of conception.

To deglutinate the fimbria, a closed 3 mm forceps is inserted into the fallopian tube through the phimotic opening. The jaws of the forceps are opened within the tube; the open forceps are withdrawn. This procedure is repeated until satisfactory.

Neosalpingostomy

Once the laparoscope is inserted, two more suprapubic trocars are placed; the suction-irrigator and grasping forceps can be introduced. The distal portion of the tube is manipulated into position with the grasper or the uterine fundus. Fluid distention of the tube using chromotubation allows identification of the avascular central point, which is generally the thinnest portion of the tube. A cruciate incision should be given using the scissor.

Neosalpingostomy also can be performed by opening the distended end of the tube and then grasping the endosalpinx with an atraumatic grasping forceps, pulling it out and back over the tube like a sleeve. The defocused laser may be used to further avert the edges. The edges of the tube are sutured to the tubal serosa using 6-0 PDS. Tubal patency is confirmed by injecting diluted indigo carmine through the cannula of the uterine manipulator. The presence of fimbrial adhesions may be assessed on close-up view of the fimbria as the dye is injected. The condition of the tubal mucosa can be evaluated by salpingoscopy.

Salpingoscopy

Until recently, it was not possible to examine the tubal mucosa endoscopically. As previously noted, the degree of tubal mucosa damage is probably the major factor in establishing a prognosis for tubal reconstructive surgery. It has been assumed that tubal patency on hysterosalpingogram (HSG) indicated tubal normality. Thus, the selection of patients who could benefit from tubal reconstructive surgery was based on preoperative HSG and laparoscopic appearance of the tubes. Although the mucosal folds can be outlined by HSG, the correlation between radiological studies and endoscopy in assessing the tubal mucosa is poor.

For salpingoscopy first laparoscopy is performed by introducing the laparoscope through the umbilicus and inserting two other accessory ports in both the iliac fossa. The tube is manipulated gently with atraumatic forceps applied to the antimesenteric serosal surface close to the fimbria. Once the fimbrial end is in the line, a 3 mm telescope is inserted through the ipsilateral accessory port and gently placed in the tubal lumen. Normal saline is infused through the Cohen cannula, which has been attached to the cervix. The saline infusion is an essential part of the procedure because it creates space and makes the anatomy of the mucosa fold more visible.

The distal end of the tube can be occluded with an atraumatic grasper if distention of the tube is inadequate. The scope is slowly and gently advanced under direct vision into the tubal infundibulum where the major and minor folds can be seen. In a normal tube, the folds are well formed, parallel to each other, and freely move in the distending fluid. The tubal lumen is followed into the ampulla by advancing the scope and carefully negotiating the bends. In the ampulla there are four to six major folds, each about 4 mm in height, with accessory folds arising from them. Between the major folds there are several minor folds approximately 1 mm in height. When the junction of ampulla and isthmus is reached, the major folds give way to three or four rounded folds. With experience, it is usually possible to follow the lumen as far as the isthmic-ampullary junction.

Salpingoscopy revealed various lesions such as synechiae and denuded areas that were unsuspected from HSG appearance, for a false negative rate of 45 percent. If the tubal mucosa seemed to have an abnormality on HSG, a normal mucosa was discovered at salpingoscopy 21 percent of the time. These data suggest that salpingoscopy more accurately indicates the condition of the tubal mucosa than HSG and that assessment of tubal status by salpingoscopy allows a better assessment of treatment options.

Currently, more infertility surgery is performed by laparoscopy than by laparotomy.

Laparoscopic salpingoscopy permits detailed examination of the ampullary portion of the tubal mucosa and is particularly useful to:

- Detect unsuspected tubal lesions not previously identified on HSG.
- Evaluate the extent of mucosal damage in a woman who has PID.
- Evaluate the status of tubal mucosa in patients who have known tubal disease with or without a hydrosalpinx.
- Decide on management of the contralateral tube in a woman with an ectopic pregnancy.
- Examine tubes before the granulocyte immunofluorescence test.

Complications from this operation are rare; however, it is possible to damage the fimbriae with the forceps, causing minor bleeding or adhesion formation. The most serious complication, perforation of the tubal mucosa, may occur when the scope is advanced blindly or with unnecessary force. Occasionally, bleeding will occur at the level of the fimbria, but usually ceases spontaneously.

Salpingectomy

There are occasions when a fallopian tube is damaged to such an extent that its removal is indicated. Circumstances that frequently require salpingectomy include pathologic conditions such as ruptured ectopic pregnancy, more than two ectopic pregnancies in the same tube, severe tubal damage, particularly if the contralateral tube is normal, severe pelvic adhesions, pain caused by recurrent hydrosalpinx, and large hydrosalpinx or torsion with nonviability of the tube.

Salpingectomy is a relatively easy procedure, requiring those instruments commonly used to perform tubal electrocoagulation for sterilization. The minimum instruments necessary are bipolar electrocoagulator, grasping forceps, scissors, and laparoscope. Once the patient is anesthetized, the laparoscope and two other ports are placed, through which the graspers and bipolar electrocoagulator are inserted. Adhesions that limit mobility of the fallopian tube are lysed and it is grasped at the isthemic portion. The most proximal portion of the isthmus is coagulated and cut using bipolar. If scissors are used, the bipolar electro-coagulator must be removed and replaced with the scissors through the same secondary trocar, or a third accessory trocar is placed. The laser generally is faster and more precise than the scissors. Cutting is performed in layers so there is less chance to cut beyond the coagulated area. Once the isthmus of the tube is transected, the mesosalpinx is alternatively coagulated and cut at intervals of 1 to 2 cm in the direction of the tubo-ovarian ligament.

Alternatives to bipolar electrocoagulation of the mesosalpinx are the automated stapling device, and Endoloop suture. The stapling device is introduced through a 12 mm trocar incision. After lysing significant adhesions and mobilizing the tube, it is pulled up and put under traction. The stapler is used from the proximal to the distal end to staple and cut the tube. One to two applications are sufficient for the entire tube. Before using the endoloop ligature, both the proximal portion of the tube and its distal attachment to the ovary are coagulated and cut. The endoloop is passed around the tube, and the mesosalpinx is ligated with one endoloop and removed. The mesosalpinx is cut above the ligature.

Once detached, the fallopian tube is removed from the pelvis through one of the 10 mm cannula or the operating channel of the laparoscope. The removal of a larger tube ruptured tubal pregnancy or hydrosalpinx, may require an endobag.

BIBLIOGRAPHY

1. Bland-Sutton B. Salpingitis and some of its effects. Lancet 1890;2:1146.
2. Hansen OH. Isolated torsion of the Fallopian tube. Acta Obstet Gynecol Scand 1970;49(1):3–6
3. Gross M, Blumstein SL, Chow LC. Isolated Fallopian tube torsion: a rare twist on a common theme. Am J Radiol 2005;185:1590–2.
4. Krissi H, Shalev J, Bar-Hava I, Langer R, Herman A, Kaplan B. Fallopian tube torsion: laparoscopic evaluation and treatment of a rare gynecological entity. J Am Board Fam Pract 2001;14(4):274–7.
5. Bernardus RE, Van der Slikke JW, Roex AJ, Dijkhuizen GH, Stolk JG. Torsion of the fallopian tube: some considerations on its etiology. Obstet Gynecol 1984;64(5):675–8.
6. Raziel A, Mordechai E, Friedler S, Schachter M, Pansky M, Ron-El R. Isolated recurrent torsion of the Fallopian tube: case report. Hum Reprod 1999;14(12):3000–3001
7. Baumgartel PB, Fleischer AC, Cullinan JA, Bluth RF. Color Doppler sonography of tubal torsion. Ultrasound Obstet Gynecol 1996;7(5):367–70.
8. Blair CR. Torsion of the fallopian tube. Surg Gynecol Obstet 1962;114:727–30.
9. American Fertility Society. The American Fertility Society classification of adnexal adhesions, distal tubal occlusion, secondary to tubal ligation, tubal pregnancies, Muèllerian anomalies, and intrauterine adhesions. Fertil Steril 1988;49:944-9.
10. Bruhat MA, Manhes H, Mage G, Pouly JL. Treatment of ectopic pregnancy by means of laparoscopy. Fertil Steril 1980;33,411-4.
11. Clasen K, Camus M, Tounaye H, Devroy P. Ectopic pregnancy: let's cut! Strict laparoscopic approach to 194 consecutive cases and review of literature on alternatives. Hum Reprod 1997;12:596-601.
12. Cropp CC, Cowell PD, Rock JA. Failure of tubal closure following laser salpingostomy for ampullary tubal ectopic pregnancy. Fertil Steril 1987;48:887-8.
13. DeCherney AH, Diamond MP. Laparoscopic salpingostomy for ectopic pregnancy. Obstet Gynecol 1987;70:948-50.
14. DeCherney AH, Kase N. The conservative surgical management of unruputured ectopic pregnancy. Obstet Gynecol 1979;54:451-5.
15. DeCherney AH, Romero R, Naftolin F. Surgical management of unruptured ectopic pregnancy. Fertil Steril 1981;35:21-4.
16. Fernandez H, Vincent SCAY, Pauthier S, Audibert F, Frydman R. Randomized trial of conservative laparoscopic treatment and methotrexate administration in ectopic pregnancy and subsequent fertility. Hum Reprod 1998;13:3239-43.
17. Fujishita A, Ishimaru T, Hideaki M, Samejima T, Matsuwaki T, Chavez RO, Yamabe T. Local injection of methotrexate dissolved in saline versus methotrexate suspensions for conservative treatment of ectopic pregnancy. Hum Reprod 1995;10:101-4.
18. Ghosh S, Mann C, Khan K, Gupta JK. Laparoscopic management of ectopic pregnancy. Semin Laparosc Surg 1999;6:68-72.
19. Is suturing necessary for laparoscopic salpingotomy? 1199
20. Hajenius PJ, Mol BWJ, Bossuyt PMM, Ankum WM, Van der Veen F. Interventions for tubal ectopic pregnancy. Cochrane Database Syst Rev 2000;2:CD000324.
21. Kawauchi H, Iino J, Ishii T, Nakai M, Kenmochi M. Laparoscopic salpingotomy for tubal pregnancy. Jpn J Gynecol Obstet Endos 1994;10(1):140. Lavy G, Diamond MP and DeCherney AH. Ectopic pregnancy: its relationship to tubal reconstructive surgery. Fertil Steril 1987;47: 543-56.
22. Lang PF, Tamusssion K, HoÈnigl W, Ralph G. Treatment of unruptured tubal pregnancy by laparoscopic instillation of hyperosmolar glucose solution. Am J Obstet Gynecol 1992;154 1216-21.
23. Lindblom B, Halin M, Lundorff P, Thorbun L. Treatment of tubal pregnancy by laparoscope-guided injection of prostaglandin F2a. Fertil Steril 1990;54:404-8.
24. Lundorff P, Thorburn J, Lindblom B. Second-look laparoscopy after ectopic pregnancy. Fertil Steril 1990;53:604-9.
25. Mecke H, Semm K, Lehmann-Willenblock E. Results of operative pelviscopy in 202 cases of ectopic pregnancy. Int J Fertil 1989;34,93-100.
26. Nelson LM, Margara RA, Winston RMK. Primary and secondary closure to ampullary salpingotomy compared in the rabbit. Fertil Steril 1986;45:292-5.
27. Pouly JL, Mahnes H, Mage G, Canis M, Bruhat MA. Conservative laparoscopic treatment of 321 ectopic pregnancies. Fertil Steril 1986;46:1093-7.

28. Reich H, Freifeld ML, McGlynn F, Reich E. Laparoscopic treatment of tubal pregnancy. Obstet Gynecol 1987;69:275-79. Semm K. Advances in pelviscopic surgery. Curr Probl Obstet Gynecol 1982;5:20-5.

29. Tulandi T, Guralnick M. Treatment of ectopic pregnancy by salpingostomy with or without tubal suturing and salpingectomy. Fertil Steril 1991;55:53-5.

30. Tulandi T, Saleh A. Surgical management of ectopic pregnancy. Clin Obstet Gynecol 1999;42:31-8.

31. Vermesh M. Conservative management of ectopic gestation. Fertil Steril 1989;51:559-67.

32. Vermesh M, Presser SC. Reproductive outcome after linear salpingostomy for ectopic gestation: a prospective 3-year follow up. Fertil Steril 1992;57:682-4.

33. Yao M, Tulandi T. Current status of surgical and nonsurgical management of ectopic pregnancy. Fertil Steril 1997;67:421-433. Submitted on October 3, 2003; accepted on January 8, 2003

30

Ureteral Injury and Laparoscopy

URETERAL INJURIES

Ureteral injury is one of the most serious complications of gynecologic surgery. Ureteral injury during laparoscopic surgery has become more common as a result of the increased number of laparoscopic hysterectomies and retroperitoneal procedures that are being performed. Consequently, prevention of ureteral injuries should be a priority during laparoscopic gynecologic surgery. When a ureteral injury does occur, quick recognition of the problem and a working knowledge of its location and treatment are essential in providing patients with optimal medical care. Detailed anatomic knowledge of the retroperitoneum is necessary to prevent ureteral injuries.

The ureters are retroperitoneal tubular structures that extend from the renal pelvis, coursing medially and inferiorly to the bladder (Fig. 30.1). Each ureter travels inferiorly along the psoasmuscle and crosses the iliac vessels at approximately the level of the bifurcation of the common iliac arteries. In females, the ureter is crossed anteriorly by the ovarian vessels as they enter the pelvis. Inferiorly, they are crossed anteriorly by the uterine artery. At this point, they enter the cardinal ligament, approximately 1.5 to 2.0 cm lateral to the cervix before their insertion into the trigone of the bladder (Fig. 30.1).

The ureters derive their blood supply from the renal artery, aorta, gonadal artery, and common iliac artery while they traverse intra-abdominally. These vessels approach the ureter from its medial side and course longitudinally within the periureteral adventitia. In the pelvis, the ureter derives its blood supply from the internal iliac artery or its branches. These vessels approach the ureter from its lateral side and also course longitudinally within the periureteral adventitia.

A significant ureteral injury is defined as any recognized or unrecognized iatrogenic trauma to the ureter that prevents it from functioning properly or effectively. The injury may lead to acute ureteral obstruction (e.g. a ureter that is inadvertently ligated)

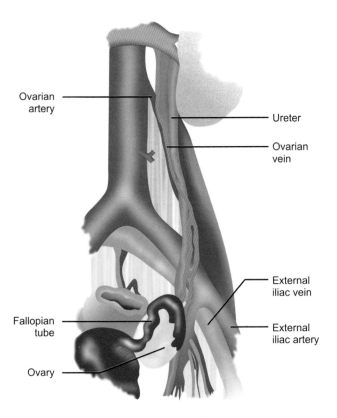

Fig. 30.1: Anatomy of ureter

Ovarian artery

Ureter

Ovarian vein

External iliac vein

External iliac artery

Fallopian tube

Ovary

or discontinuity (i.e. inadvertent ureteral resection). If an injury to the ureter has occurred and is unrecognized, it may lead to chronic ureteral obstruction (i.e. crush injury, ischemia) or the formation of fistulas.

Frequency of Ureteral Injury

The frequency of ureteral injury following gynecologic surgery is approximately 1%, with a higher percentage of injuries occurring during abdominal hysterectomies and partial vaginectomies. Patients who have received pelvic radiation or who have advanced pelvic cancers requiring extensive surgical procedures are more likely to experience a ureteral injury (Fig. 30.2).

The rate of ureteral injuries in laparoscopic procedures varies. While some physicians report that laparoscopic procedures have an equivalent rate of ureteral stricture formation secondary to ureteral injury, other authors argue that the rate of ureteral strictures is significantly higher. More research is necessary before a definitive statement can be made regarding the rates of ureteral injury during laparoscopy.

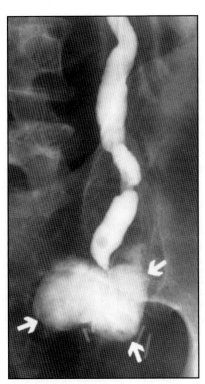

Fig. 30.2: Ureteric injury during laparoscopic hysterectomy

Etiology

The six most common mechanisms of operative ureteral injury are as follows:
- Crushing from misapplication of a clamp
- Ligation with a suture
- Transection (partial or complete)
- Angulation of the ureter with secondary obstruction
- Ischemia from ureteral stripping or electro-coagulation
- Resection of a segment of ureter
- Excessive use of Monopoler which creates remote injury of ureter.

Any combination of these injuries may occur.

Several predisposing factors have been identified in iatrogenic urologic injury. These factors include uterus size larger than 12 weeks gestation, ovarian cysts 4 cm or larger, endometriosis, pelvic inflammatory disease, prior intra-abdominal operation, radiation therapy, advanced state of malignancy, and anatomical anomalies of the urinary tract. Ureteral injuries can be either expected or unexpected, and they may be the result of carelessness or due to a technically challenging procedure.

LEVEL OF URETERAL INJURIES

Intraoperative ureteral injury may result from transection, ligation, angulation, crush, ischemia, or resection (Fig. 30.1).

There are three specific anatomic locations for potential ureteral injury during gynecologic laparoscopy:
1. At the infundibulopelvic ligament
2. At the ovarian fossa, and
3. In the ureteral canal.

Among all the ureteral injuries 14.3 percent occurred at or above the level of the pelvic brim, 11.4 percent occurred at or above the uterine artery, and 8.6 percent occurred at the level of the bladder (Fig. 30.3). The initial procedure in 20 percent of these cases was laparoscopic-assisted vaginal hysterectomy. Alterations to normal anatomy may also hinder identification of the ureters as in severe endometriosis, which may involve the ureter and also cause intraperitoneal adhesions.

Section Three

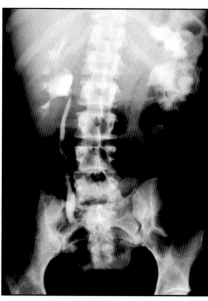

Fig. 30.3: IVP showing ureteric injury

PREVENTION OF URETERAL INJURY

Injury to the ureters can be prevented by meticulous surgical technique and adequate visualization.

Techniques to enhance visualization include:
1. Ureteral catheterization with lighted stent
   Ureteral catheterization with lighted stents have been used to assist in identifying the location of the ureters during laparoscopic surgery to help prevent iatrogenic injury. If the lighted stents are not visible during laparoscopic surgery, 4 options are available, as follows:
   - Change the intensity of the laparoscopic lighting. By dimming the lights, the light from the stent may become visible.
   - Change the camera to a different port.
   - Identify the ureter where it is visible and follow it down to the surgical field.
   - Convert to an open procedure so that the ureter can be palpated and identified.

   Although ureteral catheterization helps to identify the ureters. However, in a large review of major gynecologic surgeries, Kuno et al. found that ureteral catheterization did not substantially reduce the risk of ureteral injury. The surgeon must practice meticulous surgical technique and have intimate knowledge of the ureter's course to prevent ureteral injury.

2. Hydrodissection
   By making a small opening in the peritoneum and injecting 50 to 100 ml of lactated Ringer's or normal saline solution along the course of the ureter, one can displace the ureter laterally and create a safe plane within which to operate.
3. Preoperative intravenous pyelogram
   IVP has been used to locate the ureters in high-risk patients with potentially distorted anatomy; however, this did not decrease the risk of ureteral injury.

RECOGNITION OF URETERAL INJURY

Once a ureteral injury is suspected, the ureter must be identified to assess the severity of the injury. Ureteral injury should be suspected with the presence of hematuria or urinary extravasation. Intravenous indigo carmine may be given to aid in the diagnosis and localization of the site of injury. Unfortunately, the majority of ureteral injuries are diagnosed in the postoperative period. Patients who present with postoperative fever, flank pain, and leukocytosis should undergo evaluation for ureteral injury.

Pathophysiology

The pathophysiology of ureteral injury depends on many factors, including the type of injury and when the injury is identified. Numerous consequences may occur after ureteral injury, including spontaneous resolution and healing of the injured ureter, hydronephrosis, ureteral necrosis with urinary extravasation, ureteral stricture formation, and uremia.

Spontaneous Resolution and Healing

If the injury to the ureter is minor, easily reversible, and noticed immediately, the ureter may heal completely and without consequence. Inadvertent ligation of the ureter is an example of such an injury. If this injury is noticed in a timely fashion, the suture can be cut off the ureter without significant injury.

Hydronephrosis

If complete ligation of the ureter occurs, the urine from the ipsilateral kidney is prevented from draining into the bladder, leading to hydronephrosis and progressive

Section Three

deterioration of ipsilateral renal function. These events may occur with or without symptoms. If the urine in this obstructed system becomes infected, the patient will almost certainly become septic with pyonephrosis.

Ureteral Necrosis with Urinary Extravasation

In complete unrecognized ligation of the ureter, a section of the ureteral wall necrosis because of pressure-induced ischemia. The ischemic segment of the ureter eventually weakens, leading to urinary extravasation into the periureteral tissues. If the urinary extravasation drains into the adjacent peritoneum, urinary ascites may develop. If the urinary ascites is infected, peritonitis may ensue. If the peritoneum has remained closed, a urinoma may form in the retroperitoneum.

Ureteral Stricture

Ureteral stricture may occur when the adventitial layer of the ureter is stripped or electrocoagulated. When the adventitia, the outer layer of the ureter that contains the ureteral blood supply, is disturbed by either stripping or electrocoagulation, ischemia to a particular segment of ureter may result. Ischemic strictures of the ureter may then develop, leading to obstruction and hydronephrosis of the ipsilateral kidney.

Uremia

Uremia results when ureteral injury causes total urinary obstruction. This may result from bilateral ureteral injury or from a unilateral injury occurring in a solitarily functioning kidney. Anuria is the only immediate sign of imminent uremia. These cases require immediate intervention to preserve renal function.

Management

Depending on the type, duration, and location of the ureteral injury, surgical treatment may range from simple removal of a ligature to ureteroneocystostomy Flow chart 30.1. The most common surgical treatments for ureteral injury are simple removal of a ligature, ureteral stenting, ureteral resection and ureteroureterostomy, transureteroureterostomy, and ureteroneocystostomy

Observation

If a clamp or ligature constricting the ureter is discovered, the clamp or ligature should be removed immediately, and the ureter should be examined. If ureteral peristalsis is preserved and it is believed that minimal damage has occurred, the ureter injury may be managed with observation.

Ureteral Stenting with or without Ureterotomy

If tissue ischemia or a partial transection of the ureteral wall is suspected, a ureteral stent should be placed. The purpose of the stent, which is typically placed cystoscopically, is to act as a structural backbone onto which the healing ureter may mold. It also guarantees drainage of urine from the renal pelvis directly to the urinary bladder. It also can work as a gentle dilator since it moves slightly in an up-and-down motion, associated with breathing, as the kidney unit moves. The use of the stent is thought to minimize the rate of

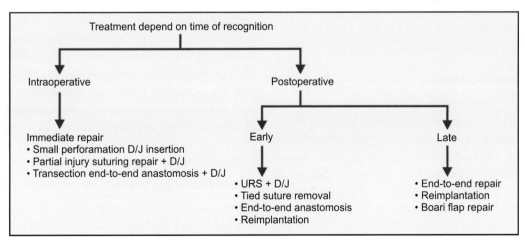

Flow chart 30.1: Treatment logarithm of ureteric injuries

obstruction of a ureteral stricture in the injured area. Alternatively, a ureterotomy may be made along the length of the injured or strictured section of ureter before placement of a stent. Davis described this technique in 1943 (the Davis intubated ureterotomy) in which a ureterotomy is made and left open over the stent. The ureter eventually heals to form a watertight closure over the stent. The stent is withdrawn 6 weeks after it is placed, as it is estimated that all ureteral healing has occurred by that time.

The principles of the Davis intubated ureterotomy have been extended to endoscopic treatments of ureteral strictures. Ureteroscopic endoureterotomy and Acucise endoureterotomy are two modalities that are used to attempt to treat the segment of strictured ureter endoscopically by a longitudinal full-thickness ureteral incision, followed by a stent placement. The success of these procedures closely resembles the success of the open Davis intubated ureterotomy, which approaches 80 percent patency at 3 years.

Ureteral Resection and Ureteroureterostomy

The establishment of an anastomosis between two ureter or between two segments of the same ureter. This end-to-end anastomosis between two portions of a transected ureter can be done by open as well as laparoscopic surgery. If extensive ischemia or necrosis is the result of an injury, the ureter injury is best treated by excising the injured segment of the ureter and re-establishing continuity with the urinary system. If the ureteral injury occurred above the pelvic brim, the simplest reconstruction is a ureteroureterostomy, a procedure that is indicated for injuries to short segments of the ureter (i.e. < 2 cm), in which an anastomosis is performed between the 2 cut edges of the ureter.

Transureteroureterostomy

Transureteroureterostomy (TUU) is a urinary reconstruction technique that is used to join one ureter to the other across the midline. It offers patients with distal ureteral obstruction an option to live without external urostomy appliances or internal urinary stents. TUU is also used in undiversion procedures when the surgeon wants to avoid the pelvis because of previous trauma, surgery, or radiation therapy. If ureteroureterostomy cannot be performed technically and the defect is too proximal in the ureter for ureteroneo-

cystostomy, transureteroureterostomy may be performed. Absolute contraindications to transureteroureterostomy include urothelial cancer, contralateral reflux, pelvic irradiation, retroperitoneal fibrosis, or chronic pyelonephritis. Stone disease, which was once considered an absolute contraindication, is now considered a relative contraindication by some urologists, based on the current ability to prevent stone formation in over 90 percent of patients with medical therapy.

Ureteroneocystostomy

An operation to implant the upper end of a transected ureter into the bladder. If the ureteral injury occurred below the pelvic brim, where visualization of the ureter is difficult and where the vesical pedicles overlie the ureter, ureteroureterostomy is often too difficult to perform. In these cases, 2 types of ureteroneocystostomy procedures are indicated, either a psoas hitch or a Boari flap, in which the bladder is mobilized to reach the easily identifiable ureter proximal to the injury. Boari flaps are contraindicated in patients with prior pelvic radiation, a history of bladder cancer, or any condition with a thick, hypertrophied bladder wall.

Preoperative Details

If consultation with a urologist is indicated intraoperatively, the urologist dictates no specific preoperative preparation. If a ureteral injury is identified after the patient is stabilized following the initial gynecologic operation, a discussion is conducted regarding the possible treatment options. Preoperative antibiotics that target urinary organisms should be administered. If patients are persistently febrile secondary to a potentially infected and obstructed renal unit, percutaneous nephrostomy on the affected side may be indicated. Pertinent radiographic studies (e.g. IVU, CT scan) may be used to help define the location of ureteral injury preoperatively.

Intraoperative Details

Ureteral Stent Placement with or without Ureterotomy

The perineum of patient should be prepared and draped in the standard sterile manner and while the patient sedated adequately or anesthetized, a cystoscope should be inserted into the bladder.

After the bladder is examined and the ureteral orifices are identified, the ureteral orifice on the side of the injury should be cannulated with a ureteral catheter. A dilute cystografin-gentamicin mixture should be injected slowly through the ureteral catheter under fluoroscopy. Fluoroscopy should be reveal the course of the ureter and identifying potential sites of injury.

A Teflon-coated guidewire should be placed under fluoroscopic guidance through the ureteral catheter and up the ureter into the renal pelvis. A double-J stent should be placed over the wire and pushed so that its proximal J-hook is placed within the renal pelvis and its distal J-hook is within the bladder. Then, the wire is pulled, and the stent position is reaffirmed fluoroscopically. Proper length of the stent can be estimated from the measured length of the ureter on retrograde pyelography from the ureteral orifice to the ureteropelvic junction. Allowing for roughly 10 percent magnification from the radiograph, subtract 2-3 cm and select that length ureteral stent. If, after placement, the stent is not well positioned because of inadequate or surplus length, it is best to replace it with a stent of proper dimensions (Fig. 30.4).

If an endoscopic ureterotomy is to be made, prior to placing the stent, retrograde pyelography should be performed to delineate the ureteral anatomy, and a Teflon-coated guidewire, acting as a safety wire, is positioned into the renal pelvis and out through the urethra.

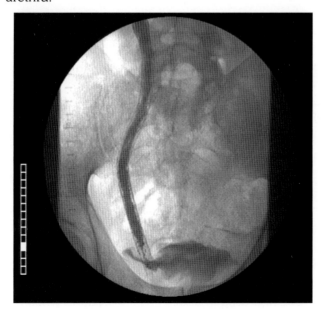

Fig. 30.4: Stent in the ureter

With ureteroscopic endoureterotomy, a rigid ureteroscope should be placed through the ureteral orifice and into the ureter lumen until the ureteral lesion can be visualized. The ureteral stricture is then cut with a probe from a number of cutting modalities, including Holmium laser or electrocautery. A full-thickness incision through the ureteral wall should be made until periureteral fat is visualized. Retrograde pyelography should be performed; extravasation of contrast outside the ureter should be seen. A wide-caliber ureteral stent should be then placed (usually 8F) in the fashion described above.

If Acucise endoureterotomy is performed, the Acucise device should be placed over the safety wire. Once position is confirmed via fluoroscopic guidance and the orientation of the cut is set, the Acucise balloon is inflated and electrocautery is instituted. The Acucise device should be withdrawn, retrograde pyelography should be performed to confirm extravasation, and a wide-caliber ureteral stent should be placed in the fashion described above.

The formal Davis intubated ureterotomy is typically performed intraoperatively only when consultation with a urologist is called for while the patient is open. In this case, the injured ureter is cut sharply in a longitudinal fashion. A stent then can be placed to the kidney and bladder through the ureteral incision.

Ureteroureterostomy

End-to-end anastomosis of the two portions of a transected ureter. If the urologist is asked to evaluate the ureteral lesion intraoperatively, further dissection of the existing exposure is often necessary, because the lack of exposure is the most likely contributor to the injury. Additional blunt and sharp dissection is often necessary to adequately identify the ureter and its course.

If the ureteral injury is discovered after the initial gynecologic procedure, the urologist must decide whether to enter through the original incision and approach the ureter transperitoneally or to make a new incision and approach the ureter using a retroperitoneal approach. Either approach is acceptable, and each has distinct advantages and disadvantages.

If one decides to enter through a previous midline incision, intraperitoneal adhesions may complicate the dissection; however, this approach spares the patient an additional incision.

In contrast, if a modified Gibson incision is made to approach the ureter retroperitoneally, the dissection may be less challenging technically because it avoids the adhesions of the peritoneal cavity, but the patient is left with an additional incision.

Regardless of the approach, a Foley catheter is placed and the patient is prepared and draped in a sterile manner.

In the transperitoneal approach, an incision is made though the scar of the old incision. The dissection is extended down to the peritoneal cavity, and once the small bowel and colon are identified, a vertical incision is made along the left side of the small bowel mesentery. Blunt dissection is performed in the retroperitoneum until the desired ureter is identified. If the inferior mesenteric artery limits the exposure, it can be divided without consequence. If the left lower ureter is the area of the injury, the sigmoid can be mobilized medially to gain adequate exposure.

In the retroperitoneal approach, after the incision is made, the external oblique, internal oblique, and transversus abdominus muscles are dissected in a muscle-splitting manner. Once the transversalis fascia is incised, take care not to enter the peritoneal cavity. The peritoneum and its contents are retracted medially, and the ureter is located in its extraperitoneal position.

The ureter is most consistently found at the bifurcation of the common iliac artery, but it is often difficult to identify, especially when dilated. Steps that can differentiate the ureter from a blood vessel with a similar appearance include pinching the structure with forceps and watching for peristalsis. If peristalsis occurs, the ureter has been identified. Additionally, a fine needle can be placed into the lumen of the questionable structure. If urine is retrieved through aspiration, the ureter has been identified; if blood is aspirated, the structure is a blood vessel.

Once the ureter is identified and dissected from its surrounding tissues, the diseased segment is excised. Take particular care not to disrupt the adventitia of the ureter, because its blood supply is contained within this layer. If difficulty is encountered in identifying the diseased segment, retrograde ureteropyelography can be performed to aid in localizing the lesion. Another option is to place a ureteral catheter cystoscopically up to the lesion; the ureteral catheter can then be palpated during the ureteral dissection.

Stay sutures are placed in each end of the ureter, and the ureter is mobilized enough so that tension-free anastomosis can be performed. Simple ureteroureterostomy is typically performed for ureteral lesions shorter than 2 cm. If the lesion is longer than 2 cm, or if it appears that the ureteral ends will not come together without tension, seek an alternative surgical approach. Options include further mobilization of the ureter, mobilization of the ipsilateral kidney, transureteroureterostomy, ureteroneocystostomy, ileal ureter interposition, or a combination of the above.

Once the ureter appears to have enough length to be anastomosed without tension, both ureteral ends are spatulated. Two 5-0 absorbable sutures are placed in through the apex of the spatulated side of one ureter and out through the nonspatulated side of the opposite ureter. Each suture is tied, and a running stitch is performed on one half of the ureter. The same steps are performed to complete the anastomosis on the opposite half of the anastomosis.

Before completion of the second half, a double-J ureteral stent is placed by first placing a 0.038-cm Teflon-coated guidewire caudally and passing a standard 7F double-J stent over the wire. The wire is pulled after the position of the distal portion of the stent is confirmed within the bladder. Next, a small hole is made within the stent, such that the wire can be passed cephalad, placed into the proximal tip of the stent, and comes out of the created hole in the side of the stent. Once the position of the cephalad tip in the renal pelvis is confirmed, the wire is pulled, leaving a well-positioned stent.

After the anastomosis is completed, a Penrose drain or a Jackson-Pratt (JP) drain is placed in the retroperitoneum and is brought out through the skin. Omentum may be retrieved from a small incision in the posterior peritoneum and can be used to wrap the repair. Adjacent retroperitoneal fat may be used. The anterior abdominal fascia and skin are closed.

Transureteroureterostomy

Transureteroureterostomy (TUU) is a urinary reconstruction technique that is used to join one ureter to the other across the midline. It offers patients with distal ureteral obstruction an option to live without external urostomy appliances or internal urinary stents. TUU is also used in undiversion procedures when the surgeon wants to avoid the pelvis because of previous trauma, surgery, or radiation therapy. A transuretero-ureterostomy is approached best via a midline incision and can be performed using both intraperitoneal and extraperitoneal approaches. A left-to-right intraperitoneal transureteroureterostomy is described.

After a Foley catheter is placed and the patient is prepared and draped in a sterile manner, a midline incision is made, and the peritoneal cavity is opened. The small bowel is packed medially, and the posterior peritoneum lateral to the sigmoid and descending colon is incised to expose the ureter. The ureter is dissected, preserving its adventitia. The diseased portion of the ureter is identified, and a clamp is placed on the ureter proximal to the diseased portion. The diseased portion of ureter is excised, a stay stitch is placed on the proximal segment of the ureter, and the distal stump is ligated. The proximal ureter is dissected for a length of approximately 9-12 cm, while the adventitial vessels are preserved.

Attention is then turned to exposing the right ureter. The ascending colon is retracted medially while an incision is made through the posterior peritoneum lateral to the colon. Blunt dissection aids in the identification of the ureter. Approximately 4-6 cm above the level of transection of the left ureter, the right ureter is exposed to make room for an anastomosis.

A retroperitoneal tunnel is created via blunt dissection, and the left ureter is pulled through the tunnel by the stay suture. When the left ureter is pulled through, taking care not to wedge the ureter between the inferior mesenteric artery (IMA) and the aorta is important, because obstruction may result. Instead, the ureter should be passed either over or under the IMA and should not be angulated or be under any tension. If the ureter is too short and a tension-free anastomosis can only be performed with the ureter firmly wedged between the IMA and the aorta, it is appropriate to consider ligation of the IMA. If this maneuver is not performed and the ureter is left firmly between the IMA and the aorta, a fibrous reaction of the ureter typically occurs, which causes an obstruction that must be treated later with a surgical procedure.

The tip of the left ureter is spatulated, and the medial wall of the right ureter is incised using a hook blade for a distance just longer than the diameter of the lumen of the left ureter. Using 4-0 or 5-0 absorbable suture material, a suture is placed at each end of the ureteral incision from the outside in. Each stitch is run over the course of one half of the anastomosis. Before finishing the second side of the anastomosis, a stent is placed along the entire right ureter using the technique described in ureteral stent placement. The 2 stitches are tied to each other.

After the anastomosis is completed, a Penrose drain or a JP drain is placed in the retroperitoneum and is brought out through the skin. Omentum or any adjacent retroperitoneal fat may be used to wrap the repair. The anterior abdominal fascia and skin are closed.

Psoas Hitch

The psoas hitch ureteral reimplantation technique has been used with great success to bridge defects in ureteral length due to injury or planned resection. Several surgical principles have been historically stressed when performing this procedure, including adequate mobilization of the bladder, fixation of the bladder to the psoas tendon before reimplantation, the use of a submucosal nonrefluxing-type ureteral anastomosis, and a 6-week delay before attempting repair after a surgical injury.

After a Foley catheter is placed and the patient is prepared and draped in a sterile manner, various incisions are acceptable, including a midline, a Pfannenstiel, or a suprapubic V-shaped incision. A midline incision is preferred if the patient has a pre-existing midline scar from a previous gynecologic operation. If entering the peritoneal cavity can be avoided, this incision is preferred.

The peritoneal reflection is dissected off the bladder. Some advocate saline installation in the subperitoneal connective tissue as a way of facilitating this portion of the dissection. If a peritoneal defect is encountered, it can be closed with a running chromic suture. Once the peritoneum is dissected off the bladder, the peritoneum can be reflected medially.

Attention is then turned to dissection and excision of the diseased ureteral segment. The diseased portion of the ureter is identified, and a clamp is placed on the ureter proximal to it. A diseased portion of ureter is excised, a stay stitch is placed on the proximal segment of the ureter, and the distal stump is ligated.

The superior pedicle of the bladder is ligated on the ipsilateral side, and the bladder wall is incised transversely, a little more than halfway around the bladder, in an oblique manner across the middle of its anterior wall at the level of its maximum diameter. When this horizontal incision is closed vertically, the effect of the incision is the elongation of the anterior wall of the bladder so that the apex of the bladder can be positioned and fixed above the iliac vessels.

After the bladder incision is made, 2 fingers are placed into the bladder to elevate it to the level of the proximal end of the ureter. If the bladder does not reach the proximal ureter, several steps can be performed for additional length. These steps include extending the bladder wall incision laterally to obtain further length, or the peritoneum and connective tissue from the pelvic and lateral walls may be dissected from the contralateral side of the bladder. This dissection may require ligation and division of the superior vesical pedicle on the contralateral side.

Once adequate mobilization of the bladder has occurred, the bladder is held against the tendinous portion of the psoas minor muscle without tension. Prolene sutures (2-0) are sutured into the bladder wall and to the tendon to fix the bladder in place.

With the bladder open, attention is turned to the ureteral reimplant. An incision is made in the bladder mucosa at the proposed site of the new ureteral orifice. A submucosal dissection occurs approximately 3 cm from the incision site so that a tunnel is created. Lahey scissors may be used to facilitate this dissection. After achieving a 3-cm tunnel length, the scissors are inverted and the tips are pushed through the bladder wall. An 8F feeding tube is passed over the scissor blades, and the stay suture on the proximal tip of the ureter is tied to the other end of the catheter so that traction on the catheter draws the ureter into the bladder. The ureteral tip is trimmed obliquely, and 4-6 absorbable sutures (4-0) are used to fix the ureter to the bladder mucosa. The ureteral adventitia is tacked to the extravesical bladder wall with several 4-0 absorbable sutures. A double-J ureteral stent may be placed at this time.

A nontunneled reimplant is also an acceptable choice in most adults if ureteral length is insufficient. The end of the ureter can be reflected back after making a small longitudinal incision from the tip proximally about 1.5 cm. This will make the end of the ureter into a nonrefluxing nipple, which is useful when there is inadequate length for an antirefluxing submucosal tunnel.

After completing the reimplant, 2 fingers are placed within the bladder, while 5 or 6 absorbable sutures (2-0) are placed within the bladder muscle, the psoas muscle, and the psoas minor tendon, paying specific attention not to suture the genitofemoral nerve. Alternatively, sutures may also take deep bites in the muscle itself. The bladder is closed with a 3-0 running absorbable suture on the mucosa and a running 2-0 suture incorporating the bladder muscle and adventitial layers. A Penrose drain or a JP drain is placed in the retroperitoneum next to the bladder closure. The anterior abdominal fascia and the skin then are closed.

Boari Flap

A Boari flap may be required to bridge long defects of the middle and lower ureter to the bladder. Laparoscopic construction of a Boari flap was performed in a patient with a ureteral stricture secondary to iatrogenic injury. The salient steps performed were spatulation of the transected ureteral end, fashioning of a Boari flap from the bladder, end-to-side anastomosis of the ureter to the flap, placement of a stent with the aid of a suction cannula, and closure of the flap over the stent. A Boari flap can be accomplished laparoscopically with minimal morbidity.

After preparing and draping the patient, a midline or Pfannenstiel incision is made. Once the transversalis fascia is incised, the ureter may be approached either transperitoneally or retroperitoneally. In the transperitoneal approach, the peritoneal cavity is entered, the sigmoid or cecum is reflected medially, the posterior peritoneum is incised, and the ureter is identified. In the retroperitoneal approach, care is taken not to enter the peritoneal cavity, the peritoneum is mobilized medially, and the ureter is identified and exposed. A stay stitch is placed in healthy ureter tissue just proximal to the injury. The remaining end of the ureter is tied off.

The peritoneum is then dissected from the wall of the bladder. This dissection may be facilitated with hydrodissection, in which saline is injected subperitoneally, separating the peritoneal layer from the muscle layers of the bladder.

The necessary length of the bladder flap (i.e. the distance between the posterior wall of the bladder and the end of the healthy proximal ureter) is measured with umbilical tape, the bladder is one half full of saline, and the length and shape of the bladder flap are planned. To measure accurately on the dome of the bladder, several stay stitches are placed at the base of the proposed bladder flap and at the apex. The bladder flap should be planned with a large base, because the base will contain the blood supply for the flap. The length of the bladder flap (i.e. the distance between the base and apex) should equal the distance between the posterior wall of the bladder and the end of the healthy proximal ureter. The width of the apex should be at least 3 times the diameter of the ureter to prevent constriction after the flap is tubularized. Avoid scarred areas of the bladder.

After proper planning, an outline of the flap is made in the bladder wall with coagulating current, and the bladder flap is remeasured. If the measurements are satisfactory, the bladder flap is cut via cutting current, and the concomitant bleeding vessels are coagulated.

After the bladder flap is turned superiorly, Lahey scissors are used to prepare a ureteral tunnel. The tunnel should be at least 3 cm long and is created by placing the Lahey scissors submucosally at the apex of the flap, tunneling the appropriate distance and coming out through the mucosa. Submucosal injection of saline may aid in this dissection. An 8F feeding tube is pulled through the tunnel by the scissors and the stay suture on the proximal ureter is tied to the feeding tube after the ureteral end is spatulated. The feeding tube is pulled toward the bladder, followed by the ureter. The stay suture is cut after the ureter has traveled completely through the tunnel.

The bladder flap is sutured to the psoas tendon of the psoas minor with a few 2-0 absorbable sutures. These sutures fix the flap in place to prevent tension on the ureteral anastomosis.

The ureter is anastomosed to the bladder mucosa with several 4-0 absorbable sutures. A few of the sutures should include the muscle layer of the bladder to fix the ureter into place. An 8F feeding tube is passed up the ureter into the renal pelvis and out through the bladder and body wall.

Before closing the bladder, a large suprapubic tube is placed, i.e. either a 22-24F Malecot or Foley. Then, the bladder is closed by approximating the bladder mucosa with a 3-0 absorbable running suture followed by a second row of running sutures, which approximates the muscularis and adventitial layers. A few absorbable sutures (5-0) can be placed to approximate the distal end of the flap to the adventitia of the ureter. If a transperitoneal approach is used, close the peritoneum and then place a Penrose or a JP drain retroperitoneally adjacent to the bladder closure. The anterior abdominal fascia and skin are closed.

Postoperative Details

Ureteral Stent

After the patient has recovered from anesthesia and is in suitable condition, the patient may be discharged with instructions to return to the clinic in 14-21 days, when the stent will be removed. The patient is discharged with 3 days of antibiotics and oral analgesics for potential bouts of discomfort from the stent.

Ureteroureterostomy, Transureteroureterostomy, Psoas Hitch and Boari Flap

Patients who underwent a transperitoneal approach are kept on a regimen of nothing by mouth (NPO) for the first day after surgery. Subsequently, signs of bowel function are monitored routinely. Once bowel sounds are present, the diet is advanced to clear liquids, and when the patient passes flatus, a regular diet is instituted.

Patients who undergo a retroperitoneal approach are started on clear liquids on the first day after surgery unless they are nauseous. Their diets are also advanced when they have passed flatus.

All patients receive a patient-controlled anesthetic (PCA) pump postoperatively unless they had an epidural catheter placed intraoperatively. They are then given an epidural pump. Oral analgesics are administered after patients tolerate a regular diet.

All patients receive a 24 hours course of intravenous antibiotics to prevent wound infections.

Patients are encouraged to ambulate on the first day after surgery. Once the pain is controlled with oral analgesics and patients are tolerating a regular diet, they are eligible for discharge, with or without their drains. If drains are not removed in the hospital, set appointments to assess patients and their drains in the clinic.

Follow-up

In patients who do not require a cystotomy, the Foley catheter or suprapubic tube is left to drain the bladder until the drain output from the Penrose or JP drain is less than 30 mL per day. If this is achieved, the Foley catheter can be removed or the suprapubic tube can be clamped, and the output from the Penrose or JP drain is monitored. If no drainage occurs, the drain can be removed. If drainage increases from the previous level, the Foley catheter is replaced, or the suprapubic tube is unclamped. After several days, the same sequence of events occurs to determine whether the ureter has healed completely. If a stent or feeding tube is used, it can be removed 7-10 days after surgery.

In patients who require cystotomy, the Foley catheter or suprapubic tube is left in place for 7-10 days after surgery, at which time cystography is usually performed. If no extravasation is observed during the cystogram, the Foley catheter or suprapubic tube can be removed. At the same time, the outputs from the Penrose or JP drain are monitored. If no drainage occurs, the drain can be removed. If drain output increases from the previous level, the Foley catheter is replaced. After several days, the same sequence of events occurs to determine whether the ureter has healed completely. If a stent is used, the stent is removed 10-14 days after surgery.

Laparoscopic surgery has become a surgical discipline in its own right. Like any other surgical technique it does involve a risk of complications. This risk of ureteral injury is related to the complexity of the laparoscopic procedure. The set-up phase for laparoscopy must never be considered banal. The methods of postoperative monitoring must be adapted to take into account the shorter hospital stay and the fact that a considerable number of ureteral injury go unnoticed intraoperatively.

CONCLUSION

• Awareness of risk factors and good experience in laparoscopy are the main factors in preventing and reducing the Ureteric injuries.

• Immediate and early diagnosis of ureteral injuries gives excellent out come and minimal morbidty. While delayed diagnosis had prolong morbidity.
• For any suspicious of Ureteric injury investigation should be done to role out the injury.
• Placement of stent is helpful specially in difficult cases reduce rate of Ureteric injury.
• Intraoperative cystoscopy during laparoscopy leads to immediate diagnosis of Ureteric injuries.
• Excessive use of diathermy near the Ureter follow by thermal injury.

BIBLIOGRAPHY

1. Alleyassin A, Khademi A, Aghahosseini M, Safdarian L, Badenoosh B, Akbari HE. Comparison of success rates in the medical management of ectopic pregnancy with single-dose and multiple dose administration of methotrexate: a prospective, randomized clinical trial. Fertil Steril 2006;85:1661–6.
2. Ankum WM, Vander Veen F, Hamerlynck HV, Lammes FB. Suspected ectopic pregnancy. What to do when human chorionic gonadotropin levels are below the discriminatory zone. Suspected ectopic pregnancy. J Reprod Med 1995;40:525–8.
3. Bender S. Fertility after tuba pregnancy. J. Obstet. Gynecol Br. Cmtth. 1956;63:400-03.
4. Boury-Heyler C, Madelenat P. Surgical treatment of 150 cases of extrauterine pregnancy. Chirurgie, 1983;109: 395–8.
5. Bouyer J, Job-Spira N, Pouly J, Coste J, Germain E, Fernandez H. Fertility following radical, conservative-surgical or medical treatment for tubal pregnancy: a population-based study. BJOG 2000;107:714–21.
6. Bruhat MA, Manhes H, Mage G, Pouly JL. Treatment of ectopic pregnancy by means of laparoscopy. Fenil. Steril 1980;33:411-4.
7. Carp MJ, Oelsner G, Serr DM, Mashiach S. Fertility after non surgical treatment of ectopic pregnancy. J Reprod Med 1986;31:119.
8. Cartwright PS. Peritoneal trophoblastic implants after surgical management pregnancy. J Reprod Med 1991;36:523–4.
9. Chapron C, Querleu D, Crepin G. Laparoscopic treatment of ectopic pregnancy: a one hundred cases study. Eur J Obstet Gynecol Reprod Biol 1991;41:187–90.
10. Clausen I. Conservative versus radical surgery for tubal pregnancy. Acta Obstet Gynecol Scand 1996;75:8–12.
11. Condous G, Okaro E, Khalid A, Timmerman DL, Zhou Y, van HS, Bourne T. The use of a new logistic regression model for predicting the outcome of pregnancies of unknown location. Hum Reprod 2004;19:1900–1910.
12. Cutler SJ, Ederer F. Maximum utilization of life table methods in analyzing survival. J Chronic Dis 1958;8:699–707.

13. D Flamant R, and Lellouch J. Clinical Trials. Academic Press, London, 1980;214–23.
14. DeChemey AH and Boyer SP. Laparoscopic salpingostomy for ectopic pregnancy. Obstet Gynecol 1987;70:948–50.
15. Dias Pereira G, Hajenius PJ, Mol BWJ, Ankum WM, Hemrika DJ, Bossuyt PMM. Fertility outcome after systemic methotrexate and laparoscopic salpingostomy for tubal pregnancy. Lancet 1999;353:724–5.
16. Donnez J and Nisolle M. Laparoscopic treatment of ampullary tubal pregnancy. J Gynecol Surg 1989;5:157–62.
17. Douglas J and Shingleton HM. Surgical management of tubal pregnancy: effect on subsequent fertility. South. Med. J 1969;62:954.
18. Dubuisson JB, Aubriot FX, Cardone V. Laparoscopic salpingectomy for tubal pregnancy. Fenil, Steril 1987;47:225–8.
19. Dubuisson JB, Aubriot EX, Foulot H et al. Reproductive outcome after laparoscopic salpingectomy for tubal pregnancy. Fenil. Steril. 1990;S3:1004–07.
20. Egarter C, Kiss H, Husslein P. Prostaglandin versus expectant management in early tubal pregnancy. Prostaglandins Leukot Essent Fatty Acids 1991;42:177–9.
21. Elmoghazy DAM and Nour-El-Dine NM. Prevention of persistent ectopic pregnancy with single dose methotrexate after surgical conservation of the tube. Abstracts of the XVI FIGO World Congress of Obstetrics and Gynecology 2000, 57.
22. El-Sherbiny MT, El G I, Mera IM. Methotrexate verus laparoscopic surgery for the management of unruptured tubal pregnancy. Middle East Fertil Soc J 2003;8:256–62.
23. Fedele L, Bianchi S, Tozzi L, Zanconato G, Silvestre V. Intramesosalpingeal injection of oxytocin in conservative laparoscopic treatment for tubal pregnancy: preliminary results. Hum Reprod 1998;13:3042–4.
24. Fernandez H, Baton C, Lelaidier C, Frydman R. Conservative management of ectopic pregnancy: prospective randomized clinical trial of methotrexate versus prostaglandin sulprostone by combined transvaginal and systemic administration. Fertil Steril 1991;55:746–50.
25. Fernandez H, Baton C. Treatment of ectopic pregnancy by transvaginal aspiration: Prospective randomized clinical trial of Methotrexate versus Sulprostone by sonographic injection followed by systemic injection. Contraception, Fertilite, Sexualite 1990;18:261–5.
26. Fernandez H, Bourget P, Ville Y, Lelaidier C, Frydman R. Treatment of unruptured tubal pregnancy with methotrexate: pharmacokinetic analysis of local versus intramuscular administration. Fertil Steril 1994;62:943–7.
27. Fernandez H, Pauthier S, Doumerc S, Lelaidier C, Olivennes F, Ville YY. Ultrasound guided injection of methotrexate versus laparoscopic salpingotomy in ectopic pregnancy. Fertil Steril 1995;63:25–9.
28. Fernandez H, Pauthier S, Sitbon D, Vincent Y, Doumerc S. Role of conservative therapy and medical treatment in ectopic pregnancy: literature review and clinical trial comparing medical treatment and conservative laparoscopic treatment. Contraception Fertilite Sexualite 1996;24:297–302.
29. Fernandez H, Yves VS, Pauthier S, Audibert F, Frydman R. Randomized trial of conservative laparoscopic treatment and methotrexate administration in ectopic pregnancy and subsequent fertility. Hum Reprod 1998;13:3239–43.
30. Foulot H, Chapron C, Morice P. et al. Failure of laparoscopic treatment for implants. Hum. Reprod, 1994;9:92-3.
31. Franklin EW, Zeiderman AM, Laemmle P. Tubal ectopic pregnancy: etiology and obstetric and gynecologic sequelae. Am, J, Obstet, Gynecol, 1973;Ill:220–5.
32. Fujishita A, Ishimaru T, Masuzaki H, Samejima T, Matsuwaki T, Ortega-Chavez RR. Local injection of methotrexate dissolved in Treatment of tubal ectopic pregnancy 317.
33. Fujishita A, Masuzaki H, Newaz KK, Kitajima M, Hiraki K, Ishimaru T. Laparoscopic salpingotomy for tubal pregnancy: comparison of linear salpingotomy with and without suturing. Hum Reprod 2004;19: 1195–1200.
34. Garbin O, de TR, de PL, Coiffic J, Lucot JP, Le-Goueff FF. Medical treatment of ectopic pregnancy; a randomized clinical trial comparing methotrexatemifepristone and methotrexate-placebo. J Gynecol Obstet Biol Reprod 2004;33:391–400.
35. Gazvani MR, Baruah DN, Alfirevic Z, Emery SJ. Mifepristone in combination with methotrexate for the medical management of tubal pregnancy: a randomized controlled trial. Hum Reprod 1998;13:1987–90.
36. Giana M. Trataments chirurgico conservative in caza digravidenza tubarica. Minerva Ginecol, 1979;30:51–99.
37. Gjelland K, Hordnes K, Tjugum J, Augensen K, Bergsjø P. Treatment of ectopic pregnancy by local injection of hypertonic glucose: a randomized trial comparing administration guided by transvaginal ultrasound or laparoscopy. Acta Obstet Gynecol Scand 1995;74:629–34.
38. Gracia CR, Brown HA, Barnhart KT. Prophylactic methotrexate after linear salpingostomy: a decision analysis. Fertil Steril 2001;76:1191–5.
39. Graczykowski JW, Mishell DR. Methotrexate prophylaxis for persistent ectopic pregnancy after conservative treatment by salpingostomy. Obstet Gynecol 1997;89:118–22.
40. Gray DT, Thorburn J, Lundorff P, Strandell A, Lindblom B. A cost-effectiveness study of a randomized trial of laparoscopy versus laparotomy for ectopic pregnancy. Lancet 1995;345:1139–43.
41. Hajenius P, Mol F, Mol B, Bossuyt P, Ankum W, Van der Veen F. Interventions for tubal ectopic pregnancy. Cochrane Database Syst Rev 2007; CD000324.
42. Hajenius PJ, Engelsbel S, Mol BWJ, Van der Veen F, Ankum WM, Bossuyt PMM. Randomized trial of systemic methotrexate versus laparoscopic salpingostomy in tubal pregnancy. Lancet 1997;350:774–9.
43. Hallatt JG. Tuba conservation in ectopic pregnancy: a study of 200 cases Am J. Obstet Gynecol 154, 1216-21.
44. Hordnes K. Reproductive outcome after treatment of ectopic pregnancy with local injection of hypertonic glucose. Acta Obstet Gynecol Scand 1997;76:703–5.
45. Hu CX, Han LX. Mifepristone in combination with methotrexate for the medical treatment of unruptured ectopic pregnancy. Acta Acadumiae Medicinae CPAPF 2003; 12:171–2.

Section Three

46. Hugues GJ. Fertility and ectopic pregnancy. Eur J Obstet Gynecol, Reprod, BioL 1980;10:361–5.
47. Intramuscular. Fertil Steril 1996;65:206–7. Colacurci N, De FP, Zarcone R, Fortunato N, Passaro M, Mollo AA. Time length of negativization of hCG serum values after either surgical or medical treatment of ectopic pregnancy. Panminerva Medica 1998;40:223–5.
48. Judlin P, Leguin T, Zaccabri A, Landes P. Avenir genital des patientes apres GEU: A propos d'une sine continue de 330 cas J Gynecol Obstet BioL Reprod. 1988;17:58-59.
49. Kaya H, Babar Y, Ozmen S, Ozkaya O, Karci M, Aydin AR. Intra tubal methotrexate for prevention of persistent ectopic pregnancy after salpingostomy. J Am Assoc Gynecol Laparosc 2002;9:464–7.
50. Klauser CK, May WL, Johnson VK, Cowan BD, Hines RS. Methotrexate for ectopic pregnancy: a randomized single dose compared with multiple dose. Obstet Gynaecol 2005;105:64S.
51. Koninckx PR, Witters K, Brosens J, Stemers N, Oosterlynck D, Meuleman C. Conservative laparoscopic treatment of ectopic pregnancies using the CO_2 laser. Br J Obstet Gynaecol 1991;98:1254–9.
52. Korhonen J, Stenman U, Ylostalo P. Low-dose oral methotrexate with expectant management of ectopic pregnancy. Obstet Gynecol 1996;88:775–8.
53. Laatikainen T, Tuomivaara L, Kaar K. Comparison of a local injection of hyperosmolar glucose solution with salpingostomy for the conservative treatment of tubal pregnancy. Fertil Steril 1993;60:80–4.
54. Landstrom G, Bryman I, Ekstrom P, Engman M, Gunnarsson J, Hjersing MM. Ectopic pregnancy: local medical treatment versus oral methotrexate therapy—a multicentre pilot study. Hum Reprod 1998;13:38.
55. Lang PF, Weiss PA, Mayer HO, Haas JG, Honigl W. Conservative treatment of ectopic pregnancy with local injection of hyperosmolar glucose solution or prostaglandin F2a: a prospective randomised study. Lancet 1990;336:78–81.
56. Langebrekke A, Somes T, Umes A. Fertility after treatment of tuba! pregnancy by laparoscopic laser surgery. Acta Obstet. Gynecol. Scand. 1993;72:547-9.
57. Langer R, Raziel A. Ron-EL, R, et al. Reproductive outcome after conservative surgery for unrupted tubal pregnancy. Fertil. Steril 1990;53:227–31.
58. Lindblom B, Lundorff P, Thorburn J. Second-look laparoscopy after ectopic pregnancy. Proceedings of the 6th annual Congress of the European Society for Gynaecological Endoscopy 1997;21.
59. Lund J. Early ectopic pregnancy -comments on conservative treatment. J Obstet Gynecol Br Empire 1955;62:70–76.
60. Lundorff P, Thorburn J, Hahlin M, Kallfelt B, Lindblom B. Laparoscopic surgery in ectopic pregnancy. A randomized trial versus laparotomy. Acta Obstet Gynecol Scand 1991;70:343–8.
61. Lundorff P, Thorburn J, Lindblom B. Fertility after conservative surgical treatment of ectopic pregnancy, evaluated in a randomized trial. Ugeskr Laeger 1993;155:3282–6.
62. Lundorff P, Thorburn J, Lindblom B. Fertility outcome after conservative surgical treatment of ectopic pregnancy evaluated in a randomized trial. Fertil Steril 1992;57:998–1002.
63. Lundorff P. Laparoscopic surgery in ectopic pregnancy. Acta Obstet Gynecol Scand 1997;164:81–4.
64. Lundorff P. Treatment of ectopics and subsequent adhesion formation. Prog Clin Biol Res 1993;381:139–47.
65. Lundorff P, Hahlin M, Sjoblom P, and Lindblom B. Persistent trophoblast after conservative treatment of tubal pregnancy: prediction and detection. Obstet. Gynecol, TI, 1991;129-133.
66. Lundorff P, Thorbum J, and Lindblom B. Fertility outcome after surgical treatment of ectopic pregnancy evaluated in a randomized trial, Fenil Sleril, 1992;57:998-1002.
67. Makinen JI, Salmi TU, Nikkanen VPJ Koskinen, EYJ. Encouraging rates of fertility after ectopic pregnancy. Int J Fenil, 1989;34:46-51.
68. Manhes H, Mage G, Pouly JL et al. Treatment, coelioscopique de la grossesse tubaire: ameliorations techniques. Presse Med 1983;12:1431.
69. Mathieu J and Soulerin A. Le pronostic obstetrical apres grossesse extra uterine. Rev Fr Gynicol. Obstet 1957;52:167–76.
70. Methotrexate. Zhongguo Zhong Xi Yi Jie He Za zhi Zhongguo Zhongxiyi Jiehe Zazhi 2002;22:417–9.
71. Mol BW, Hajenius PJ, Ankum WM, Van der Veen F, Bossuyt PM. Conservative versus radical surgery for tubal pregnancy. Acta Obstet Gynecol Scand 1996;75:866–7.
72. Mol BW, Van der Veen F, Bossuyt PM. Implementation of probabilistic decision rules improves the predictive values of algorithms in the diagnostic management of ectopic pregnancy. Hum Reprod 1999;14:2855–62.
73. Mol BWJ, Hajenius PJ, Engelsbel S, Ankum WM, Hemrika DJ, Van der Veen F. The treatment of tubal pregnancy in The Netherlands: an economic evaluation of systemic methotrexate and laparoscopic salpingostomy. Am J Obstet Gynecol 1999;181:945–51.
74. Mol BWJ, Hajenius PJ, Engelsbel S, Ankum WM, Van der Veen F, Hemrika DJ. Serum human chorionic gonadotropin measurement in the diagnosis of ectopic pregnancy when transvaginal sonography is inconclusive. Fertil Steril 1998a;70:972–81.
75. Mol BWJ, Matthijsse HM, Tinga DJ, Huynh VT, Hajenius PJ, Ankum WM, Bossuyt PM, Van der Veen F. Fertility after conservative and radical surgery for tubal pregnancy. Hum Reprod 1998b;13:1804–09.
76. Mottla GL, Rulin MC, Guzick DS. Lack of resolution of ectopic pregnancy by intratubal injection of methotrexate. Fertil Steril 1992;57:685–7.
77. Murphy AA, Nager CW, Wujek JJ, Kettel LM, Torp VA, Chin HG. Operative laparoscopy versus laparotomy for the management of ectopic pregnancy: a prospective trial. Fertil Steril 1992;57:1180–5.
78. Murphy AA. Operative laparoscopy. Fenil, Steril, 1987;47:1–18.

79. Nagamani M, London S, St Amand P. Factors influencing fertility after ectopic pregnancy. Am J, Obstet, Gynecol, 1984;149:533–5.

80. Nieuwkerk PT, Hajenius PJ, Ankum WM, Van der Veen F, Wijker W, Bossuyt PMM. Systemic methotrexate therapy versus laparoscopic salpingostomy in patients with tubal pregnancy. Part I. Impact on patients' health related quality of life. Fertil Steril 1998a;70:511–7.

81. Nieuwkerk PT, Hajenius PJ, Van der Veen F, Ankum WM, Wijker W, Bossuyt PMM. Systemic methotrexate therapy versus laparoscopic salpingostomy in tubal pregnancy. Part II Patient preferences for systemic methotrexate. Fertil Steril 1998b;7:518–22.

82. Oelsner G, Goldenberg M, Admon D, et al. Salpingectomy by operative laparoscopy and subsequent reproductive performance. Hum Reprod, 1994;9:83-6.

83. Paavonen J, Varjonen-Toivonen M, Komulainen M, Heinonen PK. Diagnosis and management of tubal pregnancy: effect on fertility outcome Int J Gynecol Obstet, 1985;23:123–33.

84. Palmer R. Resultats et indications de la chirurgie conservatrice au cours de la grossesse extra utirine. CR Soc Fr Gynecol 1972;42:317–20.

85. Peng LX. The comparison of three conservative treatments for ectopic pregnancy; analysis of 97 cases. Guangxi Med J 1997;19:752–4.

86. Ploman L, and Wicksell F. Fertility after conservative surgery in tubal pregnancy, Acta Obstet, Gynecol, Scand 1960;39:143-52.

87. Porpora MG, Oliva MM, De CA, Montanino G, Cosmi EV. Comparison of local methotrexate and linear salpingostomy in the conservative laparoscopic treatment of ectopic pregnancy. J Am Assoc Gynecol Laparosc 1996;3:271–6.

88. Pouly JL, Chapron C, Manhes H, et al. Multifactorial analysis of fertility after conservative laparoscopic treatment of ectopic pregnancy in a series of 223 patients. Fenil, Steril 1991;56:453–60.

89. Pusey J, Taylor PJ, Leader A, Pattinson HA. Outcome and effect on medical intervention in women experiencing infertility following removal of an ectopic pregnancy. Am J Obstet, Gynecol 1984;148:524–7.

90. Querleu D, Lenain F, Hennion A, et al. Feconditi apres grossesse extrauterine. Contr, Fenil, Sex, 1988;16:131–5.

91. Reich H, Jones DA, De Caprio J, et al. Laparoscopic treatment of 109 consecutive ectopic pregnancies. J Reprod, Med, 1988;33:885-90.

92. Rozenberg P, Chevret S, Camus E, de TR, Garbin O, Poncheville LL. Medical treatment of ectopic pregnancies: a randomized clinical trial comparing methotrexate-mifepristone and methotrexate-placebo. Hum Reprod 2003;18:1802–08.

93. Sadan O, Ginath S, Debby A, Rotmensch S, Golan A, Zakut HH. Methotrexate versus hyperosmolar glucose in the treatment of extrauterine pregnancy. Arch Gynecol Obstet 2001;265:82–4.

94. Saline versus methotrexate suspensions for the conservative treatment of ectopic pregnancy. Hum Reprod 1995;10:3280–3.

95. Saraj AJ, Wilcox JG, Najmabadi S, Stein SM, Johnson MB, Paulson RJ. Resolution of hormonal markers of ectopic gestation: a randomized trial comparing single dose intramuscular methotrexate with salpingostomy. Obstet Gynecol 1998;92:989–94.

96. Seifer DB, Gutmann JN, Grant WD, et al. Comparison of persistent ectopic pregnancy after laparoscopic salpingostomy at laparotomy for ectopic pregnancy. Obstet Gynecol 1993;81:378–82.

97. Sharma JB, Gupta S, Malhotra M, Arora R. A randomized controlled comparison of minilaparotomy and laparotomy in ectopic pregnancy cases. Indian J Med Sci 2003;57:493–500.

98. Shea RT, Thompson GR, Harding A. Intra-amniotic methotrexate versus CO_2 laser laparoscopic salpingotomy in the management of tubal ectopic pregnancy a prospective randomized trial. Fertil Steril 1994;62:876–8.

99. Sherman A, Langer R, Sadovsky G, Bukovsky I, Caspi E. Improved fertility following ectopic pregnancy. Fenil. Steril 1982;37:497–502.

100. Shulman A, Maymon R, Zmira N, Lotan M, Holtzinger M, Bahary C. Conservative treatment of ectopic pregnancy and its effect on corpus luteum activity. Gynecol Obstet Invest 1992;33:161–4.

101. Silva PD, Schaper AM, Rooney B. Reproductive outcome after 143 laparoscopic procedures for ectopic pregnancy. Obstet. Gynecol 1993;81:710–15.

102. Skulj V, Pavic J, Stoilkovic C et al. Conservative operative treatment of tubal pregnancy. Fenil, Steril, 1964;15:634-39.

103. Sowter MC, Farquhar CM, Gudex G. An economic evaluation of single dose systemic methotrexate and laparoscopic surgery for the treatment of unrupted ectopic pregnancy. Br J Obstet Gynaecol 2001a;108:204–12.

104. Sowter MC, Farquhar CM, Petrie KJ, Gudex G. A randomized trial comparing single dose systemic methotrexate and laparoscopic surgery for the treatment of unrupted ectopic pregnancy. Br J Obstet Gynaecol 2001b;108:192–203.

105. Stovall TG, Ling FW, Gray LA, et al. Methotraxale treatment of unrupted ectopic pregnancy: a report of 100 cases. Obsiet. Gvneeol, 1991;77:749–53.

106. Su Y, Sun Y, Ma M. Observation on treatment of ectopic pregnancy by combination therapy of Chinese herbal medicine with Mifepristone or Mol et al. 318.

107. Submitted on October 5, 2007; resubmitted on January 16, 2008; accepted on March 28, 2008.

108. Sultana CJ, Easley K, Collins RL. Outcome of laparoscopic versus traditional surgery for ectopic pregnancies. Fenil. Steril 1992;57:285–9.

109. Thorburn J, Philipson M, Linblom B. Fertility after ectopic pregnancy in relation to background factors and surgical treatment. Fenil Steril 1988;49:595–601.

110. Timonen S and Nieminen U. Tuba] pregnancy: choice of operative method of treatment. Ada Obstet, Gynecol, Scand, 1967;46:327-39.

111. Tulandi T, Guralnick M. Treatment of tubal ectopic pregnancy by salpingotomy with or without tubal suturing and salpingectomy. Fertil Steril 1991;55:53–5.

Section Three

404 **Textbook of Practical Laparoscopic Surgery**

112. Tuomivaara L and Kaupilla A. Radical or conservative surgery for ectopic pregnancy? A follow-up study of fertility of 323 patients, Fenil, Steril 1988;50:580–3.

113. Tzafettas J, Anapliotis S, Zournatzi V, Boucklis A, Oxouzoglou N, Bondis J. Transvaginal intra-amniotic injection of methotrexate in early ectopic pregnancy. Advantages over the laparoscopic approach. Early Hum Dev 1994;39:101–7.

114. Ugur M, Yesilyurt H, Soysal S, Gokmen O. Prophylactic vasopressin during laparoscopic salpingotomy for ectopic pregnancy. J Am Assoc Gynecol Laparosc 1996;3:365–8.

115. Vehaskari A. The operation of choice for ectopic pregnancy to subsequent fertility. Acta Obstet, Gynecol, Scand, 1960;39:1–7.

116. Vermesh M, Presser SC. Reproductive outcome after linear salpingostomy for ectopic gestation: a prospective 3 year follow-up. Fertil Steril 1992;57:682–4.

117. Vermesh M, Silva PD, Rosen GF, Stein AL, Fossum GT, Sauer MV. Management of unruptured ectopic gestation by linear salpingostomy: a prospective, randomized clinical trial of laparoscopy versus laparotomy. Obstet Gynecol 1989;73:400–04.

118. Wang J, Yang Q, Yu Z. Clinical study of tubal pregnancy treated with integrated traditional Chinese and Western medicine. Zhongguuo Zhong Xi Yi Jie Z Zhi 1998;18:531–3.

119. Wei FY, Chen HF. [Clinical analysis of 82 cases of ectopic pregnancy treated by methotrexate combined with traditional Chinese recipe]. Zhong Xi Yi Jie He Xue Bao 2003;1:267-92.

120. Weinstein M, Morris MB, Dutters D. Ectopic pregnancy: a new surgical epidemic. Obstet Gynecol 1983;61:698–701.

121. Yalcinkaya TM, Brown SE, Mertz HL, Thomas DW. A comparison of 25 mg/ m² vs 50 mg/m² dose of methotrexate (MTX) for the treatment of ectopic pregnancy (EP). J Soc Gynecol Invest 2000;7:179A.

122. Zilber U, Pansky M, Bukovsky I, Golan A. Laparoscopic salpingostomy versus laparoscopic local methotrexate injection in the management of unruptured ectopic gestation. Am J Obstet Gynecol 1996;175:600–02.

31 Laparoscopic Management of Ectopic Pregnancy

Laparoscopy is one of the major advancement for tubal and uterine disease. Surgical procedures for managing benign adnexal masses include aspiration, fenestration, ovarian cystectomy, unilateral or bilateral salpingo-oophorectomy and laparoscopically-assisted vaginal hysterectomy (LAVH) with or without unilateral or bilateral salpingo-oophorectomy.

Ectopic Pregnancy

The risk of ectopic pregnancy is higher in white women. It increases three to four times in women between the age of 35 and 44 compared to those from 15 to 24. About 64 percent of ectopic pregnancies occur in the ampulla where fertilization occurs. The recent increase

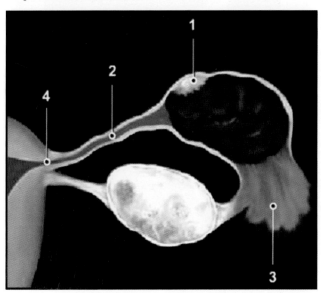

Fig. 31.1: Tubal pregnancy, 1. The ampulla, 2. The isthmus, 3. The infundibulum, 4. The intramural junctions

in incidence of ectopic pregnancy has been attributed to a greater incidence of sexually transmitted disease, delayed childbearing, previous sexual organ surgical interference and successful clinical detection. Any condition that prevents or retard migration of fertilized ovum to the uterine cavity could predispose a woman to an ectopic gestation (Fig. 31.1).

Ectopic pregnancy usually occurs 99 percent of cases in the uterine tube (Fig. 31.1). It can be found in:
1. The ampulla (64%)
2. The isthmus (25%)
3. The infundibulum (9%)
4. The intramural junction (2%)
5. Ovarian (0.5%)
6. Cervical (0.4%)
7. Abdominal (0.1%)
8. Intraligamental (0.05%).

Major contributing factors and associated relative risks for ectopic pregnancy are:
- Current use of intrauterine device (11.5%)
- Use of clomiphene citrate (10%)
- Prior tubal surgery (5.6%)
- Pelvic inflammatory disease (4.0%)
- Infertility (2.9%)
- Induced abortion (2.5%)
- Adhesions (2.4%)
- Abdominal surgery (2.3%)
- T shaped uterus (2%)
- Myoma (1.7 %)
- Progestin only contraceptives (1.6%).

If laparoscopy is planned, the location, the size, and the nature of the tubal pregnancy are ascertained. If the bleeding has ceased or can be arrested adequately, rupture tubal pregnancies can be treated successfully endoscopically. Once bleeding is controlled, the products of conception and blood clots are removed. If there is more than 1,500 cc hemoperitoneum, laparoscopic approach is contraindicated. Heparinized saline should be used in cases of large hematoma. Large ruptured ectopic require extracorporeal knotting.

A 10 mm suction instrument is used to clean the abdominal cavity. Forced irrigation with normal saline should dislodge the clot and trophoblastic tissue from the serosa of the peritoneal organs with minimal injury to these structures (Figs 31.2A to C).

For unruptured tubal pregnancy, the fallopian tubes is identified and mobilized to minimize bleeding, a 5 to 8 ml diluted solution containing 5 unit vasopressin in 20 ml of saline is injected with a 20 gauge spinal or laparoscopic needle. It should be injected in the mesosalpinx just below the ectopic and over the antemesentric surface of the tubal segment containing gestational product. The needle must not be inserted deep within a blood vessel because intravascular injection may precipitate acute arterial hypertension, bradycardia and sometime it may be fatal.

After stabilizing the tube by grasper in one hand and microelectrode in other, a linear incision is made on the antimesenteric surface extending one to two cm over the thinnest portion of tube. The fine needle tip should be used in the cutting mode, and should barely touch the tissue surface. With electrosurgery, thermal damage may spread if large tips are used on large surface areas in contact with tissue. It is important to remain aware of the location of underlying or adjacent structures. If the gynecologists are not careful there may be a chance of adjacent visceral injury (Fig. 31.3).

The pregnancy usually should protrude through the incision and slowly slips out of tube. It may be teased gently out using hydrodissection or laparoscopic atraumatic forceps. Sometimes forceful irrigation in the tubal opening can dislodge the gestation from implantation. As pregnancy is pulled out or extrudes from the tube, some of the product of conception can adhere to the implantation site by a ligamentous structure containing blood vessels. Using bipolar this structure should be coagulated before removing the tissue. Depending upon the size of the product of conception, ectopic is removed usually through a 10 mm trocar sleeve.

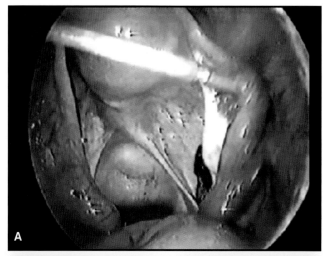

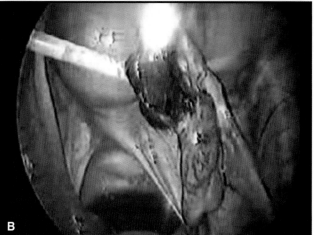

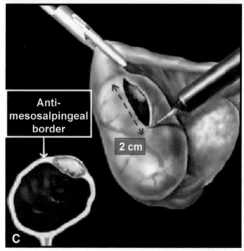

Figs 31.2A to C: Salpingotomy for unruptured ectopic pregnancy

Resection of the tubal segment containing the gestation is preferable to salpingostomy for an isthmic pregnancy or a ruptured tube or if hemostasis is difficult to obtain. Segmental tubal resection is performed by

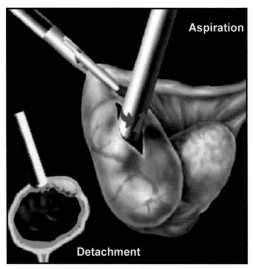

Fig. 31.3: Suction of trophoblast for unruptured ectopic pregnancy

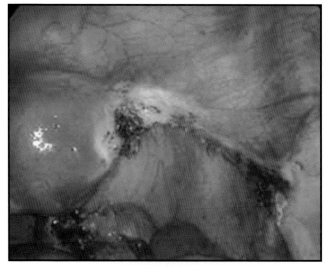

Fig. 31.4: Salpingectomy

the help of bipolar forceps or harmonic scalpel. Automatic stapling or suturing devises can be used for bloodless tubal resection. If the mesosalpinx bleeds, it should be cauterized by using bipolar forceps, particular attention given to the arcuate anatomizing branches of the ovarian and uterine arteries. Total salpingectomy is performed by progressively coagulating and cutting the mesosalpinx, beginning with the proximal portion to fimbrial end. It is separated from the uterus using bipolar coagulation and scissors (Fig. 31.4). The isolated segment containing the tubal pregnancy is removed intact or in sectioned part, through the 10 mm trocar sleeve. The product of conception can be placed in a plastic bag and removed. Multifire stapling devices for salpingectomy require a 10 mm trocar. If the tissue is bulky and can not be accommodated through cannula, endobag can be used for retrieval of tissue.

Adhesion or other pathologic processes such as endometriosis can be treated simultaneously during removal of ectopic pregnancy without significantly prolonging the operation. In one week the beta hCG should return to baseline, i.e. undetectable or very low.

If the pregnancy is interstitial it may be associated with traumatic rupture, hemorrhagic shock and there is two-fold increase in maternal mortality over other tubal pregnancies. Delayed diagnosis and increased vascularity of this make laparoscopic procedure difficult. Two to four percent of ectopic are interstitial. The anatomy of ectopic accommodates the growing

gestation, accounting for its late recognition. The traditional management is better in these case, i.e. salpingectomy with or without corneal resection and in some difficult cases hysterectomy may be necessary. Interstitial pregnancy can be suspected at the time of laparoscopy when large and asymmetrical uterus is seen.

Most patients are discharged within 48 hours. There is a higher fertility rate/intrauterine pregnancy rate in subsequent pregnancies with laparoscopic techniques (Fig. 31.5).

Laparoscopic surgery is a good option for rupture ectopic and ruptured ectopic does not necessarily

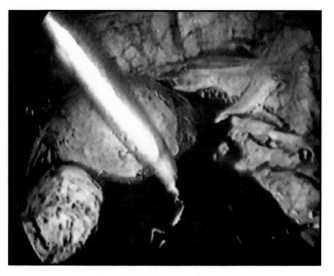

Fig. 31.5: Hemoperitoneum

Section Three

warrant a laparotomy. If the patient is hemodynamically stable and initial laparoscopic examination indicates a moderate blood loss, it may be possible to control bleeding laparoscopically and perform any indicated procedures. If the patient is in stage II or stage III shock who has a large hemoperitoneum, laparotomy is the better choice. Managing ruptured ectopic pregnancies involves examining the pelvis, localizing the ectopic, aspirating blood and clots, localizing and controlling the bleeding points, and performing either salpingectomy or in rare situations, an oophorectomy is performed concurrently.

Controlling bleeding is the most critical part of the procedure, and several methods can be attempted sequentially to achieve hemostasis:

- Identification of the bleeding point followed by careful bipolar electrodesiccation.
- Injection of vasopressin over the mesosalpinx.
- Electrodesiccation of the mesosalpinx.
- If bleeding does not stop by these means the partial or complete salpingectomy, depending on the portion of tube involved and the patient's desire for fertility.

After successfully managing the ectopic pregnancy laparoscopically, the patient can be discharged second day. The patient should come again for a serum ft-hCG one week postoperatively to ascertain resolution of the ectopic gestation. The ft-hCG level should be either undetectable or very low after one week of surgery. If it is above 20 mIU/mL, a repeat blood test is ordered one to 2 weeks later when the ft-hCG should be undetectable.

DISCUSSION

Ectopic pregnancy was first discovered in the 11th century, and until the middle of the 18th century, it was usually fatal. John Bard reported the first successful surgical intervention to treat an ectopic pregnancy in 1759.

According to Sepilian, the survival rate in the 19th century was dismal, however, in the beginning of the 20th century, improvement in blood transfusion, anesthesia, and antibiotics contributed to the decrease in the maternal mortality. Ectopic pregnancy currently is the leading cause of pregnancy-related deaths in the first trimester. Sepilian stated that ectopic pregnancy is derived from the Greek word "ektopos" meaning

out of place, and it refers to the implantation of the fertilized ovum in a location outside of the uterine cavity including the fallopian tubes, cornual or interstitial region of the uterus and fallopian tubes, cervix, ovary, and the abdominal cavity. This abnormally implanted pregnancy grows and draws its blood supply from the site of abnormal implantation, as the gestation enlarges it creates the potential for organ rupture because only the uterine cavity is designed to expand and accommodate fetal development. The arterial blood supply to the mesosalpinx provided by branches of the ovarian artery that derive directly from the aorta as well as the branches from the uterine artery that derive from the internal iliac artery, provides the fallopian tubes with a rich arterial supply that can bleed in the event of a perforated tube, to massive catastrophic hemorrhage and maternal death.

Seeber reported in 2006 from a study at the University of Pennsylvania reported that the incidence of ectopic pregnancy has increased 6-fold since 1970, and is responsible for approximately 9 percent of all pregnancy related deaths in the United States. The author further reported that a rise in the quantitative beta subunit of human chorionic gonadotropin of a maximum of 53% over two days would be required for a viable pregnancy, and a decline of 21 to 35 % in 48 hours would be mandatory for a diagnosis of spontaneous abortion.

Seeber stated that the absence of an intrauterine pregnancy above an established cut point of hCG is consistent with an abnormal pregnancy, but does not distinguish a miscarriage from an ectopic pregnancy.

Seeber stated that the symptoms of abdominal pain or pelvic pain and vaginal bleeding are the most common complaints suggestive of ectopic pregnancy. The multiple potential sites of ectopic pregnancies add to the complexity of the diagnosis. Seeber also stated that these symptoms may be erratic and variable, and in some cases, absent. Likewise, such symptoms are non-specific, and also have been associated with spontaneous abortion, cervical irritation, or trauma, and infection.

Sepelian wrote that the classic triad of amenorrhea, pain, and vaginal bleeding has been strongly associated with the clinical presentation of ectopic pregnancy. However, 50% of patients with ectopic pregnancy present without this triad. They may have symptoms associated with early pregnancy, including nausea, fatigue, lower abdominal pain, painful uterine cramping, recent dyspareunia, and shoulder pain.

Due to increased technology, most entopic are diagnosed prior to rupture. Sepilian reported that approximately 20% of ectopic patients are hemodynamically unstable at initial presentation suggesting a ruptured ectopic gestation. There is a 10-25% chance of a recurrent ectopic pregnancy.

Risk factor included progesterone intrauterine device. Increasing maternal age plays important roles in ectopic pregnancy and women age 35-44 years have a 3 to 4-fold higher chance compared to women aged 15-24 years.

Smoking may alter tubal and uterine motility, and is associated with a risk of 1.6-3.5 times more than non smokers. Other factors associated with an increased risk of ectopic pregnancies include prior abdominal surgery, a ruptured appendix, exposure to diethylstilbestrol and uterine developmental abnormalities.

Most authors list prior tubal infection. Chlamydia may be asymptomatic and untreated as well as other infectious agents associated with an increased risk of salpingitis and potential tubal damage. Sepilian stated that within the last 2 decades, there has been a more conservative surgical approach to unruptured ectopic gestation. Utilizing minimally invasive surgery, laparoscopy has become the recommended approach in most cases. Laparotomy has been usually reserved for cases where the patients have been hemodynamically unstable, or when the surgeon is inexperienced in laparoscopy.

Seeber stated that laparoscopic minimally invasive approach has become the preferred surgical approach, and laparotomy is reserved for hemodynamically unstable patients. Other situations in which the open surgical approach may be preferable include extensive pelvic adhesions where adequate visualization of the ectopic is impossible or extratubal, intra-abdominal ectopic gestation, where risk of injury to other pelvic structures is high. Bruhart reported the first laparoscopic surgery for ectopic pregnancy in 1980.

Laparoscopy vs Laparotomy in Treatment of Ectopic Pregnancies

El-Tabbakh reported the results of a trial in Kuwait from March 1999 to October 2001, involving 207 patients to compare laparoscopy vs. laparotomy for surgical treatment of ectopic pregnancy. One hundred eighty-four were treated by laparoscopy and 23 by laparotomy of the 207 patients with a diagnosis of ectopic pregnancy based on clinical symptoms, history, physical examination, positive serum beta hCG, transvaginal ultrasonography and ectopic pregnancy conformed at laparoscopy. Following surgery, patients were followed with serial quantitative beta hCG on days 4 and 7, then weekly until labels less than 20 IU/L were obtained. Those treated with laparoscopy had an overall success rate of 98.9%. Moreover, the patients treated by laparoscopy had significantly lower blood loss. Blood transfusion was required by 13% in the laparoscopically treated group compared to 23% in the laparotomy group. All patients had the ectopic pregnancy confirmed by laparoscopy and the decision to proceed with operative laparoscopy or laparotomy depended on the minimal invasive surgery experience of the surgeon on call. There were no intraoperative complications and the duration of surgery ranged from 66 minutes to 72 minutes for both groups. The Kuwait study led the author to conclude that laparoscopy treatment offered benefits superior to laparotomy with less blood loss, therefore, a reduced need for transfusion. The patients experienced less need for analgesia, and a shortened postoperative hospitalization.

Yuen's study included 105 patients in Hong Kong, there were no differences in age, parity, gestational age, and pregnancy of previous laparotomy between the groups had a diagnostic laparoscopy prior to laparotomy. The laparoscopy group had a lower incidence of hemoperitoneum (45.9% vs 75%); Yuen's study was performed in Hong Kong. Yuen stated that operative laparoscopy has the advantage of combining diagnostic and therapeutic procedures in a single operation in a better approach than laparotomy for the management of tubal pregnancy.

Xiang's study was conducted in Shanghai. Seventy two of ectopic pregnancy patients were treated laparoscopically. The author concluded that while it was more expensive than laparotomy the operating time and postoperative hospitalization were shortened. In the laparoscopy studies, the authors stressed reduced blood loss, shortened hospital stay, and reduced need for postoperative analgesia as recurrent positive findings throughout the various studies.

Seeber commented on the laparoscopic treatment of salpingostomy versus salpingectomy. Seeber noted that if salpingostomy has not resulted in improvement of subsequent pregnancy rate over salpingectomy, then she would have recommended salpingostomy for all ectopic pregnancy patients. However, she states that the data to support this contention are not clear cut. The approximate 50% subsequent pregnancy rate has been noted with either method. The rate of recurrent ectopic pregnancy appeared higher in the salpingostomy (15 to 10%). The decision to perform salpingostomy is opposed to salpingectomy is often made intraoperatively. In case of severe damage or tubal rupture, tubal conservation is not indicated. Moreover, if tubal bleeding occurs that requires extensive coagulation, then salpingectomy may be indicated due to tubal damage. The success of *in vitro* fertilization has been beneficial for those patients who have salpingectomy. The formation of shadisation postoperatively has been more extensive with laparotomy. Seeber noted that ectopic pregnancy occurs most frequently as a result of fallopian tube pathology; therefore, there is a risk of recurrence in both the affected and contralateral tube. Women who undergone salpingectomy will have a risk of subsequent ectopic pregnancy in the remaining tube.

As the surgeons gain more experience and training with laparoscopic surgery for ectopic pregnancy, it has become the preferred choice when equipment and resources are available.

Section Three

32 Laparoscopic Surgery in Pregnancy: Precautions and Complications

Since the advent of laparoscopic surgery in the 1980s, laparoscopic surgery has been popularized by surgeons throughout the world. However, routine laparoscopic surgery has been slow to catch the pregnant patient. Treatment of surgical disease in the gravid patient requires a unique and careful approach where safety of the mother and fetus are both considered.

During pregnancy due to the physiological changes that take place in the mother and considering the presence of a living fetus in utero, surgical conditions are handled with a lot of care and cautions. In past pregnancy was considered to be absolutely contraindicated for laparoscopic intervention, but with better understanding of physiology of pregnancy and improved anesthetic and laparoscopic techniques, emergency laparoscopic procedures such as, diagnostic laparoscopy for pain abdomen, appendicectomy, splenectomy, pheochromocytoma, cholecystectomy, are feasible in pregnancy. Lachman et al, have already reported 300 laparoscopic procedures during pregnancy.

The responsibility of caring for two patients during one operation and the concern over potential harm to the unborn fetus due to the pneumoperitoneum and/or instrumentation are factors that have played a role in the delay of adapting laparoscopic surgery to the pregnant patient (Fig. 32.1). However, recent evidence suggests that not only is laparoscopic surgery safe in the pregnant patient in all three trimesters, but it is also often preferable.

During pregnancy usually all surgical procedures are avoided to minimize various risks of anesthesia and procedure to mother and fetus. At times emergency

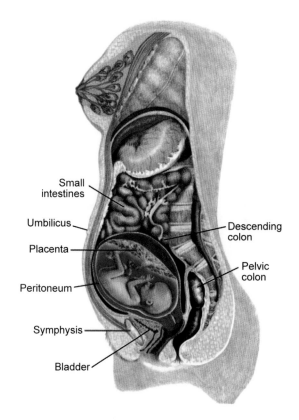

Small intestines
Umbilicus
Placenta
Peritoneum
Symphysis
Bladder
Descending colon
Pelvic colon

Fig. 32.1: Anatomical changes inside abdominal cavity during pregnancy

surgical conditions makes it absolutely necessary for intervention. With increasing progress in minimal access surgery more and more surgeons have found the skill and interest to perform the emergency procedures laparoscopically. Laparoscopy was first done in pregnancy for diagnosis and evaluation. The first laparoscopic appendicectomy in pregnancy was performed by Scheiber in 1990. The first laparoscopic cholecystectomy in laparoscopy was first done in pregnancy for diagnosis and evaluation of acute abdominal pain in 1980. The first laparoscopic appendicectomy in pregnancy was done by Weber in 1991.

However, surgical intervention in pregnant ladies needs special consideration of well-being of both mother and fetus, if intrauterine viable fetus is present, and in cases of ectopic pregnancy or heterotrophic pregnancy the pathophysiological changes brought about during pregnancy should be considered for the safety of patient (Fig. 32.2). Furthermore, with advancement of pregnancy laparoscopic diagnosis and procedures becomes more challengingly difficult as the gravid uterus displaces the organs and becomes completely an abdominal organ.

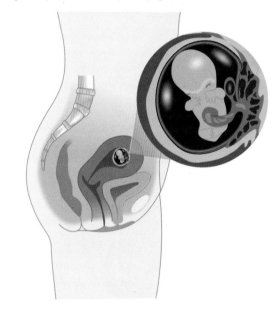

Fig. 32.2: Proper evaluation of patient is necessary to evaluate pathophysiological changes

Up to date the data on laparoscopic procedures during pregnancy are still limited, but with growing ability of minimal access surgeons the recent accumulating data shows that laparoscopic procedures such as diagnostic laparoscopy, adnexal surgery, appendicectomy, splenectomy, cholecystectomy and management of ectopic and heterotrophic pregnancies are relatively safe and effective during pregnancy, if certain precautions are taken. But of course like all surgical procedures in pregnancy there is an increased risk of certain complications with laparoscopic intervention in pregnancy.

Physiological Changes in Pregnancy

Almost all the organ systems undergo physiological changes in pregnancy. These changes should be considered during operative procedures in pregnancy.

Gastrointestinal System

Due to enlarged gravid uterus, stomach is pushed towards diaphragm and assumes a more horizontal position. The viscera like transverse, ascending and descending colon are displaced so location of abdominal pain and tenderness especially in condition like appendicitis is altered. The hormonally induced decrease lower esophageal sphincter tone causes gastroesophageal regurgitation which places the pregnant lady at higher risk of aspiration, so nasogastric tube suction and careful airway management is necessary for all pregnant patients undergoing laparoscopy.

Cardiovascular and Hematological Changes

Cardiac out put and blood volume increase by 30-40 percent, but as RBC volume does not expand by same ratio this result in physiological anemia specially noticed in the second trimester. After 20 weeks gestation, the gravid uterus compresses the aorta and inferior vena cava and may cause supine hypotension syndrome, so during surgery the patient should be positioned in lateral recumbent position to avoid vena caval compression during surgery. A vasomotor block caused by spinal anesthesia produces more sever hypotension than in nonpregnant individuals. During pregnancy WBC count increases to 12,000-14,900 per mm.

A hypercoagulable state is physiologically develops in pregnancy due to increase in fibrinogen and other coagulation factors such as factor VII, factor VIII, factor IX, and factor X. Thus the risk of thromboembolism increases in pregnancy.

Respiratory System

Due to enlarging gravid uterus gradually the chest movements are restricted. There is an increase in minute ventilation and oxygen consumption and decrease in residual volume, also mixed venous oxygen content and functional reserve capacity also decreases so the patient is prone to hypoxemia and hypocapnia. $PaCO_2$ of 28-32 mm, Ph of 7.44 and decrease bicarbonate levels are detected due to chronic respiratory alkalosis which has to be maintained during pregnancy. The patient gains more weight during pregnancy and there is more edema in soft tissues of neck, so the anesthetist may face more difficulties in airway management.

Urinary System

Hydroureter, decreased urethral peristalsis and bladder expansion increase incidence of urinary tract infection. There is an increased retention of water and electrolytes.

Other Changes

In addition to the respiratory changes, there are mild hematologic abnormalities in the pregnant patient. Levels of fibrinogen, factor VII, and factor XII are increased, whereas there are decreased levels of antithrombin III, all of which result in an increased risk of venous thromboembolism. When considering the acute abdomen in a pregnant patient, making the correct diagnosis may often be difficult. Nausea and vomiting, leukocytosis, low-grade fever, mild hypotension, and anorexia are common. The gravid uterus pushes the abdominal contents cephalad, displacing organs and inhibiting the migration of the omentum, causing altered landmarks and often distorting the clinical picture. During the second and third trimesters, the gravid uterus may cause decreased gastric motility and may lead to an increased risk of gastroesophageal reflux disease (GERD) and aspiration as well.

Fetal Consideration

Fetus is a hidden patient in the womb of the pregnant mother and its health should be considered by surgeon and anesthetist both. It is important to:
1. Maintain uteroplacental blood flow and oxygenation. Decreased uteroplacental blood flow may be due to maternal hypotension or increase in uterine artery resistance.
2. Maternal hypoxia causes fetal hypoxia and metabolic acidosis and in long term it may be fatal to infant so it should be prevented.
3. Avoid teratogenic drugs during anesthesia. Cocaine is known to have teratogenic effect so products containing cocaine should be avoided. Diazepam and Nitrous oxide are considered safe during anesthesia as no teratogenicity was detected clinically.
4. Avoid preterm labor. Try to manipulate uterus minimum as possible. Although there is an increased incidence of spontaneous abortion, premature delivery and low birth weight following anesthesia but in emergency situations operation is unavoidable.

Effects of Pneumoperitoneum in Pregnancy During Laparoscopic Procedure

In pregnant patient the pneumoperitonium increases the intra-abdominal pressure and this causes decreased inferior vena caval return to the heart, hence decreased cardiac output. With reverse Trendelenburg position decreased cardiac output is even worsened, Cardiac index decreases, and when this is combined with mothers hypoxia can cause fetal death. Increased intra-abdominal pressure also leads to decreased uterine blood flow and increase intrauterine pressure, these may in turn cause fetal hypoxia and may lead to fetal death. Pneumoperitoneum decreases the diaphragmatic movement, in pregnant lady already the movement of diaphragm is decreased due to bulky uterus, this further decrease in movement due to pneumoperitonium causes increased peak airway pressure, decrease functional reserve capacity, increased ventilation perfusion mismatch, decreased thoracic cavity compliance and increase pleural pressure.

Use of CO_2 for causing pneumoperitoneum leads to hypercarbia and further hypoxemia. The CO_2 absorbs across the peritoneum and leads to respiratory acidosis in patient and her fetus. If pCO_2 increases above 40 mm, decreased removal of CO_2 occurs leading to fetal acidosis. Fetal tachycardia and hypotension may develop as a result of fetal hypocarbia. This can be corrected by maintaining mild maternal respiratory alkalosis, by hyperventilating the mother during surgery. Monitoring maternal arterial blood gases is better than monitoring $PaCO_2$ during laparoscopic procedures.

N_2O as the gas for pneumoperitonization will not cause fetal respiratory acidosis, but it is highly combustible.

Criteria for Patient Selection

A safe laparoscopic procedure can be performed in all the three trimesters of pregnancy from 2-31 weeks.

During the first trimester there is increase risk of abortion up to 12 percent also risk of teratogenesis increases in first trimester. In the third trimester, there is a 40 percent risk of preterm labor and 30 percent risk of premature birth. Also the visualization in laparoscopic procedure is decreased due to enlarged uterus.

Therefore second trimester is considered the safest time for laparoscopic surgery in pregnancy. The risk of abortion is not increased, no risk of teratogenesis, and risk of preterm labor is only 5 percent in second trimester.

Advantages of Laparoscopy in Pregnancy

1. Short hospital stay
2. Early return to normal activities
3. Small incision, so rapid post operative recovery and less incision complications such as hernia, postoperative wound infection and pain.
4. Less uterine manipulation and hence decrease uterine irritability and fetal loss.

Risk of Laparoscopy in Pregnancy

1. More chance of uterine injury during port entry as uterus becomes an abdominal organ after first trimester (Fig. 32.3).
2. Problems associated with pneumoperitonization as discussed already.
3. CO_2 absorption causes increase CO_2 pressure and decrease arterial PH.
4. Risk of exposure to intra-abdominal smoke including carbon monoxide generated by electro-surgery and laser.

Strategies for Safe Laparoscopic Surgery in Pregnancy

1. Surgery should be done in second trimester.
2. If patient presents in late third trimester, surgery should be postponed if possible until after delivery.

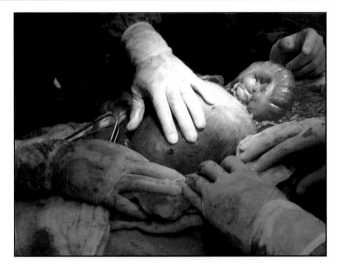

Fig. 32.3: Injury of pregnant uterus

3. Nasogastric incubation is a must in all case as there is a high risk of aspiration into the lungs.
4. Patient can be placed in dorsal lithotomy position in the first half of pregnancy, but in second half to prevent inferior vena caval compression patient is ideally placed in lateral recumbent position.
5. Hypotension should be avoided; proper fluid replacement should be done.
6. Ideal method for commencing pneumo-peritoneum is open Hasson trocar method. Placement of trocar depends on the size of gravid uterus.
7. Tocolysis is indicated if signs of uterine irritability are present.
8. Decrease operation time by using adequate number of ports, and using the most experienced surgeons.
9. Maternal hyperventilation to maintain end-tidal CO_2 Pressure at 32 mm Hg.
10. Lower CO_2 insufflations pressure of < 12 mm Hg should be used to avoid fetal acidosis.
11. Electrocautery should be used with care; the smokes containing carbon monoxide should be evacuated promptly to avoid toxic effect to fetus.
12. Entry of all instruments must be under direct vision; care should be taken to avoid injury to the gravid uterus.
13. All specimens should be removed with endobag to avoid spillage.
14. Manipulators should never be fixed to vagina or cervix.

Section Three

Society of American Gastrointestinal Endoscopic Surgery (SAGES) Recommendations:

1. Obstetrical consultation should be obtained preoperatively.
2. When possible, operative intervention should be deferred until the second trimester, when fetal risk is lowest.
3. Pneumoperitoneum enhances lower extremity venous stasis already present in the gravid patient and pregnancy induces a hypercoagulable state. Therefore pneumatic compression devices should be utilized whenever possible.
4. Fetal and uterine status, as maternal end tidal CO_2 and/or arterial blood gases, should be monitored.
5. The uterus should be protected with a lead shield if intraoperative cholangiography is a possibility.
6. Fluoroscopy should be utilized selectively.
7. Given the enlarged gravid uterus, abdominal access should be attained using an open technique.
8. Dependent positioning should be utilized to shift the uterus away from the inferior vena cava.
9. Pneumoperitoneum pressures should be kept at 10 mm Hg.
10. Further studies into methods that increase the safety of laparoscopy in pregnant patient should be done.

Discussion

Advances in laparoscopic surgery have led to development of methods to perform abdominal surgery and reduce morbidity using minimal access surgery techniques. In 1999, Lachman et al reported on a series of pregnant women undergoing 518 surgical procedures. Cholecystectomy (45%) is the most common procedures performed during pregnancy followed by adnexal surgery (34%) and appendicectomy (15%).

Operative procedures are postponed in pregnant patient until after delivery, but in acute emergency conditions even if the patient is pregnant operation should be performed.

According to the recent studies done the second trimester is ideal for laparoscopic intervention.

Most cases reported and small series indicate that laparoscopy can be safely performed during pregnancy. The incidence of prematurity and intrauterine growth restriction was reported to be higher in the open surgical group too.

Two recent studies suggest that there is no difference in fetal outcome for patient with singleton pregnancies undergoing laparoscopy or laparotomy. In one study the resultant children born after laparoscopic surgery was performed on their mother during their intrauterine life, were monitored and no evidence of developmental or physical abnormality was detected during the study period. Despite the growing clinical experience suggesting that laparoscopy is as safe as laparotomy in pregnancy, more long term clinical studies are required.

CONCLUSION

A laparoscopic access to pathology in pregnancy has many benefits for the patient but it is important that the surgeon and anesthetist both have an immense knowledge of maternal fetal physiology. An experienced surgeon can continue to perform laparoscopy safely in all trimesters by without significant increases in either maternal or fetal morbidity or mortality. Further controlled clinical studies are needed to clarify many other unknown issues, and revision may be necessary as new data appear.

BIBLIOGRAPHY

1. Adelstein S. Administered radionuclides in pregnancy. Teratology 1999;59(4):236-9.
2. Affleck DG, et al. The laparoscopic management of appendicitis and cholelithiasis during pregnancy. Am J Surg 1999;178(6):523-9.
3. Affleck DG, Handrahan DL, Egger MJ, Price RR. The laparoscopic management of appendicitis and cholelithiasis during pregnancy. Am J Surg 1999;178: 523-9.
4. Akira S, et al. Gasless laparoscopic ovarian cystectomy during pregnancy: comparison with laparotomy. Am J Obstet Gynecol 1999;180(3 Pt 1):554-7.
5. Al-Fozan H, Tulandi T. Safety and risks of laparoscopy in pregnancy. Curr Opin Obstet Gynecol 2002;14: 375-9.
6. Ames Castro M, Shipp TD, Castro EE, Ouzounian J, Rao P. The use of helical computed tomography in pregnancy for the diagnosis of acute appendicitis. Am J Obstet Gynecol 2001;184:954-7.
7. Amos JD, et al. Laparoscopic surgery during pregnancy. Am J Surg 1996;171(4):435-7.
8. Andreoli M, et al. Laparoscopic surgery during pregnancy. J Am Assoc Gynecol Laparosc 1999;6(2):229-33.

Section Three

9. Andriulli A, et al. Incidence rates of post-ERCP complications: a systematic survey of prospective studies. Am J Gastroenterol 2007;102(8):1781-8.

10. Arvidsson D, Gerdin E. Laparoscopic cholecystectomy during pregnancy. Surg Laparosc Endosc 1991;1(3):193-4.

11. Barone JE, et al. Outcome study of cholecystectomy during pregnancy. Am J Surg 1999;177(3):232-6.

12. Buser KB. Laparoscopic surgery in the pregnant patient-one surgeon's experience in a small rural hospital. 2002;6(2):121-4.

13. Canis M, et al. Laparoscopic management of adnexal masses: a gold standard? Curr Opin Obstet Gynecol 2002;14(4):423-8.

14. Clark SL, et al. Position change and central hemodynamic profile during normal third-trimester pregnancy and postpartum. Am J Obstet Gynecol 1991;164(3):883-7.

15. Conron RW Jr, et al. Laparoscopic procedures in pregnancy. Am Surg 1999;65(3):259-63.

16. Cosenza CA, Saffari B, Jabbour N, Stain SC, Carry D, Parekh D, Selby RR. Surgical management of biliary gallstone disease during pregnancy. Am J Surg 1999;178:545-8.

17. Costantino GN, et al. Laparoscopic cholecystectomy in pregnancy. J Laparoendosc Surg 1994;4(2):161-4.

18. Curet MJ. Special problems in laparoscopic surgery. Previous abdominal surgery, obesity, and pregnancy. Surg Clin North Am 2000;80(4):1093-110.

19. Curet MJ, et al. Effects of CO_2 pneumoperitoneum in pregnant ewes. J Surg Res 1996;63(1):339-44.

20. Curet MJ, et al. Laparoscopy during pregnancy. Arch Surg; 1996;131(5):546-50; discussion 550-51

21. Curet MJ, Allen D, Josloff RK, Pitcher DE, Curet LB, Miscall BG, Zucker KA. Laparoscopy during pregnancy. Arch Surg 1996;131:546-50; discussion 550-541.

22. Davis A, Katz VL, Cox R. Gallbladder disease in pregnancy. J Reprod Med 1995;40:759-62.

23. De Wilde JP, Rivers AW, Price DL. A review of the current use of magnetic resonance imaging in pregnancy and safety implications for the fetus. Prog Biophys Mol Biol 2005;87(2-3):335-53.

24. Doll R, Wakeford R. Risk of childhood cancer from fetal irradiation. Br J Radiol 1997;70:130-09.

25. Elkayam U GN. Cardiovascular physiology of pregnancy. In: Elkayam U GN (ed) Cardiac problems in pregnancy: diagnosis and management of maternal and fetal disease. Alan R Liss, New York, 1982;5.

26. Eyvazzadeh AD, Levine D. Imaging of pelvic pain in the first trimester of pregnancy. Radiol Clin North Am 2006;44(6):863-77.

27. Fallon WF Jr, et al. The surgical management of intra-abdominal inflammatory conditions during pregnancy. Surg Clin North Am 1995;75(1):15-31.

28. Fatum M, Rojansky N. Laparoscopic surgery during pregnancy. Obstet Gynecol Surv 2001;56:50-09.

29. Forsted DH, Kalbhen CL. CT of pregnant women for urinary tract calculi, pulmonary thromboembolism, and acute appendicitis. AJR Am J Roentgenol 2002;178(5):1285.

30. Friedman JD, et al. Pneumoamnion and pregnancy loss after second-trimester laparoscopic surgery. Obstet Gynecol 2002;99(3):512-3.

31. Garcia-Bournissen F, Shrim A, Koren G. Safety of gadolinium during pregnancy. Can Fam Physician 2006;52:309-10.

32. Geisler JP, et al. Non-gynecologic laparoscopy in second and third trimester pregnancy: obstetric implications. JSLS 1998;2(3):235-8.

33. Glasgow RE, et al. Changing management of gallstone disease during pregnancy. Surg Endosc 1998;12(3):241-6.

34. Glasgow RE, Visser BC, Harris HW, Patti MG, Kilpatrick SJ, Mulvihill SJ. Changing management of gallstone disease during pregnancy. Surg Endosc 1998;12:241-6.

35. Gordon MC. Maternal physiology in pregnancy. In: Gabbe SG, Niebyl JR, Simpson JL (eds) Obstetrics: normal and problem pregnancies. Churchill Livingstone, Philadelphia, 2002;63-91.

36. Graham G, Baxi L, Tharakan T. Laparoscopic cholecystectomy during pregnancy: a case series and review of the literature. Obstet Gynecol Surv 1998;53:566-74.

37. Guidelines for laparoscopic surgery during pregnancy. Surg Endosc 1998;12(2):189-90.

38. Gurbuz AT, Peetz ME. The acute abdomen in the pregnant patient: is there a role for laparoscopy? Surg Endosc 1997;11:98-102.

39. Halpern NB. Laparoscopic cholecystectomy in pregnancy: a review of published experiences and clinical considerations. Semin Laparosc Surg 1998;5(2):129-34.

40. Hiatt JR, Hiatt JC, Williams RA, Klein SR. Biliary disease in pregnancy: strategy for surgical management. Am J Surg 1986;151:263-5.

41. Hume RF, Killiam AP. Maternal physiology, in obstetrics and gynecology. In: Scott JR, KiSaia J, Hammon DB (eds) JB Lippincott, Philadelphia, 1990;93-100.

42. Hunter JG, Swanstrom L, Thornburg K. Carbon dioxide pneumoperitoneum induces fetal acidosis in a pregnant ewe model. Surg Endosc 1995;9(3):272-227; discussion 277-9.

43. Hurwitz LM, et al. Radiation dose to the fetus from body MDCT during early gestation. AJR Am J Roentgenol 2005;186(3):871-6.

44. Iafrati MD, Yarnell R, Schwaitzberg SD. Gasless laparoscopic cholecystectomy in pregnancy. J Laparoendosc Surg 1995;5(2):127-30.

45. Kammerer WS. Nonobstetric surgery during pregnancy. Med Clin North Am 1979;63:1157-64.

46. Karam PA. Determining and reporting fetal radiation exposure from diagnostic radiation. Health Phys 2000;79(5):S85-S90.

47. Kennedy A. Assessment of acute abdominal pain in the pregnant patient. Semin Ultrasound CT MR 2000;21(1):64-77.

48. Kort B, Katz VL, Watson WJ. The effect of nonobstetric operation during pregnancy. Surg Gynecol Obstet 1993;177:371-6.

49. Lachman E, et al. Pregnancy and laparoscopic surgery. J Am Assoc Gynecol Laparosc 1999;6(3):347-51.

50. Lemaire BM, van Erp WF. Laparoscopic surgery during pregnancy. Surg Endosc 1997;11:15-8.

51. Leyendecker JR, Gorengaut V, Brown JJ. MR imaging of maternal diseases of the abdomen and pelvis during pregnancy and the immediate postpartum period. Radiographics 2004;24(5):1301-16.

52. Lim HK, Bae SH, Seo GS. Diagnosis of acute appendicitis in pregnant women: value of sonography. AJR Am J Roentgenol 1992;159:539-42.

53. Lim HK, Bae SH, Seo GS. Diagnosis of acute appendicitis in pregnant women: value of sonography. AJR Am J Roentgenol 1992;159(3):539-42.

54. Lowe SA. Diagnostic radiography in pregnancy: risks and reality. Aust N Z J Obstet Gynaecol 2004;44(3):191-6.

55. Malangoni MA. Gastrointestinal surgery and pregnancy. Gastroenterol Clin North Am 2003;32(1):181-200.

56. Matsumoto T, et al. Laparoscopic treatment of uterine prolapse during pregnancy. Obstet Gynecol 1999;93 (5 pt 2):849.

57. McKellar DP, et al. Cholecystectomy during pregnancy without fetal loss. Surg Gynecol Obstet 1992;174(6):465-8.

58. McKenna DA, et al. The use of MRI to demonstrate small bowel obstruction during pregnancy. Br J Radiol 2007;80(949):11e-14e.

59. Medical radiation exposure of pregnant and potentially pregnant women. National Council on Radiation Protection and Measurements report no. 1977;54, Bethesda, MD.

60. Melgrati L et al. Isobaric (gasless) laparoscopic myomectomy during pregnancy. J Minim Invasive Gynecol 2005;12(4):379-81.

61. Menias CO, et al. CT of pregnancy-related complications. Emerg Radiol 2007;13(6):299-306.

62. Moore C, Promes SB. Ultrasound in pregnancy. Emerg Med Clin North Am 2004;22(3):697-722.

63. Muench J, et al. Delay in treatment of biliary disease during pregnancy increases morbidity and can be avoided with safe laparoscopic cholecystectomy. Am Surg 2001;67(6): 539-542; discussion 542-3.

64. Murakami T, et al. Cul-de-sac packing with a metreurynter in gasless laparoscopic cystectomy during pregnancy. J Am Assoc Gynecol Laparosc 2003;10(3):421-3.

65. Nagayama M, et al. Fast MR imaging in obstetrics. Radiographics 2002;22(3):563-80; discussion 580-2.

66. Nelson MJ, et al. Cysts in pregnancy discovered by sonography. J Clin Ultrasound 1986;14(7):509-512.

67. Nezhat FR, et al. Laparoscopy during pregnancy: a literature review. JSLS 1997;1(1):17-27.

68. Oelsner G, et al. Pregnancy outcome after laparoscopy or laparotomy in pregnancy. J Am Assoc Gynecol Laparosc 2003;10(2):200-204.

69. Oguri H, Taniguchi K, Fukaya T. Gasless laparoscopic management of ovarian cysts during pregnancy. Int J Gynaecol Obstet 2005;91(3):258-9.

70. Osei EK, Faulkner K, et al. Fetal doses from radiological examinations. Br J Radiol 1999;72(860):773-80.

71. Pucci RO, Seed RW. Case report of laparoscopic cholecystectomy in the third trimester of pregnancy. Am J Obstet Gynecol 1991;165(2):401-2.

72. Quan WL, Chia CK, Yim HB. Safety of endoscopical procedures during pregnancy. Singapore Med J 2006;47(6):525-8.

73. Qureshi WA, et al. ASGE guideline: guidelines for endoscopy in pregnant and lactating women. Gastrointest Endosc 2005;61(3):357-62.

74. Reedy MB, et al. Maternal and fetal effects of laparoscopic insufflation in the gravid baboon. J Am Assoc Gynecol Laparosc 1995;2(4):399-406.

75. Reedy MB, Kallen B, Kuehl TJ. Laparoscopy during pregnancy: a study of five fetal outcome parameters with use of the Swedish Health Registry. Am J Obstet Gynecol 1997;177:673-9.

76. Reedy MB, et al. Laparoscopy during pregnancy. A survey of laparoendoscopic surgeons. J Reprod Med 1997;42(1):33-38.

77. Rizzo AG. Laparoscopic surgery in pregnancy: long-term follow-up. J Laparoendosc Adv Surg Tech A 2003;13(1):11-15. 1924 Surg Endosc 2008;22:1917-27.

78. Rollins MD, Chan KJ, Price RR. Laparoscopy for appendicitis and cholelithiasis during pregnancy: a new standard of care. Surg Endosc 2003.

79. Romer T, Bojahr B, Schwesinger G. Treatment of a torqued hematosalpinx in the thirteenth week of pregnancy using gasless laparoscopy. J Am Assoc Gynecol Laparosc 2002;9(1):89-92.

80. Schmidt T, et al. Gasless laparoscopy as an option for conservative therapy of adnexal pedical torsion with twin pregnancy. J Am Assoc Gynecol Laparosc 2001;8(4):621-2.

81. Scott LD. Gallstone disease and pancreatitis in pregnancy. Gastroenterol Clin North Am 1992;21:803-15.

82. Shay DC, Bhavani-Shankar K, Datta S. Laparoscopic surgery during pregnancy. Anesthesiol Clin North Am 2001;19(1):57-67.

83. Society of American Gastrointestinal Endoscopic Surgeons (SAGES). Guidelines for laparoscopic surgery during pregnancy. Surg Endosc 1998;12:189-90.

84. Soriano D, et al. Laparoscopy versus laparotomy in the management of adnexal masses during pregnancy. Fertil Steril 1999;71(5):955-60.

85. State-specific changes in singleton preterm births among black and white women-United States, 1990 and 1997 MMWR Morb Mortal Wkly Rep 2000;49: 837-40.

86. Stepp K, Falcone T. Laparoscopy in the second trimester of pregnancy. Obstet Gynecol Clin North Am 2004;31(3):485-96.

87. Timins JK. Radiation during pregnancy. N J Med 2001;98(6):29-33.

88. Toppenberg KS, Hill DA, Miller DP. Safety of radiographic imaging during pregnancy. Am Fam Physician 1999;59(7):1813-18, 1820.

89. Visser BC, et al. Safety and timing of nonobstetric abdominal surgery in pregnancy. Dig Surg 2001;18(5):409-17

90. Wang CJ, et al. Minilaparoscopic cystectomy and appendectomy in late second trimester. JSLS 2002;6(4):373-75.

91. Weber AM, et al. Laparoscopic cholecystectomy during pregnancy. Obstet Gynecol 1991;78(5 Pt 2):958-9.

92. Williams JK, et al. Laparoscopic cholecystectomy in pregnancy. A case report. J Reprod Med 1995; 40(3): 243-5.

Section Three

33 Laparoscopic Management of Endometriosis

Endometriosis is a progressive, often debilitating disease, affecting 10 to 15 percent of women during their reproductive years. Among gynecologic disorder, endometriosis is surpassed in frequency only by leiomyomas. Laparoscopy and the surgical laser allowed definitive treatment following diagnosis. The debate continues as to whether laparotomy or operative laparoscopy is more effective for the treatment of endometriosis.

In women with bowel symptoms such as dyschezia, tenesmus, or cyclic rectal bleeding without any other pathology, a sigmoidoscopic examination should be done at the time of menstruation to rule out bowel involvement of endometrial implant. However, many women do not demonstrate rectal lesions, but at the time of laparoscopy significant bowel involvement is seen. It should be remembered that a negative sigmoidoscopy does not rule out bowel involvement in patients of endometriosis. In patients who have significant recto-vaginal nodularity on physical examination, a preoperative bowel preparation is necessary and antibiotics are administered the day of surgery. Gynecologist should also consult with a general surgeon experienced in laparoscopic bowel resections. A preoperative ultrasound can assess the ovaries for endometriomas. Preoperative hormonal suppressive therapy can be useful in decreasing the inflammation, bleeding, and possible postoperative adhesion formation.

The goals of surgery are to remove all implants, resects adhesion, relieve pain, and reduce the risk of recurrence and to prevent postoperative adhesion formation. It should also restore involved organs normal anatomical and physiological condition. In case of infertility restoration of tubo-ovarian relationship is essential to restore fertility.

Hysterectomy and bilateral salpingo-oophorectomy is definitive treatment of endometriosis. In advanced disease ovary may be adhered to the pelvic side wall. Ovarian dissection may increase the risk of injury to the ureter and vessels in the triangle of doom. Retroperitoneal approach is helpful in these cases and insures complete removal of ovarian tissue. It also avoid ovarian remnant syndrome.

Bilateral oophorectomy must be performed to eliminate the estrogen that sustains and stimulate the ectopic endometrium. Following hysterectomy and bilateral oophorectomy patient often require HRT. Administering the minimal effective dose of estrogen is some time associated with small risk of recurrence. HRT should begin postoperatively. Patients with residual disease may benefit from receiving progesterone from 2 to 6 months followed by combined progesterone and estrogen for additional 9 months.

Conservative surgery is indicated for women who desire pregnancy and whose disease is responsible for the symptom of pain and infertility. Surgery improves likelihood of pregnancy and offers pain relief. Twenty five percent of patients undergoing conservative operation may require subsequent operation. The rate of surgery directly depends on the extent of disease. Those who achieve pregnancy after surgery, only 10 percent require another operation. Conservative operations are cytoreductive and recurrence of symptom most likely is caused by the progression of existing pathology that was missed during laparoscopy.

Complete removal of endometriosis is difficult because of there variability in appearance and visibility. Powder burn lesions represent foci of inactive disease containing stroma and gland embedded in hemosiderin deposit. These lesions are more common in older lesion and sometime without any symptoms. When endometriosis involve uterosacral ligament, they are palpable as tender nodule and may cause dysmenorrhea and dyspareunia. Superficial endometriosis is treated optimally by electrosurgical fulguration or ablation. If large areas of peritoneum are involved with endometriosis or if a woman has recurrent endometriosis in an area previously ablated by electrosurgery or laser, it may be better to excise that entire area of peritoneum to prevent recurrence. Especially, areas with scarring or fibrosis should be excised carefully because there may be endometriosis beneath them. One concern in laser ablation or excising large areas of peritoneum is the chance of adhesion formation. Animal studies indicate that these areas are reperitonealized in 24 to 48 hours by the migration of surrounding peritoneum and that adhesion formation is low after laparoscopy. However, the surgeon should be cautious particularly when excising areas of peritoneum which are opposed by pelvic organs.

Sometime atypical lesions are seen as clear vesicle, pink vascular pattern, white scarred lesion, red lesion, yellow brown patches and peritoneal windows, which represent active endometriosis (Fig. 33.1A). These lesions secrete prostaglandin into the peritoneal fluid. The depth of endometrial implants may be related to the level of disease activity and symptoms. The peritoneum must be examined from all the angles and from different degree of illumination to see all types of lesion. The peritoneal folds must be stretched and search for small and atypical lesions. Normal appearing ovaries sometime may contain endometriosis under apparently normal cortex. By inserting the needle in the ovary small endometriosis can be identified.

All the pelvic organs are inspected thoroughly. In 15 percent of cases appendix is involved and so it should be examined. The endometriosis which has penetrated retroperitoneally, several centimeters is called an iceberg lesion. It can be detected laparoscopically by palpating areas of the pelvis and bowel with the suction irrigation probe. With the forceps or probe the endometriotic implant are examined and their size, depth and proximity to normal pelvic structure is evaluated.

The diagnostic laparoscopy may turn into operative one if the surgeon has consent. The operative procedure begins by removing adhesions if present between the bowel and pelvic organs to adequately expose the pelvic cavity. The ovaries and tube may be adhered with cul-de-sac or pelvic sidewall. These organs are freed from adhesions and chromotubated. Endometrial implants and endometriomas are resected or vaporized, and if the patient has significant central pelvic pain, uterosacral nerve ablation or presacral nerve resection is performed.

Lysis of Bowel Adhesions

Tubo-ovarian mass with bowel adhesion is common finding in extensive endometriosis. Bowel adhesions

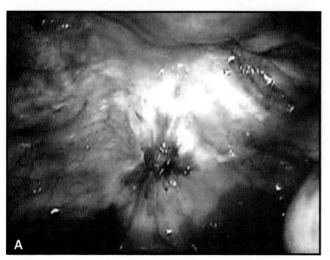
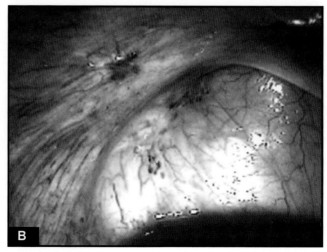

Figs 33.1A and B: Endometriosis

vary in thickness, vascularity, and cohesiveness. Some adhesions are stretched without tearing the tissue and should be excised with electrosurgery at the points of attachment to the pelvic organs. Dense adhesions are excised either with scissors or the ultrasonic dissector. The adhered structures requiring separation are pulled apart with forcers and a cleavage plane is formed. Hydrodissection is useful to identify and develop the dissection plane, which is ablated or excised, using dissecting scissors.

Peritoneal Implants

At the time of treating peritoneal endometriosis, the implants should be destroyed in the most effective and least traumatic manner to minimize postoperative adhesions and injury to retroperitoneal vessel and nerve. Although different modalities have been used, but hydrodissection and high-power fulguration or CO_2 laser are the best choices for endometriosis treatment (Fig. 33.1B).

Superficial peritoneal endometriosis may be vaporized with monopolar or bipolar current, or excised. Implants less than 2 mm are coagulated, vaporized, or excised. As lesions exceed 3 mm, vaporization or excision is needed. For lesions greater than 5 mm, deep vaporization or excisional techniques are required. If vaporization is chosen, it is important to copiously irrigate and remove the charred areas to confirm complete removal of the lesion and to avoid confusing endometriosis with a carbon deposit.

Resection of Ovarian Endometriosis

The ovaries are a common site for endometriosis. Endometrial implants or endometriomas less than 2 cm in diameter are coagulated; laser ablated, or excised using scissors, biopsy forceps, or electrodes. For successful eradication, all visible lesions and scars must be removed from the ovarian surface. Entrapment of oocytes within the luteinized ovarian follicle, as reported in experimental animal models, must be avoided. Endometriomas more than 2 cm diameter must be resected thoroughly to prevent recurrence. Draining the endometriomas or partial resection of its wall is inadequate because the endometrial tissue lining the cyst is likely to remain functional and can cause the symptoms to recur (Fig. 33.2).

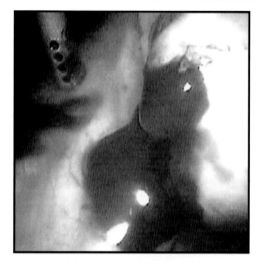

Fig. 33.2: Chocolate cyst

Many gynecologists like to perform ovarian cystoscopy and biopsy of the cyst wall before ablating the cyst. By using a double optic laparoscope, which involves the passage of a smaller operative endoscope through the channel of the main laparoscope, the ovarian cyst may be punctured, drained, the fluid sent for cytology, and the lining of inner cystic wall is visually inspected. Once it confirmed that the cyst is not malignant, its wall is ablated to a depth of 3 to 4 mm (Figs 33.3A and B).

For endometriomas over 2 cm in diameter, the cyst is punctured with aspiration needle and aspirated with the suction-irrigator probe. Deroofing of cyst wall is performed. The cyst wall should be removed by grasping its base with laparoscopic forceps and peeling it from the ovarian stroma. If peeling of the remaining wall is not possible it should be ablated using electrosurgical fulguration. When the entire cyst wall is ablated, representative biopsies are taken for histological diagnosis.

Cyst wall closure is not necessary, according to animal experiments for large defects that result from resecting endometriomas larger than 5 cm; the edges of the ovarian cortex are approximated with a single suture placed within the ovarian stroma. Fibrin sealant has been described to atraumatically approximate the edges of large ovarian defects, without adhesion formation. Although rare, some patients present with localized symptoms and severe involvement of only one ovary with disease and adhesions while the opposite ovary is normal. These patients are benefited by

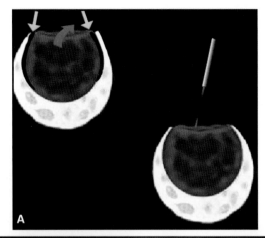

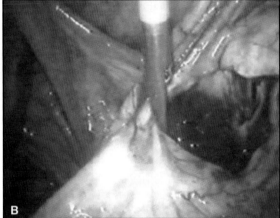

Figs 33.3A and B: Endometrioma, deroofing and marsupialization

If urinary tract endometriosis is suspected, a complete preoperative evaluation is performed, including an intravenous pyelogram, ultrasound of the kidneys, and routine blood and urine work-up. In selected cases of recurrent hematuria, cystoscopy is indicated. Superficial implants over the ureter can be treated by a variation of hydrodissection. Approximately 20 to 30 ml of Ringer's lactate is injected subperitoneally on the lateral pelvic wall; this elevates the peritoneum and backs it with a bed of fluid to prevent injury at the time of fulguration. The peritoneum is held with an atraumatic grasping forceps and peeled away with the help of suction irrigation probe. Following hydrodissection of the broad ligaments and the pelvic sidewall, many patients develop swelling of the external genitalia, most likely from the penetration of water through the inguinal canal to the labia major. This swelling resolves in most cases within 1 to 2 hours without sequelae.

The incidence of ureteral obstruction by endometriosis is low, and conventional therapy previously consisted of laparotomy followed by resection of the obstructed segment of the ureter. Laparoscopic ureteroureterostomy can be performed under direct laparoscopic observation.

The bladder wall is one of the sites least frequently involved with endometriosis. If the lesions are superficial, hydrodissection and vaporization are adequate for removal. Using hydrodissection, the areolar tissue between the serosa and muscularis beneath the implants is dissected. The lesion is circumcised with the laser and fluid is injected into the resulting defect. The lesion is grasped with forceps and dissected with the help of either sharp or electrosurgical dissection. Traction allows the small blood vessels supplying the surrounding tissue to be coagulated as the lesion is resected. Frequent irrigation is necessary to remove char, ascertain the depth of vaporization, and ensure that the lesion does not involve the muscularis and the mucosa.

Endometriosis extending to the muscularis but without mucosal involvement can be treated laparoscopically and any residual or deeper lesions may be treated successfully with postoperative hormonal therapy. When endometriosis involves full bladder wall thickness, the lesion is excised and the bladder may be reconstructed laparoscopically.

unilateral salpingo-oophorectomy. By removing the diseased ovary, the risk of disease recurrence is minimized, and the fertility potential is improved by limiting ovulation to the healthy side.

Genitourinary Endometriosis

Ureteral involvement has been reported in 1 to 11 percent of women diagnosed with endometriosis. Endometriosis of the urinary tract generally tends to be superficial but can be invasive and cause complete ureteral obstruction.

Decreased bladder capacity and stability unresponsive to conventional therapy may result from endometriosis. When bladder symptoms are present a course of danazol may be tried to see the improvement in bladder instability. Clinicians should consider endometriosis in cases of refractory and unexplained urinary complaints.

Gastrointestinal endometriosis is believed to be involved in 3 to 37 percent of women suffering from endometriosis. Endometriosis can involve rectovaginal septum, rectosigmoid colon, between the small intestine and anal canal. The symptoms are lower abdominal pain, back ache dysmenorrhea dyspareunia, diarrhea, constipation and tenesmus. Occasionally rectal bleeding is also noticed. Typically these symptoms occur cyclically at or about the time of menstruation. Surgical intervention is necessary to dissect and resect the infiltrating bowel endometriosis. Intestinal endometriosis involves the rectum and sigmoid colon in 76 percent of cases, the appendix in 18 percent and the cecum in 5 percent. Appendiceal lesion requires appendectomy. In cases of severe disease of bowel wall, resection and anastomosis is done laparoscopically. In cases of cul-de-sac endometriosis, because ureter is lateral to the uterosacral ligament, surgeons should try to separate between them. If the dissection is extended lateral to the uterosacral ligament the ipsilateral ureter should be identified by opening the overlying peritoneum and stressing it to the area of the lesion. The ureter, uterine artery and vein should be identified and bipolar forceps or titanium clips must be used if bleeding starts.

Endometriosis sometime affect diaphragm also. In these cases pleuritic shoulder or upper abdominal pain is present at the time of menses. Laparoscopy is an excellent modality to diagnose and treat diaphragmatic endometriosis. Follow-up medical treatment is necessary because extensive surgery can rupture the diaphragm. Bilateral oophorectomy is promising and further intervention may not be necessary. Three cannulas are required in the upper quadrant according to the site of lesion on diaphragm. Liver retractor is used by one port and lesions are removed using hydro-dissection and vaporization or excision. If injury to diaphragm happens it should be repaired with a 4-0 PDS. Cardiopulmonary resuscitation may be necessary after surgery.

Section Three

34 Laparoscopic Hysterectomy

Benign uterine diseases of uterus are very common and need hysterectomy and laparotomy. Most of these diseases can be performed laparoscopically. Laparoscopic assisted vaginal hysterectomy is increasingly becoming popular. Many women come to the doctor and say they want a "laser" hysterectomy. What they usually mean is a laparoscopically assisted vaginal hysterectomy or LAVH. Laparoscopically assisted vaginal hysterectomy (LAVH) is a procedure using laparoscopic surgical techniques and instruments to remove the uterus and/or tubes and ovaries through the vagina. The technique used to use lasers but now lasers have been mostly replaced by surgical clips, cautery or suturing. First laparoscopic hysterectomy was done by Reich et al in 1989. It is a technique made to replace abdominal hysterectomy.

LAPAROSCOPIC ANATOMY

The normal nulliparous uterus is approximately 8 cm in length and angled forward so the fundus lies over the posterior surface of the bladder. Uterus is all around covered with peritoneum except where the bladder touches the lower uterine segment at the anterior cul-de-sac and laterally at the broad ligament (Fig. 34.1).

Two important arteries, uterine and ovarian are of great significance in uterine surgery. The uterine arise from the internal iliac. They pass medially on the levator ani muscle, cross the ureter and ultimately divide into ascending and descending branch. The uterine artery runs in a tortuous course within the broad ligaments. The uterine arteries ascending branch terminates by anatomizing with the ovarian artery.

From anterior to posterior, following important tubular structures are found crossing the brim of true pelvis: The round ligament of the uterus, the infundibulopelvic ligament, which contains the gonadal vessels and the ureter. The ovaries and fallopian tube is found between the round ligament and the infundibulopelvic ligament (Fig. 34.2).

The ovarian ligaments run from the ovaries to the lateral border of the uterus. Ovary is attached to the pelvic side wall with infundibulopelvic ligament, which carries ovarian artery. One of the common mistakes is injury of the ureter during dissection of the

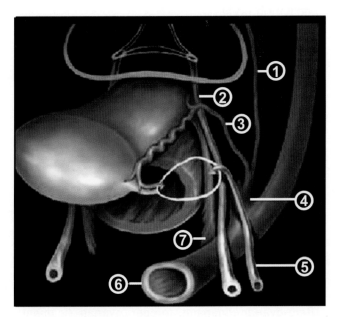

Fig. 34.1: Anatomy of uterus, 1-Umbilical artery, 2-Ureter, 3-Uterine artery, 4-Internal iliac artery, 5-Ovarian artery, 6-Common iliac artery, 7-Utero-sacral ligament

infundibulopelvic ligament. If the uterus is deviated to the contralateral side with the help of uterine manipulator infundibulopelvic ligament is spread out and a pelvic side wall triangle is created. The base of this triangle is the round ligament, the medial side is the infundibulopelvic ligament, and the lateral side is the external iliac artery. The apex of this triangle is the point at which the infundibulopelvic ligament crosses the external iliac artery. The ureter always enters medial to this triangle into the pelvis. It is visible under the peritoneum overlying the external iliac artery.

The ureters enter the pelvis in close proximity to the female pelvic organ and are at risk for injury during laparoscopic surgery of these organs. As the ureter course medially over the bifurcation of the iliac vessels, they pass obliquely under the ovarian vessels and then run in close proximity to the uterine artery.

Laparoscopy hysterectomy needs careful identification of ureter with some dissection of retroperitoneum. An incision is made in the peritoneum overlying the pelvic side wall triangle between the fallopian tube and iliac vessel.

Pelvic lymph node dissection is also necessary if gynecologist plan to perform radical laparoscopic hysterectomy. Node dissection as far distal as Cloquet's node in the femoral triangle may be included and proximally dissection may be necessary up to para-aortic lymph node.

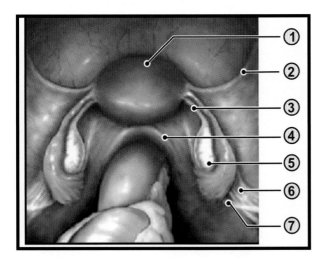

Fig. 34.2: Position of uterus, 1-Uterus, 2-Round ligament, 3-Utero-ovarian ligament (proper ovarian ligament), 4-Uterosacral ligament, 5-Ovary, 6-Suspensory ligament of the ovary, 7-Ureter

Indications of LAVH

Indications of LAVH are traditionally contraindications of vaginal hysterectomy.
Indications include:
• Previous pelvic surgery
• Endometriosis
• Previous CS
• Pelvic pain
• Suspected adnexal pathology
• Uterine myoma
• Ectopic pregnancy
• Acute or chronic pelvic inflammatory disease
• Minimum uterine mobility and limited vaginal access.

If a vaginal hysterectomy can be performed in the first place, there would be no point in adding the costs and complications of laparoscopy. Its greatest benefit is the potential to convert what would have been an abdominal hysterectomy into a vaginal hysterectomy. An abdominal hysterectomy requires both a vaginal incision and a four to six inch long incision in the abdomen, which is associated with greater post-operative discomfort and a longer recovery period than for a vaginal procedure. Another advantage of the LAVH may be the removal of the tubes and ovaries which on occasion may not be easily removed with a vaginal hysterectomy.

The most common medical reasons for performing hysterectomies include uterine fibroids (30%), abnormal uterine bleeding (20%), endometriosis (20 %), genital prolapse (15%) and chronic pelvic pain (10%). For most of these conditions, other treatments should first be considered, and hysterectomy should be reserved as a last resort.

LAVH result in a significantly shorter hospital stay, with a much more rapid return to normal activities, than total laparoscopic hysterectomy. The drug requirement to control pain and the level of pain patients experienced were also significantly less. Blood loss was not different for the two procedures (Tables 34.1 and 34.2).

Postoperative recovery times and pain levels were assessed in 37 patients with a primary complaint of pelvic pain and diagnoses of fibroid uterus, adenomyosis, and severe endometriosis who underwent LAVH. Women reported an activity level of 8.7 on a scale of 1 to 10 (10 no limits on activity)

by postoperative day 14. In another study, those undergoing abdominal hysterectomy had a mean uterine weight of 418 g compared with 150 g for those undergoing LAVH. The hospital stay after abdominal hysterectomy was 4.5 days and after LAVH 2.5 days. An important public policy issue now confronts us. As it is currently performed, LAVH is more expensive than TAH. The issue is whether the benefits of shorter convalescence and faster return to the work force, shorter hospitalization, and less need for narcotics for postoperative pain outweigh the disadvantage of the higher cost. If total health care system costs are evaluated, the short-term disability costs of 2 weeks of recovery after laparoscopic hysterectomy should be compared with disability costs of 6 to 8 weeks of recovery after abdominal hysterectomy.

For LAVH to be economically viable compared with TAH, savings in disability costs and the increased contribution to the gross domestic product must offset the increased health care costs. In the current system, insurance companies and hospitals do not share in

Table 34.1: Postoperative pain levels

Day	LAVH (n -= 19)	TAH (n= 19)	p
1	6.6	6.4	NS
3	4.4	4.3	NS
7	2.8	3.6	S
14	1.6	2.4	S
21	1.46	1.8	S
Week 6	1.35	1.4	NS

Wilcoxon's signed rank test.
Ten-point activity scale: 1 = no pain, 10 = unbearable pain.
S = significant at p < 0.005; NS = not significant at p <0.01

Table 34.2: Postoperative activity levels

Day	LAVH (n -= 19)	TAH (n= 19)	p
1	3.4	3.3	NS
3	5.4	4.4	NS
7	7.8	5.8	S
14	9.2	6.4	S
21	9.6	7.9	S
Week 6	9.95	8.5	S

Wilcoxon's signed rank test.
Ten-point activity scale: 1 = extremely limited activity, 10 = no limits on activity
S = significant at p < 0.005; NS = not significant at p <0.01

these benefits, only the costs. The economic impact of laparoscopic surgery must take into account both the cost to the hospital and insurance payers and these productivity and social issues. Insurance is based on a risk pool whereby the cost of a premium is based on the cost of treatment, not the ability of the subscriber to return to work. An economic and social cost-benefit analysis must be performed before decisions are made to modify or judge a procedure that provides substantial benefits to the patient.

Since its introduction in 1989, continued improvement of techniques will likely progress rapidly so that LAVH will be performed on an outpatient basis for many women, and will result in shorter recovery time. Thus, the increased operating room time of approximately 46 minutes is significantly outweighed by the benefits available with widespread application of this procedure.

CLASSIFICATION

Garry and Reich Classification

- Type 1 Diagnostic lap + VH
- Type 2 lap vault suspension after VH
- Type 3 LAVH
- Type 4 LH (lap ligation of uterine artery)
- Type 5 TLH
- Type 6 LSH (lap supracervical hysterectomy)
- Type 7 LHL (lap hysterectomy with lymphadenectomy)
- Type 8 LHL + O (as above + omentectomy)
- Type 9 RLH (radical lap hysterectomy)

Preoperative Measures

Patients are evaluated same as that of any major surgery. Routine preoperative test include a complete blood count with differential, serum electrolyte, bleeding time and urinalysis. More comprehensive blood studies include thrombin time, partial thrombin time, ECG, chest X-ray and endometrial biopsy. Mechanical and antibiotic bowel preparation is advised. Peglac powder 1 sachet with water a night prior to surgery is advised.

Patient Position

Patient should be in steep Trendelenburg's and lithotomy position. One assistant should remain

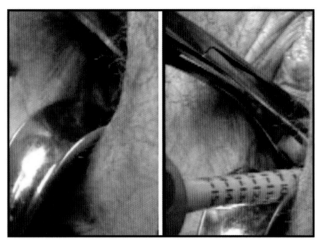

Fig. 34.3: Per-vaginal examination should be routine

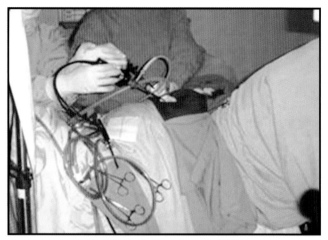

Fig. 34.4: Port position in LAVH

between the legs of patient to do uterine manipulation whenever required (Fig. 34.3).

Position of Surgical Team (Fig. 34.4)

Surgeon stand left to the patient, camera assistant should be left to the surgeon. Second assistant should be the opposite side of the body of patient. One more assistant is required between the legs to handle uterine manipulator.

Port Position

A 10 mm umbilical port for camera should be along the inferior crease. Two 5 mm ports should be placed at 5 cm away from umbilicus on either side. Sometime, accessory port at right or left iliac region may be needed according to need.

Port position should be in accordance with baseball diamond concept. If the left side of tube has to be operated, one port should be in right iliac fossa and another below left hypochondrium (Fig. 34.5).

Operative Technique

It is important throughout the procedure to be able to manipulate the uterus for optimal observation. Different types of uterine manipulators are available. Depending on the laparoscopic procedure, digital examination, probes, and sponge stick applicators are used in the cul-de-sac for identification of structures during laparoscopy. The direction and location of both ureters should be identified as much as possible (Fig. 34.6).

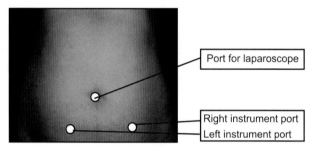

Port for laparoscope

Right instrument port
Left instrument port

Fig. 34.5: Port position for LAVH

If adenexectomy is planned, following electrodesiccation and cutting of the round ligaments, 2 to 3 cm of the uterus, the infundibulopelvic ligament is desiccated and cut, taking progressive bites of tissue starting at pelvic brim and moving towards the round ligament. If endoscopic linear stapler is used the adnexae is grasped with forceps, it is retracted medially and caudally to stretch and outline the infundibulopelvic ligament, which is grasped and secured with the stapler. Stapler is not fired until the contained tissue is identified and the ureter safety is confirmed. Once transacted the staple line should be examined closely for any possible injury and hemostasis. Following infundibulopelvic ligament transaction the adnexae and uterine fundus are retracted in the opposite direction and the tissue of the upper broad ligament, including the round ligament, is grasped, secured and cut.

The multifire GIA stapler can clamp and cut tissue efficiently. The device places six rows of small titanium staples and cuts the tissue in between, leaving three rows of staples on either side of the transected pedicle. This device leaves essentially bloodless pedicles. However, the instrument is disposable and expensive (Figs 34.7A and B).

If the adnexae is planned to preserve, the round ligament is desiccated and cut approximately 2 cm from the uterus. The anterior leaf of the broad ligament is opened towards the vesicouterine fold and bladder flap is developed. The anterior leaf of the broad ligament is grasped with forceps, elevated and dissected from the anterior lower uterine segment. The utero-ovarian ligament proximal tube and mesosalpinx are progressively dissected and cut and posterior leaf of the broad ligament is opened. Similarly, the round ligament fallopian tube and utero-ovarian ligament are grasped closed to their insertion into the uterus with endoscopic linear stapler, then secured stapled and cut. The distal end of the stapler or bipolar forceps must be kept free of the bladder and ureter (Fig. 34.8).

The uterovesical junction is identified, grasped, and elevated with forceps while being cut with scissors. The bladder pillars are identified desiccated and cut. The bladder can be completely freed from the uterus by pushing downward with the tip of a blunt probe along the vesicocervical plane until the anterior cul-de-sac is exposed completely. In patients with severe anterior cul-de-sac endometriosis, previous CS or adhesions, sharp dissection can be performed. Injecting 5 ml of indigo caramine in the patient's bladder helps to detect bladder trauma.

After dissecting the bladder from the uterus, the uterine vessels are identified desiccated and cut to free the lateral border of uterus (Figs 34.10A to D). If sutures, clips or linear staplers are used, it is important to fully skeletonize the vessel. As the uterine vessel are grasped and cut, safety and position of the ureter should be checked. Ureter injury can be completely nullified if ureteric catheter is introduced before the procedure. Cardinal ligament dissection must be

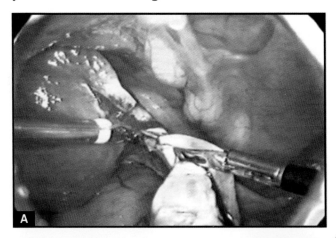

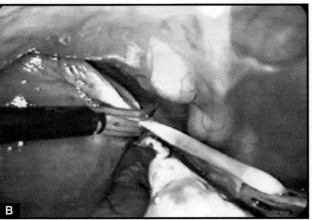

Figs 34.7A and B: Successive desiccation and dissection

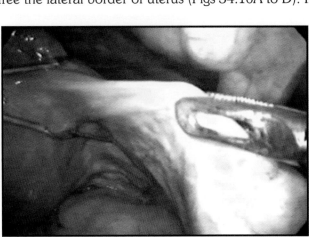

Fig. 34.6: LAVH using bipolar

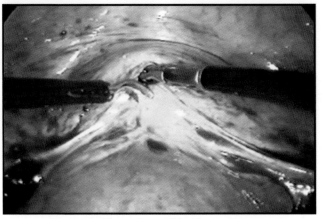

Fig. 34.8: Dissection of bladder peritoneum

carefully done as ureter and uterine artery falls just lateral to that. The linear stapler can be used only if the parametrium has been dissected with the ample margins. Once the ureter is displaced laterally, the cardinal ligament tissue closest to the cervix is electrodesiccated and transacted. Alternatively, the linear stapler can be applied both on the uterine vessels and cardinal ligament (Figs 34.11 and 34.12).

Colpotomy

A folded gauge in sponge forceps is used to mark the fornix. The vaginal wall is tented and transacted horizontally with hook electrode (Figs 34.9A to C).

Once the dissection is extended to the lower uterine segment or to the level of cardinal ligament, laparoscopic portion is temporarily terminated. Three vaginally speculum is used to get proper access for vaginal part of LAVH (Figs 34.13A to D). Once the

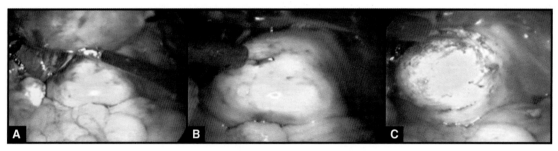

Figs 34.9A to C: Steps of colpotomy

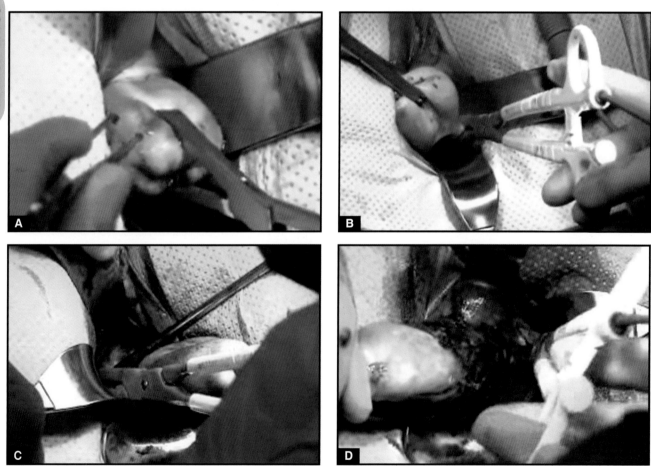

Figs 34.10A to D: Successive clamping and desiccation of uterine pedical through the vaginal route, (A) Valsaleum holding cervix, (B) Application of ligasure clamp over left uterosacral, (C) Application of ligasure over the right uterine stump, (D) Application of ligasure over the left uterine stump

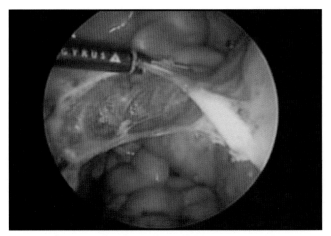

Fig. 34.11: Opening of anterior and posterior
leaf broad ligament

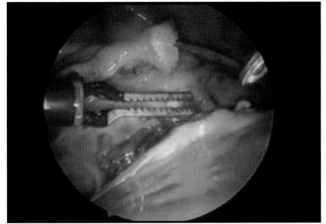

Fig. 34.12: Separation of bladder

uterus is removed, the vaginal vault is closed to ensure support of the vault; the vaginal angles are attached to the uterosacral and cardinal ligaments with 2-0 vicryl (Figs 34.14A and B). Any co-existing cystocele or rectocele is repaired. A very large fibroid uterus should be debulked by morcellation for removal vaginally. It can be combined with laparoscopic adnexal surgery, e.g. ovariectomy or adhesiolysis. Once the vaginal surgery is completed again laparoscopic inspection of the pelvis is done.

Total Laparoscopic Hysterectomy

Total laparoscopic hysterectomy requires vaginal seal to prevent gas leak. Two 4 × 4 wet sponges in the gloves can be used to insert into the vagina to prevent loss of pneumoperitoneum. By applying contralateral retraction to the uterus, vaginal wall surrounding the cervix is outlined, coagulated with the unipolar scissors or bipolar forceps and cut circumferentially until the cervix is separated. Specimen is pulled to mid vagina but not removed to preserve pneumoperitoneum. Vaginal vault is irrigated and inspected for any active bleeding. Once hemostasis is achieved, vaginal angles are sutured to the adjacent cardinal and uterosacral ligaments. Care is taken to avoid the ureter. Rest of the vaginal cuff is closed using intracorporeal knotting. Bipolar is used cautiously at the vaginal cuff to prevent tissue necrosis and subsequent wound breakdown if the sutures replaced in non-viable tissue.

The hysterectomy can be performed laparoscopically up to the uterine size of 26 weeks. These patients must have adequate hemoglobin and hematocrit. The GnRH analogue should be given if the uterus is more than 18 weeks gestational size. According to baseball diamond concept the telescopic port should be placed between umbilicus and xiphoid in the patient whose uterus is more that 18 weeks size. The secondary ports should also be placed higher than usual.

Big uterus with multiple myomas is difficult to manipulate. Sometime, 4 to 5 port may be necessary to handle this uterus. Anatomy is distorted and ureteral dissection may be necessary in these cases.

Subtotal Hysterectomy

Supracervical hysterectomy is performed to preserve libido of patient. The procedure is performed fully laparoscopically. After desiccating and cutting the uterine vessels at the level of cardinal ligaments above the uterosacral ligament, uterus is retracted and its lower segment is amputated with the scissors and unipolar cutting current. After transecting the uterus from the cervix, uterine manipulator is removed vaginally, the cervical stump is irrigated and hemostasis is achieved. The endocervical epithelium, lining the cervical canal is vaporized or coagulated with laser or electrosurgery. The rest of the endocervical canal is ablated vaginally to reduce the risk of intraepithelial cervical neoplasia. The cervical stump is closed with interrupted absorbable sutures and covered with peritoneum, which is stitched transversely with interrupted sutures. The dissected uterus is morcellated and removes through a 10 mm cannula. Mini-laparotomy or

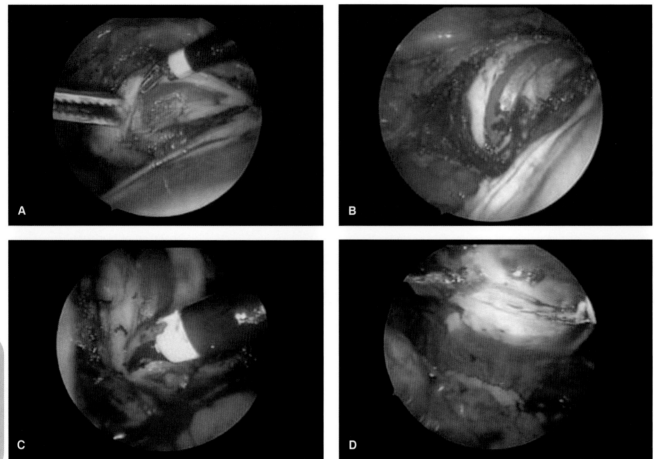

Figs 34.13A to D: Anterior and posterior colpotomy

posterior colpotomy can also be performed to remove the uterus in case of subtotal hysterectomy. These patients are advised to annual examination for Pap smear.

Ending the Procedure

One of the benefits of LAVH or TLH over NDVH is inspection of pedicles at the end of surgery. The vaginal cuff can be closed from below or above but after that pneumoperitoneum is again restored to see the pelvic and abdominal cavity. Irrigation and suction should be performed. In case of any residual bleeding it can be controlled laparoscopically. At the end pelvis is filled with 300 ml Ringer's lactate and it should be seen for change in color. Once inspection is satisfying the fluid is sucked and instrument and cannula is removed after deflating the abdominal cavity.

It has been demonstrated that TLH and LAVH are associated with a shorter hospital stay and patients require less pain medication compared to TAH. LAVH can replace most of the abdominal hysterectomy for the benign disease of uterus and with the technology available today it has definite benefit over non-descended vaginal hysterectomy.

DISCUSSION

Vaginal hysterectomy is part of repertoire of every trained gynecologist. It is considered as a feasible option to abdominal hysterectomy and many studies have shown that vaginal hysterectomy has fewer complications, short recovery, and hospital stay than laparotomy. Laparoscopic hysterectomy requires greater surgical expertise and has a steep learning curve. Randomized trials have shown advantages of laparoscopy versus laparotomy, including reduced postoperative pain, shorter hospitalization, rapid recovery and substantial financial benefits to society. The objective of performing hysterectomy laparoscopically can be achieved but the question is does this offer any advantage over vaginal route. Every mode of hysterectomy has advantages and disadvantages but the indications for each remain controversial. Good surgical practice is when the indication for hysterectomy is considered as the primary criterion for selecting the route of hysterectomy and not factors such as surgeon's choice and experience. A major determinant of the route of hysterectomy is not the clinical situation but the attitude of the surgeon. There is no need for extra training and special skills or complicated equipment for vaginal hysterectomy.

Laparoscopic hysterectomy took a long time to perform in all studies. However with increasing weight of the uterus, there was a linear increase in operating time and blood loss in hysterectomy performed vaginally which was not observed in laparoscopic assisted vaginal hysterectomy. There is no statistically significant difference in postoperative analgesia requirement, hospital stay, recovery milestones or complication rates. The biggest drawback of laparoscopic route over vaginal one is its cost due to expensive disposable instruments, prolonged operating and anesthesia time and the need for a trained senior gynecologist. For laparoscopic assisted vaginal hysterectomy to be cost effective expensive disposable instruments have to be eliminated.

Laparoscopic surgeons argue that subtotal hysterectomy can be performed laparoscopically but most randomized trials have failed to demonstrate any benefit of subtotal hysterectomy over total hysterectomy. In women who wish to retain their cervix vaginal subtotal hysterectomy described by Doderlein Kronig Technique can be performed. The disadvantage of vaginal approach is vault hematomas. The abdominal approach to hysterectomy does ensure good hemostasis under direct vision, while during the vaginal operation, the vault is closed and subsequent bleeding from the vagina between the mucosa and the peritoneum can give rise to problems, especially if a vasoconstrictor has been given that subsequently wears off. Laparoscopic approach can help check hemostasis and reduce the incidence of vault hematomas. However; this aspect needs to be evaluated in studies.

Lack of uterine descent and nulliparity, fibroid uterus, need for oophorectomy, previous pelvic surgery are no more considered as contraindications to the vaginal route. With adequate vaginal access and technical skill, and good uterine mobility, vaginal hysterectomy can easily be achieved Multiparity, lax tissues due to poor involution following multiple deliveries and lesser tissue tensile strength afford a lot of comfort to vaginal surgeon even in the presence of significant uterine enlargement. No evidence supports the use of laparoscopic hysterectomy rather than VH if latter can be performed safely. No outcomes are significantly worse for vaginal hysterectomy compared to LAVH. There are clinical situations where vaginal surgeries is not appropriate such as dense pelvic adhesions, severe endometriosis adnexal disease, when vaginal access is reduced when laparoscopic hysterectomy is indicated as it has advantages over

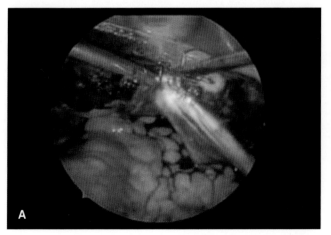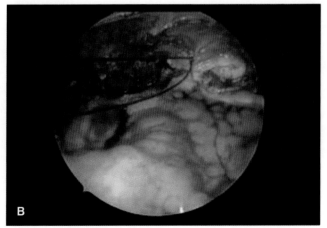

Figs 34.14A and B: Closure of vault by extracorporeal knot

the abdominal approach. Laparoscopic approach may be helpful postoperatively to rule out hemorrhage in some cases. Laparoscopic assistance should not be used to supplant inadequate skills of vaginal hysterectomy.

Lack of training in vaginal surgery is not a reason for not removing uteri vaginally. The learning curve of VH is very short compared to laparoscopic surgery, however, the current scenario in residency programs is not providing a level of surgical competency in performing difficult vaginal hysterectomies. There is a need to improve this training.

In order to compare the complication rates of different types of hysterectomies, considering an incidence of 4-5% of serious complications of hysterectomies 1460 women would be required in each arm of the study to detect 50% increase in the complication rate. Therefore, larger randomized controlled trials are required to compare different types of hysterectomies.

When the size of the uterus is greater than 16 weeks gestation there is an increase in the operative time and blood loss in VH compared to LAVH which is statistically significant.

Laparoscopically assisted vaginal hysterectomy is a useful adjunct to transvaginal hysterectomy for lysis of extensive adhesions and sometimes for certain concomitant adnexal surgery. Besides, LAVH can also secure almost all the main blood supplies to the uterus, i.e. the uterine vessels and the adnexal collaterals. Although a skilled surgeon can do transvaginal hysterectomy with a larger uterus by employing volume-reducing techniques, Kohler reported that laparoscopic coagulation hemostasis of the uterine vessels was associated with less blood loss. It may take time to achieve these goals, but they may make subsequent extirpation or volume reducing procedures easier and safer to perform. Therefore, the average operative time and estimated blood loss for the LAVH remained almost constant regardless of increasing uterine weight. Generally, the average operative time for LAVH is longer than that for transvaginal hysterectomy. It takes time to secure the uterine blood supply before extirpation and volume reducing procedures, but it also makes LAVH superior to transvaginal hysterectomy when dealing with a larger uterus. In our opinion, LAVH might be considered for a larger uterus in view of the relatively shorter operative time and less blood loss, whereas transvaginal hysterectomy is preferable for a small uterus, not only for shorter operative time and minimal wound, but also for much lower costs.

BIBLIOGRAPHY

1. Carley ME, McIntire D, Carley JM, Schaffer J. Incidence, risk factors and morbidity of unintended bladder or ureter injury during hysterectomy. Int Urogynecol J Pelvic Floor Dysfunct 2002;13:18–21.
2. Chapron C, Dubuisson JB. Laparoscopic hysterectomy. Lancet 1995;345:593. Chapron C, Dubuisson JB, Aubert V. Total laparoscopic hysterectomy: preliminary results. Hum Reprod 1994;9:2084–2089.
3. Chapron C, Fauconnier A, Goffinet F, Bre´art G, Dubuisson JB. Laparoscopic surgery is not inherently dangerous for patients presenting with benign gynaecologic pathology. Results of a meta-analysis. Hum Reprod 2002;17:1334–1342.
4. Chapron C, Laforest L, Ansquer Y, Fauconnier A, Fernandez B, Breart G and Dubuisson JB. Hysterectomy techniques used for benign disorders: results of a French multicentre study. Hum Reprod 1999;14:2464–70.
5. Chauveaud A, de Tayrac R, Gervaise A, Anquetil C and Fernandez H. Total hysterectomy for a nonprolapsed, benign uterus in women without vaginal deliveries. J Reprod Med 2002;47:4–8.
6. Cosson M, Querleu D and Crepin G Hystérectomies pour pathologies bénignes. In *Masson*. Williams et Wilkins, Paris, 1997;160.
7. Councell RB, Thorp JM Jr, Sandridge DA, Hill ST. Assessments of laparoscopic-assisted vaginal hysterectomy. J Am Assoc Gynecol Laparosc 1994;2:49–56.
8. Dandolu V, Mathai E, Chatwani A, Harmanli O, Pontari M, Hernandez E. Accuracy of cystoscopy in the diagnosis of ureteral injury in benign gynecologic surgery. Int Urogynecol J Pelvic Floor Dysfunct 2003;14:427–31.
9. Daraï E, Soriano D, Kimata P, Laplace C and Lecuru F Vaginal hysterectomy for enlarged uteri, with or without laparoscopy assistance: randomized study. Obstet Gynecol 2001;97:712–716.
10. Davies A, Vizza E, Bournas N, O'Connor H and Magos A. How to increase the proportion of hysterectomies performed vaginally. Am J Obstet Gynecol 1998;179:1008–1012.
11. Dicker RC, Greenspan JR, Strauss LT, Cowart MR, Scally MJ, Peterson HB, DeStefano F, Rubin GL, Ory HW. Complications of abdominal and vaginal hysterectomy among women of reproductive age in the United States. The Collaborative Review of Sterilization. Am J Obstet Gynecol 1982;144:841–8.
12. Dorairajan G, Rani PR, Habeebullah S, Dorairajan LN. Urological injuries during hysterectomies: a 6-year review. J Obstet Gynaecol Res 2004;30:430–5.

13. Dorsey JH, Steinberg EP and Holtz PM. Clinical indications for hysterectomy route: patient characteristics or physician preference? Am J Obstet Gynecol 1995;173:1452–60.

14. Dwyer PL, Carey MP, Rosamilia A. Suture injury to the urinary tract in urethral suspension procedures for stress incontinence. Int Urogynecol J Pelvic Floor Dysfunct 1999;10:15–21.

15. Farquhar CM, Steiner CA. Hysterectomy rates in the United States 1990–1997. Obstet Gynecol 2002;99:229–234.

16. Garry R, Fountain J, Brown J, Manca A, Mason S, Sculpher M, Napp V, Bridgman S, Gray J and Lilford R. Evaluate hysterectomy trial. A multicentre randomised trial comparing abdominal, vaginal and laparoscopy methods of hysterectomy. Health Technol Assess 2004a;8:1–154.

17. Garry R, Fountain J, Mason S, Hawe J, Napp V, Abbott J, Clayton R, Phillips G, Whittaker M, Lilford R et al. (2004b) The evaluate study: two parallel randomised trials, one comparing laparoscopy with abdominal hysterectomy, the other comparing laparoscopy with vaginal hysterectomy. BMJ 328, 129. Erratum in BMJ (2004) 328,494.

18. Gilmour DT, Das S, Flowerdew G. Rates of urinary tract injury from gynecologic surgery and the role of intraoperative cystoscopy. Obstet Gynecol 2006;107:1366–1372.

19. Gilmour DT, Dwyer PL, Carey MP. Lower urinary tract injury during gynecologic surgery and its detection by intraoperative cystoscopy. Obstet Gynecol 1999;94:883–9.

20. Gimbel H, Settnes A, Tabor A. Hysterectomy on benign indication in Denmark 1988–1998. Acta Obstet Gynecol Scand 2001;80:267–72.

21. Ha¨rkki-Siren P, Kurpi T, Sjo¨berg J, Tiitinen A. Safety aspects of laparoscopic hysterectomy. Acta Obstet Gynecol Scand 2001;80:383–91.

22. Harkki-Siren P, Sjo¨berg J, Ma¨kinen J, Heinonen PK, Kaudo M, Tomas E, Laatikainen T. Finnish national register of laparoscopic hysterectomies: A review and complications of 1165 operations. Am J Obstet Gynecol 1997;176:118–122.

23. Harkki-Siren P, Sjo¨berg J, Tiitinen A. Urinary tract injury after hysterectomy. Obstet Gynecol 1998;92:113–8.

24. Härkki-Siren P, Sjoberg J and Tiitinen A Urinary tract injuries after hysterectomy. Obstet Gynecol 1998;92:113–8.

25. Harris MB and Olive DL. Changing hysterectomy patterns after introduction Gynecol 1994;171,340–3.

26. Hurd WW, Bude RO, De Lancey JO, Pearl ML. The relationship of the umbilicus to aortic bifurcation: implications for laparoscopic technique. Obstet Gynecol 1992;80:48–51.

27. Hwang JL, Seow KM, Tsai YL, Huang LW, Hsieh BC and Lee C. Comparative study of vaginal, laparoscopically assisted vaginal and abdominal hysterectomies for uterine myoma larger than 6 cm in diameter or uterus weighing at least 450 g: a prospective randomized study. Acta Obstet Gynecol Scand 2002;81:1132–8.

28. Johns DA, Carrera B, Jones J, DeLeon F, Vincent R and Safely C. The medical and economic impact of laparoscopically assisted vaginal hysterectomy in a large, metropolitan, not-for-profit hospital. Am J Obstet Gynecol 1995;172:1709–15.

29. Johnson N, Barlow D, Lethaby A, Tavender E, Curr E and Garry R (2005a) Surgical approach to hysterectomy for benign gynaecological disease. Cochran Database Syst Rev (2): CD003677. Johnson N, Barlow D, Lethaby A, Taverder E, Curr L and Garry R (2005b) Methods of hysterectomy: systematic review and meta-analysis of randomised controlled trials. BMJ 330,1478.

30. Johnson N, Barlow D, Lethaby A, Tavender E, Curr L, Garry R. Methods of hysterectomy: systematic review and meta-analysis of randomised controlled trials. Br Med J 2005;330:1478.

31. Kadar N. Dissecting the pelvic retroperitoneum and identifying the ureters. A laparoscopic technique. J Reprod Med 1995;40:116–122.

32. Kreiker G, Bertoldi A, Sad Larcher J, Ruiz Orrico G, Chapron C. Prospective evaluation of the learning curve of total laparoscopic hysterectomy in a university hospital. J Am Assoc Gynecol Laparosc 2004;11:229–235.

33. Le´onard et al. 2010 Ou CS, Beadle E, Presthus J, Smith M. A multicenter review of 839 laparoscopic-assisted vaginal hysterectomies. J Am Assoc Gynecol Laparosc 1994;1:417–422.

34. Leonard F, Chopin N, Borghese B, Fotso A, Foulot H, Coste J, Mignon A, Chapron C. Total laparoscopic hysterectomy: preoperative risk factors for conversion to laparotomy. J Minim Invasive Gynecol 2005;12:312–317.

35. Leonard F, Chopin N, Borghese B, Fotso A, Foulot H, Coste J, Mignon A and Chapron C. Total laparoscopy hysterectomy: preoperative risk factor for conversion to laparotomy. J Minim Invasive Gynecol 2005;12:312–7.

36. Liu CY, Reich H. Complications of total laparoscopic hysterectomy in 518 cases. Gynecol Endoscopy 1994;3:203–8.

37. Ma¨kinen J, Johansson J, Tomas C, Tomas E, Heinonen PK, Laatikainen T, Kauko M, Heikkinen AM, Sjo¨berg J. Morbidity of 10 110 hysterectomy by type approach. Hum Reprod 2001;16:1473–8.

38. McMaster-Fay RA, Jones RA. Laparoscopic hysterectomy and ureteric injury: a comparison of the initial 275 cases and the last 1,000 cases using staples. Gynecol Surg 2006;3:118–21.

39. Meikle SF, Nugent EW, Orleans M. Complications and recovery from laparoscopy-assisted vaginal hysterectomy compared with abdominal and vaginal hysterectomy. Obstet Gynecol 1997;89:304–11.

40. Mteta KA, Mbwambo J, Mvungi M. Iatrogenic ureteric and bladder injuries in obstetric and gynaecologic surgeries. East Afr Med J 2006;83:79–85.

41. National Centre for Disease Control and Prevention 1997. Hysterectomy surveillance United States 1980–1993. CDC surveillance summaries, August. Mabille de Poncheville L (1998) Coeliochirurgie gynécologique en France, instantanée 1996. Résultats d'une enquête nationale. Thèse de médecine, Tours, France. Moller C, Kehlet H and Ottesen BS (1999) Hospitalization and convalescence after hysterectomy. Open or laparoscopy surgery? Ugeskr Laeger 161,4620–4624.

42. Nezhat F, Nezhat C, Admon D, Gordon S, Nezhat C. Complications and results of 361 hysterectomies performed at laparoscopy. J Am Coll Surg 1995;180:307–16.

43. O'Shea RT, Petrucco O, Gordon S, Seman E. Adelaide laparoscopic hysterectomy audit (1991–1998): realistic complications rates. Gynaecol Endoscopy 2000;9:369–372.

44. Oh BR, Kwon DD, Park KS, Ryu SB, Park YI, Presti JC Jr. Late presentation of ureteral injury after laparoscopic surgery. Obstet Gynecol 2000;95:337–339.

45. Paulson JD. Laparoscopically assisted vaginal hysterectomy. A protocol for reducing urinary tract complications. J Reprod Med 1996;41:623–628.

46. Phipps JH, Tyrrell NJ. Transilluminating ureteric stents for preventing operative ureteric damage. Br J Obstet Gynaecol 1992;99:81. Reich H, De Caprio J, McGlynn F. Laparoscopic hysterectomy. J Gynecol Surg 1989;5:213–216.

47. Ribeiro S, Reich H, Rosenberg J, Guglielminetti E, Vidali A. The value of intra-operative cystoscopy at the time of laparoscopic hysterectomy. Hum Reprod 1999;14:1727–1729.

48. Ribeiro SC, Ribeiro RM, Santos NC and Pinotti JA (2003) A randomized study of total abdominal, vaginal and laparoscopy hysterectomy. Int J Gynaecol Obstet 83,37–43.

49. Rutkow IM. Obstetric and gynecologic operations in the United States, 1979 to 1984. Obstet Gynecol 1986;67:755–759.

50. Saidi MH, Sadler RK, Vancaillie TG, Akright BD, Farhart SA, White AJ. Diagnosis and management of serious urinary complications after major operative laparoscopy. Obstet Gynecol 1996;87:272–276.

51. Shen CC, Wu MP, Kung FT, Huang FJ, Hsieh CH, Lan KC, Huang EY, Hsu TY, Chang SY. Major complications associated with laparoscopic-assisted vaginal hysterectomy: ten-year experience. J Am Assoc Gynecol Laparosc 2003;10:147–153.

52. Soriano D, Goldstein A, Lecuru F and Daraï E. Recovery from vaginal hysterectomy compared with laparoscopy-assisted vaginal hysterectomy: a prospective, randomized, multicenter study. Acta Obstet Gynecol Scand 2001;80,337–41.

53. University of York (UK) Centre for Health Economics. The management of menorrhagia. Effective healthcare 1991;1(9). Vessey MP, Villard-Mackintosh L, McPherson K, Coulter A and Yeates D. The epidemiology of hysterectomy: findings in a large cohort study. Br J Obstet Gynaecol 1992;99:402–407.

54. Vakili B, Chesson RR, Kyle BL, Shobeiri SA, Echols KT, Gist R, Zheng YT, Nolan TE. The incidence of urinary tract injury during hysterectomy: a prospective analysis based on universal cystoscopy. Am J Obstet Gynecol 2005;192:1599–1604.

55. Visco AG, Taber KH, Weidner AC, Barber MD, Myers ER. Cost-effectiveness of universal cystoscopy to identify ureteral injury at hysterectomy. Obstet Gynecol 2001;97:685–92.

56. Wattiez A, Soriano D, Cohen SB, Nervo P, Canis M, Botchorisvili R, Mage G, Pouly JL, Mille P, Bruhat MA. The learning curve of total laparoscopic hysterectomy: comparative analysis of 1647 cases. J Am Assoc Gynecol Laparosc 2002;9:339–45.

57. Wood EC, Maher P, Pelosi MA. Routine use of ureteric catheters at laparoscopic hysterectomy may cause unnecessary complications. J Am Assoc Gynecol Laparosc 1996;3:393–7.

58. Wu SM, Chao Yu YM, Yang CF and Che HL. Decision-making tree for women considering hysterectomy. J Adv Nurs 2005;51:361–8.

35 Laparoscopic Myomectomy

Fibroids are a common uterine tumor affecting 20 to 25 percent women. Fibroid develops from benign transformation of a single smooth muscle cell. The growth of myoma is dependent on many factors. Increased estrogen stimulation alone or together with growth hormone or human placental lactogen appears to be the major growth regulator of fibroid.

The severities of symptoms depend on the number of tumor, size and location. Many time they cause abdominal pressure so, urinary frequency, abdominal pain or constipation. One of the common finding is DUB due to altered blood flow through the uterus. The fibroid many time does not affect pregnancy.

In women with menorrhagia the hematocrit is used to asses the degree of anemia. Patients with large broad ligament fibroid may require an intravenous pyelogram to rule out any ureteral obstruction. For anemic patients preoperative treatment with gonadotropin releasing hormone may enable restoration of a normal hematocrit and decrease the size of myoma and thus reduce the risk of transfusion.

Intraoperatively use of dilute vasopressin helps to minimize the blood loss. Vertical uterine incision bleed less than transverse incision.

Single, vertical, anterior, midline incisions are least likely to form adhesion. Although sutures predispose to adhesions, they are often necessary to close the uterine defect.

If the endometrial cavity is entered due to large myoma a patient who subsequently becomes pregnant should undergo cesarean delivery.

Preoperative GnRH agonist has been used by some gynecologists to decrease myomas and intraoperative blood loss.

The risk of future uterine rupture is a major concern following myomectomy. The difficulty of adequately closing the layers laparoscopically and use of electrocoagulation may contribute to the risk of uterine rupture.

Uteroperitoneal fistulas may follow laparoscopic myomectomy because meticulous laparoscopic approximation of all layers is very difficult. Use of electrosurgery for hemostasis inside the uterine defect may also increase the risk of uteroperitoneal fistula formation.

The chances of postoperative adhesion are also quite high in case of laparoscopic myomectomy. A single uterine incision for removal of multiple leiomyomas and subserosal approximation of the uterine defect should be done.

Laparoscopic assisted myomectomy can reduce the chance of this complication. The suturing will be done outside so decreasing the operating time and secure layered suturing ensures uterus does not rupture in later pregnancy. Pelvic observation during the laparoscopy allows the diagnosis and treatment of any other disease like endometriosis or adhesion. The criteria for LAM are myoma greater than 5 cm, numerous myomas, requiring vigorous use of morcellator, deep intramural myoma and removal that require uterine repair with sutures.

Procedure

Pedunculated myomas are easiest to remove by just coagulating and cutting the stalk. Diluted vasopressin may be injected in the base of stalk.

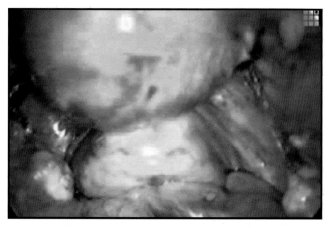

Fig. 35.1: Colpotomy

Intramural fibroid require more manipulation so dilute vasopressin should be injected to multiple site between the myometrium and the fibroid capsule (Figs 35.1 to 35.2C). An incision is made on the serosa overlying the leiomyomas using the monopolar electrode. The incision is extended until it reaches the capsule. The myometrium retracts as incision is made, exposing the tumor. Two grasping tooth forceps hold the edges of myometrium and the suction irrigator is used as blunt probe to remove covering of the leiomyomas from its capsule. The myoma crew should be inserted into the fibroid to apply traction while the suction irrigation instrument can be used as a blunt dissector. The CO_2 laser is used to further dissect capsular attachment. Vessels are electrocoagulated before being cut. After complete myoma removal the uterine defect is irrigated, bleeding points are identified and controlled with the open jaw of bipolar. If the fibroid is small and patient does not want baby, the edges of the uterine defects are approximated by coagulating the myometrium without suturing and tube ligation is performed. If the defect is deep situated, the edges of defect should be approximated by using 4-0 PDS. The repair mainly involve serosal and subserosal layer or can be in one layer. Sutures are applied at a distance of 5 mm. After repair, thorough suction and irrigation should be performed. Some gynecologist use adhesive medical glues over the suture line to prevent adhesion. Even in the hand of expert the laparoscopic myomectomy is difficult. Tumble square knot is better to use if the edges are in tension. Dundee jamming knot with continuous suturing may be used if there is not much tension followed by Aberdeen termination. Precise suturing of several layers is almost impossible laparoscopically.

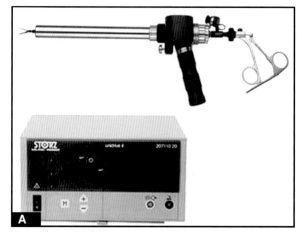

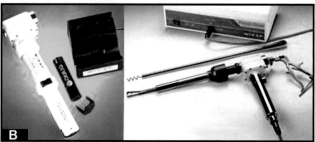

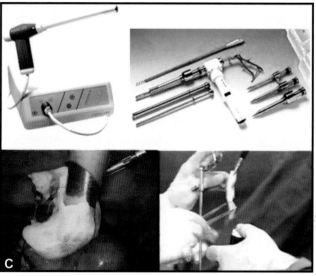

Figs 35.2A to C: Morcellator is necessary equipment for myoma tissue retrieval

Intraligamentous and broad ligament fibroid are difficult to remove due to risk of injury to ureter and uterine artery at the time of dissection. Following a thorough exposure of ureter and vessels and depending on the location of myoma, an incision is made on the anterior or posterior leaf of the broad ligament and the leiomyomas is slowly shelled as other subserosal or intramural fibroid.

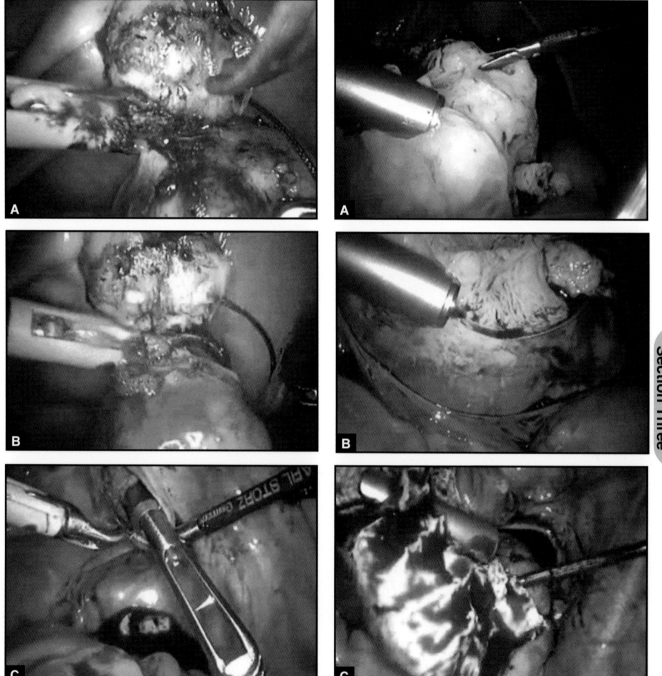

Figs 35.3A to C: Dissection of myoma

Figs 35.4A to C: Morcellation of myoma

Throughout the procedure the location of the ureter is monitored, bleeding points are controlled by bipolar. The broad ligament and peritoneum are not closed in cases of broad ligament Myoma. If postoperative bleeding is suspected, a drain should be left.

Removal of Myoma

Fibroid removal is one of the difficult and time consuming procedures. Larger myoma may be removed through posterior colpotomy (Fig. 35.3C).

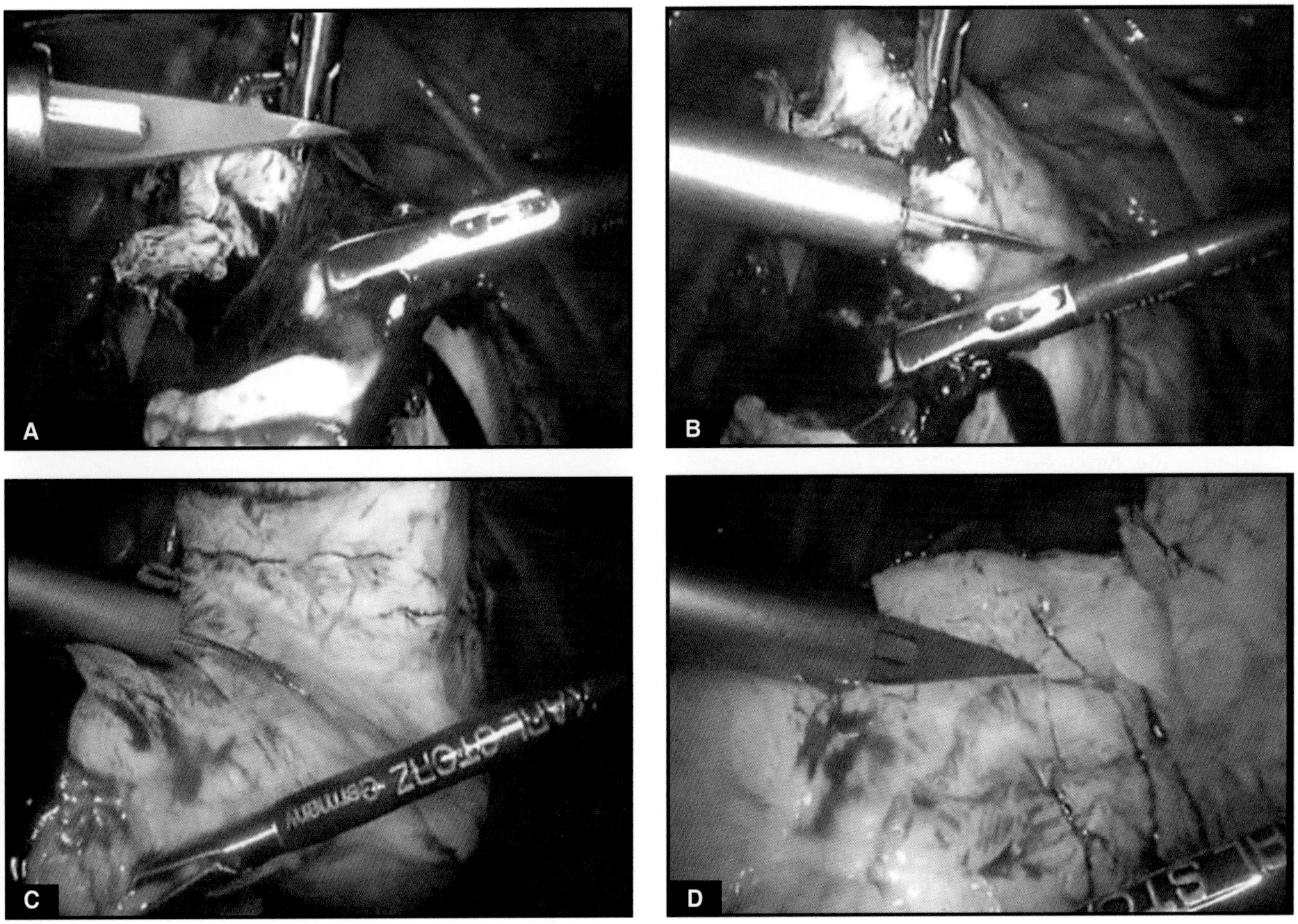

Figs 35.5 A to D: Endoknife used to divide myoma

In women with concurrent posterior cul-de-sac pathology posterior colpotomy is not safe. Medium and large size fibroid is morcellated using a morcellator (Figs 35.2A to 35.3C), scalpel (Figs 35.5A to D) or scissors. The process is ineffective for calcified myomas.

For infected tissue and in case of suspected carcinoma tissue retrieval bag should be used. Many sizes of disposable tissue retrieval bags are available and hard rim of these retrieval bags are easy to negotiate inside the abdominal cavity.

For large size gynecological tissue, colpotomy route is good for retrieval. Colpotomy can be done laparoscopically with the help of heal of hook. Counter pushing by other instruments is effective. Sponge over sponge holding forceps is inserted in posterior vaginal fornix by one assistant and surgeon cuts the vaginal fascia between both the uterosacral ligaments with the heel of hook.

Use of morcellator is another way which facilitates grinding of solid tissue and then these can be taken out without any difficulty (Fig. 35.3). Recently many companies have launched battery operated morcellator. The morcellator is important instrument for tissue retrieval in myomectomy and splenectomy (Figs 35.4A to C).

BIBLIOGRAPHY

1. Banas T, Klimek M, Fugiel A, Skotniczny K. Spontaneous uterine rupture at 35 weeks' gestation, 3 years after laparoscopic myomectomy, without signs of fetal distress. J Obstet Gynaecol Res 2005;31(6):527–30.
2. Banas T, Klimek M, Fugiel A, Skotniczny K. Spontaneous uterine rupture at 35 weeks' gestation, 3 years after laparoscopic myomectomy, without signs of fetal distress. J Obstet Gynaecol Res 2005;31(6):527–30.
3. Dubuisson J, Fauconnier A, Deffarges J, Norgaard C, Kreiker G, Chapron C. Pregnancy outcome and deliveries following laparoscopic myomectomy. Hum Reprod 2000b;15,869–73.

4. Dubuisson J, Fauconnier A, Deffarges J, Norgaard C, Kreiker G, Chapron C. Pregnancy outcome and deliveries following laparoscopic myomectomy. Hum Reprod 2000b;15:869–73.

5. Dubuisson JB, Fauconnier A, Chapron C, Kreiker G, Norgaard C. Reproductive outcome after laparoscopic myomectomy in infertile women. J Reprod Med 2000a; 45,23–30.

6. Dubuisson JB, Fauconnier A, Chapron C, Kreiker G, Norgaard C. Reproductive outcome after laparoscopic myomectomy in infertile women. J Reprod Med 2000a; 45:23–30.

7. Farmer RM, Kirschbaum T, Potter D, Strong TH, Medearis AL. Uterine rupture during trial of labour after previous cesarean section. Am J Obstet Gynecol 1991;65:996–1001.

8. Farmer RM, Kirschbaum T, Potter D, Strong TH, Medearis AL. Uterine rupture during trial of labour after previous cesarean section. Am J Obstet Gynecol 1991;65:996–1001.

9. Flamm BL, Goings JR, Liu Y, Wolde-Tsadik G. Elective repeat cesarean delivery versus trial of labor: a prospective multicenter study. Obstet Gynecol 1994;83:927–32.

10. Flamm BL, Goings JR, Liu Y, Wolde-Tsadik G. Elective repeat cesarean delivery versus trial of labor: a prospective multicenter study. Obstet Gynecol 1994;83:927–32.

11. Golan D, Aharoni A, Gonen R, Boss Y, Sharf M. Early spontaneous rupture of the post myomectomy gravid uterus. Int J Gynaecol Obstet 1990;31(2):167–70.

12. Golan D, Aharoni A, Gonen R, Boss Y, Sharf M. Early spontaneous rupture of the post myomectomy gravid uterus. Int J Gynaecol Obstet 1990;31(2):167–70.

13. Grande N, Catalano GF, Ferrari S, Marana R. Spontaneous uterine rupture at 27 weeks of pregnancy after laparoscopic myomectomy. J Minim Invasive Gynecol 2005;12,301.

14. Grande N, Catalano GF, Ferrari S, Marana R. Spontaneous uterine rupture at 27 weeks of pregnancy after laparoscopic myomectomy. J Minim Invasive Gynecol 2005;12:301.

15. Hurst BS, Matthews ML, Marshburn PB. Laparoscopic myomectomy for symptomatic uterine myomas. Fertil Steril 2005;83:1–23.

16. Hurst BS, Matthews ML, Marshburn PB. Laparoscopic myomectomy for symptomatic uterine myomas. Fertil Steril 2005;83:1–23.

17. Kumakiri J, Takeuchi H, Kitade M, Kikuchi I, Shimanuki H, Itoh S, Kinoshita K. Pregnancy and delivery after laparoscopic myomectomy. J Minim Invasive Gynecol 2005;12:241–6.

18. Kumakiri J, Takeuchi H, Kitade M, Kikuchi I, Shimanuki H, Itoh S, Kinoshita K. Pregnancy and delivery after laparoscopic myomectomy. J Minim Invasive Gynecol 2005;12:241–6.

19. Landi S, Fiaccavento A, Zaccoletti R, Barbieri F, Syed R, Minelli L. Pregnancy outcomes and deliveries after laparoscopic myomectomy. J Am Assoc Gynecol Laparosc 2003;10:177–81.

20. Landi S, Fiaccavento A, Zaccoletti R, Barbieri F, Syed R, Minelli L. Pregnancy outcomes and deliveries after laparoscopic myomectomy. J Am Assoc Gynecol Laparosc 2003;10:177–81.

21. Lieng M, Istre O, Langebrekke A. Uterine rupture after laparoscopic myomectomy. J Am Assoc Gynecol Laparosc 2004;11,92–3.

22. Lieng M, Istre O, Langebrekke A. Uterine rupture after laparoscopic myomectomy. J Am Assoc Gynecol Laparosc 2004;11:92–3.

23. Nielsen TF, Ljungblad U, Hagberg H. Rupture and dehiscence of cesarean section during pregnancy and delivery. Am J Obstet Gynecol 1989;160:569–73.

24. Nielsen TF, Ljungblad U, Hagberg H. Rupture and dehiscence of cesarean section during pregnancy and delivery. Am J Obstet Gynecol 1989;160:569–73.

25. Nkemayim DC, Hammadeh ME, Hippach M, Mink D, Schmidt W. Uterine rupture in pregnancy subsequent to previous laparoscopic electromyolysis. Case report and review of the literature. Arch Gynecol Obstet 2000;264,154–6.

26. Nkemayim DC, Hammadeh ME, Hippach M, Mink D, Schmidt W. Uterine rupture in pregnancy subsequent to previous laparoscopic electromyolysis. Case report and review of the literature. Arch Gynecol Obstet 2000;264:154–6.

27. Ozeren M, Ulusov M, Uvanik E. First-trimester spontaneous uterine rupture after traditional myomectomy: case report. Isr J Med Sci 1997;33(11):752–3.

28. Ozeren M, Ulusov M, Uvanik E. First-trimester spontaneous uterine rupture after traditional myomectomy: case report. Isr J Med Sci 1997;33(11):752–3.

29. Pelosi MA III, Pelosi MA. Spontaneous uterine rupture at thirtythree weeks subsequent to previous superficial laparoscopic myomectomy. Am J Obstet Gynecol 1997;177:1547–9.

30. Pelosi MA III, Pelosi MA. Spontaneous uterine rupture at thirtythree weeks subsequent to previous superficial laparoscopic myomectomy. Am J Obstet Gynecol 1997;177:1547–9.

31. Phelan JP, Clark SL, Diaz F, Paul RH. Vaginal birth after cesarean. Am J Obstet Gynecol 1987;157:1510–15.

32. Phelan JP, Clark SL, Diaz F, Paul RH. Vaginal birth after cesarean. Am J Obstet Gynecol 1987;157:1510–15.

33. Pisarska MD, Carson SA. Incidence and risk factors for ectopic pregnancy. Clin Obstet Gynecol 1999;42:2–8.

34. Pisarska MD, Carson SA. Incidence and risk factors for ectopic pregnancy. Clin Obstet Gynecol 1999;42:2–8.

35. Roopnarinesingh S, Suratsingh J, Roopnarinesingh A. The obstetric outcome of patients with previous myomectomy or hysterotomy. West Indian Med J 1985;34:59–62.

36. Roopnarinesingh S, Suratsingh J, Roopnarinesingh A. The obstetric outcome of patients with previous myomectomy or hysterotomy. West Indian Med J 1985;34:59–62.

37. Seinera P, Farina C, Todros T. Laparoscopic myomectomy and subsequent pregnancy: results in 54 patients. Hum Reprod 2000;15:1993–6.

38. Seinera P, Farina C, Todros T. Laparoscopic myomectomy and subsequent pregnancy: results in 54 patients. Hum Reprod 2000;15:1993–6.

Section Three

39. Stringer NH, Strassner HT, Lawson L, Oldham L, Estes C, Edwards M and Stringer EA. Pregnancy outcomes after laparoscopic myomectomy with ultrasonic energy and laparoscopic suturing of the endometrial cavity. J Am Assoc Gynecol Laparosc 2001;8:129–36.

40. Stringer NH, Strassner HT, Lawson L, Oldham L, Estes C, Edwards M, Stringer EA. Pregnancy outcomes after laparoscopic myomectomy with ultrasonic energy and laparoscopic suturing of the endometrial cavity. J Am Assoc Gynecol Laparosc 2001;8:129–36.

36 Laparoscopic Management of Stress Incontinence

Genuine stress incontinence is the involuntary loss of urine which occurs when the intravesical pressure exceeds the maximum urethral pressure in the absence of a detrusor contraction. The preferred therapy for genuine stress incontinence is surgery. Urinary incontinence is becoming more prevalent as the population ages. A significant improvement in the psychological status of these patients after the successful surgical cure of stress incontinence has been demonstrated.

In genuine stress incontinence the proximal urethra is displaced outside the abdominal cavity. Stress incontinence then results from inadequate transmission of increases in intra-abdominal pressure to the proximal urethra. The urethra has in fact lost its retropubic position due to attenuated support. As a result, coughing will produce an immediate increase in intravesical pressure but not a concomitant increase

in intraurethral pressure, and a dribble of urine results. More than 160 types of operations are available to correct stress urinary incontinence, an optimal approach has not been developed. The Burch procedure is considered by many to be the gold standard for surgical treatment of genuine stress incontinence (Fig. 36.1).

The Burch procedure requires the elevation of the anterior wall of the vagina to the level of the origin of the paravaginal fascia by suspension from Cooper's ligaments (iliopectineal ligaments). A properly performed Burch procedure cures 93 percent.

Laparoscopic Anatomy

The space of Retzius lies between the vesicoumbilical fascia posteriorly and the posterior rectus sheath and pubic bone, anteriorly. This is the space first entered in Burch suspension.

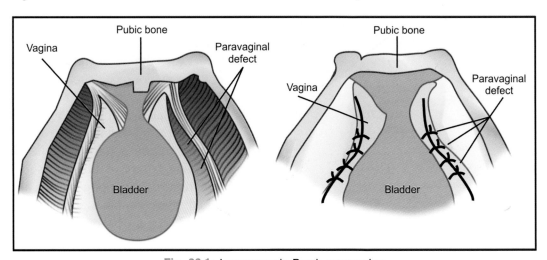

Fig. 36.1: Laparoscopic Burch suspension

Preoperative Evaluation

Postmenopausal women should receive at least 3 months of estrogen replacement therapy. Preoperative evaluation includes history, physical, gynecologic, and neurologic examinations. The routine tests include stress test, Q-tip test, urinalysis, urine culture and sensitivity. All women should undergo an urodynamic evaluation, with emphasis on voiding time, voiding volume, and post-void residual urine volume. Stress incontinence is diagnosed by a positive stress test in the absence of simultaneous detrusor contractions or pressure equalization on the stress urethral closure pressure profile.

Operative Technique

Following the induction of general endotracheal anesthesia, a Foley's catheter should be applied in the bladder. A 10 mm operative video laparoscope is inserted infraumbilical and three 5 mm accessory trocars are inserted according to baseball diamond concept.

300 cc of methylene blue solution is placed into the bladder to keep the bladder weighted down and to allow the clear delineation of the dome of the bladder. Three port techniques is used one in umbilicus and two 5 cm lateral and slightly below the umbilicus.

The anterior abdominal wall peritoneum 3 to 5 cm above the symphysis pubis is cut and pulled down. To enter the space of Retzius intra-abdominally, the umbilical ligaments are identified laterally (Fig. 36.2).

The space of Retzius is developed using blunt and CO_2 dissection of fibrofatty tissue. Care is taken to avoid obturator nerve and aberrant obturator vessel injury.

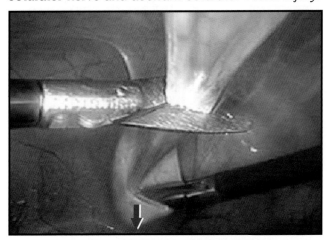

Fig. 36.2: Peritoneal incision in midline

The midline trocar entry and anatomic landmarks, including the round ligament from the internal ring, are used to avoid bladder entry. Blunt dissection, hydrodissection, and the CO_2 laser for sharp dissection are used to expose the retropubic space. Surgeon should stay close to the back of the pubic bone, dropping the anterior bladder wall, vaginal wall, and urethra downward. Dissection is limited over the urethra in the mid-line, to approximately 2 cm lateral to the urethra to protect its delicate musculature. An assistant should introduce one finger on each side of the catheterized urethra, elevating the lateral vaginal fornix. The overlying fibrofatty tissue is cleared laparoscopically from the anterior vaginal wall. The bladder is dissected medially from the paravaginal fascia from lateral to medial. Blunt dissection with atraumatic grasper is continued until the urethrovesical junction becomes apparent and the white glistening tissue of the paravaginal fascia appears.

Bladder muscle fibers of the urethrovesical junction should not be damaged at the time of dissection. Bleeding if happens in this area is controlled only with bipolar electrocoagulation because; monopolar current can cause perforation of bladder of stricture of urethra. Retropubic dissection is continued until Cooper's ligament is clearly exposed. Dissection in the space of Retzius is difficult in patients who have undergone previous laparotomy. Pneumoperitoneum pressure provides exposure of the space and its contents out to the obturator nerve (Figs 36.3A and B).

The space of Retzius also can be entered with a pre-peritoneal approach just like transabdominal preperitoneal hernia surgery. The balloon dissector consists of a cannula, balloon system. The dissector is inserted through a 10 mm infraumbilical incision. It is advanced between the rectus muscle and the anterior surface of the posterior rectus sheath to the symphysis pubis. The dissector's external sheath is removed, and the balloon is inflated with approximately 500 ml of saline solution. During inflation, the balloon unrolls sideways and exerts a perpendicular force that separates tissue layers. A blunt dissection of the connective tissues is propagated as the balloon expands. Full dissection takes about one minute but surgeon should keep the balloon inflated for 5 minute to achieve proper hemostasis. Lateral pressure of balloon will stop capillary bleeding if kept for 5 minutes.

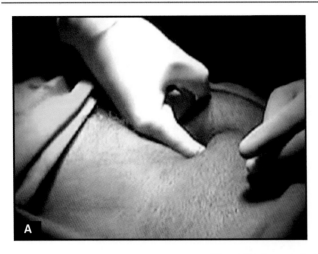
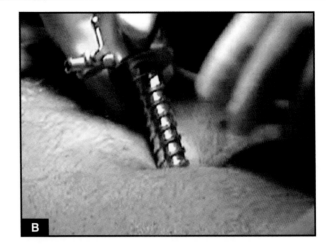

Figs 36.3A and B: Extraperitoneal approach

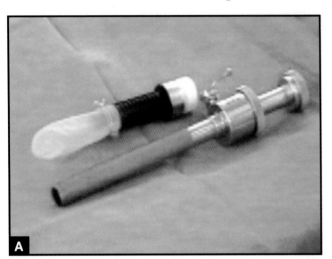
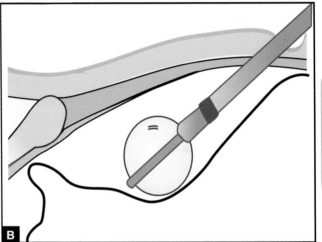

Figs 36.4A and B: Balloon dilatation

When maximal volume is reached, the balloon is deflated and removed through the incision (Figs 36.4A and B).

The dissected space is insufflated with CO_2 at a pressure of 8-10 mm Hg. The predefined shape of the balloon, its non-elastomeric material, and the incompressible character of the saline assure a large, relatively bloodless working space of predictable size and shape. The space is adequate for identification of pertinent landmarks and unencumbered manipulation of endoscopic surgical instruments.

After complete dissection, the paravaginal fascia is identified as glistening fascia over the finger of assistant. Using a needle holder a suture placed over the paravaginal fascia at the level of the urethrovesical junction, approximately 1 to 1.5 cm from the urethra

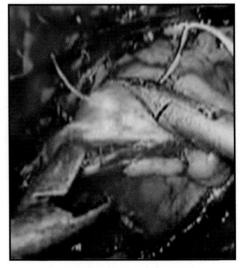

Fig. 36.5: Suturing of paravaginal fascia

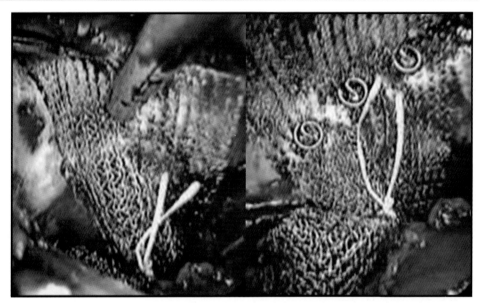

Fig. 36.6: Mesh fixed with Cooper's ligament

(Fig. 36.5). The urethrovesical junction can be identified easily because of the Foley bulb with the catheter under gentle traction. This suture is placed perpendicular to the vaginal axis to include approximately 0.5 to 1 cm of tissue.

The complete vaginal fascia should be taken so that it will not cut through. Precaution should be taken that suture does not penetrate the vaginal mucosa. Once the suture is placed over the paravaginal fascia, the suture is fixed to Cooper's ligament or the midline of the symphysis pubis.

The suture is tied either intracorporeal or extra-corporeally with the help from an assistant who lifts the vagina upward and forward. The urethra is observed carefully to prevent it from being compressed against the pubic bone. This same suturing technique is repeated on the opposite side, the aim is to create a platform on which the bladder neck can rest. If the suspension is not enough with one suture, a second and rarely, a third set of sutures can be placed along the base of the bladder proximally.

After taking suture on both sides, cystoscopy should be performed to ensure that there is no suture pierced in the bladder, cystoscopy also help to assess the urethrovesical junction angle, and to check ureteral patency.

Proline mesh can be used instead of direct suture for bladder neck suspension. Medially over paravaginal fascia, mesh is fixed by sutures and laterally over Cooper's ligament it should be fixed with the help of Protak or Anchor. One of the advantages of mesh is that after some time it gives very good platform for bladder neck due to fibrosis developed through the mesh (Fig. 36.6).

Once the procedure is finished the pneumo-peritoneum pressure is decreased and the retropubic space is evaluated. If there is any bleeding, it is controlled with bipolar electrocoagulation. The peritoneal defect may be left open to heal spontaneously, or, if it is large, it should be closed laparoscopically with three to four interrupted or purse string sutures. The laparoscope is withdrawn from the abdomen and the procedure concluded. The Foley's catheter should be left in place for 2 to 3 days. If there is any fear of detrusor instability or bladder injury, the Foley's should be in place for one week or more.

Intercourse should be avoided for 6 to 8 weeks postoperatively and the patients are advised to avoid heavy lifting or strenuous exercise for at least 2 months.

BIBLIOGRAPHY

1. Alcalay M, Monga A, Stanton SL. Burch colposuspension: a 10–20 year follow up. Br J Obst Gynaecol 1995;102:740–5.
2. Ankardal M, Ekerydh A, Crafoord K, et al. A randomised trial comparing open Burch colposuspension using sutures with laparoscopic colposuspension using mesh and staples

in women with stress urinary incontinence. Br J Obst Gynaecol 2004;119:974–81.

3. Bo K, Talseth T, Holme I. Single blind, randomised, controlled trial of pelvic floor exercises, electrical stimulation, vaginal cones and no treatment in management of genuine stress incontinence in women. BMJ 1999;318:487–93.

4. Boyles SH, Webber AM, Meyn L. Procedures for urinary incontinence in the United States 1979–1997. Am J Obstet Gynecol 2003;189:70–5.

5. Burch JC. Urethro-vaginal fixation to Cooper's ligament for correction of stress incontinence, cystocoele and prolapse. Am J Obstet Gynecol 1961;81:281–90.

6. Burton G. Five year prospective randomised urodynamic study comparing open and laparoscopic colposuspension. Neurourol Urodyn 1999;18:295–6.

7. Cardozo L, Drutz HP, Baygani SK, Bump RC. Pharmacological treatment of women awaiting surgery for stress urinary incontinence. Obstet Gynecol 2004;104:511–19.

8. Cardozo LD, Cutner AA. Surgical management of stress incontinence. Contemporary reviews in obstetrics and gynaecology. 1992;4:36-41.

9. Chaliha C, Stanton SL. Complications of surgery for genuine stress incontinence. Br J Obst Gynaecol 1999;106:1238–45.

10. Delorme E. Transobturator urethral suspension: a mini invasive procedure on the treatment of stress urinary incontinence in women. Prog Urol 2001;11:1306–13.

11. Duckett JRA. The use of periurethral injectables in the treatment of genuine stress incontinence. Br J Obst Gynaecol 1998;105:390–6.

12. Eckford SD, Abrams P. Para-urethral collagen implantation for female stress incontinence. Br J Urol 1991;68:586-9.

13. Foldspang A, Mommsen S. Overweight and urinary incontinence in women. Ugeskr Laeger 1995;157:5848–51.

14. Gorton E, Stanton SL, Monga A, et al. Periurethral collagen injection: a long-term follow-up study. Br J Urol Int 1999; 84:966-71.

15. Groutz A, Gordon D, Woman I, Jaffa AJ, David MP, Lessing JB. Tension-free vaginal tape for stress urinary incontinence: is there a learning curve? Neurourol Urodyn 2002;21:470-2.

16. Henalla SM, Hall V, Duckett JR, et al. A multicentre evaluation of a new surgical technique for urethral bulking in the treatment of genuine stress incontinence. Br J Obst Gynaecol 2000;107:1035-9.

17. Hilton P, Mayne C. The Stamey endoscopic bladder neck suspension: a clinical and urodynamic investigation including actuarial follow up over four years. Br J Obstet Gynaecol 199;98:1141-9.

18. Huang KH, Kung FT, Liang HM, Huang LY, Chang SY. Concomitant surgery with tension free vaginal tape. Acta Obstet Gynecol Scand 2003;82:948–53.

19. Iosif CF, Bekassy Z, Ryhdestrom H. Prevalence of urinary incontinence in middle age women. Int J Gynecol Obstet 1980;26:255–9 N Christofi and A Hextall Which procedure for incontinence?

20. Iosif CF, Bekassy Z. Prevalence of genitourinary symptoms in the menopause. Acta Obstet Gynecol Scand 1984;63:257–60.

21. Jarvis GJ, Hall S, Stamp S, Millar DR, Johnson A. An assessment of urodynamic examination in incontinent women. Br J Obst Gynaecol 1980;87:893–6.

22. Jarvis GJ. Surgery for genuine stress incontinence. Br J Obst Gynaecol 1994;101:371–4.

23. Jolleys JV. Reported prevalence of urinary incontinence in a general practice. BMJ 1988;296:1300–2.

24. Khullar V, Cardozo LD, Abbott D, Anders K. GAX collagen in the treatment of urinary incontinence in elderly women: a two year follow-up. Br J Obstet Gynaecol 1997;104:96-9.

25. Kligman AM, Armstrong RC. Histological response to intradermal zyderm and zyplasy (gluteraldehyde cross-linked) collagen in humans. J Dermat Surg Oncol 1986;12:351-7.

26. Kondo A, Kato K, Saito M, et al. Prevalence of hand washing incontinence in females in comparison with stress and urge incontinence. Neurourol Urodyn 1990;19:330–1.

27. Mommsen S, Foldspang A. Body mass index and adult urinary incontinence. World J Urol 1994;12:319–22

28. Monga AK, Robinson D, Stanton SL. Peri-urethral collagen injections for genuine stress incontinence: a two year follow-up. Br J Urol 1995;76:156-60.

29. Mukherjee K, Constantine G. Urinary stress incontinence in obese women: tension free vaginal tape is the answer. BJU Int 2001;88:881–3.

30. National Institute for Clinical Excellence. Guidance on the Use of TVT for Stress Incontinence. Technology Appraisal Guidance No. 56. London: NICE, February 2003.

31. National Institute for Clinical Excellence. Interventional Procedures Review of Transobturator Tape Insertion for Stress Urinary Incontinence. London: NICE, March 2004.

32. Pickard R, Reaper J, Wyness L, Cody DJ, McClinton S, N'Dow J. Periurethral injection therapy for urinary incontinence in women. Cochrane Database Syst Rev 2003;(2):CD003881.

33. Rekers H, Drogendijk AC, Valkenburg H, et al. Urinary incontinence in women from 35 to 79 years of age: prevalence and consequences. Eur J Obstet Gynecol Reprod Biol 1992;43:229–34.

34. Schultheiss D, Hofner K, Oelke M, Grunewald V, et al. Percutaneous bladder neck suspension with bone anchors: an improvement in the therapy of female stress urinary incontinence. Neurourol Urodyn 1998;17:457-58.

35. Ulmsten U, Petros P. Intravaginal salingoplasty: an ambulatory surgical procedure for the treatment of female urinary incontinence. Scand J Urol Nephrol 1995;29:75-82.

36. Ulmsten U, Henriksson L, Johnson P, Varhos G. An ambulatory surgical procedure under local anaesthesia for treatment for female urinary incontinence. Int Urogynecol J 1996;7:81–6.

37. Van Kerrebroeck P, Abrams P, Lange R, et al. Duloxetine urinary incontinence study group. Br J Obst Gynaecol 2004;111:249–57.
38. Vancaillie T, Schuessler W. Laparoscopic bladderneck suspension. J Laparoscopic Surg 1991;3:169–73.
39. Vetter NJ, Jones DA, Victor CR. Urinary incontinence in the elderly at home. Lancet 1981;ii:1275–7.
40. Ward K, Hilton P. Prospective multicentre randomised trial of tension free vaginal tape and colposuspension for primary urodynamic stress incontinence: two year follow-up. Am J Obstet Gynecol 2004;190:324–31.
41. Ward K, Hilton P. Prospective multicentre randomised trial of tension free vaginal tape and colposuspension as primary treatment for stress incontinence. BMJ 2002;325:67–70.

Section Three

37 Minimally Invasive Sling Operation for Stress Incontinence

TENSION FREE VAGINAL TAPE

Stress Urinary Incontinence or Genuine Stress Incontinence is a problem of the urinary bladder where the urethral sphincter weakens and as a result, cannot prevent the flow of urine through it when the intra-abdominal pressure rises such as in coughing, sneezing, lifting something heavy or even standing or walking.

There are several causes of urethral sphincter weakness, most common being:

• Unattended pregnancy and childbirth
• Frequent heavy lifting
• Estrogen deficiency or menopause
• Obesity

Urinary incontinence is reported by 14 percent of women, and urodynamic stress incontinence, the involuntary leakage of urine during increased abdominal pressure in the absence of a detrusor contraction is diagnosed in over half of the women presenting to hospital with urinary incontinence. Systematic reviews have shown that colposuspension has the best surgical results when compared with other treatments for urodynamic stress incontinence, with cure rates of up to 90 percent in women who have had no previous surgery for incontinence, although there are only limited data from randomized trials on which to base clinical practice. Although colposuspension remains the most popular choice for the treatment of stress incontinence, some authors have reported less than half of patients remaining dry and free of complications long term. Complications include hemorrhage, hematoma, bladder injury, and urinary tract infection. Up to 20 percent of women may develop *de novo* detrusor over activity; voiding dysfunction has been reported in 3 percent to 32 percent of women, and surgery for vaginal prolapse may be required in 2.5 percent to 26.7 percent after the procedure.

Minimally invasive suburethral sling procedures have become a mainstay for the surgical treatment of stress urinary incontinence in women. Transvaginal Tape is a minimally invasive procedure for women who suffer from stress urinary incontinence. In Transvaginal Tape, the urinary bladder and urethra are repaired, strengthened and returned to its original position in the pelvis. Tension free vaginal tape (also known as TVT) was first introduced in Sweden in the mid 1990's by Ulf Ulmsten and Papa Petros. The American Urological Association (AUA) has established a task force to determine the most effective operations for the treatment of stress urinary incontinence. They concluded the most curative operations as published in the worldwide medically indexed literature were the: Burch urethral suspension procedure and the suburethral sling operation. Cure rates for both procedures were found to fall routinely between 80-90 percent. The TVT operation is a "sling" operation and its cure rate falls within the international standards of cure for other types of sling procedures. The tension free vaginal tape procedure is a relatively recent treatment for stress incontinence.

A polypropylene tape is inserted suburethrally under local anesthesia with sedation. The procedure is thought to work by providing a pubourethral "neoligament." Increased intra-abdominal pressure results in a kink at the point of fixation, which prevents urine flow (Fig. 37.1).

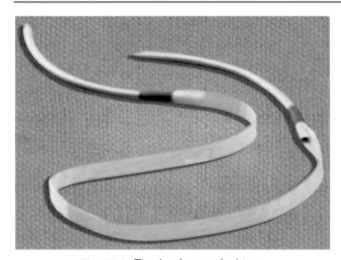

Fig. 37.1: Tension free vaginal tape

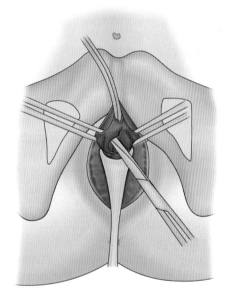

Fig. 37.2: Abdominal and vaginal incision for TVT

Surgical Technique

The patient should be placed in the lithotomy position taking care to avoid hip flexion greater than 60°. The procedure can be carried out under local anesthesia, but it can also be performed using regional or general anesthesia. The extent of dissection is minimal, i.e. a vaginal midline entry with a small paraurethral dissection to initially position the needle and two suprapubic skin incisions.

Using forceps, grasp the vaginal wall at each side of the urethra. Using a small scalpel, make a sagittal incision about 1.5 cm long starting approximately 1.0 cm from the outer urethral meatus. This incision will cover the mid-urethral zone and will allow for subsequent passage of the sling (tape). With a small pair of blunt scissors, two small paraurethral dissections (approximately 0.5 cm) are made so that the tip of the needle can then be introduced into or passed through the paraurethral dissection (Fig. 37.2).

Then, two abdominal skin incisions of 0.5-1 cm are made one on each side of the midline just above the symphysis not more than 4-5 cm apart. Incision placement and needle passage near the midline and close to the back of the pubic bone are important to avoid anatomic structures in the inguinal area and lateral pelvic sidewall.

The TVT rigid catheter guide is inserted into the channel of the Foley catheter (18 French). The handle of the guide is fixed around the catheter, proximal to its widening. The purpose of the guide is to move the bladder neck and urethra away from where the tip of the needle will pass into the retropubic space (Fig. 37.3).

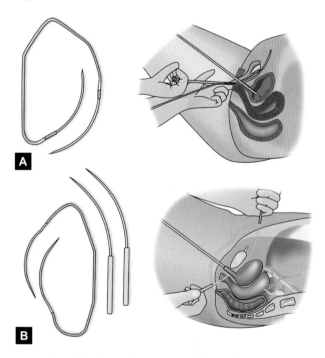

A

B

Figs 37.3A and B: Passage of needle through retropubic space

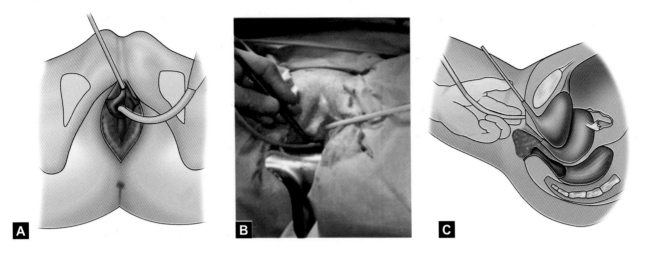

Figs 37.4A to C: Safe entry of needle with use of urethral catheter guide

Via use of the Foley catheter and the rigid catheter guide, the urethra and bladder are moved contralaterally to the side of the needle passage. During this maneuver, the bladder should be empty. Using the introducer, the needle is passed paraurethrally penetrating the urogenital diaphragm. Insertion and passage are controlled by using the long or index finger in the vagina under the vaginal wall on the ipsilateral side and fingertip control on the pelvic rim. The curved part of the needle should rest in the palm of the "vaginal" hand.

If you are right handed this means that the left hand generally is the one to be used for needle guidance (Fig. 37.4). With the other hand, grip the handle of the introducer gently. Now introduce the needle tip into the retropubic space. Once again, observe that this should be done by the palm of the vaginal hand and with the needle tip horizontally, i.e. in the frontal plane. After passage of the urogenital diaphragm, you will feel that the resistance is significantly reduced. Immediately aim the tip of the needle towards the abdominal midline and lower the handle of the introducer thereby pressing the tip of the needle against the back of the pubic bone. Now, move the needle tip upwards to the abdominal skin incision, keeping in close contact with the pubic bone all the way. When the needle tip has reached the abdominal incision, cystoscopy is performed to confirm bladder integrity. The bladder must be emptied after the first cystoscopy. Disarticulate the reusable introducer and pull the remaining portion of the TVT needle through the abdominal incision. The procedure is then repeated on the other side.

The needles are then pulled upward to bring the tape (sling) loosely, i.e. without tension, under the midurethra. Cut the tape close to the needles. Now, adjust the tape so that leakage is reduced allowing a few drops of urinary leakage to occur under stress. For this, use patient feedback, i.e. coughing with a full bladder (approximately 300 ml) and keep the vaginal incision temporarily closed by a gentle grip with small forceps (Fig. 37.5).

The plastic sheaths that surround the tape are then removed (Fig. 37.6). To avoid putting tension on the tape, a blunt instrument (scissors or forceps) should be placed between the urethra and the tape during removal of the plastic sheaths (Fig. 37.7).

Premature removal of the sheath may make subsequent adjustments difficult. After proper adjustment of the tape, close the vaginal incision. The abdominal ends of the tape are then cut and left in subcutis. Do not suture them. Suture the skin incisions. Empty the bladder. Following this procedure, postoperative catheterization is not typically required. The patient should be encouraged to try to empty the bladder 2-3 hours after the operation.

Transobturator Tape

When tension-free vaginal tape (TVT) was first introduced into clinical practice in the mid- to late 1990s, the gold standard surgical procedure in the treatment of stress urinary incontinence was the Burch colposuspension. Several randomised controlled trials have compared the efficacy and safety of these two procedures and shown that TVT has a lower morbidity

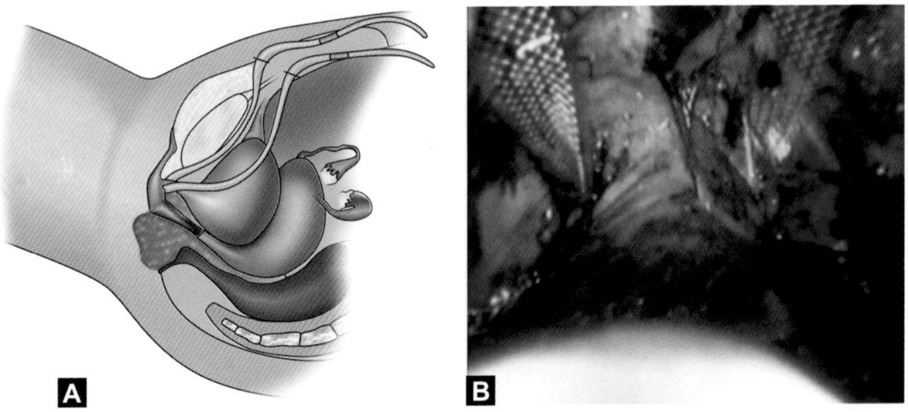

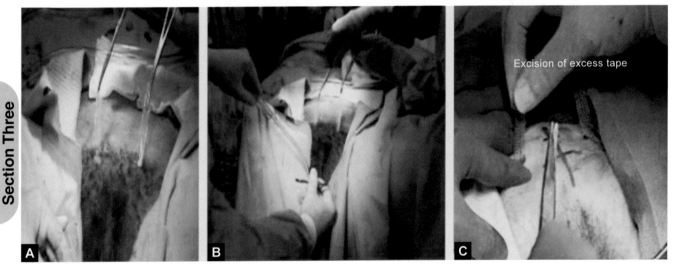

Figs 37.5A and B: Completed application of tape with laparoscopic view

Figs 37.6A to C: Removal of plastic tape with cutting the excessive mesh

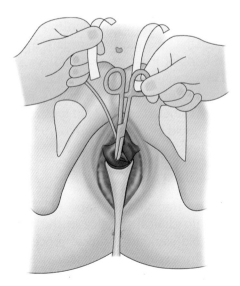

Fig. 37.7: Scissors or forceps should be placed between the urethra and the tape

rate and equal or superior efficacy at mid-term follow-up. TVT has gradually replaced the colposuspension as the first choice procedure, especially now that the long term results (5-7 year outcome) are known (81.3 percent and 82 percent cure rate).

There are, however, concerns over the safety of TVT. A Finnish series of 1455 women treated for stress urinary incontinence demonstrated several vascular injuries (venous lacerations were the most frequent injury reported), while Zilbert et al reported a case of right external iliac artery injury. In addition, two deaths due to serious vascular injuries have been reported to the manufacturers, as have bowel perforations. Most of these complications are related to the penetration of the retropubic space. In order to avoid these complications, but keep the principle of a minimally invasive procedure to reinforce the structures supporting the urethra, Delorme described the transobturator tape (TOT). In this technique a 2 cm incision is made through the vagina over the urethra, and a tunnel created out to the obturator foramen on either side. A trocar is then passed from the thigh fold through the obturator foramen from the outside to the inside and brought round through the vaginal incision. A multifilament microporous tape is then fed through the trocar and brought through the obturator foramen. The procedure is repeated on both side and the tape left under no tension under the midurethra. De Leval et al described a further modification to the surgical technique, which allows the passage of a trocar and tape through the obturator foramen from inside to out. The authors felt that this further reduced any risk of damage to the urethra and bladder; however, the long-term safety of this type of procedure is not known.

The tension-free vaginal tape has revolutionized the surgical treatment of stress urinary incontinence but remains an abdominal procedure with all of the potential complications therein. The transobturator tape procedure described here produces the same end result, i.e. a tension-free tape left under the midurethra, but without the risks of an abdominal procedure.

Bladder perforation is the most common complication occurring during the TVT procedure, with the incidence reported as between 0.8 percent and 21 percent. However, with the TOT procedure, the risk of bladder perforation is significantly reduced (Fig. 37.8).

Functional Theories and Comparison with Tension-free Vaginal Tape

DeLancey's theories on pelvic support for the bladder and urethra help to explain the mechanism of action of the transobturator tape in the treatment of stress urinary incontinence, in that the position of the tape is similar to that of the natural hammock supporting the urethra. The TOT procedure using polypropylene tape satisfies most of the requirements for effective surgery.

In the medium-term the results are satisfactory and, unlike the retropubic tape (TVT), the purely perineal location of the transobturator tape minimizes the risk of trauma to the bladder, intestine, major vessels and nerves (Figs 37.9A and B).

Operative Technique

Patient should be positioned in dorsal lithotomy with hips hyperflexed with buttock flush to the edge of

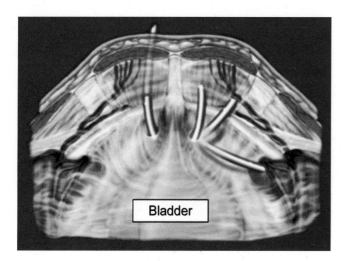

Fig. 37.8: Injuries in TVT procedure

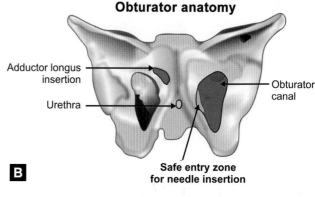

Figs 37.9A and B: Pelvic anatomy demonstrating obturator foramen

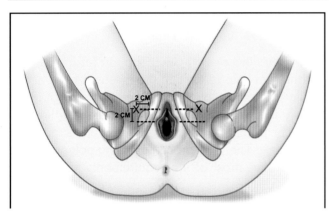

Fig. 37.10: Position the patient, mark thigh exit point and make vaginal midline incision

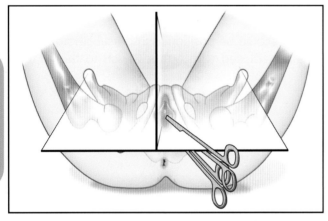

Fig. 37.11: Dissect to the obturator membrane and perforate obturator membrane

the table. Make the exit points by tracing a horizontal line at the level of the urethral meatus, and a second line parallel and 2 cm above the first line. Locate the exit points on the second line, 2 cm lateral of the folds of the thigh. Using Allis clamps for traction make a 1 cm midline vaginal incision starting 1 cm proximal to the urethral meatus (Fig. 37.10).

After initiating sharp dissection, continue by using a "push-spread" technique preferably using pointed curved scissor (Fig. 37.11). The path of the lateral dissection should be oriented at a 45° angle from the midline, with the scissors oriented on the horizontal plane. Continue dissection towards the "junction" between the body of the pubic bone and the inferior pubic ramus and perforate the obturator membrane.

Winged guide should be inserted into the dissected trace and through the obturator membrane. Insert the TOT device tip with the helical pressure into the dissected tract following the channel of the winged guide. Push the direction of TOT device inward traversing, and perforating the obturator membrane. Once in the TOT needle is in position, winged guide should be withdrawn (Fig. 37.12).

Once the winged guide has been removed, move the handle of TOT needle towards the midline to a near-vertical position. Then rotate the handle of the helical passer counter clock wise for patient's right side and clockwise for patient's left side (Fig. 37.13).

The point of the helical passer should exit near the previously determined exit points. Slight skin manipulation may be required particularly in obese patients (Fig. 37.14).

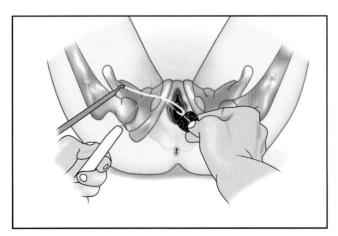

Fig. 37.12: Insert winged guide and helical passer and then remove winged guide

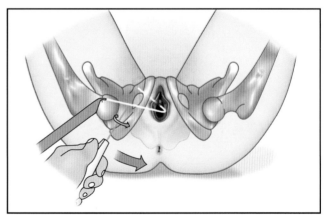

Fig. 37.13: Rotate helical passer while moving the handle into midline

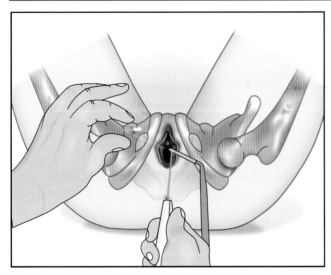

Fig. 37.14: Facilitate passage of tot through skin incision

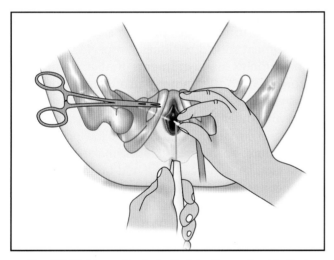

Fig. 37.15: Grasp tip of plastic tube then retract helical passer by reverse rotation

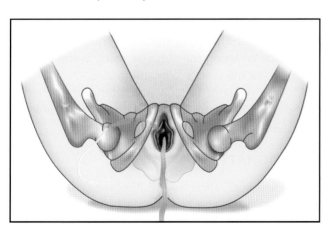

Fig. 37.16: Pull plastic tube and tape completely through the skin

When the tip of the plastic tube appears and passes at the skin opening, grasp the extreme point of the tip with a clamp and, while stabilizing the tube near the urethra, remove the Helical Passer by a reverse rotation of the handle (Fig. 37.15).

After removing the helical passer the plastic tube should be pulled completely through the skin until the tape appears (Fig. 37.16).

Same procedure of TOT mesh insertion should be repeated for other side keeping in mind that there should not be twisting of mesh in the midline (Fig. 37. 17).

When the tape is in position, the plastic sheath that covers the tape should be removed. One blunt instruments (e.g. Scissors or Forcep) should be placed between the urethra and the tape during removal of a plastic sheath, or use other suitable means during sheath removal, to avoid positioning the tape with

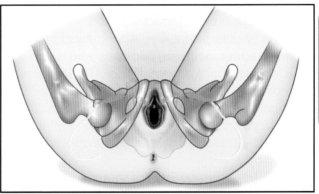

Fig. 37.17: Steps of introduction of mesh should be repeated on patient's other side

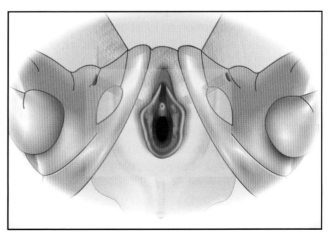

Fig. 37.18: Adjust the tape, remove plastic sheath and close incision

Section Three

tension. Following tape adjustment, close the vaginal incisions. Cut the tape ends at the exit points just below the skin on the inner thigh. Close the skin incisions with suture or surgical skin adhesive (Fig. 37.18). Surgeon should remember that "Looser is Better than Tighter".

CONTRAINDICATIONS OF TVT AND TOT

As with any suspension surgery, these sling procedure should not be performed in pregnant patients. Additionally, because the prolene polypropylene mesh will not stretch significantly, it should not be performed in patients with future growth potential including women with plans for future pregnancy.

WARNINGS AND PRECAUTIONS

- Do not use TVT or TOT procedure for patients who are on anti-coagulation therapy.
- Do not use TVT or TOT procedure for patients who have a urinary tract infection.
- Users should be familiar with surgical technique for bladder neck suspensions and should be adequately trained in the TVT or TOT implantation procedure before employing these devices. It is important to recognize that TVT or TOT is different from a traditional sling procedure in that the tape should be located without tension under mid-urethra.
- Acceptable surgical practice should be followed for the TVT or TOT procedure as well as for the management of contaminated or infected wounds.
- The TVT or TOT procedure should be performed with care to avoid large vessels, nerves, bladder and bowel. Attention to local anatomy and proper passage of needles will minimize risks especially in TVT.
- Retro pubic bleeding may occur postoperatively. Observe for any symptoms or signs before releasing the patient from hospital.
- Cystoscopy should be performed to confirm bladder integrity or recognize a bladder perforation.
- Do not remove the plastic sheath until the tape has been properly positioned.
- Ensure that the tape is placed with minimal tension under mid-urethra.
- Prolene mesh in contaminated areas should be used with the understanding that subsequent infection may require removal of the material.

- The patient should be counseled that future pregnancies may negate the effects of the surgical procedure and the patient may again become incontinent.
- Since no clinical experience is available with vaginal delivery following the TVT or TOT procedure, in case of pregnancy delivery via caesarean section is recommended.
- Postoperatively the patient is recommended to refrain from heavy lifting and/or exercise (i.e. cycling, jogging) for at least three to four weeks and intercourse for one month. The patient can return to other normal activity after one or two weeks.
- Should dysuria, bleeding or other problems occur, the patient is instructed to contact the surgeon immediately?
- All surgical instruments are subject to wear and damage under normal use. Before use, the instrument should be visually inspected. Defective instruments or instruments that appear to be corroded should not be used and should be discarded.
- As with other incontinence procedures, de novo detrusor instability may occur following the TVT procedure. To minimize this risk, make sure to place the tape tension-free in the mid-urethral position.
- Punctures or lacerations of vessels, nerves, bladder or bowel may occur during needle passage and may require surgical repair.
- Transitory local irritation at the wound site and a transitory foreign body response may occur. This response could result in extrusion, erosion, fistula formation and inflammation.
- As with all foreign bodies, Prolene mesh may potentiate an existing infection. The plastic sheath initially covering the Prolene mesh is designed to minimize the risk of contamination.
- Over correction, i.e. too much tension applied to the tape, may cause temporary or permanent lower urinary tract obstruction.

BIBLIOGRAPHY

1. Andersson G, Johansson JE, Garpenholt O, Nilsson K. Urinary incontinence prevalence, impact on daily living and desire for treatment: a population-based study. Scand J Urol Nephrol. 2004;38:125-130.
2. Andonian S, Chen T, St-Denis B, Corcos J. Randomized clinical trial comparing suprapubic arch sling (SPARC) and

tension-free vaginal tape (TVT): one-year results. Eur Urol. 2005;47:537-41.

3. Brophy MM, Klutke JJ, Klutke CG. A review of the tension-free vaginal tape procedure: outcomes, complications, and theories. Curr Urol Rep 2001;2:364-9.

4. Brown JS, Vittinghoff E, Wyman JF, et al. Urinary incontinence: does it increase risk for falls and fractures? Study of Osteoporotic Fractures Research Group. J Am Geriatr Soc 2000;48:721-5.

5. Burgio KL, Ives DG, Locher JL, Arena VC, Kuller LH. Treatment seeking for urinary incontinence in older adults. J Am Geriatr Soc 1994;42:208-12.

6. Chaliha C, Stanton SL. The ethnic cultural and social aspects of incontinence a pilot study. Int Urogynecol J Pelvic Floor Dysfunct 1999;10:166-170.

7. Cindolo L, Salzano L, Rota G, Bellini S, D'Afiero A. Tension-free transobturator approach for female stress urinary incontinence. Minerva Urol Nefrol 2004;56:89-98.

8. Costa P, Grise P, Droupy S, Monneins F, Assenmacher C, Ballanger P, et al. Surgical treatment of female stress urinary incontinence with a trans-obturator-tape (TOT) Uratape: short term results of a prospective multicentric study. Eur Urol 2004;46:102-6.

9. Dargent D, Bretones S, George P, Mellier G. Insertion of a sub-urethral sling through the obturating membrane for treatment of female urinary incontinence. Gynecol Obstet Fertil 2002;30: 576-82.

10. De Leval, J. Novel surgical technique for the treatment of female stress urinary incontinence: transobturator vaginal tape inside-out. Eur Urol 2003;44:724-30.

11. DeLancey JO. Structural support of the urethra as it relates to stress urinary incontinence: the hammock hypothesis. Am J Obstet Gynecol 1994;170:1713-20.

12. Delorme E, Droupy S, de Tayrac R, Delmas V. Transobturator tape (Uratape): a new minimally invasive procedure to treat female urinary incontinence. Eur Urol 2004;45:203-7.

13. Delorme E. Transobturator urethral suspension: mini invasive procedure in the treatment of stress urinary incontinence in women. Prog Urol 2001;11:1306-13.

14. Diokno AC, Burgio K, Fultz NH, Kinchen KS, Obenchain R, Bump RC. Medical and self-care practices reported by women with urinary incontinence. Am J Manag Care. 2004;10:69-78.

15. Dugan E, Roberts CP, Cohen SJ, et al. Why older community-dwelling adults do not discuss urinary incontinence with their primary care physicians. J Am Geriatr Soc 2001;49: 462-5.

16. Fultz NH, Fisher GG, Jenkins KR. Does urinary incontinence affect middle-aged and older women's time use and activity patterns? Obstet Gynecol 2004;104: 1327-34.

17. Goldberg RP, Kwon C, Gandhi S, Atkuru LV, Sand PK. Urinary incontinence after multiple gestation and delivery: impact on quality of life. Int Urogynecol J Pelvic Floor Dysfunct. 2005;16:334-6.

18. Grodstein F, Fretts R, Lifford K, Resnick N, Curhan G. Association of age, race, and obstetric history with urinary symptoms among women in the Nurses' Health Study. Am J Obstet Gynecol 2003;189:428-34.

19. Hagen S, Hanley J, Capewell A. Test-retest reliability, validity, and sensitivity to change of the urogenital distress inventory and the incontinence impact questionnaire. Neurourol Urodyn 2002;21:534-9.

20. Harvey MA, Kristjansson B, Griffith D, Versi E. The Incontinence Impact Questionnaire and the Urogenital Distress Inventory: a revisit of their validity in women without a urodynamic diagnosis. Am J Obstet Gynecol 2001;185:25-31.

21. Heit M, Blackwell L, Thomas S, Ouseph R. Prevalence and severity of urinary incontinence in kidney transplant recipients. Obstet Gynecol 2004;103:352-8.

22. Hermieu JF, Messas A, Delmas V, Ravery V, Dumonceau O, Boccon-Gibod L. Bladder injury after TVT transobturator. Prog Urol 2003;13:115-7.

23. Holroyd-Leduc JM, Straus SE. Management of urinary incontinence in women: clinical applications. JAMA. 2004;291:996-9.

24. Kinchen KS, Burgio K, Diokno AC, Fultz NH, Bump R, Obenchain R. Factors associated with women's decisions to seek treatment for urinary incontinence. J Women's Health (Larchmt) 2003;12:687-98.

25. Kuuva N, Nilsson CG. A nationwide analysis of complications associated with the tension-free vaginal tape (TVT) procedure. Acta Obstet Gynecol Scand 2002;81:72-7.

26. Lagace EA, Hansen W, Hickner JM. Prevalence and severity of urinary incontinence in ambulatory adults: an UPRNet study. J Fam Pract 1993;36:610-4.

27. Lukban JC. Suburethral sling using the transobturator approach: a quality-of-life analysis. Am J Obstet Gynecol. 2005;193:2138-43.

28. Melville JL, Delaney K, Newton K, Katon W. Incontinence severity and major depression in incontinent women. Obstet Gynecol 2005;106:585-92.

29. Melville JL, Katon W, Delaney K, Newton K. Urinary incontinence in US women: a population-based study. Arch Intern Med 2005;165:537-42.

30. Muir TW, Tulikangas PK, Fidela Paraiso M, Walters MD. The relationship of tension-free vaginal tape insertion and the vascular anatomy. Obstet Gynecol 2003;101:933-6.

31. Nilsson CG, Falconer C, Rezapour M. Seven-year follow-up of tension-free vaginal tape procedure for treatment of urinary incontinence. Obstet Gynecol 2004;104:1259-62.

32. Novielli KD, Simpson Z, Hua G, Diamond JJ, Sultana C, Paynter N. Urinary incontinence in primary care: a comparison of older African-American and Caucasian women. Int Urol Nephrol 2003;35:423-8.

33. Nygaard I, Turvey C, Burns TL, Crischilles E, Wallace R. Urinary incontinence and depression in middle-aged United States women. Obstet Gynecol 2003; 101:149-56.

34. Paraiso MF, Walters MD, Karram MM, Barber MD. Laparoscopic Burch colposuspension versus tension-free vaginal tape: a randomized trial. Obstet Gynecol 2004;104:1249-58.

35. Peyrat L, Boutin JM, Bruyere F, Haillot O, Farfak H, Lanson Y. Intestinal perforation as a complication of tension-free vaginal tape procedure for urinary incontinence. Eur Urol 2001;39:603-5.

Section Three

36. Reymert J, Hunskaar S. Why do only a minority of perimenopausal women with urinary incontinence consult a doctor? Scand J Prim Health Care. 1994;12: 180-3.

37. Sampselle CM, Harlow SD, Skurnick J, Brubaker L, Bondarenko I. Urinary incontinence predictors and life impact in ethnically diverse perimenopausal women. Obstet Gynecol 2002;100:1230-8.

38. Sandvik H, Seim A, Vanvik A, Hunskaar S. A severity index for epidemiological surveys of female urinary incontinence: comparison with 48-hour pad-weighing tests. Neurourol Urodyn 2000;19:137-45.

39. Shaw C, Tansey R, Jackson C, Hyde C, Allan R. Barriers to help seeking in people with urinary symptoms. Fam Pract. 2001;18:48-52.

40. Shumaker SA, Wyman JF, Uebersax JS, McClish D, Fantl JA. Health-related quality of life measures for women with urinary incontinence: the Incontinence Impact Questionnaire and the Urogenital Distress Inventory: Continence Program in Women (CPW) Research Group. Qual Life Res 1994;3:291-306.

41. Thom D. Variation in estimates of urinary incontinence prevalence in the community: effects of differences in definition, population characteristics, and study type. J Am Geriatr Soc 1998;46:473-80.

42. Thom DH, Haan MN, Van Den Eeden SK. Medically recognized urinary incontinence and risks of hospitalization, nursing home admission and mortality. Age Ageing 1997;26:367-74.

43. Thom DH, van den Eeden SK, Ragins AI, et al. Differences in prevalence of urinary incontinence by race/ethnicity. J Urol. 2006;175:259-64.

44. Ulmsten U, Henriksson L, Johnson P, Varhos G. An ambulatory surgical procedure under local anesthesia for treatment of female urinary incontinence. Int Urogynecol J Pelvic Floor Dysfunct 1996;7:81-5.

45. van Brummen HJ, Bruinse HW, van de Pol G, Heintz AP, van der Vaart CH. The effect of vaginal and cesarean delivery on lower urinary tract symptoms: what makes the difference? Int Urogynecol J Pelvic Floor Dysfunct. doi:10.1007/s00192-006-0119-5. Accessed July 24, 2006.

46. Ward KL, Hilton P; UK and Ireland TVT Trial Group. A prospective multicenter randomized trial of tension-free vaginal tape and colposuspension for primary urodynamic stress incontinence: two-year follow-up. Am J Obstet Gynecol 2004;190:324-31.

47. Zilbert AW, Farrell SA. External iliac artery laceration during tension-free vaginal tape procedure. Int Urogynecol J Pelvic Floor Dysfunct 2001;12:141-3.

38

Laparoscopic Sacral Colpopexy

Vaginal vault prolapse occurs when the apex of the vagina descends below the introitus. It is sequelae of incorrectly performed hysterectomy and occurs due to disruption of the ligaments that maintain vaginal support. Numerous surgical techniques have been proposed to prevent and correct this condition, including abdominal sacral colpopexy with interposition of a mesh between the prolapsed vaginal vault and anterior surface of the sacrum. Traditionally open surgical procedure usually requires a midline abdominal incision and extensive bowel manipulation.

Indications

Symptomic Prolapse

1. Feeling of pelvic heaviness or full and low back pain
2. Perception of lump at the opening of the vulva
3. Mucosal erosion.

The advantages of a laparoscopic sacral colpopexy include a better view of the pelvis, precise hemostasis, smaller incision and less manipulation of the viscera. Sacral colpopexy involves placing a Hammock of polypropylene mesh between the prolapsed vaginal vault and the anterior surface of the sacrum. Multiple permanent sutures attach one end of the mesh to the apex of the vaginal vault and the opposite end to either the hollow of the sacrum or to the sacral promontory.

Operative Procedure

Mechanical and antibiotic bowel preparation is given prior to the night of surgery. The vagina is thoroughly cleansed with an antiseptic before the procedure. The laparoscope is placed through the umbilicus and other instruments through three suprapubic 5 mm accessory trocars. The patient is placed in a steep Trendelenburg's position and tilted to the left to move the bowel away from the operating field.

Before starting procedure, diagnostic laparoscopy is performed. The vagina is pushed up by a sponge on a ring forceps in the vaginal vault and adhesiolysis is performed as necessary. Peritoneum and connective tissue are removed from the vaginal apex until the vaginal fascia and scar are identified. While holding the vaginal apex with grasping forceps, the vesical peritoneum over the vaginal apex is incised using blunt dissection, hydrodissection or scissors. The bladder is dissected from the anterior vaginal wall and the rectum from the posterior vaginal wall to expose approximately 4 cm of the vaginal vault. If a button whole is made by

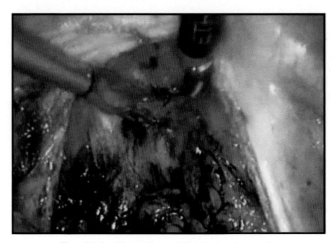

Fig. 38.1: Dissection of levator ani muscle

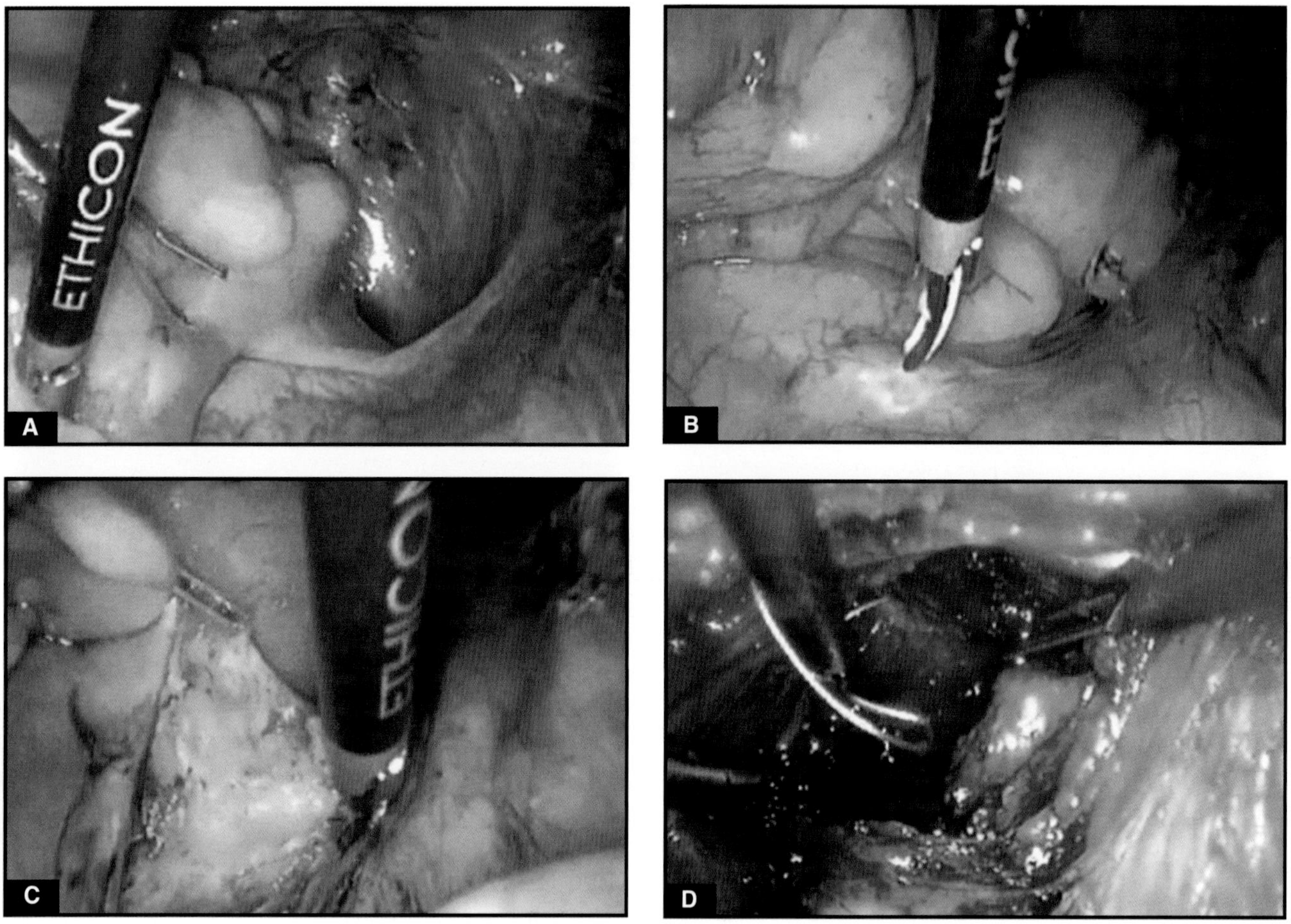

Figs 38.2A to D: Dissection of peritoneum over sacral promontory

mistake in the vagina, an inflated surgical glove is placed in the vagina to help maintain pneumoperitoneum.

If a coexisting enterocele is found, the repair is performed laparoscopically by excising the sac followed by a modified Moschcowitz posterior cul-de-sac obliteration. After identifying the ureter, the lateral peritoneum is elevated, and the suture placed through the peritoneum, passed through the cul-de-sac base, the opposite side of the peritoneum, and the anterior rectosigmoid colon serosa. A continuous purse string suture is placed (Fig. 38.1.)

The posterior parietal peritoneum is lifted with grasping forceps and the anterior sacral fascia exposed (Figs 38.2A to D). Care is taken to avoid injuring the presacral vessels. Bleeding is controlled with bipolar electrodesiccation suture or clips. The peritoneal incision is extended downward to the vagina through the presacral space. The presacral space is entered

through a vertical peritoneal incision at the right pararectal area using hydrodissection combined with the bipolar; this can be replaced by any cutting modality that the surgeon chooses. The following anatomic landmarks are identified to avoid bowel, ureter, and vessel injury: The right ureter, internal iliac artery and vein, descending colon, and presacral vessels. The sigmoid colon is reflected laterally to avoid injury to vessels in the sigmoid mesentery.

The central 5 mm trocar above the symphysis pubis is replaced with a 10 mm trocar. The polypropylene mesh is rolled and introduced into the abdomen through the 10 mm suprapubic port. Three to five 1-0 nonabsorbable polybutilate coated polyester sutures are placed in a single row in the vaginal wall apex from one lateral fornix to the other. Each suture is placed through one end of the polypropylene mesh and tied loosely using extracorporeal or intracorporeal knot (Figs 38.3A to D).

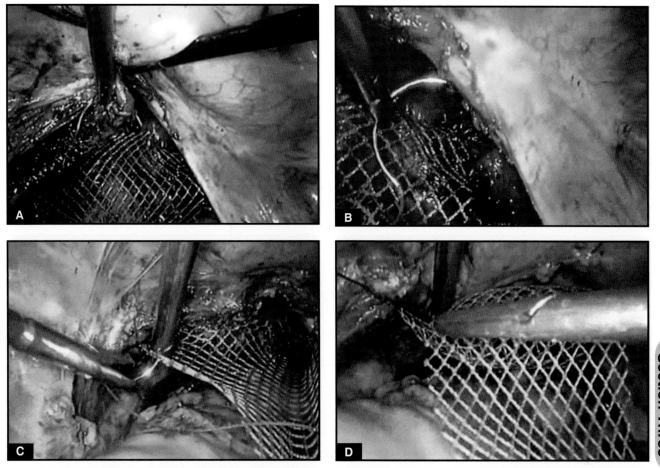

Figs 38.3A to D: A and B-Fixation of mesh to levator ani, C and D-Fixation of mesh with uterosacral ligament

In most cases, other supportive measures in the lower vagina were necessary such as anterior and posterior colporrhaphy for the lower and middle third of the vagina (Figs 38.4A to C). Partial vaginectomy was necessary in two patients, and this was done vaginally, with the mesh sutured to the posterior vaginal wall and placed intraperitoneal before closing the vaginal cuff (Figs 38.5A to C).

Two permanent sutures or staples are placed in the periosteum of the sacrum approximately 1 cm apart in the midline over S-3 and S-4 (Figs 38.6A to D). Care is taken to avoid vascular injury to paravertebral and perforating blood vessels in this area. Hemostasis is difficult even by laparotomy because of retraction of the severed vessels. The mesh is adjusted to hold the vaginal apex in the correct anatomic position without being tight. The excess mesh is trimmed from the strap. The peritoneum is closed over the strap using multiple interrupted sutures or clips (Fig. 38.7). Postoperatively, patients remain in bed for 24 hours.

They are advised to avoid intercourse for 2 months. Their diet is advanced as tolerated and a mild laxative is prescribed to prevent constipation.

Vaginal vault prolapse results from poor support of ligaments that normally maintain vaginal position. Several operative techniques are available to correct this problem. Abdominal colpopexy by suspending a mesh Hammock between the prolapsed vault and sacrum has been reported with good results. The laparoscopic modification of this operation combines the advantages of several procedures. Proper anatomic relationships are restored by correcting enterocele, reconstructing paracolpium fibers, and directing the vaginal axis toward S-3 or S-4 by evenly distributing tension over vaginal vault, and the posterior cul-de-sac is obliterated using a Moschcowitz technique.

A laparoscopic approach has achieved favorable results with minimal blood loss, reduced hospitalization, and rapid recovery. An overall decrease in complications such as wound infection

Section Three

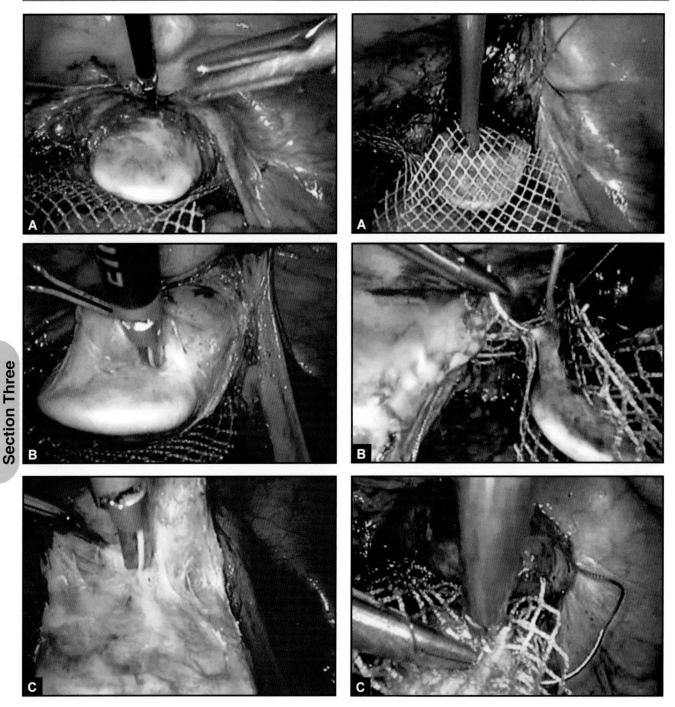

Figs 38.4A to C: Dissection of bladder

Figs 38.5A to C: Fixation of another mesh over vaginal cuff

and dehiscence, deep vein thrombophlebitis, and small bowel ileus was noted compared to laparotomy. Important patient selection factors include an ability to tolerate prolonged general anesthesia and pneumoperitoneum.

Vesicovaginal Fistula Repair

Vesicovaginal fistulas are treated by different surgical techniques depending on their cause and location. Small vesicovaginal fistulas unresponsive to nonsurgical management usually are repaired easily.

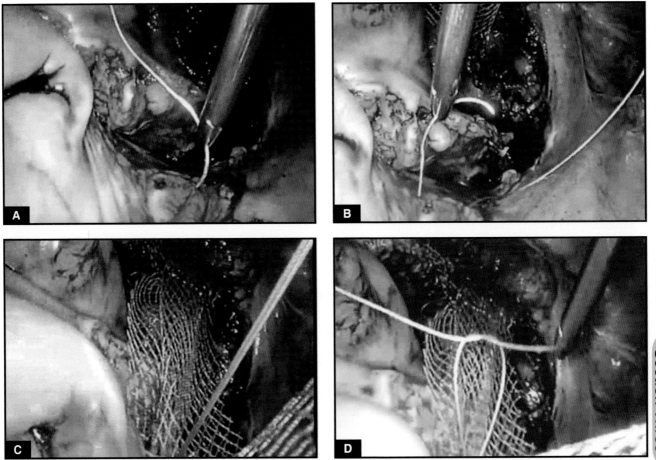

Figs 38.6A to D: Fixation of the mesh with anterior longitudinal ligament

The edges of the fistula are removed and the defect is closed. Latzko's technique is the most commonly used vaginal approach in which some fistulas are surrounded by severe fibrosis and are close to the bladder neck or urethral meatus. Lee and coworkers recommended an abdominal approach for fistulas in the upper part of a narrow vagina, multiple fistulas, those associated with other pelvic abnormalities, and fistulas close to the ureter. A combined abdominal and vaginal approach has been recommended in some instances.

Technique

The basic principles for fistula repair include suitable equipment and lighting, adequate exposure, excision of fibrous tissue from the edges of the fistula, approximation of the edges without tension, the use of suitable suture material, and efficient postoperative bladder drainage.

A 10 mm infraumbilical incision is made for the insertion of the operative laparoscope coupled with the CO_2 laser. Three 5 mm trocars are inserted in the lower abdomen for the suction irrigator probe, grasping forceps, and the bipolar forceps. A simultaneous cystoscopy is performed and both ureters are catheterized to aid in their identification and protection during excision and closure of the fistula. A ureteral catheter is pulled through the fistula into the vagina to facilitate identification during excision.

A digital rectovaginal examination is performed to exclude rectal involvement. Using the CO_2 laser, an opening is made in the vagina, avoiding the bladder and rectum. An inflated glove in the vagina helps maintain pneumoperitoneum.

The anterior vaginal wall is elevated with a grasping forceps, and the fistula is identified with the help of the previously inserted catheter. It also delineates the posterior bladder wall. The bladder is filled with water, and a cystotomy is performed above the fistula using the CO_2 laser. The water is evacuated as the bladder is distended by the pneumoperitoneum from the cystotomy. The fistula tract, vesicovaginal space, and ureters are observed laparoscopically. The vesicovaginal space is developed laparoscopically using the CO_2 laser and hydrodissection. The bladder is freed posteriorly from the vaginal wall. The bladder fistula is identified, held with a grasping forceps, and excised using the CO_2 laser. Adequate bladder dissection and mobilization are performed to eliminate tension upon suturing.

Initially, the vaginal wall opening of approximately 1.5 cm is closed with one layer of interrupted polyglactin suture. Then, the vesical defect is repaired in one layer with four interrupted 1-0 endoknot polyglactin sutures (Ethicon) using extracorporeal knotting. It is important to close the defects in the vagina and bladder separately. Hemostasis of the vesicovaginal space and fistula area is essential. A peritoneal flap is obtained superior and lateral to the bladder dome close to the round ligament and diverted toward the bladder base. The flap is used to separate the vesicovaginal space, and it is secured with two interrupted polyglactin sutures. The dissected peritoneal area heals secondarily. No intraperitoneal drainage is used. Following the procedure, a suprapubic catheter is inserted and ureteral catheters are removed.

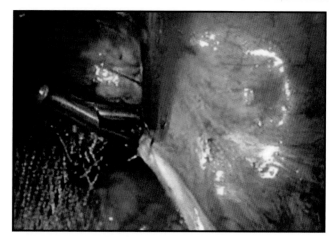

Fig. 38.7: Peritonization of mesh

CONCLUSION

Laparoscopy can be an alternative to laparotomy in managing several disorders. The exposure and magnification afforded by video laparoscopy provide direct access to the fistula. The videocystoscope enhances the access, eliminating the need for bladder dome incision for exposure. The fistula is resected under direct observation without ureteral trauma. An edge-to-edge approximation of the resected fistula is preformed without difficulty. The magnification and exposure allow meticulous and atraumatic bladder dissection and fistula resection. The bladder capacity is not reduced significantly. There is no tension in the repair and it is vascularized.

39
Essentials of Hysteroscopy

DEFINITION

Hysteroscopy is a procedure used to view the inside of the uterus through a telescope-like device called a hysteroscope. The hysteroscope is placed in the vagina and introduced into the uterus (Fig. 39.1).

INDICATIONS

- Abnormal uterine bleeding
- Infertility
- Recurrent pregnancy loss
- Abnormal hysterosalpingogram revealing intrauterine adhesions, polyps, fibroids, septum
- Possible intrauterine foreign bodies.

CONTRAINDICATIONS

- Pregnancy
- Heavy uterine bleeding
- Pelvic inflammatory disease
- Cervical malignancy
- Recent uterine perforation

History (Figs 39.2A and B)

- First hysteroscope with cystoscope of desormeaux by Pantaleoni 1869
- First hysteroscope with built in lens to magnify the image.

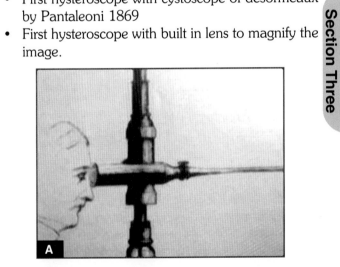

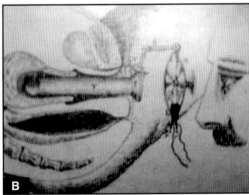

Figs 39.2A and B: History of hysteroscopy, A-First hysteroscope with cystoscope of desormeaux by Pantaleoni, B-First hysteroscope with built in lens to magnify the image

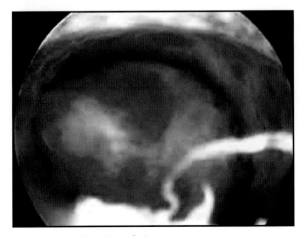

Fig. 39.1: Submucous myoma

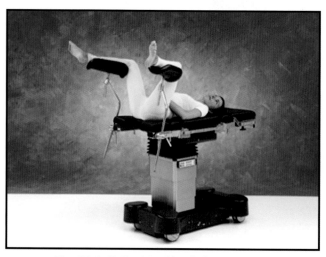

Fig. 39.3: Patient position in hysteroscopy

DELIVERY DEVICES

- Maximum recommended intrauterine operating pressure is 150 mm Hg
- Intrauterine pressure is a function of inflow pressure and outflow pressure
- Inflow pressure may be produced by gravity, pressured cuffs with (pressure) gauges, or approved pumps.

DISTENDING MEDIA

- Group A: Isotonic ionic solutions (Normal saline, Ringer's lactate)
- Group B: 5% Dextrose in water
- Group C: 1.5% Glycine, sorbitol, cytal
- Group D: Hyskon (32% dextran70).

FLUID MONITORING

It is the role of the circulating nurse to maintain a flow sheet record of inflow and outflow of hysteroscopic media during the case.

For groups A, B and C, the inflow and outflow must be estimated for every 500 cc of fluid used and measured at the conclusion of each bag of distending media.

For group D, the inflow and outflow must be measured for every 100 cc of fluid used.

The operating surgeon will be informed of fluid balance status as it is recorded on the flow sheet. Spillage should be avoided.

Use of a table drape to collect excess fluid for accurate recording of fluid output is required.

EXCESSIVE FLUID ABSORPTION

The recommended volume of input to output discrepancy at which point the surgeon must assess serum electrolytes (especially sodium concentration) is:
Group A: 1 liter
Group B: 1 liter
Group C: 1 liter
Group D: 250 ml.

Once these volumes of discrepancy have been reached, serum electrolytes must be obtained and the operating surgeon has the option of:

Terminating the case: Awaiting the results of the electrolyte levels and proceeding accordingly.

Administering Lasix IV and judiciously proceeding with the case until the results are available.

Resectoscope

- The *resectoscope* has been used for male prostate surgery for over 50 years.
- The resectoscope with a built in wire loop or other shape device uses high-frequency electrical current to cut or coagulate tissue (Fig. 39.4).

Procedure

Patient position is shown in Figure 39.3. Inside of the uterus is a potential cavity, like a collapsed air-dome, it is necessary to fill (distend) it with either a liquid or a gas (carbon dioxide) in order to see.

Diagnostic hysteroscopy and simple operative hysteroscopy can usually be done in an office setting. More complex operative hysteroscopy procedures are done in operating room setting (Fig. 39.5).

The volumes that are recommended in this section are not based on established "standards of care" since such standards have not yet been clearly formalized. For example, many surgeons use 1 liter as a cut off for D5W while others use 3 liters. There is no established limit for the volume of D5W that can safely be given as an IV solution being directly infused into the circulation of a healthy person. No reports of major

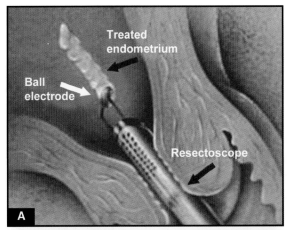

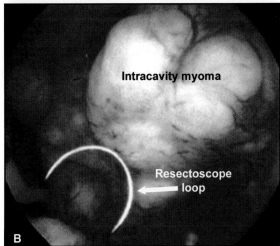

Figs 39.4A and B: (A) Ball electrodem (B) Resectoscopic loop

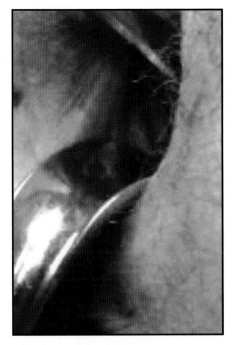

Fig. 39.5: Vaginal speculum

morbidity associated with the use of D5W have been reported in the literature.

Additional patient assessment following a large volume discrepancy between input and output may immediately involve determination of serum electrolytes. If a significant time has passed since the (presumed) absorption of fluid, other clinical parameters (if available) may become more informative (evidence of tissue edema, an increase in cardiac output associated with volume overload, change in pulse oximetry or ventilation parameters, change in patient temperature if room temperature fluid is used.

Use a resectoscope with continuous flow and a loop electrode to perform most of hysteroscopic surgery. Any of the irrigation system for distending media available today is not sufficiently accurate. They are not rapid in response (so as to maintain a constant pressure), affordable, and easy to use. At present, many

gynecologists use a simple system of placing a blood pressure cuff around each one liter bag of normal saline solution to be used and apply 150 mm Hg pressure as measured on a gauge attached to the cuff to the pressure cuff. This is connected to the inflow port on the resectoscope and flow is then adjustable using a stop cock on this port. Outflow from the resectoscope is via tubing that connects directly to a suction canister under full wall suction. The outflow port also has a stopcock that can be used to adjust the outflow.

The circulating nurse's primary responsibility during the operative hysteroscopy is to maintain pressure on the pressure cuff and watch the inflow and outflow balance. The nurse might appropriately report this balance to the surgeon and anesthesiologist every 15 minutes or whenever there is a significant volume of use (500 cc).

The resectoscope's monopolar electrocautery loop is attached to an electrical generator with variable power (wattage) settings. For any given power setting selected, there are also various blends of cutting or coagulation that can be chosen. Use blend 1 which applies current 80% of the time and gives just a little coagulation as compared to pure cutting. For most resectoscopic use 50-80 watts on blend 1 and coagulate bleeders (if not initially controlled with the blend 1 settings) using 50 watts at pure coagulation.

Once the hysteroscopic portion of the case is completed, a final tabulation of inflow and outflow volumes for the distending media is done. Direct your attention to the laparoscopy once the hysteroscopy is complete. A uterine manipulator is placed through the cervix.

Laparoscope should be inserted now. For this Veress needle is introduced. Insufflation of the abdomen with CO_2 gas so as to create a pneumoperitoneum is accomplished after "confirming the proper placement" of the Veress needle.

Once the pneumoperitoneum is created, the Veress needle is replaced by a trocar and sleeve. The diameter of the umbilical (main) trocar is 10-12 mm so that this instrument can cause considerable injury if not placed properly and atraumatically into the abdominal cavity. The presence of adhesions (scar) that elevates the bowel to the anterior abdominal wall is a consistent source of concern for laparoscopic surgeons.

If abundant adhesions are anticipated such that the surgeon believes that the complication rate with the blind Veress needle and trocar insertion is unacceptably high, then "open laparoscopy" may be chosen. Hasson introduced this technique in which the direct insertion of the trocar without the creation of a prior pneumoperitoneum is accomplished by performing a cut down under direct observation of the layers of the abdominal wall. Suture holds the layers of the inner abdominal wall (fascia and peritoneum) to the trocar sleeve to prevent the release of gas through the incision site during the case. Extreme care must be exercised in making the peritoneal incision since bowel injury to adherent bowel may occur under direct observation as well.

Accessory trocar sites are usually required during the laparoscopic case. Typically, use two additional sites for placement of 5 mm (or uncommonly 10 mm) trocars in the suprapubic midline and left lower quadrant. All accessory trocars have the advantage of being able to be inserted under direct observation so injury is less common. One injury associated with placement of the accessory trocars is laceration of the deep inferior epigastric vessels (which may be difficult

to see either directly or via transillumination). Injury to the inferior epigastric vessels can be consistently avoided by placement of the additional trocars either lateral to the internal inguinal ring or medial to the umbilical ligaments (two structures that are usually easy to identify under direct laparoscopic observation).

Tools that are selected for the performance of the laparoscopic surgery should allow the surgeon to minimize postoperative adhesion formation. The surgical principles as discussed above are very important in terms of achieving the desired outcome. Gentle tissue handling during laparoscopy takes a great deal of time to develop. Avoidance of bleeding with gentle tissue handling is important and so is careful hemostasis using (selective) bipolar cautery. Continuous irrigation and aspiration of the tissues to remove char and minimize drying should be second nature to the laparoscopic infertility surgeon. Use of cutting instruments that minimize lateral tissue damage is also a primary concern.

Once the case has been completed, the instruments are removed from the abdomen allowing for the efflux of CO_2 gas. Usually take additional 5 or so minutes to move the abdominal wall and contents about with only one remaining trocar sleeve in place to try to allow any trapped gas to escape. Incisions are closed with subcuticular stitches so as to avoid cosmetically unpleasant "railroad" type skin scars. The fascia is closed on any incision in the fascia greater than 5 mm. In the immediate postoperative recovery time period common problems include nausea and vomiting, most likely related to the CO_2 gas or the narcotic pain medications used perioperatively. Zofran is often the most effective anti-emetic agent for post-laparoscopic vomiting. The nausea and vomiting does not typically persist for more than 12 hours postoperatively.

Shoulder pain due to retained CO_2 gas, which if trapped under the diaphragm (at base of the lungs) causes irritation of the phrenic nerve to cause the sensation of shoulder pain. Lying on one's abdomen with a pillow under the hips and lower abdomen (or the knee chest position) may allow the CO_2 gas to recollect in the pelvis rather than under the lungs and reduce this discomfort.

Subcutaneous crepitance (crackling) under the skin over the abdomen and extending superiorly to the chest and neck or inferiorly to the buttocks and thighs is typically a minor complication due to escape of the gas into the abdominal wall. A rare patient develop a very low blood pressure (not related to blood loss) and usually responds immediately to a bolus of IV solution.

Incisional pain is usually mild but the internal (visceral) pain after surgery can be intense and may require narcotics or anti-inflammatory agents. Reportedly a heating pad applied to the abdomen may also be helpful.

If a large volume of fluid is left in the abdomen at the conclusion of the case then leakage through the incision sites is common for up to 2 days.

The surgeon should be called if there is a fever (greater than 100 degrees) or chills, heavy or prolonged vaginal bleeding, heat or swelling of the incision sites, frequency or burning on urination, severe pelvic pain, persistent nausea or vomiting, faintness or dizziness, inability to spontaneously urinate.

Postoperative urinary retention occurs more often in cases that last longer than 2 hours. If the patient is not able to void within 4-5 hours postoperative (and after removal of the Foley's catheter) then she should be straight catheterized for the residual volume of urine and she should try to void spontaneously once again. Do not allow patients to go home until either they can void spontaneously or they have an indwelling Foley's catheter placed (for about 1 day).

Complications of Operative Hysteroscopy

- Trauma
  - Cervical laceration
  - Uterine perforation
  - Injury to intra-abdominal viscera-rectum, bladder, intestine.
- *Intravasation:* Predisposing factors for venous intravasation of distending media:
  - Uterine tuberculosis
  - Submucous tumor
  - Hypoplastic uterus
  - Recently traumatized uterine cavity
  - Proximal tubal obstruction

  - Excessive pressure of instillation
  - Infection.
- Exacerbate latent salpingitis
- PID
- Febrile reaction
- Bleeding
- Peritonitis.

Safety Measures

Dilatation of the Cervix

The cervix must be dilated in order to enter the hysteroscope into the uterine cavity. Most resectoscope has an outer sheath diameter of about 9 mm so that cervical dilation using mechanical dilators must be at least this amount. It is optimal to avoid over dilation of the cervix since leakage of the distending media through the cervix and around the hysteroscope (especially under pressures of about 150 mm Hg) then becomes possible.

Some cervical canals are difficult to negotiate with dilators. Different dilators have a variable amount of curvature to choose from. It is possible to perforate the lower uterine segments during dilation. Clinical situations in which perforation is more common include dilation of the pregnant uterus, fibroid uterus, uterus of a women exposed to DES in utero, uterus after exposure to prostaglandins for cervical ripening, and infected uterus. Many cases of perforation occur at the onset of dilation and the subsequent dilators then continue to open the perforation site.

Occasionally, a rent in the lower uterine segment occurs during dilation. It is thought that rapid dilation or a difficult dilation involving a stenotic inflexible cervix may enhance the frequency of these tears. It is possible for a tremendous amount of distending media to become intravasated through these rents and into the large vessels of the lower uterine region if they are transacted.

Cervical incompetence following hysteroscopic surgery is rarely reported but theoretically possible. The cervix is composed of a tough fibro connective tissue and smooth muscle. Closure of the internal os of the cervix is the general rule even following manual dilatation of up to 15 mm.

Section Three

Bleeding

The pressure maintained in the uterine cavity may (but generally should not) exceed both the venous and the arterial pressures so that active blood flow from transacted vessels may not become apparent until the uterus is deflated. At lesser pressures, bleeding can be identified and usually controlled. If there is excessive bleeding following destructive procedures such as endometrial ablation, it can be frequently controlled by tamponade using an inflated Foley's catheter balloon (10-30 ml for up to 16 hours) in the uterus. Sometimes the excessive flow can be controlled with estrogens hormonal therapy (if due to denuding the lining).

Excessive Intravasation of Distending Media or CO_2 Gas

Whenever vessels are transacted during hysteroscopic surgery and either fluid or gas is entered into the uterine cavity under pressure there is a possibility of intravasation (entry of these substances into the circulation).

D5W (5% Dextrose in water) is a good distending media for diagnostic hysteroscopy. Major complications with this solution are very rare. In fact, there are no reports in the world literature of major morbidity or mortality with the use of D5W at hysteroscopy. Possible complications include water intoxication (a reduction in serum osmolality) with a dilutional reduction in sodium concentration, volume overload (when the circulating volume in the vascular system exceeds the ability of the heart to adequately pump this volume and the excess fluid typically begins to collect in the tissues of the lungs, hypothermia (significant reduction in body temperature) if room temperature solutions are used without warming the patient with devices like a "Bair Hugger," and hyperglycemia (significant excess in circulating glucose concentration that may not be rapidly metabolized if the patient has insulin resistance or diabetes mellitus).

The major complication that most hysteroscopic surgeon's focus on avoiding is water intoxication. The risk of water intoxication from D5W in a healthy woman with normal renal function is very low, since the kidneys can typically produce in excess of

1000 cc of dilute urine in response to a decrease in serum osmolarity.

Adhesions

Following hysteroscopic surgery, there is a chance of adhesion (scar) formation. If significant electrocoagulation is used within the uterine cavity in the infertility patient with intraoperative estrogen IV (25 or 50 mg of Premarin) and at least a 30 day course of higher dose Premarin postoperatively (1.25 mg or preferably 2.5 mg if tolerated) should be used.

Burn Injury to the Bowel

When resectoscopic electrosurgery is performed in the area of the uterine ostia (near the entry site of the fallopian tubes) there is a chance of thermal injury to adjacent tissue outside the uterine cavity. This is because the uterine wall in these regions is very thin and heat from the cautery can travel through the uterine wall and burn adjacent bowel.

Infection

Endometritis is uncommon after operative hysteroscopy and antibiotics are usually not "routinely" given. The potential benefits of antibiotics outweigh their risks when exposure to infection occurs.

Hysteroscopy in Abnormal Uterine Bleeding (Fig. 39.6)

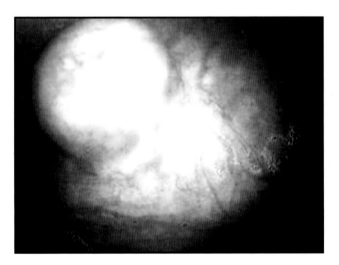

Fig. 39.6: Submucous myoma

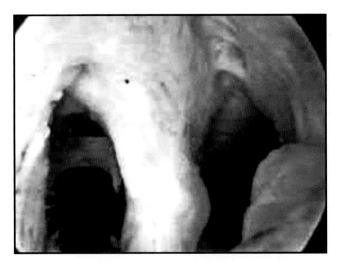

Fig. 39.7: Septate uterus

Hysteroscopy in Cases of Infertility

Diagnostic laparoscopy in hyteroscopy shown in Figures 39.7 to 39.12.

Tubal Cause of infertility

To clarify tubal cause of infertility:

Ureteric catheter used to cannulate tube

- Intracavitary pressure rises
- Flow rate falls
- Salpingo-catheterization not possible
- Inability to induce contraction of tubal angle (Post-inflammatory fibrosis)
- Combined laparoscopy and hysteroscopy used for tubal patency test and therapeutic options.

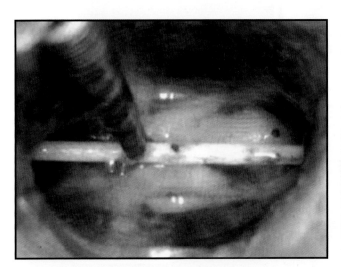

Fig. 39.8: Forgotten IUD

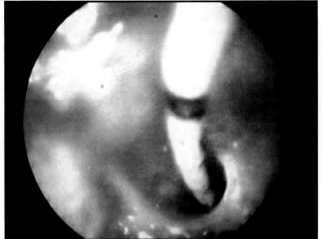

Fig. 39.9: Salpingo-catheterization

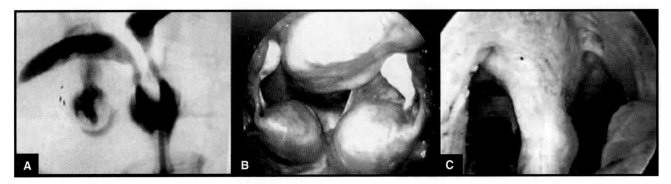

Figs 39.10A to C: Bicornuate uterus

Hysteroscopic Correlation and Diagnosis

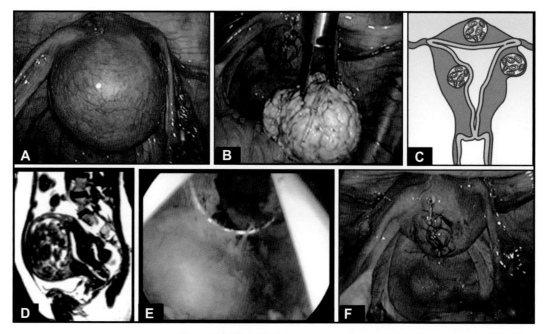

Figs 39.11A to F: Intramural myoma

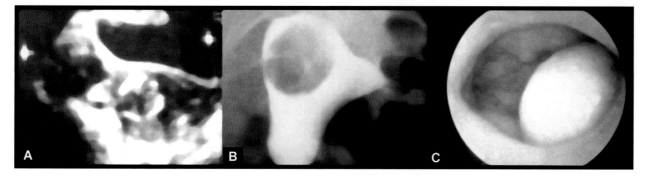

Figs 39.12A to C: Submucous myoma

Contraindications of Hysteroscopy

- Absolute
  - Adnexal and endometrial infection
- Relative
  - Menstruation
  - Cone biopsy of cervix
  - Pelvic irradiation
  - Cardiac and pulmonary diseases
  - Scarred uterus and adhesions.

BIBLIOGRAPHY

1. Acunzo G, Guida M, Pellicano M, Tommaselli GA, Di Spiezio Sardo A, Bifulco G, Cirillo D, Taylor A, Nappi C. Effectiveness of auto-cross-linked hyaluronic acid gel in the prevention of intrauterine adhesions after hysteroscopic adhesiolysis: a prospective, randomized, controlled study. Hum Reprod 2003;18:1918–21.
2. Agostini A, Cravello L, Bretelle F, Shojai R, Roger V, Blanc B. Risk of uterine perforation during hysteroscopic surgery. J Am Assoc Gynecol Laparosc 2002;9:264–7.

Section Three

3. Alborzi S, Parsanezhad ME, Mahmoodian N, Alborzi S, Alborzi M. Sonohysterography versus transvaginal sonography for screening of patients with abnormal uterine bleeding. Int J Gynaecol Obstet 2007;96:20–3.

4. Aydeniz B, Gruber IV, Schauf B, Kurek R, Meyer A, Wallwiener D. A multicenter survey of complications associated with 21,676 operative hysteroscopies. Eur J Obstet Gynecol Reprod Biol 2002;104:160–64.

5. Baumann R, Magos AL, Kay JD, Turnbull AC. Absorption of glycine irrigating solution during transcervical resection of endometrium. BMJ 1990;300:304–5.

6. Benecke C, Kruger TF, Siebert TI, Van der Merwe JP, Steyn DW. Effect of fibroids on fertility in patients undergoing assisted reproduction. A structured literature review. Gynecol Obstet Invest 2005;59:225–30.

7. Berkeley AS, DeCherney AH, Polan ML. Abdominal myomectomy and subsequent fertility. Surg Gynecol Obstet 1983;156:319–22.

8. Bernard G, Darai E, Poncelet C, Benifla JL, Madelenat P. Fertility after hysteroscopic myomectomy: effect of intramural fibroids associated. Eur J Obstet Gynecol Reprod Biol 2000;88:85–90.

9. Bettocchi S, Ceci O, Di Venere R, Pansini MV, Pellegrino A, Marello F, Nappi L. Advanced operative office hysteroscopy without anaesthesia: analysis of 501 cases treated with a 5 Fr. bipolar electrode. Hum Reprod 2002;17:2435–8.

10. Bettocchi S, Ceci O, Nappi L, Di Venere R, Masciopinto V, Pansini V, Pinto L, Santoro A, Cormio G. Operative office hysteroscopy without anesthesia: analysis of 4863 cases performed with mechanical instruments. J Am Assoc Gynecol Laparosc 2004;11:59–61.

11. Bettocchi S, Nappi L, Ceci O, Selvaggi L. What does 'diagnostic hysteroscopy' mean today? The role of the new techniques. Curr Opin Obstet Gynecol 2003;15:303–8.

12. Bonnamy L, Marret H, Perrotin F, Body G, Berger C, Lansac J. Sonohysterography: a prospective survey of results and complications in 81 patients. Eur J Obstet Gynecol Reprod Biol 2002;102:42–7.

13. Botsis D, Papagianni V, Makrakis E, Aravantinos L, Creatsas G. Sonohysterography is superior to transvaginal sonography for the diagnostic approach of irregular uterine bleeding in women of reproductive age. J Clin Ultrasound 2006;34:434–9.

14. Bradley LD. Abnormal uterine bleeding. Nurse Pract 2005;30:38–42.

15. Bradley LD. Complications in hysteroscopy: prevention, treatment and legal risk. Curr Opin Obstet Gynecol 2002;14:409–15.

16. Bronz L, Suter T, Rusca T. The value of transvaginal sonography with and without saline instillation in the diagnosis of uterine pathology in pre and postmenopausal women with abnormal bleeding or suspect sonographic findings. Ultrasound Obstet Gynecol 1997;9:53–8.

17. Brooks PG, Loffer FD, Serden SP. Resectoscopic removal of symptomatic intrauterine lesions. J Reprod Med 1989;34:435–7.

18. Brooks PG. Resectoscopic fibroid vaporizer. J Reprod Med 1995;40:791–5.

19. Buttram VC, Jr, Reiter RC. Uterine leiofibroidta: etiology, symptomatology, and management. Fertil Steril 1981;36:433–45.

20. Campo S, Campo V, Gambadauro P. Short-term and long-term results of resectoscopic myomectomy with and without pretreatment with GnRH analogs in premenopausal women. Acta Obstet Gynecol Scand 2005;84:756–60.

21. Cheng YM, Lin BL. Modified sonohysterography immediately after hysteroscopy in the diagnosis of submucous fibroid. J Am Assoc Gynecol Laparosc 2002;9:24–8.

22. Cheong Y, Ledger WL. Hysteroscopy and hysteroscopic surgery. Obstet Gynecol Reprod Med 2007;17:99–104.

23. Cicinelli E, Romano F, Anastasio PS, Blasi N, Parisi C, Galantino P. Transabdominal sonohysterography, transvaginal sonography, and hysteroscopy in the evaluation of submucous fibroids. Obstet Gynecol 1995;85:42–7.

24. Clark TJ, Mahajan D, Sunder P, Gupta JK. Hysteroscopic treatment of symptomatic submucous fibroids using a bipolar intrauterine system: a feasibility study. Eur J Obstet Gynecol Reprod Biol 2002;100:237–42.

25. Corson SL, Brooks PG, Serden SP, Batzer FR, Gocial B. Effects of vasopressin administration during hysteroscopic surgery. J Reprod Med 1994;39:419–23.

26. Corson SL, Brooks PG. Resectoscopic myomectomy. Fertil Steril 1991; 55:1041–4.

27. Corson SL. Hysteroscopic diagnosis and operative therapy of submucous fibroid. Obstet Gynecol Clin North Am 1995;22:739–55.

28. Cravello L, Agostini A, Beerli M, Roger V, Bretelle F, Blanc B. Results of hysteroscopic myomectomy. Gynecol Obstet Fertil 2004;32:825–8.

29. Darwish A. Modified hysteroscopic myomectomy of large submucous fibroids. Gynecol Obstet Invest 2003;56:192–6.

30. Derman SG, Rehnstrom J, Neuwirth RS. The long-term effectiveness of hysteroscopic treatment of menorrhagia and leiofibroids. Obstet Gynecol 1991;77:591–4.

31. Di Spiezio Sardo et al. 118

32. Dodson MG. Use of transvaginal ultrasound in diagnosing the etiology of menometrorrhagia. J Reprod Med 1994;39:362–72.

33. Donnez J, Gillerot S, Bourgonjon D, Clerckx F, Nisolle M. Neodymium: YAG laser hysteroscopy in large submucous fibroids. Fertil Steril 1990;54:999–1003.

34. Donnez J, Jadoul P. What are the implications of fibroids on fertility? A need for a debate? Hum Reprod 2002;17:1424–30.

35. Donnez J, Nisolle M, Clerckx F, Gillerot S, Saussoy P. Hysteroscopic myomectomy. In: Donnez J, Nisolle M (eds). An Atlas of Laser Operative Laparoscopy and Hysteroscopy. London: Parthenon Publishing, 1994;323–35.

36. Donnez J, Nisolle M, Grandjean P, Gillerot S, Clerckx F. The place of GnRH agonists in the treatment of endometriosis and fibroids by advanced endoscopic techniques. Br J Obstet Gynaecol 1992;99(Suppl. 7):31–3.

37. Donnez J, Nisolle M, Grandjean P, Gillerot S, Clerckx F. The role of GnRH agonists in the endoscopic treatment of endometriosis and fibrofibroids. Contracept Fertil Sex 1993;21:59–62.
38. Donnez J, Polet R, Smets M, Bassil S, Nisolle M. Hysteroscopic myomectomy. Curr Opin Obstet Gynecol 1995;7:311–6.
39. Donnez J, Schrurs B, Gillerot S, Sandow J, Clerckx F. Treatment of uterine fibroids with implants of gonadotropin-releasing hormone agonist: assessment by hysterography. Fertil Steril 1989;51:947–50.
40. Emanuel MH, Hart A, Wamsteker K, Lammes F. An analysis of fluid loss during transcervical resection of submucous fibroids. Fertil Steril 1997;68:881–6.
41. Emanuel MH, Wamsteker K, Hart AA, Metz G, Lammes FB. Long -term results of hysteroscopic myomectomy for abnormal uterine bleeding. Obstet Gynecol 1999;93:743–8.
42. Emanuel MH, Wamsteker K. The Intra Uterine Morcellator: a new hysteroscopic operating technique to remove intrauterine polyps and fibroids. J Minim Invasive Gynecol 2005;12:62–6.
43. Emanuel MH, Wamsteker K. Uterine leiomyomas. In: Brosens I, Wamsteker K (eds). Diagnostic Imaging and Endoscopy in Gynecology. London: WB Saunders, 1997;185–98.
44. Farquhar C, Ekeroma A, Furness S, Arroll B. A systematic review of transvaginal ultrasonography, sonohysterography and hysteroscopy for the investigation of abnormal uterine bleeding in premenopausal women. Acta Obstet Gynecol Scand 2003;82:493–504.
45. Farrugia M, McGurgan P, McMillan DL, O'Donovan PJ. Recent advances in electrosurgery (Chap 18). In: O'Donovan PJ, Dowens E (eds). Advances Di Spiezio Sardo et al. 116 in Gynaecological surgery, 1st edn. London: Greenwich Medical Media, 2002.
46. Farrugia M, McMillan L. Versapoint™ in the treatment of the focal intra-uterine pathology in an outpatient clinic setting. Ref Gynecol Obstet 2000;7:169–73.
47. Fedele L, Bianchi S, Dorta M, Brioschi D, Zanotti F, Vercellini P. Transvaginal ultrasonography versus hysteroscopy in the diagnosis of uterine submucous fibroids. Obstet Gynecol 1991;77:745–8.
48. Fedele L, Vercellini P, Bianchi S, Brioschi D, Dorta M. Treatment with GnRH agonists before myomectomy and the risk of short-term fibroid recurrence. Br J Obstet Gynaecol 1990;97:393–6.
49. Fernandez H, Sefrioui O, Virelizier C, Gervaise A, Gomel V, Frydman R. Hysteroscopic resection of submucosal fibroids in patients with infertility. Hum Reprod 2001;16:1489–92.
50. Fried FA, Hulka JF. Transuterine resection of fibroids: a new approach to the management of submucous fibroids in selected patients. J Urol 1987;138:1256–7.
51. Fukuda M, Shimizu T, Fukuda K, Yomura W, Shimizu S. Transvaginal hysterosonography for differential diagnosis between submucous and intramural fibroid. Gynecol Obstet Invest 1993;35:236–9.
52. Gallinat A. Hysteroscopic treatment of submucous fibroids using the Nd:YAG laser and modern electrical equipment. In: Leuken RP, Gallinat A (eds). Endoscopic Surgery in Gynecology. Berlin: Demeter Verlag, 1994;72–88.
53. Gallinat A. The Master Resectoscope. J Minim Invasive Gynecol 2005;12:S31–S32.
54. Garcia CR, Tureck RW. Submucosal leiofibroids and infertility. Fertil Steril 1984;42:16–9.
55. Gianaroli L, Gordts S, D'Angelo A, Magli MC, Brosens I, Cetera C, Campo R, Ferraretti AP. Effect of inner myometrium fibroid on reproductive outcome after IVF. Reprod Biomed Online 2005;10:473–7.
56. Giatras K, Berkeley AS, Noyes N, Licciardi F, Lolis D, Grifo JA. Fertility after hysteroscopic resection of submucous fibroids. J Am Assoc Gynecol Laparosc 1999;6:155–8.
57. Glasser MH, Zimmerman JD. The HydroThermAblator system for management of menorrhagia in women with submucous fibroids: 12- to 20-month follow-up. J Am Assoc Gynecol Laparosc 2003;10:521–7.
58. Glasser MH. Endometrial ablation and hysteroscopic myomectomy by electrosurgical vaporization. J Am Assoc Gynecol Laparosc 1997;4:369–74.
59. Goldenberg M, Sivan E, Sharabi Z, Bider D, Rabinovici J, Seidman DS. Outcome of hysteroscopic resection of submucous fibroids for infertility. Fertil Steril 1995;64:714–6.
60. Goldrath MH, Fuller TA, Segal S. Laser photovaporization of endometrium for the treatment of menorrhagia. Am J Obstet Gynecol 1981;140:14–9.
61. Guida M, Acunzo G, Di Spiezio Sardo A, Bifulco G, Piccoli R, Pellicano M, Cerrota G, Cirillo D, Nappi C. Effectiveness of auto-crosslinked hyaluronic acid gel in the prevention of intrauterine adhesions after hysteroscopic surgery: a prospective, randomized, controlled study. Hum Reprod 2004;19:1461–4.
62. Gutmann JN, Corson SL. GnRH agonist therapy before myomectomy or hysterectomy. J Minim Invasive Gynecol 2005;12:529–37.
63. Hallez JP. Myomectomies by endo-uterine resection. Curr Opin Obstet Gynecol 1996;8:250–6.
64. Hallez JP. Single-stage total hysteroscopic myomectomies: indications, techniques, and results. Fertil Steril 1995;63:703–8.
65. Hamou J. Electroresection of fibroids. In: Sutton C, Diamond MP (eds). Endoscopic Surgery for Gynecologists. London: WB Saunders, 1993;327–30.
66. Haney AF. Clinical decision making regarding leiofibroidta: what we need in the next millennium. Environ Health Perspect 2000;108 (Suppl. 5):835–9.
67. Hart R, Molnar BG, Magos A. Long term follow up of hysteroscopic myomectomy assessed by survival analysis. Br J Obstet Gynaecol 1999;106:700–5.
68. Hickey M, Farquhar CM. Update on treatment of menstrual disorders. Med J Aust 2003;178:625–9.
69. Hricak H. MRI of the female pelvis: a review. AJR Am J Roentgenol 1986;146:1115–22.

70. Hunt JE, Wallach EE. Uterine factors in infertility—an overview. Clin Obstet Gynecol 1974;17:44–64.

71. Indman PD. Hysteroscopic treatment of menorrhagia associated with uterine leiofibroids. Obstet Gynecol 1993;81:716–20.

72. Indman PD. Hysteroscopic treatment of submucous fibroids. Clin Obstet Gynecol 2006;49:811–20.

73. Indman PD. Use of carboprost to facilitate hysteroscopic resection of submucous fibroids. J Am Assoc Gynecol Laparosc 2004;11:68–72.

74. Isaacson K. Hysteroscopic myomectomy: fertility-preserving yet underutilized. OBG Manag 2003;15:69–83.

75. Istre O, Bjoennes J, Naess R, Hornbaek K, Forman A. Postoperative cerebral oedema after transcervical endometrial resection and uterine irrigation with 1.5% glycine. Lancet 1994;344:1187–9.

76. Jansen FW, Vredevoogd CB, van Ulzen K, Hermans J, Trimbos JB, Trimbos-Kemper TC. Complications of hysteroscopy: a prospective, multicenter study. Obstet Gynecol 2000;96:266–70.

77. Kanaoka Y, Hirai K, Ishiko O. Microwave endometrial ablation for an enlarged uterus. Arch Gynecol Obstet 2003;269:30–32.

78. Kanaoka Y, Hirai K, Ishiko O. Microwave endometrial ablation for menorrhagia caused by large submucous fibroids. J Obstet Gynaecol Res 2005;31:565–70.

79. Keltz M, Varasteh N, Levin B, Neuwirth R. Pregnancy rates following hysteroscopic polypectomy, myomectomy, and a normal cavity in infertile patients. Prim Care Update Ob Gyns 1998;5:168.

80. Kolankaya A, Arici A. Fibroids and assisted reproductive technologies: when and how to act? Obstet Gynecol Clin North Am 2006;33:145–52.

81. Laifer-Narin SL, Ragavendra N, Lu DS, Sayre J, Perrella RR, Grant EG. Transvaginal saline hysterosonography: characteristics distinguishing malignant and various benign conditions. AJR Am J Roentgenol 1999;172:1513–20.

82. Lasmar RB, Barrozo PR, Dias R, Oliveira MA. Submucous fibroids: a new presurgical classification to evaluate the viability of hysteroscopic surgical treatment–preliminary report. J Minim Invasive Gynecol 2005;12:308–11.

83. Lasmar RB, Barrozo PR. Histeroscopia: uma abordagem pra'tica. Vol 1, Medsi, Rio de Janeiro, 2002. 121–142. pp. Brazil.

84. Leone FP, Bignardi T, Marciante C, Ferrazzi E. Sonohysterography in the preoperative grading of submucous fibroids: considerations on three-dimensional methodology. Ultrasound Obstet Gynecol 2007;29:717–8.

85. Leone FP, Lanzani C, Ferrazzi E. Use of strict sonohysterographic methods for preoperative assessment of submucous fibroids. Fertil Steril 2003;79:998–1002.

86. Lethaby A, Vollenhoven B, Sowter M. Efficacy of pre-operative gonadotrophin hormone releasing analogues for women with uterine fibroids undergoing hysterectomy or myomectomy: a systematic review. BJOG 2002;109:1097–1108.

87. Lethaby A, Vollenhoven B, Sowter M. Pre-operative GnRH analogue therapy before hysterectomy or myomectomy for uterine fibroids. Cochrane Database Syst Rev 2001;2:CD000547.

88. Lin B, Akiba Y, Iwata Y. One-step hysteroscopic removal of sinking submucous fibroid in two infertile patients. Fertil Steril 2000;74:1035–8.

89. Litta P, Vasile C, Merlin F, Pozzan C, Sacco G, Gravila P, Stelia C. A new technique of hysteroscopic myomectomy with enucleation in toto. J Am Assoc Gynecol Laparosc 2003;10:263–70.

90. Loffer FD. Endometrial ablation in patients with fibroids. Curr Opin Obstet Gynecol 2006;18:391–3.

91. Loffer FD. Hysteroscopic endometrial ablation with the Nd:Yag laser using a nontouch technique. Obstet Gynecol 1987;69:679–82.

92. Loffer FD. Improving results of hysteroscopic submucosal myomectomy for menorrhagia by concomitant endometrial ablation. J Minim Invasive Gynecol 2005;12:254–60.

93. Loffer FD. Preliminary experience with the VersaPoint bipolar resectoscope using a vaporizing electrode in a saline distending medium. J Am Assoc Gynecol Laparosc 2000;7:498–502.

94. Loffer FD. Removal of large symptomatic intrauterine growths by the hysteroscopic resectoscope. Obstet Gynecol 1990;76:836–40.

95. Maher PJ, Hill DJ. Transcervical endometrial resection for abnormal uterine bleeding—report of 100 cases and review of the literature. Aust N Z J Obstet Gynaecol 1990;30:357–60.

96. Maher PJ. Endoscopic management of fibrofibroidta. Rev Gynecol Pract 2003;3:41–5.

97. Marziani R, Mossa B, Ebano V, Perniola G, Melluso J, Napolitano C. Transcervical hysteroscopic myomectomy: long-term effects on abnormal uterine bleeding. Clin Exp Obstet Gynecol 2005;32:23–6.

98. Mazzon I, Sbiroli C. Miomectomia. In: Mazzon I, Sbiroli C (eds). Manuale di Chirurgia Resettoscopica in Ginecologia. Torino, Italy: UTET, 1997;191–217.

99. Mazzon I. Nuova tecnica per la miomectomia isteroscopica: enucleazione con ansa fredda. In: Cittadini E, Perino A, Angiolillio M, Minelli L (eds). Testo-Atlante di Chirurgia Endoscopica Ginecologica. Palermo, Italy: COFESE Ed, 1995, cap XXXIIIb. Hysteroscopic myomectomy 117.

100. Mencaglia L, Tantini C. GnRH agonist analogs and hysteroscopic resection of fibroids. Int J Gynaecol Obstet 1993;43:285–88.

101. Munoz JL, Jimenez JS, Hernandez C, Vaquero G, Perez Sagaseta C, Noguero R, Miranda P, Hernandez JM, De la Fuente P. Hysteroscopic myomectomy: our experience and review. JSLS 2003;7:39–48.

102. Murakami T, Shimizu T, Katahira A, Terada Y, Yokomizo R, Sawada R. Intraoperative injection of prostaglandin F2alpha in a patient undergoing hysteroscopic myomectomy. Fertil Steril 2003;79:1439–41.

103. Murakami T, Tachibana M, Hoshiai T, Ozawa Y, Terada Y, Okamura K. Successful strategy for the hysteroscopic myomectomy of a submucous fibroid arising from the uterine fundus. Fertil Steril 2006;86:1513. e19–22.

104. Murakami T, Tamura M, Ozawa Y, Suzuki H, Terada Y, Okamura K. Safe techniques in surgery for hysteroscopic myomectomy. J Obstet Gynaecol Res 2005;31:216–23.

105. Nappi C, Di Spiezio Sardo A, Greco E, Guida M, Bettocchi S, Bifulco G. Prevention of adhesions in gynaecological endoscopy. Hum Reprod Update 2007;13:379–94.

106. Narayan R, Rajat Goswamy K. Treatment of submucous fibroids, and outcome of assisted conception. J Am Assoc Gynecol Laparosc 1994;1:307–11.

107. Neuwirth RS, Amin HK. Excision of submucus fibroids with hysteroscopic control. Am J Obstet Gynecol 1976;126:95–9.

108. Neuwirth RS. A new technique for and additional experience with hysteroscopic resection of submucous fibroids. Am J Obstet Gynecol 1978;131:91–4.

109. Neuwirth RS. Hysteroscopic management of symptomatic submucous fibroids. Obstet Gynecol 1983;62:509–11.

110. Neuwirth RS. Hysteroscopic submucous myomectomy. Obstet Gynecol Clin North Am 1995;22:541–58.

111. Ng EH, Ho PC. Doppler ultrasound examination of uterine arteries on the day of oocyte retrieval in patients with uterine fibroids undergoing IVF. Hum Reprod 2002;17:765–70.

112. Oliveira FG, Abdelmassih VG, Diamond MP, Dozortsev D, Melo NR, Abdelmassih R. Impact of subserosal and intramural uterine fibroids that do not distort the endometrial cavity on the outcome of in vitro fertilization-intracytoplasmic sperm injection. Fertil Steril 2004;81:582–7.

113. Pace S. Transcervical resection of benign endocavitary lesions. Gynecol Endosc 1993;2:165–9.

114. Parazzini F, Vercellini P, De Giorgi O, Pesole A, Ricci E, Crosignani PG. Efficacy of preoperative medical treatment in facilitating hysteroscopic endometrial resection, myomectomy and metroplasty: literature review. Hum Reprod 1998;13:2592–7.

115. Parent B, Barbot J, Guedj H, Nordarian P. Hysteroscopic resection of uterine fibroids (in French). In: Parent B, Barbot J, Guedj H, Nordarian P (eds). Hysteroscopie Chirurgicale. Laser et Techniques Classiques. Paris, France: Masson, 1994.

116. Perez-Medina T, Bajo JM, Martinez-Cortes L, Castellanos P, Perez de Avila I. Six thousand office diagnostic-operative hysteroscopies. Int J Gynaecol Obstet 2000;71:33–8.

117. Perino A, Chianchiano N, Petronio M, Cittadini E. Role of leuprolide acetate depot in hysteroscopic surgery: a controlled study. Fertil Steril 1993;59:507–10.

118. Phillips DR, Nathanson HG, Meltzer SM, Milim SJ, Haselkorn JS, Johnson P. Transcervical electrosurgical resection of submucous leiofibroids for chronic menorrhagia. J Am Assoc Gynecol Laparosc 1995;2:147–53.

119. Polena V, Mergui JL, Perrot N, Poncelet C, Barranger E, Uzan S. Long-term results of hysteroscopic myomectomy in 235 patients. Eur J Obstet Gynecol Reprod Biol 2007;130:232–7.

120. Preutthipan S, Theppisai U. Hysteroscopic resection of submucous fibroid: a result of 50 procedures at Ramathibodi Hospital. J Med Assoc Thai 1998;81:190–94.

121. Pritts EA. Fibroids and infertility: a systematic review of the evidence. Obstet Gynecol Surv 2001;56:483–91.

122. Propst AM, Liberman RF, Harlow BL, Ginsburg ES. Complications of hysteroscopic surgery: predicting patients at risk. Obstet Gynecol 2000;96:517–20.

123. Richards PA, Richards PD, Tiltman AJ. The ultrastructure of fibrofibroidtous myometrium and its relationship to infertility. Hum Reprod Update 1998;4:520–25.

124. Romer T, Schmidt T, Foth D. Pre- and postoperative hormonal treatment in patients with hysteroscopic surgery. Contrib Gynecol Obstet 2000;20:1–12.

125. Romer T. Benefit of GnRH analogue pretreatment for hysteroscopic surgery in patients with bleeding disorders. Gynecol Obstet Invest 1998;45 (Suppl 1):12–20.

126. Saidi MH, Sadler RK, Theis VD, Akright BD, Farhart SA, Villanueva GR. Comparison of sonography, sonohysterography, and hysteroscopy for evaluation of abnormal uterine bleeding. J Ultrasound Med 1997;16:587–91.

127. Salim R, Lee C, Davies A, Jolaoso B, Ofuasia E, Jurkovic D. A comparative study of three-dimensional saline infusion sonohysterography and diagnostic hysteroscopy for the classification of submucous fibroids. Hum Reprod 2005;20:253–7.

128. Seoud MA, Patterson R, Muasher SJ, Coddington CC, III. Effects of fibroids or prior myomectomy on in vitro fertilization (IVF) performance. J Assist Reprod Genet 1992;9:217–21.

129. Serden SP, Brooks PG. Treatment of abnormal uterine bleeding with the gynecologic resectoscope. J Reprod Med 1991;36:697–9.

130. Shokeir TA. Hysteroscopic management in submucous fibroids to improve fertility. Arch Gynecol Obstet 2005;273:50–54.

131. Smets M, Nisolle M, Bassil S, Donnez J. Expansive benign lesions: treatment by laser. Eur J Obstet Gynecol Reprod Biol 1996;65:101–5.

132. Smith DC, Uhlir JK. Myomectomy as a reproductive procedure. Am J Obstet Gynecol 1990;162:1476–9.

133. Somigliana E, Vercellini P, Daguati R, Pasin R, De Giorgi O, Crosignani PG. Fibroids and female reproduction: a critical analysis of the evidence. Hum Reprod Update 2007;13:465–76.

134. Stamatellos I, Apostolides A, Tantis A, Stamatopoulos P, Bontis J. Fertility rates after hysteroscopic treatment of submucous fibroids depending on their type. Gynecol Surg 2006;3:206–10.

135. Stamatellos I, Bontis J. Hysteroscopic myomectomy. Eur Clinics Obstet Gynecol 2007;3:17–23.

136. Starks GC. CO2 laser myomectomy in an infertile population. J Reprod Med 1988;33:184–6.

137. Sudik R, Husch K, Steller J, Daume E. Fertility and pregnancy outcome after myomectomy in sterility patients. Eur J Obstet Gynecol Reprod Biol 1996;65:209–14.

138. Surrey ES, Minjarez DA, Stevens JM, Schoolcraft WB. Effect of myomectomy on the outcome of assisted reproductive technologies. Fertil Steril 2005;83:1473–9.

139. Sutton C. Hysteroscopic surgery. Best Pract Res Clin Obstet Gynaecol 2006;20:105–37.

140. Takeda A, Manabe S, Hosono S, Nakamura H. Preoperative evaluation of submucosal fibroid by virtual hysteroscopy. J Am Assoc Gynecol Laparosc 2004;11:404–9.

141. Taskin O, Sadik S, Onoglu A, Gokdeniz R, Erturan E, Burak F, Wheeler JM. Role of endometrial suppression on the frequency of intrauterine adhesions after resectoscopic surgery. J Am Assoc Gynecol Laparosc 2000;7:351–4.

142. Trew GH. Hysteroscopy and hysteroscopic surgery. Curr Obstet Gynaecol 2004;14:183–90.

143. Tulandi T, al-Took S. Endoscopic myomectomy. Laparoscopy and hysteroscopy. Obstet Gynecol Clin North Am 1999;26:135–48.

144. Tulandi T. Modern surgical approaches to female reproductive tract. Hum Reprod Update 1996;2:419–27.

145. Turner RT, Berman AM, Topel HC. Improved demonstration of endometrial polyps and submucous fibroids using saline-enhanced vaginal sonohysterography. J Am Assoc Gynecol Laparosc 1995;2:421–5.

146. Ubaldi F, Tournaye H, Camus M, Van der Pas H, Gepts E, Devroey P. Fertility after hysteroscopic myomectomy. Hum Reprod Update 1995;1:81–90.

147. Valle RF, Baggish MS. Hysteroscopic myomectomy. In: Baggish MS, Valle RF, Guedj H (eds)., Hysteroscopy. Visual Perspectives of Uterine Anatomy, Physiology and Pathology Diagnostic and Operative Hysteroscopy, 3rd edn. Philadelphia: Lippincott Williams and Wilkins, a Wolters Kluwer business, 2007;385–404.

148. Valle RF. Hysteroscopic removal of submucous leiofibroids. J Gynecol Surg 1990;6:89–96.

149. Van Dongen H, Emanuel MH, Smeets MJ, Trimbos B, Jansen FW. Follow-up after incomplete hysteroscopic removal of uterine fibroids. Acta Obstet Gynecol Scand 2006;85:1463–7.

150. Varasteh NN, Neuwirth RS, Levin B, Keltz MD. Pregnancy rates after hysteroscopic polypectomy and myomectomy in infertile women. Obstet Gynecol 1999;94:168–71.

151. Vercellini P, Zaina B, Yaylayan L, Pisacreta A, De Giorgi O, Crosignani PG. Hysteroscopic myomectomy: long-term effects on menstrual pattern and fertility. Obstet Gynecol 1999;94:341–7.

152. Verkauf BS. Myomectomy for fertility enhancement and preservation. Fertil Steril 1992;58:1–15.

153. Vidal JJ. Patolog1'a tumoral del cuerpo uterino. In: Usandizga JA, De la Fuente PY (eds). Tratado de Ostetricia y Ginecolog1'a Tomo II. Interamericana, 1998;373.

154. Vilos GA, Abu-Rafea B. New developments in ambulatory hysteroscopic surgery. Best Pract Res Clin Obstet Gynaecol 2005;19:727–42.

155. Walker CL, Stewart EA. Uterine fibroids: the elephant in the room. Science 2005;308:1589–92.

156. Wamsteker K, Emanuel MH, de Kruif JH. Transcervical hysteroscopic resection of submucous fibroids for abnormal uterine bleeding: results regarding the degree of intramural extension. Obstet Gynecol 1993;82:736–40.

157. West JH, Robinson DA. Endometrial resection and fluid absorption. Lancet II 1989;1387–8.

158. Wheeler JM, Taskin O. Second-look office hysteroscopy following resectoscopy: the frequency and management of intrauterine adhesions. Fertil Steril 1993;60:150–56.

159. Wieser F, Tempfer C, Kurz C, Nagele F. Hysteroscopy in 2001: a comprehensive review. Acta Obstet Gynecol Scand 2001;80:773–83.

160. Williams CD, Marshburn PB. A prospective study of transvaginal hydrosonography in the evaluation of abnormal uterine bleeding. Am J Obstet Gynecol 1998;179:292–8.

161. Wortman M, Dagget A. Hysteroscopy myomectomy. J Am Assoc Gynecol Laparosc 1995;3:39–46.

162. Yang JH, Lin BL. Changes in myometrial thickness during hysteroscopic resection of deeply invasive submucous fibroids. J Am Assoc Gynecol Laparosc 2001;8:501–5.

163. Yaron Y, Shenhav M, Jaffa AJ, Lessing JB, Peyser MR. Uterine rupture at 33 weeks' gestation subsequent to hysteroscopic uterine perforation. Am J Obstet Gynecol 1994;170:786–7.

Section Three

Laparoscopic Urology

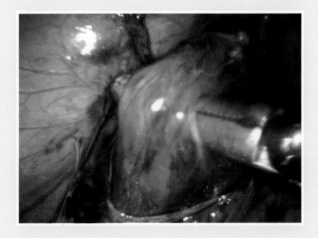

40 Laparoscopic Urological Procedure

Laparoscopic urological surgery can be divided into three areas:

1. Diagnostic
2. Extirpative
3. Reconstructive.

Because much of urologic surgery is reconstructive, and because radiologic imaging techniques continue to refine the accuracy of urologic diagnoses, the role of laparoscopy in urologic practice has decreased in the past few years. However, there are specific areas of urologic surgery in which laparoscopic applications have expanded. Laparoscopy is used extensively in pediatric urology for the diagnosis and operative correction of undescended testicles as well as the laparoscopic removal of obstructed or poorly functioning kidneys. Another major surgery is laparoscopic adrenalectomy for both benign and malignant conditions of the adrenal gland.

LAPAROSCOPIC NEPHRECTOMY

Several obstacles are preventing laparoscopic Nephrectomy technique from being more widely embraced. The first is the time factor which is considerably longer than for an open nephrectomy. The second is the handling of the renal pedicle. Clayman and coworkers have used titanium clips to secure the renal artery and vein. Ehrlich and coworkers used an endoscopic linear stapler to secure the pedicle. Despite the fact that Clayman and coworker's group did not report any significant intraoperative or postoperative bleeding because of inadequate pedicle control, many urologists are uneasy with this aspect of the operation. The third and perhaps most serious concern is the applicability of this technique to cases of renal malignancy. Currently, the adrenal gland is not included in the laparoscopic radical nephrectomy; although this exclusion is probably more a theoretical concern in lower pole and midpole tumors, it would be a limiting factor in upper pole tumors.

Tumor spillage during any laparoscopic procedure is an obvious practical concern. Several reports documented tumor implantation during laparoscopy. Clayman and coworkers tried to solve this problem by developing an entrapment system for the kidney and the lymph nodes. These systems consist of impermeable bags inserted through the laparoscopic trocar. The surgical specimen is placed within the bag or pouch and a drawstring around the opening of the bag allows for closure and acts as a handle to remove the pouch from the abdominal cavity through the laparoscopic trocar. In nephrectomy, the renal specimen is fragmented and aspirated using a especially designed electrical tissue morcellator placed through the neck of the kidney sack. The development of this type of technology decreases but does not eliminate the potential for tumor spillage. Undoubtedly, more work is needed to address the concern of tumor implantation, if this technique is to be applied to malignant renal tumors.

Operative Technique

After induction of general anesthesia, a occlusion balloon catheter is passed up the ureter of the kidney to be removed. A bladder drainage catheter is also used as well as a nasogastric tube. The patient is placed in a supine position. A Veress needle is placed at the umbilicus, and a carbon dioxide pneumoperitoneum is created in the usual manner. Then two 11 mm laparoscopy ports are placed, one at the umbilicus and one immediately subcostal along the midclavicular line. A 5 mm port is also placed in the midclavicular line, 2 to 3 cm below the level of the umbilicus. The patient is then placed in the lateral decubitus position and secured to the operating table. Two 5 mm ports are placed in the anterior axillary line, one on a level with the umbilicus and one off the tip of the eleventh or twelfth rib.

Dissection commences by incising the line of Toldt and resecting the colon medially. The ureter is then identified and secured with a 5 mm locking forceps. The lower pole lateral surfaces, upper pole lateral surfaces, and upper pole of the kidney are dissected free. The adrenal gland is left in place. The kidney is then lifted upward, which places the renal hilum on traction. The renal artery and vein are then dissected. Three endosurgical clips are placed on the distal portion of each vessel, and two clips are placed on the proximal portion of each vessel; an endoscopic scissors is then used to divide the vessels.

The ureter is divided between two clips and the kidney is free. An impermeable nylon surgical sack is introduced through a 11 mm port. Three 5 mm graspers are used to open the mouth of the sack, and the kidney is pushed into the open sack. The drawstrings on the sack are grasped by a 5 mm forceps and pulled through the 11 mm umbilical port, thereby closing the neck of the sack on the kidney. The mouth of the sack is then brought out through the skin, and the metal shaft of the electrical tissue morcellator is introduced into the sack. The morcellator is activated, and the renal tissue is fragmented and aspirated. When all the renal tissue is removed, the empty sack is removed from the abdomen. The port sites are closed in the standard fashion.

In the two cases of transitional cell carcinoma, the ureter was dissected down to the bladder, and a laparoscopic GIA stapler was used to include the distal ureter and a cuff of bladder. Clayman and coworkers and Gaur and coworkers also described a retroperitoneal approach to laparoscopic nephrectomy. A key advance to this approach has been the use of a retroperitoneal balloon dissector that facilitates the development of working space within the retroperitoneal space.

LAPAROSCOPIC VARICOCELECTOMY

Laparoscopic varicocele ligation has been performed by many urologists, and reports from several medical centers have been published. The data suggest that laparoscopic varicocele ligation is therapeutically superior to open surgical and radiographic (embolization) techniques. Laparoscopic varicocelectomy appears to reduce postoperative morbidity. Whether it is necessary to identify and preserve the testicular artery during laparoscopic varicocelectomy remains controversial. Loughlin and Brooks reported on the use of a laparoscopic Doppler probe that they believe, facilitates the identification and preservation of the testicular artery. Matsuda and coworkers claim that the testicular artery does not have to be preserved; they clip the testicular artery and veins en bloc. Further multicenter experience is needed to resolve whether the testicular artery should be preserved during laparoscopic varicocele ligation. Because the testicular artery is preserved during open surgical repair or radiographic embolization procedures we generally preserve the testicular artery during varicocelectomy.

Operative Technique

The technique of laparoscopic varicocele ligation is straightforward. The procedure is usually performed using general anesthesia A urethral catheter is placed to empty the bladder, and a Veress needle is placed at the umbilicus to inflate the peritoneal cavity with carbon dioxide. Alternatively, Hassons technique can be performed at the inferior margin of the umbilicus, and the trocar can be placed into the peritoneum under direct vision. Three laparoscopic ports are placed for varicocelectomy according to baseball diamond concept.

The intra-abdominal vas deferens can be identified as structure joining the spermatic cord above the internal inguinal ring (Fig. 40.1). The gonadal vessels are visualized easily in the retroperitoneum. The posterior peritoneum is excised with cautery, laser, or endoscopic scissors. The gonadal vessels are then mobilized; however, reliably identifying the spermatic artery and its branches is sometimes difficult through the laparoscope (Figs 40.2A and B). Therefore, many surgeons prefer to use the laparoscopic Doppler probe to facilitate identification of the spermatic artery during laparoscopic varicocele ligation. The Doppler probe is

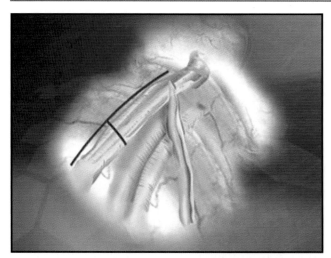

Fig. 40.1: Laparoscopic varicocelectomy

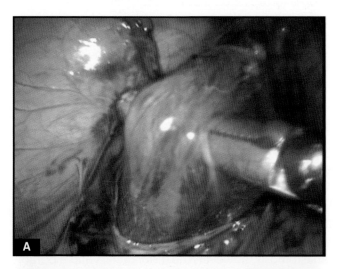

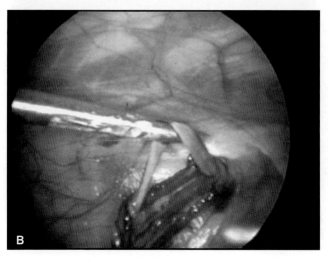

Figs 40.2A and B: The spermatic vein is identified

28.58 cm long and fits through a 5 mm laparoscopic port. After identifying the gonadal artery, the surgeon isolates the gonadal vein or veins using blunt dissection with atraumatic graspers.

Endoscopic clip applier is used to secure it or intracorporeal suturing is used to ligate the gonadal vein or veins while sparing the artery (Fig. 40.3).

LAPAROSCOPIC RETROPERITONEAL NODE DISSECTION

The laparoscopic retroperitoneal node dissection in the management of testicular cancer is still not very frequently performed. Increased operating time is a consideration in applying laparoscopic techniques to a procedure. As with pelvic node dissection, the question has also been raised as to the completeness of the laparoscopic retroperitoneal node dissection. Laparoscopic dissection of the nodal tissue behind the aorta and vena cava is difficult laparoscopically.

Laparoscopic retroperitoneal node dissection appears, at least for now, best applied to patients without evidence of bulky disease in the retroperitoneum who would otherwise be candidates for observation rather than surgical exploration. Although the laparoscopic procedure does not currently appear to be as thorough a dissection as the open node dissection, it offers the opportunity to have some pathologic documentation of nodal status in patients considered for observation. The technique for laparoscopic retroperitoneal node dissection has not

Section Four

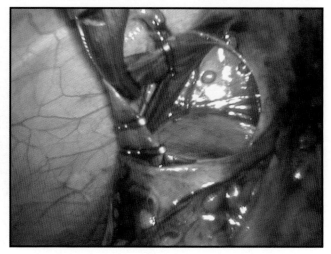

Fig. 40.3: Clips applied around spermatic vein

been standardized and is still evolving; therefore, the reader is referred to the case reports for the authors individual techniques.

LAPAROSCOPIC MANAGEMENT OF LYMPHOCELES

Lymphoceles are not uncommon after renal transplantation; an incidence of 0.6 to 18 percent has been reported. It can also occur after pelvic lymphadenectomy, and an incidence of 5.6 percent has been reported in this circumstance . Most of these patients are asymptomatic and do not require much aggressive treatment. When the lymphocele becomes symptomatic or is associated with fever and potential infection, however, drainage of the lymphocele is indicated. Several investigators have reported successful laparoscopic drainage of lymphoceles.

Operative Technique

The technique of lymphocele drainage is described as follows. After the induction of general endotracheal anesthesia, the surgeon places a urethral catheter to drain the bladder, and a nasogastric tube is then inserted. A Veress needle is inserted into the peritoneal cavity in the left upper quadrant to avoid the transplant allograft. A pneumoperitoneum is achieved in the usual manner, and 10 mm trocar sheath is inserted through the same site into the peritoneal cavity. The video endoscope is placed through this port, and two additional 5 mm ports are inserted under direct vision in the periumbilical area in the right upper quadrant at the level of the midclavicular line.

The abdomen is carefully inspected, and the renal transplant and associated lymphocele are visualized. They appear as two extrinsic bulges in the retroperitoneum. The lymphocele is distinguishable by its superolateral location to the graft and the soft consistency on probing. The lymphocele also transmits light readily when the light source is placed at its wall. The patient is placed in Trendelenburg's position to allow the small bowel to fall cephalad and to facilitate the visibility of the lymphocele. The lymphocele is then entered using electrocautery. The peritoneum and its attached lymphocele wall are grasped, and the incision is extended circumferentially using laparoscopic scissors. An ellipse of lymphocele wall is removed, thereby creating a window. After careful marsupia-

lization of the edges of the window, the lymphocele is inspected, and all internal loculations are lysed and excised to create a single cavity. At the end of surgery the cavity is irrigated and inspected for adequate hemostasis prior to the usual completion of the laparoscopic procedure.

LAPAROSCOPIC URETEROLYSIS

Usually the patient underwent laparoscopic ureterolysis via a transperitoneal approach. An external ureteral stent should be placed to help identify the ureter as is done with laparoscopic nephrectomy. The ureter is identified by close up vision of telescope and then successfully mobilized laparoscopically. Laparoscopic biopsy forceps should be used to obtain multiple biopsy specimens of the periureteral tissue. Laparoscopic ureterolysis is not a very frequently performed procedure. Additional experience will help determine how applicable laparoscopic ureterolysis will become in the future.

LAPAROSCOPIC ILEAL CONDUIT

In many centers, laparoscopic surgeons are performing laparoscopic ileal loop conduit. This procedure is commonly performed for palliation of obstruction in old man with fibrosarcoma of the prostate. The ileal loop itself is fashioned laparoscopically using endoscopic stapling devices. To perform the ureteral anastomosis, however, the distal ureters and a portion of the conduit has to be brought in through a trocar site, and an extracorporeal, hand-sewn, ureteroileal anastomosis is performed on each side.

The report emphasizes the limitation of laparoscopic instrumentation at this time. Laparoscopic suturing is cumbersome, and the ureteroileal anastomosis could not have been completed easily laparoscopically. Until either tissue welding techniques or better suturing techniques are available, only limited applications are available for laparoscopic reconstructive surgery such as that outlined in this case report.

LAPAROSCOPIC PELVIC LYMPHADENECTOMY

Laparoscopic pelvic lymphadenectomy has the potential to aid in the staging of prostate cancer. Most urologists embrace the philosophy that if the pelvic lymph nodes are involved in prostate cancer, cure cannot be achieved with radical prostatectomy or radiation therapy, and hormonal therapy is indicated in these patients for palliation.

Vascular injuries are most common complication during dissection. Adherence to good laparoscopic technique and familiarity with the anatomy are the most reliable ways to avoid complications.

Operative Technique

The pneumoperitoneum is established in the standard manner. Trocar placement is then performed. The size and location of trocar sites for the procedure vary with the surgeon's preference. Most use the diamond configuration. An alternative used by some surgeons is the so called fan configuration for trocar placement. This configuration allows the surgeon and the surgical assistant to manipulate instruments with both hands during the dissection. It is also helpful in obese patients or in those with a prominent urachus. The size of the trocars used at each site may vary. A 10 mm port is usually placed in the umbilicus for the laparoscope. An additional 10 mm port is placed in at least one other site for tissue removal. Another 10 mm port is used for the endoscopic clip applier. Usually, 5 mm ports are used for the remaining trocar sites. After completion of trocar placement, the laparoscopic landmarks for pelvic node dissection are identified. These landmarks include the medial umbilical ligament (remnant of the obliterated umbilical artery), urachus, bladder, vas deferens, iliac vessels, spermatic vessels, and internal ring. The next maneuver is to incise the posterior peritoneum parallel and lateral to the medial umbilical ligament . Early identification of the ureter is important to avoid ureteral injury. The vas deferens is then divided to facilitate operative access to the obturator space. Using primarily blunt dissection, the iliac vein and artery are identified. The nodal tissue overlying the external iliac vein is then teased medially to expose the internal obturator muscle. A laparoscopic vein retractor can be used to retract the external iliac vein laterally and permit easier, more complete dissection of the nodal tissue beneath the vein. The dissection proceeds with removing tissue off the vein distally until Cooper's ligament and the pubic bone are identified.

Electrosurgery is used to fulgurate small vessels and lymphatics, and the distal extent of the packet is freed from the pubic bone. The packet is pulled proximally and freed from the underside of the pubic bone. At this point, the obturator nerve is identified. Because nodal tissue can be quite bulky and difficult to grasp, adequate forceps can ensure a more reliable grasp of the specimen. With blunt dissection, the obturator nerve is cleaned off proximally, and endoscopic clips are used to divide the distal portion of the dissection. At the completion of the laparoscopic pelvic lymphadenectomy, the iliac artery, vein, pubic bone, and obturator nerve can be seen clearly. The field is checked for hemostasis, and the dissection is performed in an identical manner on the opposite side. The trocars are removed, and the puncture sites are closed in the usual manner.

BIBLIOGRAPHY

1. Berends FJ, den Hoed PT, Bonjer HJ, Kazemier G, van Riemsdijk I, Weimar W, et al. Technical considerations and pitfalls in laparoscopic live donornephrectomy. Surg Endosc 2002;16:893-8.
2. Buell JF, Lee L, Martin JE, Dake NA, Cavanaugh TM, Hanaway MJ, et al. Laparoscopic donor nephrectomy vs open live donor nephrectomy: a quality of life and functional study. Clin Transplant 2005;19:102-9.
3. De Klerk M, Keizer KM, Claas FH, Witvliet M, Haase-Kromwijk BJ, Weimar W. The Dutch national living donor kidney exchange program. Am J Transplant 2005;5:2302-5.
4. Dunker MS, Bemelman WA, Slors JF, van Duijvendijk P, Gouma DJ. Functional outcome, quality of life, body image, and cosmesis in patients after laparoscopicassisted and conventional restorative proctocolectomy: a comparative study. Dis Colon Rectum 2001;44:1800-7.
5. Govani MV, Kwon O, Batiuk TD, Milgrom ML, Filo RS. Creatinine reduction ratio and 24-hour creatinine excretion on posttransplant day two: simple and objective tools to define graft function. J Am Soc Nephrol 2002;13:1645-9.
6. Guillonneau B, Jayet C, Tewari A, Vallancien G. Robot assisted laparoscopic nephrectomy. J Urol 2001;166:200–01.
7. Horgan S, Vanuno D, Sileri P, Cicalese L, Benedetti E. Robotic-assisted laparoscopic donor nephrectomy for kidney transplantation. Transplantation 2002;73:1474–9.
8. Hoznek A, Hubert J, Antiphon P, Gettman M, Hemal AK, Abbou CC. Robotic renal surgery. Urol Clin North Am 2004;31:731–6.
9. Hsu THS, Su L, Ratner LE, Kavoussi LE. Renovascular complications of laparoscopic donor nephrectomy. Urology 2002;60:811–5.
10. Ingelfinger JR. Risks and benefits to the living donor. N Engl J Med 2005;353:447-9.

Section Four

11. Johansson M, Thune A, Nelvin L, Stiernstam M, Westman B, Lundell L. Randomized clinical trial of open versus laparoscopic cholecystectomy in the treatment of acute cholecystitis. Br J Surg 2005;92:44-9.

12. Joshi GP. Anesthesia for minimally invasive surgery: laparoscopy, thoracoscopy, hysteroscopy. Anesthesiol Clin North America 2001;19:89–105.

13. Kok NF, Alwayn IP, Lind MY, Tran KT, Weimar W, Ijzermans JN. Donor nephrectomy: mini-incision muscle-splitting open approach versus laparoscopy. Transplantation 2006;81:881-7.

14. Kuang W, Ng CS, Matin S, Kaouk JH, El-Jack M, Gill I. Rhabdomyolysis after laparoscopic donor nephrectomy. Urology 2002;60:911(i)–911(ii).

15. Leventhal JR, Deeik RK, Joehl RJ, Rege RV, et al. Laparoscopic live donor nephrectomy – is it safe? Transplantation 2000;70:602–6.

16. Lewis GR, Brook NR, Waller JR, Bains JC, Veitch PS, Nicholson ML. A comparison of traditional open, minimal-incision donor nephrectomy and laparoscopic donor nephrectomy. Transpl Int 2004;17:589-95.

17. Lind MY, Hazebroek EJ, Hop WC, Weimar W, Jaap Bonjer H, IJzermans JN. Right-sided laparoscopic live-donor nephrectomy: is reluctance still justified? Transplantation 2002;74:1045-8.

18. Lind MY, Liem YS, Bemelman WA, Dooper PM, Hop WC, Weimar W, et al. Live donor nephrectomy and return to work: does the operative technique matter? Surg Endosc 2003;17:591-5.

19. London E, Rudich S, McVicar J, Wolfe B, Perez R. Equivalent renal allograft function with laparoscopic versus open live donor nephrectomies. Transplant Proc 1999;31:258–60.

20. Majeed AW, Troy G, Nicholl JP, Smythe A, Reed MW, Stoddard CJ, et al. Randomised, prospective, single-blind comparison of laparoscopic versus small-incision cholecystectomy. Lancet 1996;347:989-94.

21. Najarian JS, Chavers BM, McHugh LE, et al. 20 years or more of follow-up of living kidney donors. Lancet 1992;340(8823):807–10.

22. Nogueira JN, Cangro CB, Fink JC, et al. A comparison of recipient renal outcomes with laparoscopic versus open live donor nephrectomy. Transplantation 1999;67:722–8.

23. Novotny MJ. Advanced urologic laparoscopy. Laparoscopic live donor nephrectomy. Urol Clin North Am 2001;28:127–35.

24. Oyen O, Andersen M, Mathisen L, Kvarstein G, Edwin B, Line PD, et al. Laparoscopic versus open living-donor nephrectomy: experiences from a prospective, randomized, single-center study focusing on donor safety. Transplantation 2005;79:1236-40.

25. Perry KT, Freedland SJ, Hu JC, Phelan MW, Kristo B, Gritsch AH, et al. Quality of life, pain and return to normal activities following laparoscopic donor nephrectomy versus open mini-incision donor nephrectomy. J Urol 2003;169:2018-21.

26. Philosophe B, Kuo PC, Schweitzer EJ, et al. Laparoscopic versus open donor nephrectomy. Comparing ureteral complications in the recipients and improving the laparoscopic technique. Transplantation 1999;68:497–502.

27. Ratner LE, Ciseck LJ, Moore RG, Cigarroa FG, Kaufman HS, Kavoussi LR. Laparoscopic live donor nephrectomy. Transplantation 1995;60:1047-9.

28. Ratner LE, Mongomery RA, Maley WR, et al. Laparoscopic live donor nephrectomy: the recipient. Transplantation 2000; 69:2319–23.

29. Rodrigo E, Ruiz JC, Pin˜ era C, et al. Creatinine reduction ratio on post-transplant day two as criterion in defining delayed graft function. Am J Transplant 2004;4:1163–9.

30. Simforoosh N, Basiri A, Tabibi A, Shakhssalim N, Hosseini Moghaddam SM. Comparison of laparoscopic and open donor nephrectomy: a randomized controlled trial. Br J. Urolog Int 2005;95:851-5.

31. Smets EM, Garssen B, Cull A, de Haes JC. Application of the multidimensional fatigue inventory (MFI-20) in cancer patients receiving radiotherapy. Br J Cancer 1996;73:241-5.

32. Srivastava A, Tripathi DM, Zaman W, Kumar A. Subcostal versus transcostal mini donor nephrectomy: is rib resection responsible for pain related donor morbidity. J Urol 2003;170:738-40.

33. Subramonian K, DeSylva S, Bishai P, Thompson P, Muir G. Acquiring surgical skills: a comparative study of open versus laparoscopic surgery. Eur Urol 2004;45:346–51.

34. Sundqvist P, Feuk U, Ha¨ ggman M, Persson AEG, Stridsberg M, Wadstro¨ m J. Hand-assisted retroperitoneoscopic live donor nephrectomy in comparison to open and laparoscopic procedures: a prospective study on donor morbidity and kidney function. Transplantation 2004;78:147–53.

35. Sung GT, Gill IS. Robotic renal and adrenal surgery. Surg Clin North Am 2003;83:1469–82.

36. Troppmann C, Ormond DB, Perez RV. Laparoscopic (vs open) live donor nephrectomy: a UNOS database analysis of early graft function and survival. Am J Transplant 2003; 3:1295–1301.

37. Wadstrom J. Hand-assisted retroperitoneoscopic live donor nephrectomy: experience from the first 75 consecutive cases. Transplantation 2005;80:1060-6.

38. Ware JE, Snow KK, Kosinski M, Gandek B. SF-36 health survey. Manual and interpretation guide. Boston, MA: Health Institute, New England Medical Center, 1993.

39. Wolf JS Jr, Merion RM, Leichtman AB, Campbell DA Jr, Magee JC, Punch JD, et al. Randomized controlled trial of hand-assisted laparoscopic versus open surgical live donor nephrectomy. Transplantation 2001;72:284-90.

40. Yang SL, Harkaway R, Badosa F, Ginsberg P, Greenstein MA. Minimal incision living donor nephrectomy: improvement in patient outcome. Urology 2002;59:673-7.

41. Yilmaz S, Paavonen T, Havry P. Chronic rejection of rat allografts. II. The impact of prolonged ischaemia time on transplant histology. Transplantation 1992;53:823–7.

Section Four

Pediatric Laparoscopy

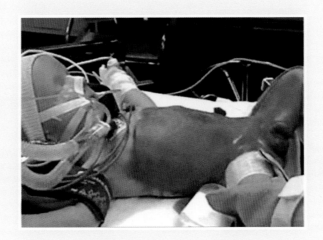

41 Laparoscopic Pediatric Surgery

"There are no great discoveries or advances
as long as there are unhappy children in the world".
-Albert Einstein

LAPAROSCOPY IN INFANTS AND CHILDREN

When wide spread use of laparoscopy and thoracoscopy in adult patients occurred in the first part of the 1990s, it did not transfer into widespread application in the pediatric population for a number of reasons. One of the strong reason was the fact that pediatric surgeons did not have a commonly performed procedure, such as cholecystectomy, in which to refine their endoscopic skills. The most common intra-adominal procedure performed in infants and children is appendectomy and fundoplication, and it is difficult initially to learn these skills. In addition, the small intra-abdominal working space in infants and young children makes the operations more difficult and time consuming. Children seem to recover more rapidly than adults, because of the fact that there is no underlying heart or lung disease (Fig. 41.1). In the early 1990s, it was unclear whether there would be further benefits to an already faster healing process and recovery time. The main advantage of laparoscopy is the fact that it enables a magnified view of the abdominal cavity and the treatment of more than one pathology, even if located in different parts of the abdominal cavity, without enlarging the abdominal incision as in case of open surgery, and during the same anesthesia. Moreover, the laparoscopy permits identification and treatment of clinically silent

pathologies or discovery of a rare associated pathology while performing surgery for a different indication.

Many of the leaders in pediatric surgery were not skilled in this new technology and, therefore, pediatric surgeons finishing their training program were not being trained in this laparoscopic approach. When information and documentation of the benefits of minimal access surgery have been published, this technology is used more today as compared to the mid-1990s. Intra-abdominal procedures such as fundoplication, splenectomy, appendectomy, and cholecystectomy are being commonly performed by pediatric surgeons. In addition, many pediatric surgeons use diagnostic laparoscopy through a known unilateral inguinal hernia sac to determine whether there is a contralateral patent processus vaginalis, which might indicate the need for contralateral repair under

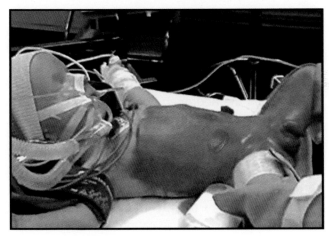

Fig. 41.1: All the vital parameter should be strictly monitored in pediatric age group

the same anesthesia. Laparoscopic primary pull through procedures in the neonatal period for correction of Hirschsprung's disease are popular among many pediatric surgeons. The cutting edge of laparoscopy in pediatric surgery is procedures such as intestinal resection for Crohn disease and colectomy with J-pouch reconstruction for ulcerative colitis. In the chest, many operations in children are applicable for the thoracoscopic route as thoracoscopic repair of esophageal atresia with tracheoesophageal fistula, but the thoracoscopic approach remains in its infancy with this congenital anomaly at this time.

A number of pediatric surgeons utilizes laparoscopic fundoplication following open gastrostomy in children. Regarding recurrence of gastroesophageal reflux following partial anterior fundoplication, many of these recurrences can simply be converted to a Nissen fundoplication with good results. Usually there is much less inflammation and adhesion formation following the initial laparoscopic procedure than occurs following an open operation.

Laparoscopic Appendicectomy in Children

Below the age of 1 year, the port for the telescope is inserted through the abdominal wall 1 cm to the left of the umbilicus. In small children, the umbilical ring is too loose to keep the trocar airtight. In older children the umbilicus is chosen for the telescopic port. Before advancing the trocar, a skin incision is made slightly smaller than the trocar in order to secure gas tight skin closure around the trocar shaft. Too small incision is risky because it results in too forceful trocar insertion. A Veress needle is inserted and CO_2 is insufflated up to an intra-abdominal pressure of 12 mm mercury. The smaller the child, the slow the insufflation flow rate should be. With practice, the pressure can be estimated by palpating the abdomen. Insufflation and pressure control are executed through valves at the trocars. A second and third trocar is inserted in the right lower hypochondria and left iliac fossa according to base ball diamond concept. Its site is chosen by pressing the abdominal wall from outside. In pediatric age the surgeon should try to stay lateral to the umbilical ligaments. Trocars may get caught in a ligament and may therefore be difficult to advance. The right trocar is used for the grasper forceps and also to take in the

appendix for later removal. In children up to 8-10 years, the appendix will usually fit a 7.5 mm trocar. If the child is over 10, a 10 mm port suffices. A 5 mm trocar in the left lower abdomen will provide access for the cautery, scissors and a second forceps. Expiratory capnography is mandatory for the anesthesiologist in all children. They are prepared to ventilate with decreased residual functional capacities, decreased tidal volumes, and increased frequencies during laparoscopy.

Urinary catheters and nasogastric tubes or drainages were never used. The fascia was approximated with a single absorbable suture. The appendix stump was simply ligated with a Roeder's or Meltzers knot just like adult patient. No purse string or Z suture is required. In the beginning, laparoscopy took considerably longer than an open approach (up to 90 min vs 25 min). Practice decreased the time consumed, which is now nearly identical to that required for open procedures (25 min).

Other Causes of Pain Abdomen in Pediatric Age Group

Hydatids can easily be exposed and removed laparoscopically. We have seen a few cases in pediatric group that mimicked acute appendicitis. The ovaries can be trapped within dense adhesions; sometimes other additional signs of previous inflammatory processes are demonstrated as well. Such adhesions can be transacted laparoscopically, although we are not sure it is worth the trouble. A Meckel's diverticulum can be identified and removed by laparoscopy. Congenital and acquired adhesions and ligaments are also found frequently in childrens. New aspects may be added to clinical symptoms. Laparoscopy can be used in children with incidentally discovered inguinal hernia.

Laparoscopic Cholecystectomy in Children

Laparoscopic cholecystectomy is the procedure of choice for the treatment of adults with gallbladder stone disease. However, cholelithiasis is rare in children; for this reason, it is difficult to evaluate the validity of this procedure in a large case series of pediatric patients. The presence of gallbladder stones is generally idiopathic in children, and their discovery is sometimes incidental during a sonographic exam performed to search for other abdominal pathologies. However, there are well-known predisposing factors to the developing gallbladder stones in children. Among infants affected by hemolytic disease hemolytic anemia, for instance the incidence of gallbladder stones is much higher than the normal population. Its reported incidence ranges from 10 to 40 percent in various series. The management of children with cholelithiasis requires great caution; an accurate hematological study is always necessary to detect a possible underlying hematological disease. In cases of gallstones discovered incidentally, an accurate follow-up is suggested, since a spontaneous resolution of the pathology is possible. Generally, noncalcified gallbladder stones in children disappear within 3-6 months. By contrast, surgery is needed for calcified stones in both nonsymptomatic and symptomatic children. Laparoscopic cholecystectomy rather than open cholecystectomy is the procedure of choice in symptomatic infants. Laparoscopy in infants should be performed using very small instruments (3 or 5 mm in diameter). Technically, this approach is similar to the one employed for adults, although careful consideration of a child's anatomical difference is essential to avoid complications. It is important to keep in mind that in pediatric patients there may be biliary tree anomalies, such as gallbladder duplication, ductal abnormalities, accessory bile duct, or accessory cystic artery. These findings do not represent a contraindication to the laparoscopic procedure if the surgeon is able to perform a delicate and accurate dissection of the elements at the level of Calot's triangle. Bile duct injuries, which are often reported in adults, are very rare in children maybe due to more clear anatomy and less fat. The junction between the cystic duct and the common bile duct is much more visible in children, due to the scarcity of fatty tissue and adhesions at the level of Calot's triangle at this age. This improved visualization makes the dissection of the cystic duct easier and less dangerous than in adult patients. The presence of common bile duct stones in children is an extremely rare event in the pediatric population. At any rate, the presence of jaundice, dilatation of the biliary tree at ultrasonography, alkaline phosphatase and total bilirubin above the normal range by >5 mg/dl, and/or a history of pancreatitis are indications for a cholangiography or an ERCP. In addition, we believe that intraoperative cholangiograms can also be performed in infants.

With respect to the ERCP, the sequential approach of endoscopic sphincterectomy and stone extraction followed by laparoscopic cholecystectomy is a safe and effective method in children as well as adults. One important advantage is that laparoscopic cholecystectomy in children can be associated, if necessary, with other technical procedures, such as the closure of a peritoneal vaginal duct in cases of inguinal hernia; thus, a second operation or another incision can be avoided. However, if another procedure is required, laparoscopic expertise on the part of the surgeon is fundamental to avoid additional morbidity. We performed a concomitant splenectomy in infants affected by spherocytosis and one with thalassemia. Based on our experience, laparoscopic cholecystectomy is as valid and effective a procedure in pediatric patients as it is in adults. In children, it is important to perform a complete preoperative evaluation to search for the possible coexistence of hematological disease.

Laparoscopic Splenectomy in Children

The preliminary results and the retrospective comparison help establish the safety and efficacy of laparoscopic splenectomy in children. Although the peritoneal cavities of the children are limited, there are no special risks in the pediatric patients. As many splenectomies are now being performed for cytopenic/anemic disease in children, pediatric patients requiring splenectomy may benefit from this minimally access approach. Decreased postoperative pain and recovery time are anticipated in these patients, just as for thousands of patients undergoing laparoscopic splenectomy.

Absolute contraindications to laparoscopic splenectomy include contraindications to general anesthesia. Extensive inflammation and adhesions in the left upper quadrant may be a relative contraindication because of the increased possibility of hemorrhage. Significant splenomegaly may also be a relative contraindication caused by increased difficulty of dissection and the need for more complex extraction procedures. A large spleen compared to small abdomen is a problem in pediatric laparoscopic splenectomy. Especially in patients with HS, the spleen size is usually large.

Bleeding tendency is a contraindication to laparoscopic procedures. Many patients requiring splenectomy are coagulopathic from thrombocytopenia or qualitative platelet dysfunction. Preoperative use of intravenous IgG should be considered for the patients with ITP. The response to IgG is generally as efficacious as the response to steroids with the added advantage of fewer associated side effects.

The surgeon performing splenectomy must be cognizant of this fact and have a low threshold for conversion to an open procedure in the event of a hemorrhage that is not easily visualized or controlled through the operating ports. As LS is an advanced technique, we recommend that anyone attempting the procedure be fully experienced in laparoscopic surgical techniques and instrumentation. Understanding the limitations of minimal access surgery, in addition to possessing the ability to convert to the open procedure to assure safe splenectomy and patient safety, is also important. Laparoscopic Splenectomy may prove at least as safe as the open approach if performed by experienced surgeons.

The disadvantage is increased operative time. However, this may diminish with experience and introduction of the Endocatch II. With more experience and advances in technology, laparoscopic splenectomy may become easier, and surgeon may be able to reduce their operative time and anesthetic risks. Several other aspects of the operative technique developed in pediatric patients deserve emphasis. Early mobilization of the spleen significantly increases the difficulty of exposing the hilum. The splenic artery and vein are individually clipped and divided, and a linear stapler is not necessary in pediatric patients. As superior branches of the short gastric vessels are difficult to clip at the early phase of procedure, those branches should be left and divided at the end. Accessory spleen should be searched in patients with hematologic disease requiring splenectomy for hypersplenism. Although these may occur within the attaching ligaments of the spleen and in the mesentery and omentum, they most frequently occur in the hilum along the splenic vessels. Four accessory spleens were found in our series, and they were successfully removed under laparoscopic guidance. The magnified view afforded during laparoscopy can allow for easier identification of accessory spleens, especially in the hilar region. The inability to identify accessory spleens by palpation is one limitation of laparoscopic surgery.

Thorough evaluation for accessory splenic tissue is essential intraoperatively. Traditional splenectomy, performed through a midline or subcostal incision, is associated with a number of complications, including hemorrhage, atelectasis, pneumonia, ileus, subdiaphragmatic abscess, and incisional hernias. These may prolong the hospital stay and convalescence.

Because the small incisions of laparoscopic surgery are less painful than upper abdominal incisions, patients use fewer narcotics, have fewer respiratory complications, and have improved return of pulmonary function. Patients treated laparoscopic splenectomy ambulated the same day, and a decrease in postoperative hospital stay was seen compared to those who underwent open surgery. Most of the patients returned to unrestricted activities within 1 week after being discharged.

Laparoscopic Repair of Pediatric Hernia

The first use of laparoscopy in cases of inguinal hernia in children was for diagnosis. Laparoscopic or transinguinal laparoscopic evaluation for a contralateral patent vaginalis process has been previously reported as a means of avoiding metachronous hernias. In these cases, the internal examination has been performed by laparoscopic technique, placing the optical trocar through the umbilicus. The main problem is to decide whether or not to treat the contralateral hernia sac immediately. Is the contralateral vaginalis process wide and deep enough to be responsible in the short-term for a metachronous contralateral hernia?

During laparoscopy for inguinal hernia repair, surgeon often encounter an unexpected bilateral hernia. This situation underscores the importance of laparoscopy as a means of improving the diagnosis of bilateral hernias. Femoral hernias are often misdiagnosed and treated as inguinal hernias. Thus, laparoscopic groin exploration is valuable means of evaluating children with presumed recurrent inguinal hernias. Less than 1 percent of all groin masses seen in children are due to femoral hernias. Because these hernias are so uncommon, they are often overlooked, misdiagnosed, or even treated as inguinal hernias. In fact, the correct diagnosis of femoral hernia is often made at the time of groin re-exploration for a presumed recurrent inguinal hernia. The laparoscopic approach may offer better diagnostic ability than conventional open exploration because all potential hernial defects in both groins can be examined under direct laparoscopic vision. Furthermore, unilateral or simultaneous bilateral tension free repair can be done using the laparoscopic technique. Laparoscopy is helpful to diagnose a femoral hernia. It enables an accurate identification of the nature of the groin defect. However, the technical details of laparoscopic femoral hernia repair are still under discussion, even in adult series. The role of laparoscopy in the management of suspected recurrent pediatric hernias has been described. For patients with a patent processus vaginalis, laparoscopy is efficient for diagnosis and treatment.

Which laparoscopic procedure is most efficient in pediatric surgery cases?

- Ligature alone of the hernia sac without dividing the peritoneum. It has a high recurrence rate; this may due to the use of absorbable sutures or to the continuity of the peritoneum, which is left intact. Furthermore, the risk of injury to the vas or the vessels from the needle running under the peritoneum without previous dissection seems to be high.
- Performing the procedure without ligature of the hernia sac while only dividing the peritoneum on the site of the inner inguinal ring, seems to be enough to avoid early complications and to achieve a low recurrence rate. But it may lead to intraperitoneal adhesions.
- To avoid such adhesions, many surgeon operate the patent process vaginalis just like open surgery. The vaginalis process is divided by separating the sac, which remains in the scrotal pouch or in the labia majora, and the peritoneum at the internal inguinal ring. This procedure does not require opening of the inguinal canal. Dissection of the vas and spermatic vessels is done at the level of the internal inguinal ring, where these elements are more easy to spare from the peritoneum, whereas more adhesions may be encountered in the inguinal canal. The peritoneum is ligated. At the end of the

procedure, one should pay close attention to the testis position, so as to avoid a secondary occurrence at an ectopic site. Pain and discomfort resolve very quickly.

Laparoscopic herniorrhaphy in children is gaining increasing acceptance in pediatric surgery. The essential step in the conventional method for inguinal hernia repair in children is the simple ligation of the hernial sac without narrowing the open ring (Figs 41.4A to C). The internal inguinal ring is reached by opening the inguinal canal and dissecting the hernial sac from the cord structures. Postoperatively, the major damage from which the patient has to recover is not the ligature of the hernial sac, but the trauma of access itself. Therefore, the clinical goal is to leave the abdominal wall as intact as possible. Laparoscopy is most appropriate for this purpose to gain access to the abdominal cavity in order to close the inner inguinal ring from within.

The laparoscopic repair of pediatric hernia requires 2 mm instruments; the use of larger instruments would lead to an increase in the size of the incision that would make it equivalent to a conventional groin incision (Fig. 41.2). Bilateral inguinal hernias, as well as indirect and direct hernias, are of no concern in laparoscopic herniorrhaphy. There is no difference between the access and treatment for unilateral and bilateral laparoscopic hernia repair and the laparoscopic repair of a direct hernia. Needle for intracorporeal suturing is introduced through abdominal wall in case of pediatric patient (Figs 41.3A and B).

Because it remains unclear whether a small open processus vaginalis develops subsequently into a

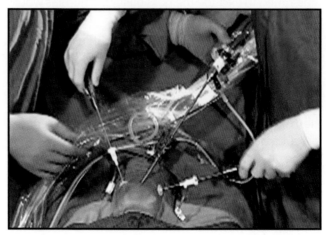

Fig. 41.2: Port position for pediatric appendicectomy

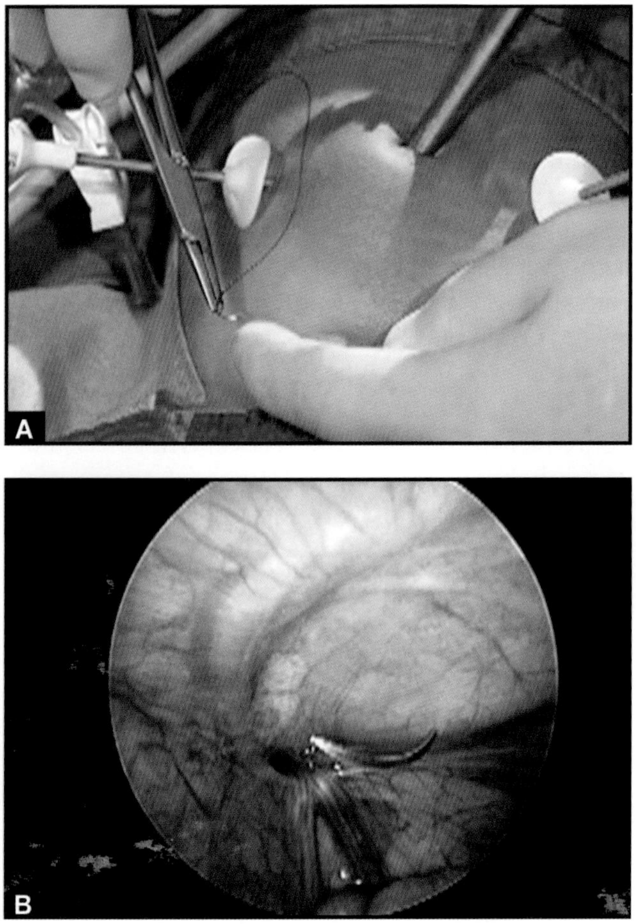

Figs 41.3A and B: Needle should be introduced percutaneous in pediatric age group

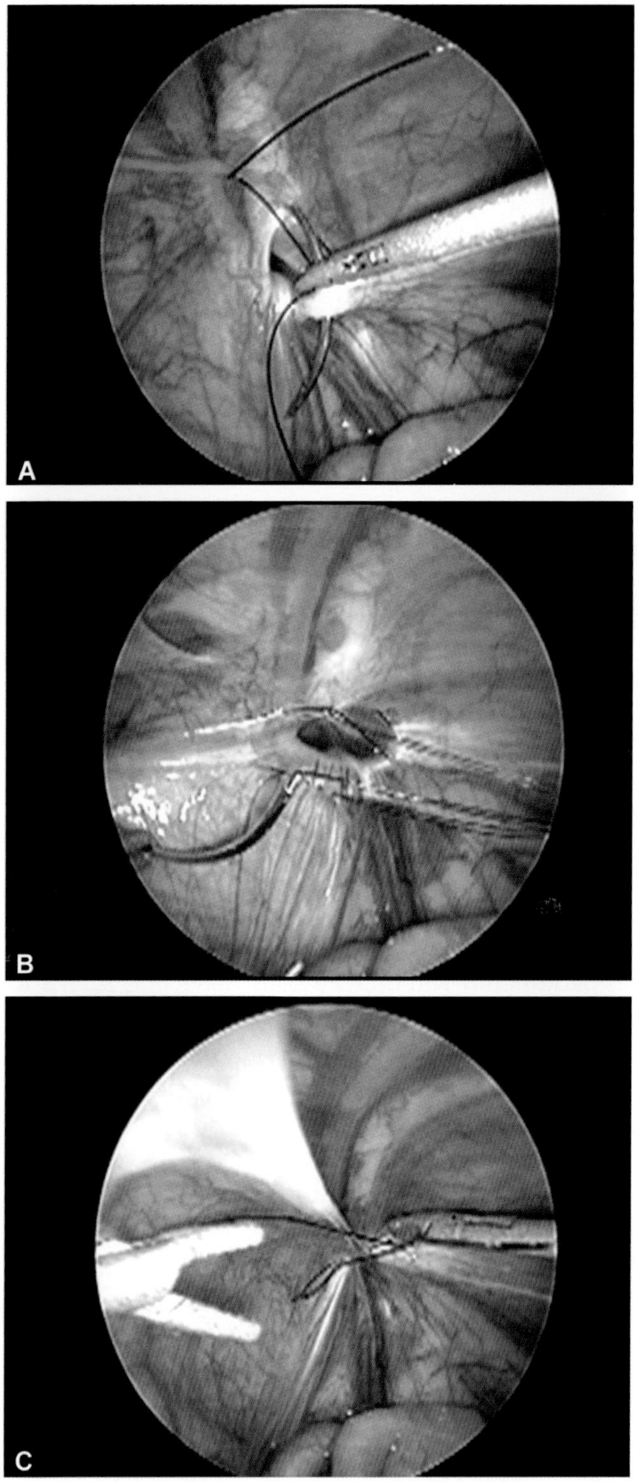

Figs 41.4A to C: Purse string suture for pediatric inguinal hernia repair

hernia, we choose to close open inner inguinal rings down to a 2 mm width whether they are unilateral or bilateral. In many of patients, the contralateral side was found to be open as well; by closing these openings, it is assumed to exclude the possibility that hernias would occur.

The recurrence rate of inguinal hernias in children is slightly higher with laparoscopic herniorrhaphy than with the conventional technique. In patients with recurrences after laparoscopic herniorrhaphy, the surgeon has an undisturbed anatomy for groin incision; the risk of an injury to the vas deferens, subsequent testicular atrophy, and the risk of superior displacement of the testicle seem less likely. In cases of hernia recurrence after conventional hernia repair, laparoscopy allows us to clearly differentiate an indirect hernia from a direct one. Direct inguinal hernias in children are not that rare. The cosmetic results are excellent. Once the technique of intracorporeal suturing in a limited space is mastered, laparoscopic herniorrhaphy is safe, reproducible, and technically easy for experienced laparoscopists. If there is any uncertainty about the contralateral side, whether it is a direct or an indirect hernia, and in cases of inguinal hernia recurrence, the laparoscopic procedure is highly preferable as a primary technique that combines diagnosis and the potential for immediate treatment.

Laparoscopic Pediatric Fundoplication

Gastroesophageal fundoplication currently is one of the three most common major operations performed on infants and children by pediatric surgeons. With the advent of laparoscopic surgery, the number of gastroesophageal fundoplications has virtually exploded. Morbidity always was substantial with this operation, and laparoscopy has not changed this.

In recent years, laparoscopic Nissen fundoplication has been performed with increasing frequency in pediatric patients with symptomatic GER because it causes minimal trauma to the abdominal wall and supposedly eases patient recovery. Initial experience demonstrates that Nissen fundoplication can be accomplished successfully and safely using the laparoscopic approach in very small babies suffering from severe GER. Infants and children who are candidates for antireflux procedure differ in many aspects from the adult population. In adults, GER is typically associated with hiatal hernia and is usually unrelated to any other abnormality. In children, on the other hand, there is usually no hiatal hernia, but clinically significant GER is often associated with neurological impairment, metabolic abnormality, or some other severe underlying disease. Therefore, even after successful surgical resolution of GER, these babies often remain very sick due to their primary disease.

Many children undergoing antireflux operation are at increased risk because of chronic parenchymal lung damage due to recurrent episodes of pneumonia and because they are often severely malnourished. Operative risk is especially high in children with familial dysautonomia. Concomitant impairment of gastrointestinal motility is also unique to the pediatric population. In particular, impairment of the swallowing mechanism and delayed gastric emptying should be taken into account by the surgeon. Hence, when the swallowing mechanism is impaired, gastrostomy should be constructed for postoperative feeding or fluid administration to prevent persistent aspirations. Likewise, the surgeon should consider pyloroplasty when there is preoperative evidence of delayed gastric

emptying. In this case, it is usually preferable to do an open procedure, although a pyloroplasty can be accomplished through a small laparotomy incision at the end of the laparoscopic procedure. There are several technical concerns in laparoscopic Nissen fundoplication that are unique to infants and small children. Because the operating space is very small, it is necessary to use especially designed short instruments and to handle them with great care. To prevent dislocation, the trocars need to be secured to the skin by stitches.

The pneumoperitoneum should be maintained at pressures as low as 10 mm Hg. Elevation of pressure may cause difficulty in ventilation, with resultant hypercarbia. It is sometimes necessary even in pediatric age group to increase the pneumoperitoneum pressure temporarily, for example during suturing, and to immediately deflate the abdomen if expiratory CO_2 increases or any difficulty in ventilation is encountered. At the same time, the minimal fat around the esophagus in these small babies and the absence of hiatus hernia make the definition of the dissection planes clearer. Thus, the dissection itself, including mobilization of the esophagus, identification of the vagus nerves, and construction of the fundic wrap are easier in small children than in adults. Furthermore, it is usually unnecessary to divide the short gastric vessels to achieve a tension-free wrap. Small children who need an antireflux operation often suffer from chronic lung disease, which makes them especially susceptible to postoperative lung complications. The laparoscopic approach seems to minimize these complications. The minimal trauma to the upper abdominal wall in this approach results in less impairment of respiration and thus minimizes the need for narcotics and sedatives postoperatively is pediatric patients.

Recent reports suggested that recovery was smoother following laparoscopic antireflux operations than after open procedures, with comparable short-term results. Laparoscopic Nissen fundoplication is feasible and safe in very small children and infants and that it appears to offer some advantages over the standard open technique.

LAPAROSCOPIC PEDIATRIC UROLOGY

The major advances in laparoscopic urologic surgery began with pediatric applications. Laparoscopy has raised great interest in the past few years in the field of pediatric urology. It has evolved from a simple diagnostic maneuver to complex operative procedures. With respect to current indication for laparoscopy in pediatric urology, several well-established clinical procedures like treatment of varicocele, nonpalpable testis, the current data suggest that laparoscopic surgery is a safe and feasible technique in pediatric urology if performed by expert surgeons, and that it certainly will develop further in the next few years.

The first laparoscopic urologic applications were in the localization of an impalpable undescended testicle. This technique became the definitive diagnostic and first operative step in management of this condition. Laparoscopy offered a 97 percent chance of finding a testicle or proving its absence. Recent advances in endoscopic and accessory instrumentation have allowed the urologist to expand the role of laparoscopy in the pediatric population. In some respects, children may be better suited for laparoscopic procedures than adults because of their decreased intra-abdominal and retroperitoneal fat.

The main problem in pediatric laparoscopic urology is the choice of the most suitable way to reach the urinary tract. Until a few years ago, the transperitoneal route was the only route to the kidney and the urinary tract. In general, surgeons prefer the transperitoneal approach at the beginning of their experience in pediatric laparoscopic urology because of the well-known and wide peritoneal chamber. Usually, four to five ports are necessary and, after the colic angle is detached and Told's fascia is opened, the kidney and upper urinary tract are easily identifiable. The lower urinary tract, the testis, and the spermatic vessels also can be treated using this approach. Retroperitoneoscopy, also called lumboscopy, follows all the criteria of open renal surgery, respecting the integrity of the peritoneal cavity.

Currently, laparoscopy has been used in pediatric urology for:
1. Localization and evaluation of impalpable undescended testicles
2. Gonadal examination and biopsy in patients with intersex disorders
3. Orchiectomy for undescended testicles
4. Diagnosis and treatment of pediatric inguinal hernias
5. Staged orchiopexy

6. Spermatic vein ligation in patients with a varicocele
7. Retarded testicular growth
8. Nephrectomy
9. Nephroureterectomy
10. Pyeloplasty.

There are several important factors to consider when operating in the pediatric patient. First, there is a relatively short distance between the anterior abdominal wall and the great vessels. Thus, the margin for error in pediatric laparoscopy is inversely proportional to the age and size of the patient. Trocars and needles must not be passed too deeply to avoid vascular injury. Also, the child has a thinner abdominal fascia requiring less pressure to introduce the Veress needle and trocars into the abdomen. In addition to this, the pelvic anatomy differs in infants and young children. A large portion of the bladder is located outside the bony pelvis. Prompt decompression of the bladder with a catheter before a Veress needle is essential to avoid a bladder perforation. Also, much less carbon dioxide gas is required in the child, as the peritoneal cavity is small compared to that of an adult.

Children's dimensions are well suited to laparoscopy. Landmarks are readily identifiable and palpable. For example, the bifurcation of the great vessel as well as the sacral promontory are usually easily felt. In addition, abdominal or pelvic masses are easily detected in most children.

LAPAROSCOPY FOR THE IMPALPABLE UNDESCENDED TESTICLE OR INTERSEX EVALUATION

Cryptorchidism is the most common disorder of male sexual differentiation, affecting 0.8 percent of infants at one year of age, 3 percent of full-term newborns, and 21 percent of premature babies. Approximately 20 percent of undescended testicles are nonpalpable, either in the scrotum or in the inguinal area, and in 20 to 50 percent of children with nonpalpable testis, the testis is absent. Early investigation and treatment of nonpalpable testis is essential to decrease the incidence of infertility and to allow adequate follow-up for possible testicular malignancies.

Diagnostic laparoscopy is indicated for patients with nonpalpable testis or an intersex problem. After a thorough physical examination has been accomplished, laparoscopy may be used and has a direct impact on any subsequent surgical procedure. For example, if the testis is absent and blind ending vessels are seen, an open exploration can be avoided. If, however, a testicle is present, the precise location with laparoscopy determines the optimal incision for any open procedure. If an orchiopexy is considered, the first part of a Fowler-Stephens procedure may be performed laparoscopically. This results in minimal manipulation of the testicle. Furthermore, if the testicle is dysplastic, it may be removed laparoscopically.

A testicle that cannot be located and palpated on careful physical examination of the inguinal or scrotal areas, is defined as *nonpalpable*. In such a case, intra-abdominal location, true agenesis, the "vanishing testis," hypoplasia, and ascent of a canalicular testicle on examination are all possibilities that have to be investigated.

Abdominal inspection starts with assessment of the insertion site to evaluate the safety of using a 5 mm port, and continues with evaluation of the spermatic vessels and vas deferens on the normal side. Only the affected side is assessed, and the spermatic vessels and vas deferens are followed to the internal inguinal ring. When both, the spermatic vessels and the vas deferens meet and enter the internal inguinal ring, the intervention is concluded. If a small intra-abdominal testis is observed, two additional trocars are inserted in the two sides of the lower abdomen, and laparoscopic orchiectomy is performed after clipping of the spermatic vessels and the vas deferens. When an apparently normal testis is observed inside the abdomen, the spermatic vessels are clipped as high as possible from the testicle, in order to avoid inadvertent production of ischemia. In this way, the first stage of the Fowler-Stephens procedure is accomplished. In the second stage, performed six months later, the laparoscope is inserted as in the first stage. When an atrophic testis is found, laparoscopic orchiectomy is performed, as described before. When a normal sized intra-abdominal testicle is observed, laparoscopic guided orchiopexy follows, without difficulty. In this way, fruitless inguinal explorations are avoided.

Laparoscopy has gradually become the gold standard for the diagnosis and proper treatment of the nonpalpable testis in children. At diagnosis, laparoscopy allows precise location of an undescended testicle and is the only diagnostic modality capable of establishing the definitive diagnosis of testicular absence. Laparoscopy precisely defines the intra-abdominal anatomy with an accuracy rate of 99 percent.

Complications following laparoscopy for diagnosis and treatment of intra-abdominal testicles are infrequent. Pre-peritoneal insufflation is undoubtedly the most common, and may be as high as 5 percent. More serious complications, including intestinal or vascular injuries, as well as injuries to the urinary bladder and ureter, have been reported but are rare. They may be reduced or avoided by the "open" introduction of a Hasson blunt trocar, thus avoiding blind puncture with a Veress needle.

Operative Technique

After placement of the Veress needle into the abdominal cavity, insufflation is begun. During insufflation, the intra-abdominal pressure should rise slowly at a rate of 0.5 liter/minute in pediatric patient and the abdomen of the child should become diffusely tympanic. Most children require carbon dioxide volumes between 0.5 and 2.0 liters. Following proper insufflation, the Veress needle is removed and trocars are placed. When placing trocars, it is important not to advance these too deeply in the abdomen in order to avoid injury to the underlying bowel and vascular structures. After placement of the umbilical 10 mm trocar, the laparoscope is introduced into the abdominal cavity. Actual pressure of 10 mm Hg suffices for diagnostic procedures. For more complex procedures, pressure of 12 to 15 mm Hg is desirable and allows for better maintenance of an adequate pneumoperitoneum.

The abdomen is inspected in the midline between the obliterated umbilical arteries in the urachus. On the pelvic side wall, the spermatic vessels may be seen coursing towards the internal inguinal ring. If a testicle is palpable in the scrotum, the vas deferens on that side is usually quite obvious as it travel through the inguinal ring to the retrovesical recess. In most children, the external iliac vessels are easily seen as there is minimal extraperitoneal pelvic fat. The cord structures may be further identified by placing slight traction on the spermatic cord and pulling down on the descended testicle. This will cause a dimpling of the peritoneum and the spermatic vessels are easily seen near the internal ring. Indirect hernias and patent processus vaginalis may also be noted.

After inspecting the side of the normal testicle, attention is focused on the side with the undescended, impalpable gonad. If a patent processus vaginalis is noted, gonads or remnants may be present distally. However, absence of a patent processus does not eliminate the possibility of a gonadal remnant in the inguinal area. If the cord structures are seen extending through the inguinal ring with a patent processus, the testicle may not be visible initially. Gentle pressure on the external canal will push a canalicular testicle back through the internal ring. Although canalicular testes may be managed with a standard, open inguinal orchidopexy, the benefit of laparoscopy in these cases is to assess cord length and testicular mobility. This will have a direct impact on the planned surgical approach.

During diagnostic laparoscopy an atraumatic grasper may be placed under direct vision to allow manipulation of bowel loops. In most cases, only two ports are needed. If the testicular absence is suspected the inspection is accomplished by direct observation of blind ending spermatic vessels. Often the vas may end blindly at the same site or nearby, but it is the determination of the spermatic vessels that is pathognomonic for a nonexistent gonad. In those patients with a blind ending vas, it is important that inspection be carried as high up along the side wall towards the lower pole of the kidney as possible. If blind ending vessels are not seen, close observation of this area is necessary. Laparoscopic inspection of the lower pole of the kidney suffices to rule out rare, high-placed gonads. Inspection of the abdominal cavity is not necessary in these patients whose spermatic vessels are blind ending, in order to declare testicular absence.

In patients with an intersex condition biopsy should be taken from dysplastic gonad or it may be removed. A biopsy may be accomplished with a biopsy needle passed directly into the abdomen under laparoscopic control. If an orchiectomy is to be performed, the dysplastic gonad is isolated. The spermatic vessels are identified and clipped. The vessels are then cut and the stump inspected to insure adequate hemostasis. If a testicle is seen, it may be brought down into the scrotum with a Fowler-Stephens procedure. When performing a Fowler-Stephens procedure, the technique is similar to removing a testicle. Once the testicle is clearly identified, the dissection is limited to the cephalad surface of the testicle to identify the spermatic artery.

This dissection will not disturb the vessels of the vas deferens, which will form the major blood supply of the testicle. Initially the spermatic artery is identified and a window is created around the vessel. A clip applier is placed through a 10 mm trocar site that has access to the spermatic artery. Two clips are placed proximal and two clips distally on the artery. The artery is then cut with scissors. In some circumstances, electrocautery may be used to coagulate the spermatic artery before the vessel is cut. This maneuver is the first step of a Fowler-Stephens procedure and can be accomplished with minimal amount of interabdominal dissection. During next stage of surgery the testicle is brought down into the scrotum on its enhanced blood supply. This two-stage procedure has been successful not only in patients with long vasal loops but also in patients with high abdominal testis and short vas deferens.

In some patients, an impalpable testicle may be proximal to the internal ring in such a way that its vessels allow adequate mobilization. In these instances, a single-stage orchidopexy may be performed. This is done laparoscopically using three ports. Two 5 mm ports are placed in a lateral position and one 10 mm trocar in the midline. A peritoneal incision lateral to the spermatic cord is made. The spermatic cord is rolled medially and elevated from the retroperitoneal tissues. The gubernaculums is opened adjacent to the patent processus vaginalis. The anterior peritoneum of the gubernaculum is then opened laterally. If a loop of the vas deferens is identified, it is reflected in the cephalad direction. The testicle is grasped and the gubernacular attachments are cauterized and divided. The vas deferens is then mobilized by opening the peritoneum medially. With adequate dissection, the testicle will be able to be moved around the pelvis.

A small transverse skin incision is created at the base of the hemiscrotum and carried down through Dartos fascia. A subcutaneous pouch is created and the testicle is pulled down into the pouch. A small clamp is passed through the canal that has been developed into the peritoneal cavity. The gubernacular reflections of the lower pole of the testis can then be grasped and the testicle brought down the hemiscrotum without tension. The testicle is secured in the Dartos pouch and the skin incision is closed. The Foley's catheter and nasogastric tube may be removed in the operating room. Patients are usually given oral antibiotics for 24 hours and discharged from the hospital on the same day. Diets are advanced as tolerated.

Laparoscopy now constitutes the reference technique for the diagnosis and treatment of the nonpalpable testis. It is a simple procedure, allowing a definitive diagnosis and two stage relocation without increasing the risk of testicular atrophy. Diagnostic laparoscopy also identifies the specific location of the intra-abdominal testicle, facilitating the development of an optimal surgical strategy. The good results reported in most series have established the laparoscopic management of the nonpalpable testis as "state-of-the-art," with results superior to those achieved with open surgical techniques regarding morbidity, complication rate, and length of hospital stay.

OTHER LAPAROSCOPIC PEDIATRIC UROLOGICAL PROCEDURES

Many other pediatric conditions may be treated using the laparoscopy. If nephrectomy in the pediatric patient is planned, a retroperitoneal approach may have a distinct advantage in certain older children. Laparoscopic pyeloplasty for ureteropelvic junction obstruction has also been performed with very encouraging result. Bladder autoaugmentation, another innovative procedure, is performed by incising the detrusor muscle to increase the capacity of the bladder. Other laparoscopic pediatric procedures such as hernia repairs and partial nephrectomy also have been performed. In pediatric laparoscopy, the greatest risk of complications occurs at the time of access. Some surgeon have eliminated this risk by using the Hasson trocar technique rather than the Veress needle technique. In children, the peritoneal space is small and the surgeon should be familiar with working in a smaller environment. The safety of pediatric laparoscopy is well established and more and more pediatric surgeons are now a days switching over to laparoscopy.

Laparoscopic Pediatric Nephrectomy

It is perhaps the most popular urologic indication for the laparoscopic procedure. The first cases reported in the international literature were managed using the transperitoneal approach, but the subsequent reports of nephrectomy in children, were based on retroperitoneoscopy. In children, the indications denote exclusively benign diseases such as multicystic or dysplastic kidneys causing renal hypertension, nonfunctioning kidneys associated with reflux nephropathy or obstructive uropathy, xanthogranulomatosis, pyelonephritis, protein losing nephropathy, and occasionally, nephrolithiasis or nephropathy causing uncontrollable hypertension. The relative contraindications are malignant renal tumors, previous intra-abdominal or retroperitoneal surgery, renal trauma attributable to poor endoscopic vision into the perinephric hematoma, severe cardiopulmonary disease or severe coagulopathy, and morbid obesity with a high positioned kidney attributable to difficult renal access retroperitoneally.

In cases of vesicoureteral reflux associated with a grossly refluxing megaureter, the ureter must be sectioned near the ureterovesical junction at the level of the bladder, whereas in the absence of a grossly refluxing megaureter, the ureter can be divided either by electrocautery or between ligatures or clips at a convenient distance from the renal tissue. The extraction of the kidney can be achieved by using endobag.

Stone Removal

Retroperitoneoscopic stone removal is another procedure that presents several advantages for children. The indications are large stones entrapped at the level of the pelvis unresponsive to medical treatment. Three ports are generally necessary, one for the telescope, two for the working instruments, and sometimes a fourth trocar for a retractor to lift the renal parenchyma. The first step of the operation is to place a uretheral probe first via cystoscopy then lumboscopy. The pelvis then is opened with scissors, after which the stone extracted and removed with an endobag.

Renal Biopsy

Renal biopsy can be performed with only one trocar, using a 10 mm operative telescope with an operative channel to introduce the biopsy instrument, if necessary, another 5 mm port can be introduced.

Adrenalectomy

Resection of the adrenal glands can be performed laparoscopically or via retroperitoneoscopy. It has various advantages over conventional open surgery. With regard to tumor size, in cases of adrenal masses smaller than 5 - 6 cm, laparoscopy or lumboscopy provides an excellent access route. If the mass is larger than 6 cm, the open approach is preferable. Although the specific indications will continue to be defined, they generally include adrenal benign cysts, pheochromocytoma, adenoma, and aldosteronoma. In the case of neuroblastoma or other malignant tumors affecting children, it is preferable to adopt an open approach. A good knowledge of the adrenal pathophysiology and surgical anatomy is fundamental to the success of this procedure. Moreover, it is important to keep in mind the potential bleeding risk during dissection, especially on the right side, where the dissection may be more difficult because of the short adrenal vein and proximity of the vena cava.

Dismembered Pyeloplasty

Open pyeloplasty has been widely accepted as the surgical treatment of choice for pyeloureteral junction obstruction in children. The success rate for this procedure exceeds 90 percent. With the rapid advent of minimally access surgical techniques, laparoscopic dismembered pyeloplasty through a transperitoneal route has been described for both adults and children. Although the procedure is technically demanding and requires advanced laparoscopic surgical suturing techniques for meticulous pelviureteric anastomosis, encouraging results projecting success rates comparable with those achieved through an open approach have been reported. The first laparoscopic dismembered pyeloplasty used to treat ureteropelvic junction obstruction was described in 1992. Since that, other reports have been published describing the use of either laparoscopy or lumboscopy.

The first step of the procedure is to identify the pyeloureteral junction and the planned line of pelvic

reduction. A 4/0 polydioxanone suture over a straight needle then is passed percutaneously through the abdominal wall to the upper pole of the renal pelvis, then passed back through the abdominal wall again at the same point. This serves as a "hitch stitch" to stabilize and present the pelvis. The pyeloureteral junction is dismembered, the pelvis trimmed, and the upper ureter spatulated. Pelviureteric anastomosis then is performed using continuous 6/0 polydioxanone sutures for infants and younger children and 5/0 polydioxanone sutures for older patients. A double pigtail transanastomotic ureteric stent usually is left in situ for a few weeks postoperatively. Certainly, well performed laparoscopy and intracorporeal suturing and knotting are necessary in the performance of this procedure. Currently, videosurgical pyeloplasty is performed only in few centers with extensive experience in pediatric laparoscopic urology.

Bladder Autoaugmentation

Bladder autoaugmentation by seromyotomy via laparoscopic technique has been used in selected cases to treat poor bladder capacity. This technique is easy to perform using laparoscopy, but in pediatric urology an enterocystoplasty or a gastrocystoplasty generally is preferred for the treatment of patients with decreased bladder capacity.

Ureteral Re-implantation

The bladder is first drained and then insufflated with carbon dioxide to 10 -12 mm Hg pressure. The bladder is anchored to the anterior abdominal wall with one or two separated stitches inserted percutaneously under cystoscopic guidance. Under cystoscopic vision, a camera port is first inserted over the dome of the bladder. Two other working ports with an umbrella mechanism then are inserted on either side of the bladder's lateral wall over the suprapubic skin crease. The refluxing ureter is isolated and dissected free as with the Cohen procedure. The ureteric hiatus is repaired with interrupted 5/0 polydioxanone sutures. After the creation of a submucosal channel, a ureteroneocystostomy is performed according to the Cohen procedure using separated 6/0 stitches. A urethral catheter is left in situ only for 24 hours postoperatively.

Excision of Prostatic Utricles

The prostatic utricles, an enlarged diverticulum in the posterior urethra of males, was first described by Englisch in 1874. Although most prostatic utricles are asymptomatic and do not need any surgical intervention. Some patient manifest symptoms as a result of infection or enlarged utricles and have been associated with recurrent urinary tract infections, stone formation, disturbed urination, recurrent epididymitis, infertility, and neoplastic degeneration. Surgical excision is the recognized treatment of choice. Surgical access to the prostatic utricle always has been a major hurdle because it lies deep within the pelvis. The first step in the operation consists of a cystourethroscopy for cannulation of the prostatic utricle. The cystoscope is left *in situ* inside the prostatic utricle to facilitate subsequent identification during laparoscopy.

The bladder dome is hitched upward to the anterior abdominal wall by a 4/0 PDS suture inserted percutaneously under laparoscopic vision. The peritoneal reflection is incised using electrocautery, starting immediately behind the bladder. The prostatic utricle is easily identified with the guidance of illumination from the cystoscope. Using a 5 mm ultrasonic scalpel, the prostatic utricle is completely mobilized and divided at its confluence with the urethra. The urethral defect is either closed by intracorporeal suturing using fine vicryl, or simply by coagulation. The excised prostatic utricle is removed through the supraumbilical camera port.

Complicated Urachal Disease

The urachus is a obliterated fibrous cord extending from the allantoic duct remnant at the umbilicus to the apex of the bladder. Traditional surgical management of benign urachal disease involves the radical excision of all anomalous tissue with a cuff of bladder tissue via the open approach. Some authors advocate the use of such aggressive surgery only for persistent and recurrent cases. However, there is the potential for malignant change and a high-risk of recurrent symptoms in conservatively managed cases. The laparoscopic approach to the complete excision of urachal abnormalities is performed via a three-port approach. The cyst is identified and removed with a cuff of bladder dome. The bladder defect is closed in two layers, and the indwelling urinary catheter is removed after 2 days.

Laparoscopic procedures have evolved greatly in pediatric urology during the past few years. With time and greater experience, surgeons began to prefer retroperitoneoscopy for cases of urologic pathology, despite the major difficulties associated with the smaller operating chamber. Moreover, lumboscopy meets all the criteria of open renal surgery, according to which all urologic interventions are performed via the retroperitoneal route without transgressing the abdominal cavity. One main problem with retroperitoneal approach is that access to the bladder base or the ureterovesical junction may be difficult in older children. In addition, the retroperitoneal approach does not allow a thorough search of the peritoneal cavity for a small dysplastic and ectopic kidney, nor does it accommodate a complex ureterocele excision or bladder base reconstruction. To overcome these problems a selective approach to the diseased kidney and ureter depending on the involved pathology is necessary. The position of the diseased kidney, the presence or absence of a refluxing ureter, and the need for ureterocelectomy and bladder base reconstruction are the main determining factors. Nephrectomy for non-functioning reflux nephropathy kidneys or duplex moiety necessitating resection of a grossly dilated megaureter, especially in children older than 5 years preferably is undertaken via a lateral extraperitoneal approach. Finally, nephrectomy for small dysplastic kidneys associated with ureteric ectopia and urinary incontinence as well as complex duplex excision with extensive ureterocelectomy and lower urinary tract reconstruction should be performed via a transperitoneal laparoscopic approach. The possible urologic indications for laparoscopic surgery can be divided into diagnostic, ablative, and reconstructive procedures. For cases of nonpalpable testis, laparoscopy is considered a better diagnostic examination and operative procedure for an orchidopexy. With regard to operative laparoscopic urologic procedures, most well-established clinical indications concern ablative procedures. To date, laparoscopic nephrectomy seems to be the procedure most frequently applied in pediatric urology.

The rapid advent of robotic technology will greatly enhance the dexterity and precision control of surgical manipulation in a small confined space of pediatric patient. It may significantly shorten the learning curve for advanced laparoscopic procedures.

BIBLIOGRAPHY

1. Allen SR, Lawson L, Garcia V, Inge TH. Attitudes of bariatric PEDIATRICS Volume 118, Number 1, July 2006 307 Downloaded from www.pediatrics.org by on March 31, 2009 surgeons concerning adolescent bariatric surgery (ABS). Obes Surg 2005;15:1192–5.

2. Ancona E, Anselmino M, Zanicnotto G, et al. Esophageal achalasia: laparoscopic versus conventional open Heller-Dor operation. Am J Surg 1995;170:265-70.

3. Antonoff MB, Kreykes NS, Saltzman DA, Acton RD. American Academy of Pediatrics Section on Surgery hernia survey revisited. J Pediatr Surg 2005;40:1009–14.

4. Apelgren KN, Molnar RG, Kisala JM. Laparoscopic is no better than open appendectomy. Am Surg 1995;61:240-43.

5. Baker LA, Docimo SG, Surer I, et al. A multi-institutional analysis of laparoscopic orchidopexy. BJU Int. 2001;87:484–9.

6. Barkun JS, Wexler MJ, Hinchey EJ, Thibeault D, Meakins JL. Laparoscopic versus open inguinal herniorrhaphy: preliminary results of a randomized controlled trial. Surgery. 1995;118:703-10.

7. Cass DL. Ovarian torsion. Semin Pediatr Surg. 2005;14:86–92.

8. Chan KL, Hui WC, Tak PK. Prospective randomized singlecenter, single-blind comparison of laparoscopic vs open repair of pediatric inguinal hernia. Surg Endosc. 2005;19:927–32.

9. Chen LE, Langer JC, Dillon PA, et al. Management of late-stage parapneumonic empyema. J Pediatr Surg. 2002;37:371-4.

10. Coran AG, Teitlebaum DH. Recent advances in the management of Hirschsprung's disease. Am J Surg. 2000;180:382-7.

11. Diamond IR, Langer JC. Laparoscopic-assisted versus open ileocolic resection for adolescent Crohn disease. J Pediatr Gastroenterol Nutr 2001;33:543-7.

12. Diaz DM, Gibbons TE, Heiss K, Wulkan ML, Ricketts RR, Gold BD. Antireflux surgery outcomes in pediatric gastroesophageal reflux disease. Am J Gastroenterol. 2005;100:1844–52.

13. Dubois F, Icard P, Berthelot G, Levard H. Coelioscopic cholecystectomy—preliminary report of 36 cases. Ann Surg. 1990;211:60-62.

14. Eshraghi N, Farahmand M, Soot SJ, Rand-Luby L, Deveny CW, Sheppard BC. Comparison of outcomes of open versus laparoscopic Nissen fundoplication performed in a single practice. Am J Surg. 1998;175:371-4.

15. Esposito C, Corcione F, Garipoli V, Ascione G. Pediatric laparoscopic splenectomy: are there real advantages in comparison with the traditional open approach? Pediatr Surg Int. 1997;12:509-10.

16. Gans SL, Berci G. Advances in endoscopy of infants and children. J Pediatr Surg. 1971;6:199-233.

17. Gans SL, Berci G. Peritoneoscopy in infants and children. J Pediatr Surg. 1973; 8:399-405.

18. Georgeson KE, Inge TH, Albanese CT. Laparoscopically assisted anorectal pull-through for high imperforate anus: a new technique. J Pediatr Surg. 2000;35:927–30; discussion 930–31.

19. Georgeson KE. Laparoscopic-assisted total colectomy with pouch reconstruction. Semin Pediatr Surg. 2002;11:233–6.

20. Gibeily GJ, Ross MN, Manning DB, Wherry DC, Kao TC. Late-presenting appendicitis. Surg Endosc. 2003;17:725–9.

21. Gilchrist BF, Lobe TE, Schropp KP, et al. Is there a role for laparoscopic appendectomy? J Pediatr Surg. 1992;27:209-14.

22. Goldstein AM, Cho NL, Mazziotti MV, Zitsman JL. Pneumatically assisted laparoscopic reduction of intussusception. Pediatr Endosurg Innov Tech. 2003;7:33–7.

23. Golub R, Siddiqui F, Pohl D. Laparoscopic versus open appendectomy: a metaanalysis. J Am Coll Surg. 1998;186:545-53.

24. Gorsler CM, Schier F. Laparoscopic herniorrhaphy in children. Surg Endosc. 2003;17:571–3.

25. Grewal H, Sweat J, Vazquez WD. Laparoscopic appendectomy in children can be done as a fast-track or same-day surgery. JSLS. 2004;8:151–4.

26. Hall NJ, Van Der Zee J, Tan HL, Pierro A. Meta-analysis of laparoscopic versus open pyloromyotomy. Ann Surg. 2004;240:774–8.

27. Horgan S, Holterman MJ, Jacobsen GR, et al. Laparoscopic adjustable gastric banding for the treatment of adolescent morbid obesity in the United States: a safe alternative to gastric bypass. J Pediatr Surg. 2005;40:86–90; discussion 90–91.

28. Ikeda H, Ishimaru Y, Takayasu H, Okamura K, Kisaki Y, Fujino J. Laparoscopic versus open appendectomy in children with uncomplicated and complicated appendicitis. J Pediatr Surg. 2004;39:1680–85.

29. Inge TH, Krebs NF, Garcia VF, et al. Bariatric surgery for severely overweight adolescents: concerns and recommendations. Pediatrics. 2004;114:217.

30. Iwanaka T, Arai M, Yamamoto H, et al. No incidence of portsite recurrence after endosurgical procedure for pediatric malignancies. Pediatr Surg Int. 2003;19:200–03.

31. Johnson AB, Peetz ME. Laparoscopic appendectomy is an acceptable alternative for the treatment of perforated appendicitis. Surg Endosc. 1998;12:940-43.

32. Kadamba P, Habib Z, Rossi L. Experience with laparoscopic adrenalectomy in children. J Pediatr Surg. 2004;39:764–7.

33. Kato Y, Yamataka A, Miyano G, et al. Tissue adhesives for repairing inguinal hernia: a preliminary study. J Laparoendosc Adv Surg Tech A. 2005;15:424–8.

34. Kenyon TA, Lenker MP, Bax TW, Swanstrom LL. Cost and benefit of the trained laparoscopic team: a comparative study of a designated nursing team vs a nontrained team. Surg Endosc. 1997;11:812-4.

35. Kia KF, Mony VK, Drongowski RA, et al. Laparoscopic vs open surgical approach for intussusception requiring operative intervention. J Pediatr Surg. 2005;40:281-4.

Section Five

36. Kim SS, Lau ST, Lee SL, Waldhausen JH. The learning curve associated with laparoscopic pyloromyotomy. J Laparoendosc Adv Surg Tech A. 2005;15:474–7.

37. Koyle MA, Oottamasathien S, Barqawi A, Rajimwale A, Furness PD 3rd. Laparoscopic Palomo varicocele ligation in children and adolescents: results of 103 cases. J Urol. 2004;172(4 pt 2):1749–52; discussion 1752.

38. Laerman LA, Grimes DA. Rapid hospital discharge following laparoscopy for ectopic pregnancy: a promise unfulfilled? West J Med. 1997;167:145-8.

39. Lawrence K, McWhinnie D, Goodwin A, et al. Randomized controlled trial of laparoscopic versus open repair of inguinal hernia: early results. BMJ. 1995;311:981-5.

40. Lejus C, Delile L, Plattner V, et al. Randomized, single-blinded trial of laparoscopic versus open appendectomy in children: effects on postoperative analgesia. Anesthesiology. 1996;84:801-6.

41. Martin LC, Puente I, Sosa JL, et al. Open versus laparoscopic appendectomy: a prospective randomized comparison. Ann Surg. 1995;222:256-62.

42. Meehan JJ, Georgeson KE. The learning curve associated with laparoscopic antireflux surgery in infants and children. J Pediatr Surg. 1997;32:426-9.

43. Memon MA, Fitzgibbons RJ Jr. Assessing risks, costs and benefits of laparoscopic hernia repair. Ann Rev Med. 1998;49:95-109.

44. Muehlstedt SG, Pham TQ, Schmeling DJ. The management of pediatric appendicitis: a survey of North American pediatric surgeons. J Pediatr Surg. 2004;39:875–9; discussion 875–9.

45. Ortega AE, Hunter JG, Peters JH, Swanstrom LL, Schirmer B. A prospective, randomized comparison of laparoscopic appendectomy with open appendectomy. Am J Surg. 1995;169:208-13.

46. Parikh MS, Shen R, Weiner M, Siegel N, Ren CJ. Laparoscopic bariatric surgery in super-obese patients (BMI_50) is safe and effective: a review of 332 patients. Obes Surg. 2005;15:858–63.

47. Ransom SB, McNeely SG, White C, Diamond MP. A cost-effectiveness evaluation of laparoscopic disposable versus nondisposable infraumbilical cannulas. J Am Assoc Gynecol Laparosc. 1996;4:25-8.

48. Reddy VS, Phan HH, O'Neill JA, et al. Laparoscopic versus open splenectomy in the pediatric population: a contemporary single-center experience. Am Surg. 2001;67:859–63; discussion 863–4.

49. Richards KF, Fisher KS, Flores JH, Christensen BJ. Laparoscopic Nissen fundoplication: cost, morbidity and outcome compared with open surgery. Surg Laparosc Endosc. 1996;6:140-43.

50. Rothenberg SS. Laparoscopic intestinal resection. Semin Pediatr Surg. 2002;11:211–6.

51. Rothenberg SS. The first decade's experience with laparoscopic Nissen fundoplication in infants and children. J Pediatr Surg. 2005;40:142–6; discussion 147.

52. Sandoval C, Strom K, Stringel G. Laparoscopy in the management of pediatric intraabdominal tumors. JSLS. 2004;8:115–8.

53. Somme S, Rodriguez JA, Kirsch DG, Liu DC. Laparoscopic versus open fundoplication in infants. Surg Endosc. 2002;16:54–6.

54. Southern Surgeons Club. A prospective analysis of 1518 laparoscopic cholecystectomies. N Engl J Med. 1991;324:1073-4.

55. Spurbeck WW, Davidoff AM, Lobe TE, Rao BN, Schropp KP, Shochat SJ. Minimally invasive surgery in pediatric cancer patients. Ann Surg Oncol. 2004;11:340–43.

56. Spurbeck WW, Prasad R, Lobe TE. Two-year experience with minimally invasive herniorrhaphy in children. Surg Endosc. 2005;19:551–3.

57. Templeman C, Fallat ME, Blinchevsky A, Hertweck SP. Noninflammatory ovarian masses in girls and young women. Obstet Gynecol. 2000;96:229–33.

58. Watson DI, Coventry BJ, Chin T, Fill PG, Malycha P. Laparoscopic versus open splenectomy for immune thrombocytopenic purpura. Surgery. 1997;121:18-22.

59. Wenner J, Graffner H, Lindell G. A financial analysis of laparoscopic and open cholecystectomy. Surg Endosc. 1995;9:702-5.

Section Five

SECTION

6

Miscellaneous

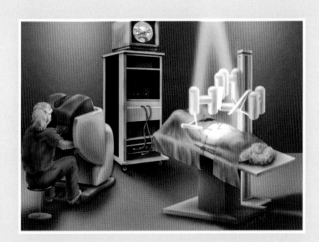

Other Minimal Access Surgical Procedures

TWO PORT CHOLECYSTECTOMY

Laparoscopic cholecystectomy is the gold standard for the treatment of gallstone disease. The operation is routinely performed using four or three ports of entry into the abdomen. At Laparoscopy Hospital we frequently perform cholecystectomy by two port method using modified extracorporeal knot (Fig. 42.1).

With this technique we can give traction over the gallbladder in any direction for proper exposure. This new innovative two-port method of gallbladder removal can be used only for simple uncomplicated cholelithiasis cases by experienced surgeon, but it has definite advantage over conventional three or four port cholecystectomy in two port cholecystectomy fundus is retracted by help of strategically passed suture (Figs 42.2 and 42.3).

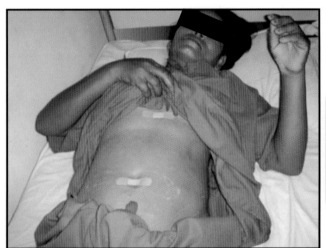

Fig. 42.1: Port position for two port cholecystectomy

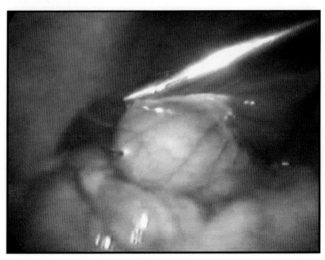

Fig. 42.2A

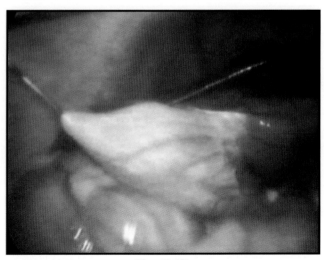

Fig. 42.2B

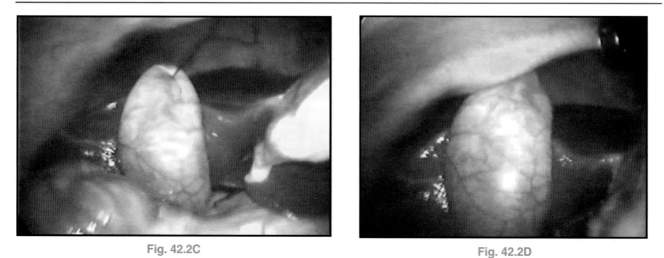

Fig. 42.2C   Fig. 42.2D

Figs 42.2A to D: Fundus is retracted up with the help of needle and thread passed through intercostals space under vision

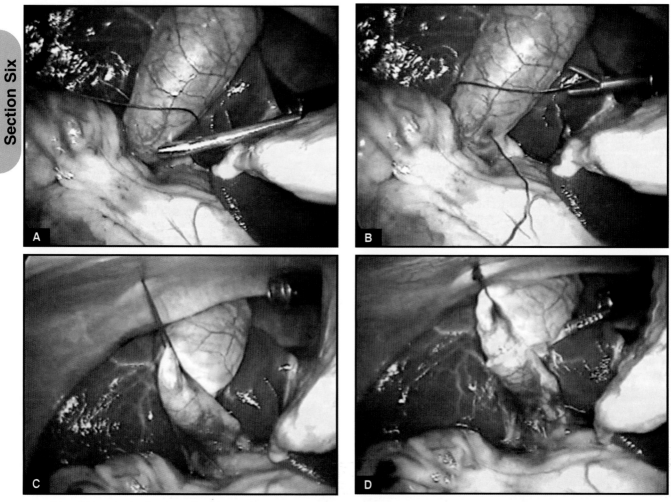

Figs 42.3A to D: Another vicryl is applied over Hartsman pouch to provide anterolateral traction. Any leak from the gallbladder is irrigated and sucked nicely with help of suction irrigation instrument

Once the proper exposure of cystic pedicle is achieved maryland is used for dissection (Figs 42.4A to D).

Extracorporeal knot can be applied for cystic duct without any problem after nice dissection of cystic pedicle (Figs 42.5A to D).

The knot which is tied over the cystic pedicle is used to pull the neck of the gallbladder up and with the help of hook GB is separated from the liver (Figs 42.6A to 42.7D).

Patients undergoing cholecystectomy by two port method had a better resumption of diet and less postoperative pain. Two-port cholecystectomy is technically feasible and may further improve the surgical outcomes in terms of postoperative pain and better cosmetic value. The two port cholecystectomy should be performed by experienced laparoscopic surgeon because skilled choreographic hand movement is very important in this surgery. Bimanual skill and correct interpretation of anatomy is must before proceeding for this technique. We don't recommend two port cholecystectomy as a routine procedure.

Ending of the Operation

The instruments and ports are removed. Telescope should be removed leaving gas valve of umbilical port open to let out all the gas. At the time of removing umbilical port, telescope should be again inserted and umbilical port should be removed over the telescope to prevent any entrapment of omentum. The wound is then closed with suture. Vicryl should be used for rectus and unabsorbable intradermal or stapler for skin.

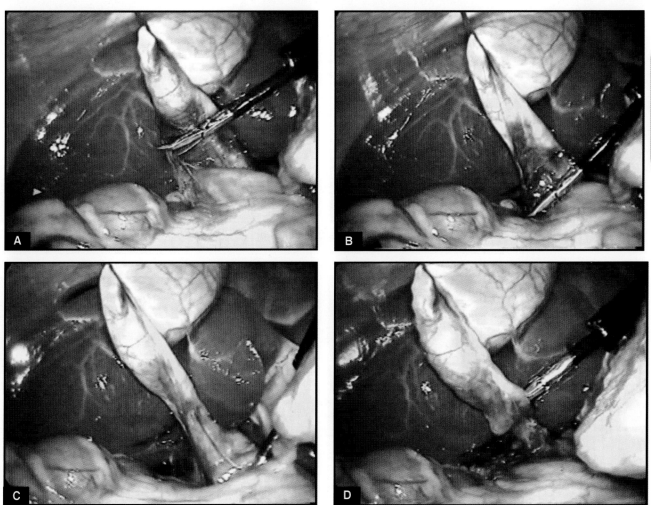

Figs 42.4A to D: Dissection of cystic pedicle is performed by maryland

Section Six

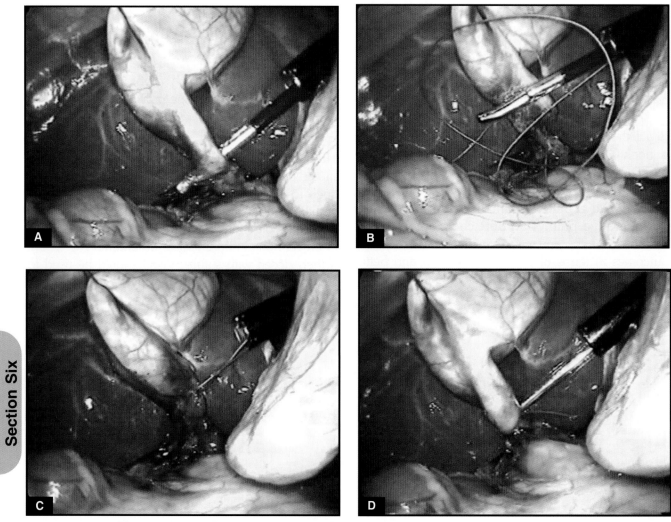

Figs 42.5A to D: Clip or extracorporeal Meltzer knot is applied over cystic artery and duct

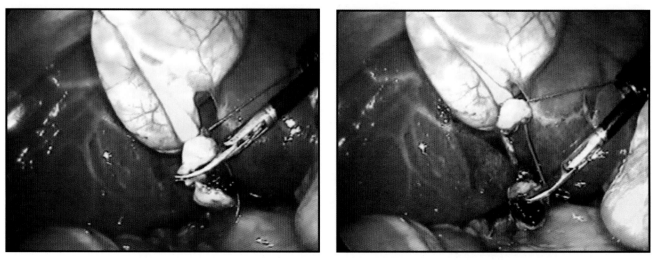

Fig. 42.6A   Fig. 42.6B

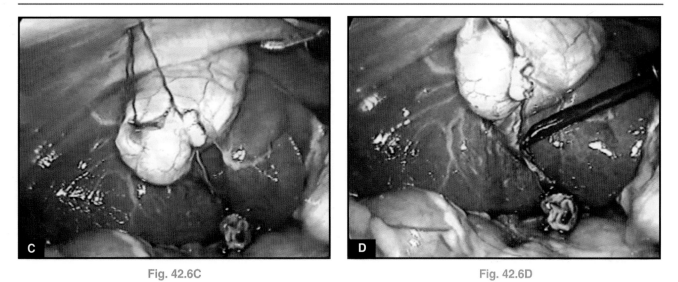

Fig. 42.6C   Fig. 42.6D

Figs 42.6A to D: The extracorporeal knot of cystic duct is used to pull the neck up and to expose bed of the gallbladder

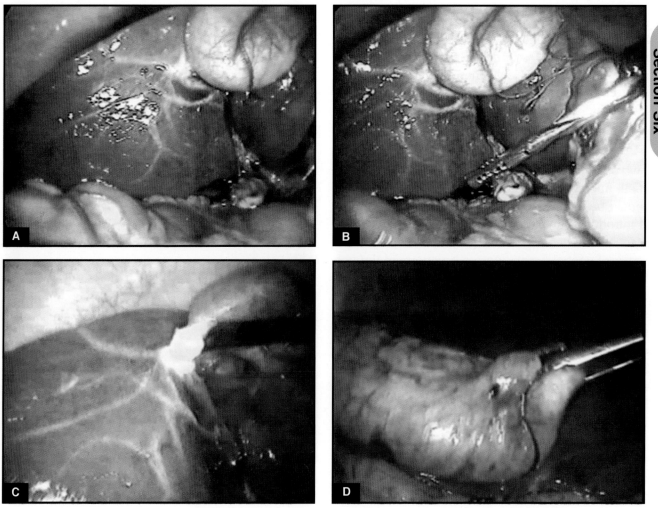

Figs 42.7A to D: Any leak should be sucked and gallbladder is separated with the help of hook

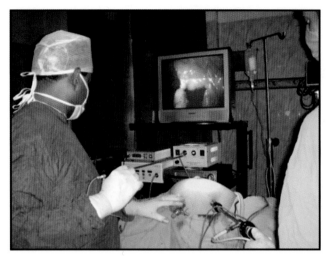

Fig. 42.8

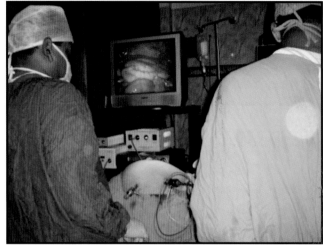

Fig. 42.9

Figs 42.8 and 42.9: Access is done through the palmar's point and 45° Azimuth angle is kept for second-port

A single suture is used to close the umbilicus and upper midline fascial opening. Many laparoscopic surgeons routinely leave this fascial defect without ill effect. Some surgeon likes to inject local anesthetic agent over port site to avoid postoperative pain. Sterile dressing over the wound should be applied.

TWO PORT REPAIR OF VENTRAL HERNIA

Two port ventral hernia is one of the option in case of small uncomplicated ventral hernia surgery. Patient should be under general anesthesia, nasogastric tube is introduced and there should not be any organomegaly if surgeon is planning two port laparoscopic repair of ventral hernia. Access is performed through Palmer's point. Veress needle or open technique both can be used for access from the palmar's point. All the safety indicators should be used and checked at the time of access. Ten mm port should be introduced carefully through Palmer's point. It should be introduced perpendicular not oblique towards anus to avoid injury of splenic flexor of colon. Telescope should be introduced and the size extent and content of hernia is assessed.

After initial assessment of ventral hernia one more port is introduced according to base ball diamond concept but keeping the azimuth angle (angle between telescope and instrument 45°) (Figs 42.8 and 42.9).

Content of hernia is reduced and adhesiolysis should be performed for any possible omental or bowel adhesion. Size of the mesh is selected in such a way that, at least it should cover 4 cm all around beyond the healthy margin of defect. One mm wide, just skin deep stab incision should be given at all the four corner of mesh.

Twelve cm long proline is tied around three corner of the mesh and one of the remaining corner should be tied through the needle and thread introduced through one of the stab wound of skin (Fig. 42.10). The thread which was introduced percutaneously will help to stabilize the mesh and it will act as the third port (Fig. 42.11).

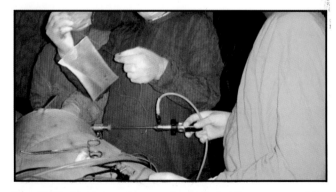

Fig. 42.10: Twelve cm long proline is tied at three corner of the mesh keeping 6 cm long pair of free suture at each end

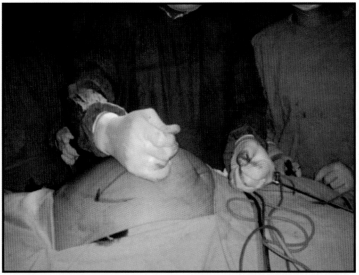

Fig. 42.11: Each pair of suture is pulled out through the same skin incision but different rectus and muscle layer

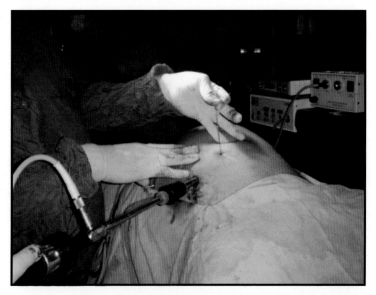

Fig. 42.12: Both end of suture is tied outside the skin. Skin is lifted to slip the knot subcutaneously

Both the end of proline is pulled out through the same skin puncture side but keeping rectus and peritoneum in between.

The end of both the thread should be ligated using tumble square knot and it should be slipped inside skin depth before locking to avoid loosening. This two port technique can be accomplished with the help of Anchor or Protack or Tacker if patient can afford. Two port technique using proline is safe and economical method of performing laparoscopic repair of ventral hernia. Although using strategically placed knot we have performed one port repair of ventral hernia also with the help of suture passer but if adhesions are present one port technique is not possible. Two port techniques should be included in the practice of repair of ventral hernia surgery laparoscopically because in case of any difficulty the third port can be introduced any time without any difficulty (Fig. 42.12).

Retroperitoneoscopy

Traditionally, laparoscopic surgeries are performed by transperitoneal approach following establishment of pneumoperitoneum by closed technique using the Veress needle or by the open mini-laparotomy. The parietal peritoneum is then secondarily incised and dissected to obtain access to the retroperitoneal target organs like kidneys, ureters, adrenals, and lymph nodes. Transperitoneal laparoscopy, although seemingly expeditious, invites the potential calamities of possible vascular and bowel injuries. On the other hand, retroperitoneal laparoscopy has its own difficulty due to working in a contained limited space. However, with technical refinements, several recent reports of successful retroperitoneoscopic surgeries have proved the feasibility and distinct advantages of this approach.

HISTORICAL PERSPECTIVE

Retroperitoneoscopy has experienced a delayed development and acceptance compared with peritoneoscopy. Difficulties in providing adequate visualization and room for surgical maneuvering as well as concerns about deleterious effects of insufflating the retroperitoneal space account for this retarded progression. Although pneumoretroperitoneum has been used safely for more than 50 years to aid in radiographic visualization of the kidneys and adrenals, the conjunctive use of endoscopes has only recently been attempted.

Retroperitoneoscopy through the flank in a human was pioneered by Wickham, who performed an extraperitoneal laparoscopic ureterolithotomy in 1978.

Earliest techniques, termed pelviscopy, utilized a telescope to bluntly dissect within the pelvic retroperitoneum to sample pelvic lymph nodes. The obvious disadvantage of such technique has been the difficulty in exposing the obturator nodes, precluding the performance of an adequate staging lymphadenectomy. In the initial series reported by Hald and Rasmussen, many of the patients had no lymph nodes found in their surgical specimen. With refinements of surgical techniques, subsequently more complete pelviscopic node dissections have been reported.

SURGICAL TECHNIQUE

Probably the most important initial step in retroperitoneoscopy is the expansion and distention of the retroperitoneal space by an expanding balloon device. A balloon device modified fingers of a latex rubber glove is tied off, and the glove is secured over the distal end of the sheath of cannula (Fig. 42.13).

The device is placed in the retroperitoneum and expanded by injecting saline. Special trocars are available with transparent balloons at their inner end that can be inflated with air or fluid to allow laparoscopic visibility of retroperitoneum through the clear distended balloon.

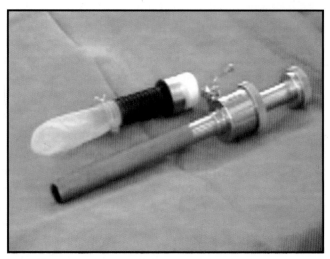

Fig. 42.13: Finger of glove over sheath of cannula

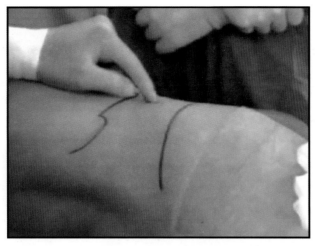

Fig. 42.14: Place for primary trocar insertion in
retroperitoneoscopy

Retroperitoneoscopy Through the Flank

This approach is applicable to surgery on adrenals, kidneys, and upper ureters. The patient is placed in a lateral decubitus position with slight forward tilt. A small incision is made about 2 cm below the twelfth rib, just lateral to the sacrospinalis. The incision is deepened through the fused lamellae of lumbar fascia to enter the perinephric space (Fig. 42.14).

The space is further dissected by blunt digital exploration. The expanding device is introduced into the retroperitoneal space and about 800-1000 ml saline are injected to inflate the balloon. The balloon is then deflated and removed (Figs 42.15A and B).

Laparoscope in 11 mm trocar is introduced into the retroperitoneal space and carbon dioxide insufflation is continued to maintain a pressure of about 14 mm Hg. With the posterior parietal peritoneum pushed away by the expanding device, the retroperitoneal space is widely opened by continued insufflation, and subsequent working ports are established under camera vision. The number and location of accessory ports are determined by the surgical procedure to be undertaken. However, it is usually advisable to keep the ports posterior to the anterior axillary line to avoid puncture of the lateral peritoneal reflection. During laparoscopic dissection it is often helpful to move the laparoscope to the anterior ports for better visibility as the situation may dictate (Fig. 42.16).

Retroperitoneoscopy: Anterolateral

For surgery on mid and lower ureters and for internal spermatic vein ligation, the retroperitoneoscopy is performed by a small incision at McBurney's point. The external oblique aponeurosis is incised, and underlying fibers of the internal oblique and transverse muscles of the abdomen are split to reach the extraperitoneal space. Following careful digital dissection, the expanding device is introduced and inflated in the retroperitoneum (Figs 42.17 to 42.18B).

Retroperitoneoscopy for Pelvic Lymph Node

Pelvic retroperitoneoscopy is ideal for bilateral staging pelvic lymph node dissection and bladder neck suspension procedures. A small midline incision is made about 2 cm below the umbilicus. The linea alba is opened, and underlying extraperitoneal space is developed by digital dissection behind the rectus muscle of the abdomen. The expanding device is introduced and expanded by injecting about 1200 ml saline solution. The balloon is decompressed and re-moved. The laparoscope is introduced with high-flow carbon dioxide insufflation. Anatomic landmarks of the symphysis pubis, superior pubic rami, bladder neck, and external iliac vein pulsations in the pelvis are easily identified. Complete bilateral staging lymph-adenectomy is accomplished by en bloc dissection of the fibrofatty lymphatic tissue from the triangular area

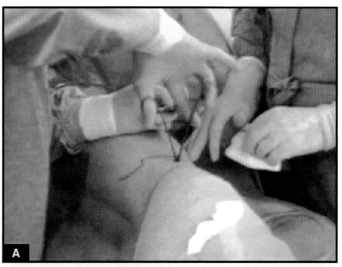

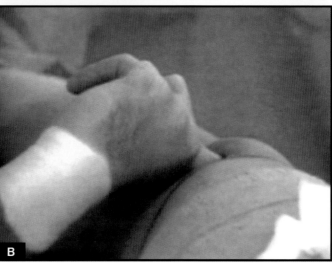

Figs 42.15A and B: Finger dissection of retroperitoneal space

bounded laterally by the external iliac vein, proximally by the hypogastric artery, and inferiorly by the endopelvic fascia (Figs 42.19 to 42.20B).

Conclusion

The pioneering concept of retroperitoneal expansion by Gaur and coworkers has led to the resurgence of retroperitoneoscopy. Artificial balloon expansion creates the necessary space and retraction of neighboring viscera, so that subsequent insufflation can maintain the open space for surgical maneuvering. In a way, this technique simulates the steps of dissection and retraction traditionally used during open surgery.

Aside from preventing the potential hazards of transperitoneal access and intraperitoneal dissection, there are certain distinct advantages of retroperitoneoscopy in patient positioning, intestinal retraction, anatomic approach to the renal hilum, and postoperative wound drainage. For retroperitoneal approaches to the adrenals, kidneys, and ureters the patient is placed in the lateral decubitus position, as opposed to the supine position for laparoscopy. The intestines contained within the intact peritoneal envelope remain displaced during retroperitoneal dissection, thereby avoiding extensive colonic mobilization and constant retraction of bowel. During nephrectomy, the renal hilum is approached from the posterior aspect, allowing easier

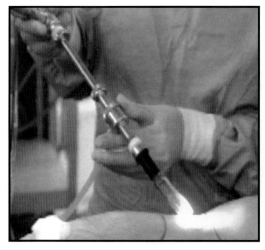

Fig. 42.16: Laparoscope with balloon cannula system

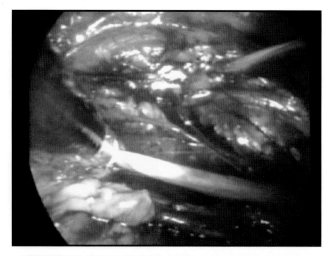

Fig. 42.17: Ureter as seen during retroperitoneoscopy

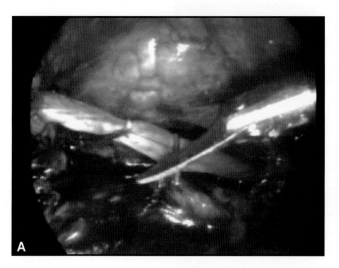

A

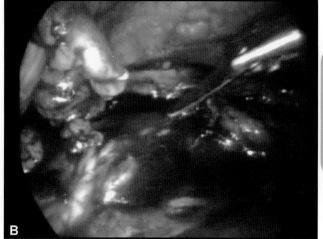

B

Figs 42.18A and B: Two clips are applied over ureter and cut in between

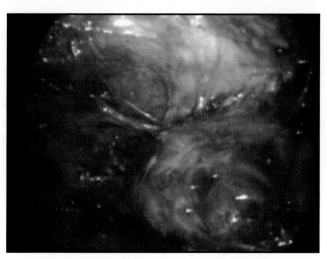

Fig. 42.19: Posterior dissection of left kidney

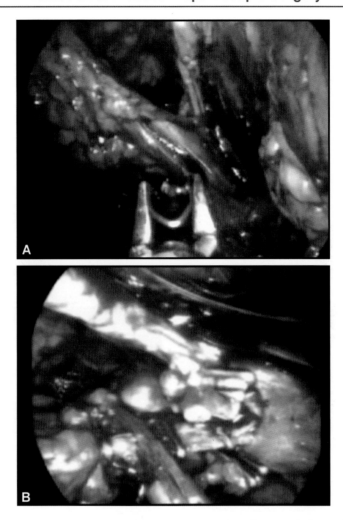

Figs 42.20A and B: Dissection of hilum of kidney and application of clips before cutting

initial control of the renal arteries. Similarly exposure of other retroperitoneal structures such as the adrenal gland in the right side is relatively easier than with the anterior approach.

The closed extraperitoneal space allows more effective postoperative drainage, especially following reconstructive and reparative surgery such as pyeloplasty, partial nephrectomy, pyelolithotomy, and ureterolithotomy. The perceived difficulties of surgical dissection of kidneys and adrenal glands in a restricted environment during retroperitoneoscopy has not proved true with the present technique or initial balloon expansion. However, organ entrapment, especially of large specimens, in the limited space is difficult.

The anterolateral extraperitoneal approach allows access for ureterolithotomy on the lower ureter at and above the pelvic inlet. Internal spermatic vein ligation extraperitoneally is done for treatment of varicocele. The extraperitoneal dissection appears, however, to be more extensive, and such an approach will not be suitable for bilateral varicocele surgery.

In the pelvis, the excellent anatomic appearance of the bladder, bladder neck, and symphysial structures makes the extraperitoneal approach ideally suited for procedures such as laparoscopic bladder-neck suspension and surgery for urachal pathologies. The majority of bladder diverticula are located posterolaterally and are therefore not often amenable to extraperitoneal excision.

For the bilateral staging pelvic lymphadenectomy the extraperitoneal approach has proved its safety and feasibility. The lymph node dissection is anatomically precise, simulating the standards of open pelvic lymphadenectomy.

The advantage of retroperitoneal CO_2 insufflation is that by avoiding CO_2 contact with the peritoneal membrane, there is less hypothermia and reduced postoperative pain from diaphragmatic irritation. In conclusion, retroperitoneoscopy offers another viable option in the developing field of laparoscopy. The surgical indications that warrant an extraperitoneal approach in open surgery hold true for retroperitoneoscopy as well. As a minimally invasive technique, retroperitoneoscopy emulates the established standards and principles of open urologic procedures without compromising surgical efficiency and patient safety.

MINIMAL ACCESS NECK SURGERY

One of the newest frontiers is in minimally invasive soft tissue surgery performed outside an established body cavity. The neck has been one of the soft tissue spaces of considerable interest, and endoscopic or endoscopic-assisted techniques have recently been used to perform both thyroidectomy and parathyroidectomy. Several technical advances have facilitated the development of these new procedures, including the availability of balloon dilator for making artificial space, external lifts, ultrasonic coagulators, and smaller 2-3 mm diameter endoscopic instrumentation.

Background

In whole world thyroidectomy and parathyroidectomy are the two most commonly performed endocrine surgical procedures. The most common indication for thyroidectomy is a solitary nodule that is not clearly benign on fine-needle biopsy. Parathyroidectomy is most commonly performed for primary hyperparathyroidism, in which a single enlarged gland or adenoma accounts for maximum number of cases. The principles of neck exploration for these two disorders are well established, and the morbidity of operation is low when carried out by an experienced minimal access surgeon. Unlike many open abdominal operations, recovery is also rapid and most patients are discharged from the hospital the day after surgery and return to unlimited physical activity within fortnight.

Already many surgeons are attempting to perform thyroidectomy and parathyroidectomy through smaller and smaller open incisions to achieve better cosmetic results. However, as open incisions become smaller, surgical exposure, access, ease of dissection, and even safety may be compromised. Further evidence is that parathyroidectomy, for example, is viewed as an invasive procedure by patients and by referring endocrinologists is the reluctance of many individuals with asymptomatic or minimally symptomatic disease to undergo a definitive and curative operation despite the cumulative risks of hyperparathyroidism over time, including osteoporosis and other metabolic sequelae.

In parathyroid surgery, there has also been interest in a focused, unilateral exploration of the neck rather than the accepted gold standard of bilateral neck exploration with identification and biopsy of all four parathyroids. Exploration of both sides of the neck avoids the problem of missed multiple adenomas or asymmetric hyperplasia, which can occur in up to 5 to 15% of cases and eliminates the need for preoperative localization studies. However, the advantages of unilateral neck exploration are that it results in less dissection, operative times are shorter. There may also be fewer injuries to the recurrent laryngeal nerve and the other parathyroid glands from leaving the contralateral neck undisturbed. Improvements in the accuracy of parathyroid imaging, such as 99mTc sestamibi scanning and intraoperative assessment of curative resection with the quick parathyroid hormone assay have led to better outcomes from and wider application of the unilateral approach. These considerations become increasingly important in the current economic environment in health care.

Under these circumstances, minimal access approach to neck exploration may offer certain possible benefits, including improved visualization due to magnification, better cosmesis, less trauma to the neck musculature, less pain, and a more rapid recovery. Disadvantages of this approach might include longer operative times, increased hospital costs, possible risk of injury to the recurrent laryngeal nerve, potential tumor spillage, inability to localize the parathyroids, and adverse effects of neck insufflation. Consideration of an endoscopic approach to neck exploration, at the least, presents several challenges from an anatomic standpoint. Unlike the abdominal cavity, in which there is an easily distensible space for laparoscopy, the area that must be expanded and maintained to allow endoscopic access in the neck is composed of only potential spaces between soft tissue and muscle planes and the trachea. The thyroid and parathyroid glands are situated within the pretracheal space and are covered by the strap muscles anteriorly and laterally, which also limits exposure and access.

The absence of a discrete anatomic compartmental boundary in the neck adds further problems if insufflation is used because of the potential for gaseous diffusion subcutaneously and into the mediastinum. The thyroid and parathyroids are also highly vascular structures and are intimately related to the recurrent laryngeal nerve and inferior thyroid artery. Further, the location of the parathyroids, especially the inferior glands, is often variable.

Several technologic advances have been necessary to facilitate the development of endoscopic neck exploration. Miniature 2-3 mm endoscopic instruments have been constructed suitable for smaller working space and the more delicate structures in the neck. Many balloon space maker devices have been invented, just like used in laparoscopic hernia repair, could be adapted to create a working space. Gasless laparoscopy has been used with mechanical lifts and retractors to maintain the working space and thus eliminate the need for insufflation of the neck. Ultrasonic coagulators and small clip appliers may be more appropriate for obtaining hemostasis in the neck rather than monopolar cautery. Endoscopic ultrasound also aid in intraoperative localization of the parathyroid adenoma, which is localized preoperatively by sestamibi scanning. These considerations led our group to first explore the possibility of an endoscopic approach to neck exploration in an experimental animal model.

Endoscopic Parathyroidectomy

Endoscopic parathyroidectomy in humans was first performed successfully by Gagner in 1995. The patient had familial hyperparathyroidism and initially presented with acute pancreatitis for which he required laparoscopic pancreaticojejunostomy with stone extraction as well as laparoscopic cholecystectomy. A preoperative sestamibi scan showed four-gland uptake consistent with generalized parathyroid hyperplasia, and a subtotal parathyroidectomy was performed endoscopically. Access to the neck was obtained with four 5 mm ports placed 1 cm above the clavicle and sternal notch. Exposure was achieved by insufflation of the subplatysmal space with 15 mm Hg2+ pressure, which was maintained throughout the operation. Operative time was 5 hours and intraoperatively the patient experienced tachycardia and hypercarbia. Postoperatively, he had subcutaneous emphysema from the eyelids to the scrotum. He recovered uneventfully, however, and was discharged on the fourth postoperative day with a normal serum calcium level.

Since this initial report, endoscopic parathyroidectomy has been carried out by a small number of surgeons using either low-level gas insufflation of the neck or external retractors without CO_2 gas. Gagner has excised parathyroid adenomas in several cases, but uses a lower CO_2 insufflation pressure (7 to 10 mm Hg2+) to reduce the adverse effects of this technique. Duluq has also successfully performed endoscopic parathyroidectomy in several patients with low-level (7 mm Hg2+) CO_2 insulation for exposure. Norman and Albrink attempted parathyroidectomy in four patients after preoperative localization with sestamibi imaging. Initial access to the pretracheal space was achieved via a 1.5 cm incision, but CO_2 at a low insulation pressure (8 mm Hg2+) was used to maintain a working space. Although the parathyroid adenoma was visualized in three of the four cases, endoscopic excision was successful in only two patients, and only one normal parathyroid was identified out of these four explorations. At the conclusion of the endoscopic procedure, all patients were converted to open exploration via a 3.5 cm incision, through which the ipsilateral remaining parathyroids, both normal and adenomatous, were identified and either biopsied or removed. Postoperatively, there was subcutaneous air in the anterior neck, but no other sequela of CO_2 insulation were noted.

We recently performed endoscopic parathyroidectomy in two patients with primary hyperparathyroidism using a gasless technique. Preoperative localization of the parathyroid adenoma was carried out with 99mTc sestamibi scanning, which identified abnormal uptake in the left neck of both patients. Following the induction of general anesthesia, the parathyroid adenoma was more precisely localized with transcutaneous ultrasound and in each case was posterior to the thyroid lobe. A 1.5 cm incision was then made at the sternal notch, and the strap muscles were divided in the midline to enter the pretracheal space under direct vision. In the first patient, a modified space maker balloon was inserted into this space and inflated to 60 ml volume. After removal of the balloon, a working space was maintained with a handheld S-shaped retractor. The strap muscles were further separated from the left lobe of the thyroid and the thyroid was retracted medially with a Babcock clamp placed through the open insertion site. Endoscopic visualization was achieved with a 3 mm 30° arthroscope. Two 4 mm ports were placed in the neck anterior to the sternocleidomastoid muscle.

A normal inferior parathyroid was identified and biopsied, and the adenoma was localized to the superior position with the aid of laparoscopic ultrasound. The enlarged gland was posterior to the thyroid lobe and wedged between two branches of the inferior thyroid artery and the recurrent laryngeal nerve, which led to a lengthy and tedious dissection. Excision was accomplished by blunt dissection with 3 mm endoscopic instruments and the ultrasonic scalpel. Small ligaclips placed through the open insertion site were used to ligate the vascular pedicle. The second patient was approached in a similar fashion, but a small lift ring attached to a mechanical retractor was used to maintain exposure. A left superior adenoma was removed that weighed 1.7 g. The recurrent laryngeal nerve and inferior thyroid artery were identified during the dissection, but it is difficult o locate the inferior parathyroid despite careful examination of the region of the thyrothymic ligament. Total operative time in our two patients has averaged approximately 4 hours. Exposure was suboptimal at times due to the small space, and there was difficulty in retracting the strap muscles laterally and the thyroid gland medially. Very small amounts of bleeding or fluid accumulation obscured the operative field and required frequent sponging through the open insertion site. Manipulation and retraction of the parathyroid with the small instruments was sometimes difficult as well. Parathyroid tissue was confirmed in all specimens and serum calcium levels have been normal postoperatively.

Miccoli used an endoscopic-assisted approach in approximately 20 patients. Handheld retractors are used to maintain exposure, and the dissection has been carried out with one or two lateral ports. A brief period of insufflation is used initially to aid in expanding the pretracheal space, but the remainder of the operation is carried out, with gasless retraction. Preliminary results have been favorable, but not all patients have had a normal ipsilateral parathyroid identified. Confirmation of successful excision of the parathyroid adenoma was made intraoperatively with use of the quick parathyroid hormone assay.

Alternatives to Endoscopic Parathyroidectomy

Minimally invasive or less invasive approaches to parathyroidectomy have been described recently that do not require endoscopic techniques or instrumentation. Norman and Chheda performed parathyroidectomy through a minimal 2-3 cm open incision after precise preoperative localization of the adenoma with sestamibi imaging. The technique used for parathyroid localization is analogous to that used for sentinel node mapping with radiolymphoscintigraphy. 99mTc sestamibi scanning is carried out 3 hours prior to surgical exploration. The operation is then directed with an 11 mm Neoprobe, which is used to scan and quanti-tate radioactivity in all four quadrants of the neck. A 2-3 cm incision is made over the site of maximal gamma activity, and the adenoma is excised through this minimal incision. The authors have used this technique in 14 patients, 13 of whom had adenomas and one who was correctly predicted to have parathyroid hyperplasia. The adenomas were located operatively on average in just 19 minutes. Nine cases were carried out under local anesthesia, and 11 (79%) patients were discharged the same day as surgery. Serum calcium levels were normal postoperatively and there were no operative complications.

This approach is potentially very attractive because it requires minimal dissection and can be carried out under local anesthesia as strictly as outpatient procedure. Both operative and recovery times should be short, which may result in lower hospital costs despite the use of preoperative scintigraphic localization. Frozen section examination by pathology may also become unnecessary if, after excision, all radioactivity is confined to the resected specimen. The limitations of this approach currently are that neither the ipsilateral parathyroid nor the recurrent laryngeal nerves have been routinely identified in these dissections. Further, the accuracy of "sentinel" mapping of the parathyroid adenoma must be confirmed by other investigators.

Thoracoscopic Parathyroidectomy

Video-assisted thoracoscopy should be considered as an alternative to median sternotomy in patients with ectopic mediastinal parathyroid adenomas. Prim and coworkers reported the use of thoracoscopic techniques to successfully excise mediastinal parathyroids in four patients with persistent hyperparathyroidism after failed cervical exploration. All glands were localized preoperatively by a combination of radio nuclide scintigraphy and CT scan. The location of the abnormal glands in these four cases included the aortopulmonary window, near the ascending aorta, the aortic arch, and the region of the main pulmonary artery. Three thoracoscopic ports were used, including a 10 mm initial access port placed in the midaxillary line at the sixth intercostal space. Operative times averaged 3.25 hours and all patients became normocalcemic postoperatively, although one patient with secondary hyperparathyroidism developed recurrent hypercalcemia 9 months after surgery. A subxiphoid laparoscopic approach has also been used to excise a mediastinal parathyroid adenoma , but this technique would appear to provide access to glands in the anterior mediastinum only.

Endoscopic Thyroidectomy

Endoscopic excision of the thyroid is more technically demanding because of the more complex blood supply and the intimate relationship of the thyroid gland to the recurrent laryngeal nerve. A lateral approach is used in which three laparoscopic trocars are placed in the subplatysmal space along the anterior border of the sternocleidomastoid muscle from the jugular notch to the angle of the mandible. Both low pressure CO_2 and a wall lifter inserted at the jugular trocar site are used to maintain a working space. Division of the strap muscles is necessary to access the thyroid. The thyroid vessels are divided with clips, and an ultrasonic dissector is used to dissect the thyroid from the recurrent laryngeal nerve. In addition, both parathyroids are identified and preserved, as is the external branch of the superior laryngeal nerve.

Conclusion

Early experience with endoscopic neck exploration prevents any definitive conclusions about its role in the management of patients with either hyperparathyroidism or thyroid disorders. Published experiences have to date been limited to small case reports, and results and outcomes have not been reported in detail. The minimally invasive open approach of "sentinel" parathyroidectomy reported by Norman and Chheda has much to commend it, including accurate localization, rapid operative times, and improved cosmesis, and it is an outpatient operation that can be performed under local anesthesia.

Although the laparoscope provides optical magnification of important neurovascular structures, including the recurrent laryngeal nerve, better methods for exposure and retraction of the strap muscles and thyroid would greatly facilitate visualization and dissection. Improved instruments are needed that allow safe manipulation of the parathyroid to lower the risk of parathyroid rupture as well as to speed the operative dissection. Suction and irrigation devices designed specifically for small spaces such as the neck would help maintain a dry operative field. Surgeons will also need flexibility in the exposure and operative approach to deal successfully with variations in parathyroid anatomy.

Patient selection should be careful for endoscopic approach until there is further experience and improved operative technique. Individuals, who are obese, have a nodular goiter, have had previous neck surgery, or who are likely to have generalized parathyroid hyperplasia should not be considered as a good candidate for an endoscopic exploration. Despite these limitations and challenges, the search for less invasive means for performing neck exploration will undoubtedly continue, and has already led to renewed interest in a unilateral operative approach in patients with primary hyperparathyroidism.

MINIMAL ACCESS SURGERY IN ORTHOPEDIC SURGERY

Introduction

Conventional (open) methods results in high amount of morbidity. To reduce the morbidity during the secondary injury, i.e. the surgical procedures while opening to reach the site of pathology, encourage the clinician to use the minimal access surgery or endoscopic techniques in orthopedic surgery. Minimal access surgery with endoscope in orthopedic practice useful in the following fields:

1. Arthroscopic surgery in sports-related injuries and other pathologies in shoulder, elbow, wrist, hip, knee, foot and ankle
2. Arthroscopic assisted surgery in orthopedic trauma
3. Spine surgery
4. Benign bone tumors.

Arthroscopy is a minimally invasive surgical procedure in which a physical examination of the interior of a joint is performed using an arthroscope, a type of endoscope that is inserted into the joint through a small incision. The advantage of arthroscopy over traditional open procedures is that the joint does not have to be opened up fully and surgery is performed with two small incisions - one for the arthroscope and other for the surgical instruments. This reduces the recovery time for the patient and may increase the

rate of surgical success due to lesser trauma to the connective tissue. It is especially useful for professional athletes, who frequently injure joints and require faster healing. There is also less scarring, because of the smaller incisions. In procedures where endoscope or arthroscope is used, the advantage increase manifold by providing magnified view. The advantages of magnification and minimal scarring are extended also to the management of fracture fixation, carpal tunnel release at wrist joint and spinal surgeries. As technology becomes more and more advanced, a greater number of minimally invasive surgical interventions have evolved. With the increase in proficiency of arthroscopic or endoscopic surgery, surgeons are now using the same technique for intramedullary lesion and tumor surgery also.

Clinical effectiveness of MAS procedures over open procedures was proven beyond doubt. Hundreds of controlled randomized trials of procedures using the MAS techniques were published in the 1970's and 1980's. The advantages of minimal access surgery over conventional open surgery are listed in Table 42.1.

In an era of rising health care costs, minimal access surgery offers a significant economic advantage over conventional open surgery. Decreased hospital time, decreased rehabilitation time, and a rapid return to normal activities all add up to a significant 'savings' in economic and social costs. Many surgical procedures require a combination of both minimal invasive and open techniques. Therefore, the use of minimal access surgery must be tempered with knowledge of its limitations.

History

Medical endoscopy for internal organs has begun in the early 1800s by Bozzini. In 1918, Prof Kenji Takagi reported the arthroscopic examination in cadaveric knee at Tokyo University with the a cystoscope. Dr Eugene Bircher was the first to perform and publish the first arthroscopy on live patients, to diagnose tuberculosis. Initially internal examination was done by direct visualization through the eye piece till the advent of fiber optic light source and camera. On the other hand, the surgical skills in arthroscopy surgery has improved with fine instrumentation. Since then the developments in arthroscopy have become many fold.

As with any other surgical technique, arthroscopic surgery continues to evolve, improvements in fiberoptics, video reproduction and miniaturization, it will enhance and widen its application. During the past two decades, arthroscopic procedures have been replacing traditional, more invasive orthopedic surgical procedures. Today arthroscopy is being done in almost all joints. High performance athletes need a minimal surgical exposure for a faster recovery and quick return to the field with very minimal morbidity. Recently, training simulators (virtual reality) have come into vogue to teach the skills necessary for arthroscopy especially the knee.

ARTHROSCOPIC SURGERY IN SPORTS RELATED INJURIES AND OTHER PATHOLOGY

Knee Joint

Diagnosis

Knee arthroscopy with the advantage of direct and magnified view inside joint, makes it an excellent diagnostic tool. Its diagnostic accuracy rate of 95% has considerable advantages, as compared with the 75% accuracy rate of clinical evaluation alone. The high sensitivity of MRI for arthroscopically remediable lesions in cases of internal derangement of the knee indicates that it could be used as a screening test before arthroscopy. Comparison of magnetic resonance imaging and arthroscopy confirmed the higher accuracy of magnetic resonance imaging in the diagnosis of internal derangement but the results for articular cartilage lesions were much less good. Intra-

Table 42.1: The benefits of MAS in orthopedics

a. Less painful
b. Faster rehabilitation
c. Better visualization of the pathology
d. Shorter hospitals stay
e. Cheaper (long-term)
f. Aesthetic
g. More precise

articular fracture, chondral injury, meniscal and ligamentous injuries (partial or complete) can be diagnosed and treated simultaneously.

Trauma

Anatomic reduction, typically obtained by direct visualization through an arthrotomy and internal fixation (open reduction and internal fixation), is the traditional treatment method for displaced intra-articular condylar fractures of the distal femur and proximal tibia. Arthroscopic assisted reduction and internal fixation, of a displaced, malrotated intra-articular fracture fragment involving the tibia or femur has benefits of decreased blood loss, shortened operative time, excellent intra-articular visualization, decreased soft tissue dissection, and shortened postoperative recovery.

Ligamentous Injury

In acute ligamentous injuries, arthroscopy has limited or no role for repair of these ligamentous structures. Once the acute stage subsides, the ligamentous structures can be reinforced or reconstructed. Arthroscopic assisted ligamentous reconstruction is the gold standard treatment for ruptured ligament.

Meniscal Injury

Meniscal tear.

Chondral Injury

According to recent research, up to 10 to 12% of individuals present with chondral injuries. When symptomatic, chondral lesions manifest as swelling and knee pain. The loss of cartilage may be partial or complete, and it may affect one or multiple locations. Nonsurgical treatment modalities include analgesics, knee brace and physiotherapy. Surgical treatment varies from arthroscopic debridement to implantation of autologous chondrocytes beneath a periosteal patch covering the lesion. Autologous chondrocyte transplantation has a durable outcome for as long as 11 years.

Osteoarthritis

Arthroscopic debridement in early osteoarthritic patients may provide early symptomatic relief to pain. The long-term results are comparable with conservative management.

Hip Joint

Hip arthroscopy is technically demanding, with a steep learning curve, and requires special distraction tools and operating equipment. Access to the hip joint is difficult because of the resistance to distraction resulting from the large muscular envelope, the strength of the iliofemoral ligament, and the negative intra-articular pressure. This operation should not be done without specific education in its methods. Hip arthroscopy allows thorough visualization of the acetabular labrum, femoral head, and acetabular chondral surfaces as well as of the fovea, ligamentum teres, and adjacent synovium. Microsurgical tools developed specifically for arthroscopic hip surgery can be used to provide the least intrusive means of diagnosis and treatment of conditions involving the above mentioned structures (Table 42.2).

No radiographic study, including high-contrast gadolinium-enhanced arthrography-magnetic resonance imaging, is entirely sensitive or specific for the diagnosis of labral tears or chondral lesions. Thus, a high level of clinical suspicion based on the patient's symptoms and positive physical findings is paramount for the clinician to recognize subtle abnormalities in the hip joint.

Ankle Joint

The advantages and experiences of arthroscopy in large joints were extended to the small joints like ankle and wrist. Arthroscopy of the ankle is a relatively new discipline but has in recent years been increasingly applied to the diagnostic and therapeutic treatment of ankle disorders . Indications for arthroscopy in ankle joint are as follow in Table 42.3.

30°, wide angles, 2.7 mm arthroscope with a 3.5 mm shaver is used for ankle joint. Ankle joint is also distended, maximum up to 50 mm Hg pressure with the help of pump. To distract the ankle joint ankle strap can also be used for manual traction. Standard portals are anteromedial, medial to the tibialis anterior tendon, and located about 5 mm proximal to the medial malleolus and anterolateral, just lateral to the peroneus tertius tendon. Initial arthroscopy is performed with the scope in the anteromedial portal, but for the majority of the case, this portal will be used for instrumentation. Possible complications with anterior approach are injury to greater saphenous nerve and vein and injury to the dorsal lateral branch of the peroneal nerve.

Recent studies suggest that, with the patient in the prone position, arthroscopic equipment may be introduced into the posterior aspect of the ankle without gross injury to the posterior neurovascular structures.

Shoulder Joint

The shoulder joint is well encapsulated with muscular covering throughout its circumference. Open surgical procedures leads to bleeding and high morbidity, hence minimal access procedures are preferred with the use of arthroscope. Indications for shoulder arthroscopy are enumerated in Table 42.4.

Beach chair position is comfortable for both the patient and the surgeon as it allows free access to shoulder joint and the option of converting to an open procedure. Standard portals for shoulder joint are posterior, anterior and lateral. Complication for shoulder arthroscopy and its position are brachial plexus strain and hypoglossal nerve injury.

Elbow

Arthroscopic surgery for elbow joint is still in primitive stage and limited to arthroscopic synovectomy. Arthroscopic synovectomy is a reliable procedure to alleviate pain in early grades of rheumatoid arthritis. The fundamental of arthroscopy is visualization and access. Visualization and access to the ulnohumeral and radiocapitellar articulation is rather difficult. Recent study has come out with a joint jack to widen the ulnohumeral joint space to work better posteriorly.

Wrist

Wrist arthroscopy is the third most common joint after knee and shoulder joint to be examined by arthroscope.

MINIMAL ACCESS SURGERY IN ORTHOPEDIC TRAUMA

Opening of the fracture site during exposure further jeopardize the vascularity at the fracture site which adversely effects the healing at the fracture site. The involvement intra-articular fracture needs minimal tissue stripping to further jeopardize the vascularity. This principle leads to the foundation of the minimal access surgical principle in orthopedic trauma surgery. This principle helps to maintain the biology around the fracture site, so this fixation is also known as biological fixation. Biological fixation or minimal access surgery is extremely useful at the site of fractures with comminution, or areas with doubtful vascularity.

SPINE SURGERY AND ARTHROSCOPY

Spinal surgeries are thought to be risky due to the vicinity of the important structures and high vascularity (venous plexus) around the spine. The conventional (open) exposure to reach the site of pathology needs

wide exposure which in turns lead to large amount of morbidity and prolongs the period of recovery especially in the thoracic spine surgeries. The advantage of endoscopy like precision, magnification and small incision for exposure has lead to the endoscopic spinal surgery to the great advantage than conventional open procedure.

The endoscope allows the surgeon to use a "keyhole" incision to access the herniated disk. Muscle and tissue are dilated rather than being cut when accessing the disk. This leads to less tissue destruction, less postoperative pain, quicker recovery times, earlier rehabilitation, and avoidance of general anesthesia. Thermal annuloplasty is an adjunctive procedure that uses bipolar electrothermal energy (radiofrequency and/or laser) to ablate or depopulate the sensitized pain nociceptors in the annulus, ablate any inflammatory/granulation tissue that has grown into the annulus, and to shrink and tighten the stretched or torn collagen fibers of the annulus.

Scoliosis is a three-dimensional problem. The aim of surgery is to try to restore the normal contour of the back from both the front view and the side view. A technique to assist in getting a maximum of correction with a minimum of scar and morbidity by releasing the contacted anterior tissue with the use of the endoscope to go into the chest (similar to the way surgeons take out gallbladders now) in front where the actual vertebra are and take out the disks in front thus relaxing up the spine so we can get better correction and the fusion in back. This method goes in through the chest using three or four small incisions to reach the front of the spine. Once inside the chest the spine is clearly visible and "soft" tissues can be cleaned off exposing the spine. The discs are easily seen and can be removed.

 Table 42.2: Indications for hip arthroscopy

1. Labral tears
2. Loose bodies
3. Acetabular and femoral head chondral flap lesions
4. Foreign body removal
5. Synovial chondromatosis
6. Collagen diseases with impinging synovitis
7. Crystalline hip arthropathies
8. Ruptured or impinging ligamentum teres
9. Capsular shrinkage (Ehlers-Danlos syndrome)
10. Post-traumatic conditions (e.g. Pipkin fracture)
11. After total hip arthroplasty
12. Osteonecrosis (early stages prior to collapse)
13. Extra-articular conditions

 Table 42.3: Indications for ankle arthroscopy

1. Soft tissue   – Soft tissue impingement
              – Synovitis (diagnosis and biopsy)
              – Arthrofibrosis
2. Osteochondral defect of the talus
3. Intra-articular fracture and occult intra-articular injury
4. Arthrodesis of ankle joint

 Table 42.4: Indications for shoulder arthroscopy

1. Soft tissue   – Soft tissue impingement
              a. Synovitis (diagnosis and biopsy)
              b. Arthroscopic-assisted lysis of adhesion
2. Arthroscopic-assisted subacromial decompression (ASAD) and acromioplasty
3. Arthroscopic reconstruction (Bankart lesion repair, slap lesions)

BONE ENDOSCOPY AND TUMORS

With the increasing experience of seeing inside the soft cavities like joint, the same arthroscope is now used to see inside the bony cavities. The initial results are equal than the open surgical procedure with added advantages of minimal invasive, no immobilization, quick hospital discharge, minimal chances of pathological fracture and very small surgical scar. This is especially useful for benign cystic lesion of bone like giant cell tumor, simple bone cyst or enchondroma. With the endoscopic technique, curettage of the cystic lesion and filling of the cavity by mersalized autologous bone or bone cement can be done effectively. This minimal invasive technique allows the lesion to heal at much faster rate and with minimal scaring. This technique is being in practice for the management of these cystic lesion in soft bones or in cancellous bones.

BIBLIOGRAPHY

1. Abbou CC, Cicco A, Gasman D, et al. Retroperitoneal laparoscopic versus open radical nephrectomy. J Urol. 1999;161(6):1776-80.
2. Abolyosr A. Laparoscopic versus open orchidopexy in the management of abdominal testis: a descriptive study. Int J Urol 2006;13(11):1421–4.
3. American Society of Anesthesiologists. New classification of physical status. Anesthesiology. 1963;24(1):111.
4. Argos Rodriguez MD, Unda Freire A, Ruiz Orpez A, Garcia Lorenzo C. Diagnostic and therapeutic laparoscopy for nonpalpable testis. Surg Endosc 2003;17:1756–8.
5. Ashton RC Jr, McGinnis KM, Connery CP, Swistel DG, Ewing DR, DeRose JJ Jr. Totally endoscopic robotic thymectomy for myasthenia gravis. Ann Thorac Surg 2003;75:569–71.
6. Azagra JS, Goergen M, Gilbart E, Jacobs D. Laparoscopic anatomical (hepatic) left lateral segmentectomy—technical aspects. Surg Endosc. 1996;10(7):758-61.
7. Baba S, Ito K, Yanaihara H, Nagata H, Murai M, Iwamura M. Retroperitoneoscopic adrenalectomy by a lumbodorsal approach: clinical experience with solo surgery. Word J Urol 1999;17:54–8.
8. Berkmen F, Alagol H. Germinal cell tumors of the testis in cryptorchids. J Exp Clin Cancer Res 1998;17(4):409–12.
9. Bisgaard T, Klarskov B, Trap R, Kehlet H, Rosenberg J. Pain after microlaparoscopic cholecystectomy. A randomized double blind controlled study. Surg Endosc 2000;14:340–44.
10. Bode CO, Nwawolo CC, Giwa-Osagie OF. Surgical education at the West African College of Surgeons. World J Surg 2008;32:2162–6.
11. Carmignani L, Morabito A, Gadda F, Bozzini G, Rocco F, Colpi GM. Prognostic parameters in adult impalpable ultrasonographic lesions of the testicle. J Urol 2005;174(30):1035–8.
12. Chandrasekharam VV. Laparoscopy vs inguinal exploration for the nonpalpable undescended testis. Ind J Pediatric 2005;72:1021–3.
13. Charny CK, Jarnagin WR, Schwartz LH, et al. Management of 155 patients with benign liver tumors. Br J Surg. 2001;88(6):808-13.
14. Cheah WK, Lenzi JE, So JB, Kum CK, Goh PM. Randomized trial of needlescopic versus laparoscopic cholecystectomy. Br J Surg 2001;88:45–7.
15. Cherqui D, Husson E, Hammoud R, et al. Laparoscopic liver resections: a feasibility study in 30 patients. Ann Surg. 2000;232(6):753-62.
16. Cherqui D, Rahmouni A, Charlotte F, et al. Management of focal nodular hyperplasia and hepatocellular adenoma in young women: a series of 41 patients with clinical, radiological and pathological correlations. Hepatology. 1995;22(6):1674-81.
17. Cherqui D. Laparoscopic liver resection. Br J Surg. 2003;90(6):644-6.
18. Cleary K, Nguyen C. State of the art in surgical robotics: clinical applications and technology challenges. Comput Aided Surg 2001;6:312–28.
19. Cortes D, Thorup J, Visfeldt J. Multinucleated spermatogonia in cryptorchid boys: a possible association with an increased risk of testicular malignancy later in life? APMIS 2003;111(1):25–30.
20. Cortez D, Thorup J, Peterson BL. Testicular neoplasia in undescended testes of cryptorchid boys-does surgical strategy have an impact on the risk of invasive testicular neoplasia? Turk J Pediatr 2004;46 Suppl:35–42.
21. Corvin S, Sturm W, Anastasiadis A, Kuczyk M, Stenzl A. Laparoscopic management of adult nonpalpable testicle. Urol Int 2005;75(4):337–9.
22. Cuschieri A, Shimi S, Banting S, Nathanson LK, Pietrabissa A. Intraoperative cholangiography during laparoscopic cholecystectomy. Routine vs selective policy. Surg Endosc 1994;8:302–5.
23. Delaunay L, Bonnet F, Cherqui D, Rimaniol JM, Dahan E, Atlan G. Laparoscopic cholecystectomy minimally impairs postoperative cardiorespiratory and muscle performance. Br J Surg. 1995;82(3):373-6.
24. DeRose JJ Jr, Swistel DG, Safavi A, Connery CP, Ashton RC Jr. Mediastinal mass evaluation using advanced robotic techniques. Ann Thorac Surg 2003;75:571–3.
25. Desai CS, Prabhu RY, Supe AN. Laparoscopic orchidectomy for undescended testis in adults. J Postgrad Med 2002;48;25–6.
26. Descottes B, Glineur D, Lachachi F, et al. Laparoscopic liver resection for benign liver tumors: results of a multicenter European experience. Surg Endosc. 2003;17(1):23-30.
27. Descottes B, Lachachi F, Sodji M, et al. Early experience with laparoscopic approach for solid liver tumors: initial 16 cases. Ann Surg. 2000;232(5):641-5.
28. Dunlap KD, Wanzer L. Is the robotic arm a cost-effective surgical tool? Assoc Oper Room Nurs J 1998;68:265–72.

29. El-Anany F, Gad El-Moula M, Abdel Moneim A, Abdallah A, Takahashi M, Kanayama H, et al. Laparoscopy for impalpable testis: classification-based management. Surg Endosc 2007;21(3):449–545.

30. Elder JS. Ultrasonography is unnecessary in evaluating boys with a non palpable testis. Pediatrics 2002;110(4):748–51.

31. Farges O, Jagot P, Kirstetter P, Marty J, Belghiti J. Prospective assessment of the safety and benefit of laparoscopic liver resections. J Hepatobiliary Pancreat Surg. 2002;9(2):242-8.

32. Farrer JH, Walker AH, Rajfer J. Management of the postpubertal cryptorchid testis: a statistical review. J Urol 1985;134:1071–6.

33. Fong Y, Jarnagin W, Conlon KC, Dematteo R, Dougherty E, Blumgart LH. Handassisted laparoscopic liver resection. Arch Surg. 2000;135(7):854-9.

34. Ford TF. The undescended testis in adult life. Br J Ur 1985; 57(2);181–4.

35. Gagner M, Rheault M, Dubuc J. Laparoscopic partial hepatectomy for liver tumor [abstract]. Surg Endosc. 1992;6(2):99.

36. Hamdorf JM, Hall JC. Acquiring surgical skills. Br J Surg 2000;87:28–37.

37. Hrebinko RL, Bellinger MF. The limited role of imaging techniques in managing children with undescended testes. J Urol 1993;150:458–60.

38. Hu¨scher CG, Lirici MM, Chiodini S. Laparoscopic liver resections. Semin Laparosc Surg. 1998;5(3):204-10.

39. IHPBA Brisbane 2000 terminology of liver anatomy and resections. HPB Surg. 2000;2(3):333-339.

40. Ivanov A, Dewey C, Fahlenkamp D, Luning M. MRT in nonpalpable testes. Rofo 1994;160(3);249–53.

41. Jarnagin WR, Gonen M, Fong Y, et al. Improvement in perioperative outcome after hepatic resection: analysis of 1803 consecutive cases over the past decade. Ann Surg. 2002;236(4):397-407.

42. Kammula US, Buell JF, Labow DM, Rosen S, Millis JM, Posner MC. Surgical management of benign tumors of the liver. Int J Gastrointest Cancer. 2001;30(3):141-6.

43. Kaneko H, Takagi S, Shiba T. Laparoscopic partial hepatectomy and left lateral segmentectomy: technique and results of a clinical series. Surgery. 1996;120(3):468-75.

44. Katkhouda N, Hurwitz M, Gugenheim J, et al. Laparoscopic management of benign solid and cystic lesions of the liver. Ann Surg. 1999;229(4):460-66.

45. Kavoussi LR, Moore RG, Adams JB, Partin AW. Comparison of robotic versus human laparoscopic camera control. J Urol 1995;154:2134–6.

46. Kneebone R, ApSimon D. Surgical skills training: simulation and multimedia combined. Med Educ 2001;35:909–15.

47. Kondraske GV, Hamilton EC, Scott DJ, Fischer CA, Tesfay ST, Taneja R, Brown RJ, Jones DB. Surgeon workload and motion efficiency with robot and human laparoscopic camera control. Surg Endosc 2002;16:1523–7.

48. Kucheria R, Sahai A, Sami TA, et al. Laparoscopic management of cryptorchidism in adults. Eur Urol 2005;48(3):453–7.

49. Laurent A, Cherqui D, Lesurtel M, Brunetti F, Tayar C, Fagniez PL. Laparoscopic liver resection for subcapsular hepatocellular carcinoma complicating chronic liver disease. Arch Surg. 2003;138(7):763-9.

50. Le Bartz G, Petit T, Ravasse P. Is there any interest to perform ultrasonography in boys with undescended testis? Arch Pediatr 2006;13(5):426–8.

51. Leggett PL, Churchman-Winn R, Miller R. Minimizing ports to improve laparoscopic cholecystectomy. Surg Endosc 2000;14:32–6.

52. Lesurtel M, Cherqui D, Laurent A, Tayar C, Fagniez PL. Laparoscopic versus open left lateral hepatic lobectomy: a case-control study. J Am Coll Surg. 2003;196(2):236-42.

53. Leung KF, Lee KW, Cheung TY, Leung LC, Lau KW. Laparoscopic cholecystectomy: two-port technique. Endoscopy 1996;6:505–7.

54. Lomanto D, De Angelis L, Ceci V, Dalsasso G, So J, Frattaroli FM, Muthiah R, Speranza V. Two-trocar laparoscopic cholecystectomy: a reproducible technique. Surg Laparosc Endosc Percutan Tech 2001;11:248–51.

55. Mcheik JN, Levard G. Laparoscopic treatment of the non palpable testis. Results. Prog Urol 2002;12(2):294–7.

56. Menconi GF, Melfi FAM, Givigliano F, Angeletti CA. Robotic pulmonary lobectomy: early operative experience and preliminary clinical results. Eur Surg 2002;34:173–6.

57. Merola S, Weber P, Wasielewski A, Ballantyne GH. Comparison of laparoscopic colectomy with and without the aid of a robotic camera holder. Surg Laparosc Endosc Percutan Tech 2002;12:46–51.

58. Moher D, Schulz KF, Altman DG. The CONSORT statement: revised recommendations for improving the quality of reports of parallel-group randomised trials. Lancet 2001;357:1191–4.

59. Morgan JA, Thornton BA, Peacock JC, Hollingsworth KW, Smith CR, Oz MC, Argenziano M. Does robotic technology make minimally invasive cardiac surgery too expensive? A hospital cost analysis of robotic and conventional techniques. J Card Surg 2005 May–Jun;20:246–51.

60. Morino M, Morra I, Rosso E, Miglietta C, Garrone C. Laparoscopic vs open hepatic resection: a comparative study. Surg Endosc. 2003;17(12):1914-8.

61. Nijs SM, Eijsbouts SW, Madern GC, Leyman PM, Lequin MH, Hazebroek FW. Non palpable testes: is there a relationship between ultrasonographic and operative findings? Pediatr Radiol 2007;37(4):374–9.

62. Panait L, Doarn CR, Merrell RC. Applications of robotics in surgery. Chirurgia (Bucur) 2002;97:549–55.

63. Perniceni T, Slim K. What are the validated indications for laparoscopy in digestive surgery? Gastroenterol Clin Biol. 2001;25(4)(suppl):B57-B70.

64. Poon CM, Chan KW, Ko CW, Chan KC, Lee DW, Cheung HY, Lee KW (2002) Two-port laparoscopic cholecystectomy: initial results of a modified technique. J Laparoendosc Adv Surg Tech A 12:259–62.

65. Poon RT, Fan ST, Lo CM, et al. Improving perioperative outcome expands the role of hepatectomy in management of benign and malignant hepatobiliary diseases: analysis of 1222 consecutive patients from a prospective database. Ann Surg. 2004;240(4):698-710.

66. Raina V, Shukla NK, Gupta NP, et al. Germ cell tumours in uncorrected cryptorchid testis at Institute Rotary Cancer Hospital, New Delhi. Br J Cancer 1995;71:380–2.

67. Ramachandran CS, Arora V. Two-port laparoscopic cholecystectomy: an innovative new method for gallbladder removal. J Laparoendosc Adv Surg Tech A 1998;8:303–8.

68. Rangarajan M, Jayakar SM. Laparoscopic orchidectomy for the adult impalpable testis—experiences in a rural teaching hospital. Surg Endosc 2007;21(1):66–9.

69. Rau HG, Buttler E, Meyer G, Schardey HM, Schildberg FW. Laparoscopic liver resection compared with conventional partial hepatectomy—a prospective analysis. Hepatogastroenterology. 1998;45(24):2333-8.

70. Ruurda JP, Hanlo PW, Hennipman A, Broeders IA. Robot-assisted thoracoscopic resection of a benign mediastinal neurogenic tumor: technical note. Neurosurgery 2003;52:462–4.

71. Satar N, Bayazit Y, Doran S. Laparoscopy in the management of impalpable testicle. Acta Chir Belg 2005;105(6):662–6.

72. Shin D, Lemack GE, Goldstein M. Induction of spermatogenesis and pregnancy after adult orchiopexy. J Urol 1997;158:2242.

73. Siemer S, Humke U, Hildebrandt U, Karadiakos N, Ziegler M. Diagnosis of non palpable testes in childhood: comparison of magnetic resonance imaging and laparoscopy in a prospective study. Eur J Pediatr Surg 2000;10(2):114–8.

74. Soper NJ, Brunt LM, Kerbl K. Laparoscopic general surgery. N Engl J Med. 1994;330(6):409-19.

75. Soper NJ, Dunnegan DL. Routine versus selective intraoperative cholangiography during laparoscopic cholecystectomy 1992.

76. Terkivatan T, de Wilt JHW, de Man RA, et al. Indications and long-term outcome of treatment for benign hepatic tumors. Arch Surg. 2001;136(9):1033-8.

77. Vibert E, Perniceni T, Levard H, Denet C, Shahri NK, Gayet B. Laparoscopic liver resection. Br J Surg. 2006;93(1):67-72.

78. Waseem T. Technologic advances in robotic. J Coll Physicians Surg Pak 2005;15:559–61.

79. Weimann A, Ringe B, Klempnauer J, et al. Benign liver tumors: differential diagnosis and indications for surgery. World J Surg. 1997;21(9):983-91.

80. Welvaart K, Tijssen JGP. Management of the undescended testis in relation to the development of cancer. J Surg Oncol 2006;17;3:219–23.

81. Wolverson MK, Houttuin E, Heiberg E, Sundaram M, Shields JB. Comparison of computed tomography with high-resolution realtime ultrasound in the localization of the impalpable undescended testis. Radiology 1983;146(1):133–6.

82. Yoshino I, Hashizume M, Shimada M, Tomikawa M, Tomiyasu M, Suemitsu R, Sugimachi K. Thoracoscopic thymomectomy with the da Vinci computer- enhanced surgical system. J Thorac Cardiovasc Surg 2001;122:783–5.

Section Six

43 Minimal Access Bariatric Surgery

LAPAROSCOPIC TREATMENT FOR MORBID OBESITY

The most frequently performed gastric procedures for morbid obesity today include the Roux-en-Y gastric bypass (RYGB) and vertical banded gastroplasty. However, four basic approaches have been traditionally used for the treatment of obesity. The first operation done for obesity was the jejunoileal bypass. This operation was aimed to bypass 90% of the jejunum and ileum to induce malabsorption. This operation was abandoned due to a high incidence of severe complications such as hepatic failure, cirrhosis, nephropathy, and numerous other metabolic complications. The gastroplasty was developed to limit the amount of oral intake per meal. This operation involves partitioning the stomach into a small upper pouch that empties through a restricted stoma. The vertical banded gastroplasty is the most popular version of the gastroplasty. The third approach to obesity is Roux-en-Y gastric bypass. This operation also involves formation of a small upper gastric pouch that is anastomosed to a Roux-en-Y jejunal limb. The operation both limits oral intake per meal as well as induces dumping syndrome. Lastly, the partial biliopancreatic bypass induces a selective maldigestion and malabsorption. This operation involves a partial gastrectomy and diversion of the biliary and pancreatic secretions to the distal 50 cm of ileum; it is primarily performed in the "super" obese population (BMI > $60 \, \text{kg/m}^2$). The most recent development has been the modification of the adjustable silicone gastric band

developed by Kuzmak. This gastric banding device has been modified for laparoscopic placement and is a form of gastric restriction or gastroplasty.

Results of Different Bariatric Surgery

The goals of surgery are to induce and maintain weight loss. Outcome from surgery is usually expressed as the amount or percent of excess weight lost. Several trials have compared the effect of gastric restriction versus gastric bypass. Subsequently several trials have confirmed that Roux-en-Y gastric bypass results in more weight loss compared with Gastric Banding. The early complications following Roux-en-Y gastric bypass operation for obesity include subphrenic abscess or leak from an anastomosis or staple line. This complication is usually amenable to percutaneous aspiration and drainage, however, a small number of patients will require reoperation. The majority of early postoperative complications are minor wound infections and seromas. Late complications of the Roux-en-Y gastric bypass include vitamin B_{12} and iron deficiency. On the other hand, vitamin B_{12} and iron deficiency anemia is uncommon after vertical banded gastroplasty. Incisional hernia is another complication of morbidly obese patients undergoing laparotomy. Other late complications include failure to lose weight, late weight regain, and outlet stenosis. Staple line disruption has been a common problem and has prompted the use of four rows of staples instead of two. Another approach has been to divide the stomach to produce an isolated gastric pouch.

Laparoscopic Vertical Banded Gastroplasty

To perform laparoscopic vertical banded gastroplasty the patient is placed in reverse Trendelenburg's position with the legs separated in low stirrups. The surgeon stands between the patient's legs. An alternative approach is to place the patient supine with a footrest in the reverse Trendelenburg's position. The surgeon stands on the patient's right side with an assistant on the left. Five trocars are placed in the standard manner for gastric surgery. The telescope is placed through the 10 mm mid epigastric port, and the liver retractor is placed through a right subcostal port (Figs 43.1A and B).

There are two operating ports, one in each paramedian position (right, 10 to 33 mm; left, 15 mm). A window is created at the lesser curve of the stomach in an avascular plane using harmonic shears. The posterior stomach wall is freed of any adhesions. An alternative approach to the lesser sac is made by dividing the gastroepiploic vessels along the greater curvature. A 32 F dilator is placed via the mouth into the stomach. A site on the anterior stomach 4 to 5 cm from the gastroesophageal junction and 3 cm from the lesser curve is marked with the electrocautery. This site will be the center of the circular stapler. The right paramedian port is upsized to a 33 mm port to allow introduction of the circular stapling device. The anvil of the circular stapler is then placed posterior to the stomach. The pointed trocar is inserted through the stomach at the site previously marked with the cautery. The stapler is then connected and fired (Fig. 43.1C).

The attachments from the diaphragm to the fundus of the stomach are divided, and the fundus is dissected inferiorly using blunt technique. A linear 60 mm, four-row, noncutting stapler is introduced through the left paramedian port. The stapler is inserted through the circular window along the dilator and fired. A linear cutter is applied lateral to the previously placed rows of staples. At the circular window a strip of polypropylene or polytetrafluoroethylene (1.5 × 5 cm) is brought around the stoma. The band is sutured into place around the dilator. A nasogastric tube is not mandatory with this procedure.

Laparoscopic Roux-en-Y Gastric Bypass

Patient positioning and port placement is as for other gastric procedures. The dissection starts at the fundus of the stomach with division of the phrenicogastric ligament. The fundus is mobilized in an inferior direction by blunt dissection. On the anterior wall of

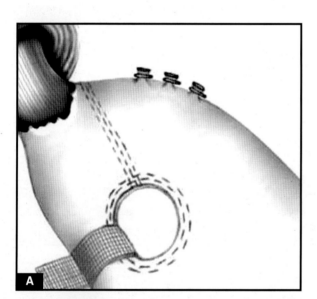

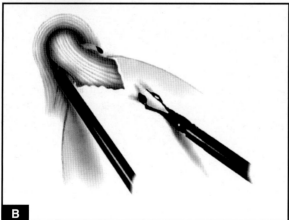

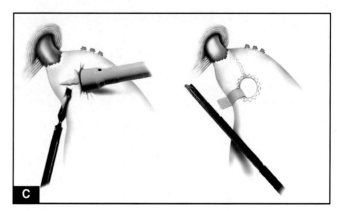

Figs 43.1A to C: Laparoscopic vertical banded gastroplasty

the stomach, an electrocautery mark is made 4 to 5 cm distal to the angle of His to serve as a landmark for the size of the gastric pouch. The lesser omentum is then opened adjacent to the mark at 4 to 5 cm inside the nerve of Laterjet. Dissection is carried through the lesser sac to an opening near the angle of His. The medial subcostal port is changed to an 18 mm port and a straight four-row cutting 60 mm stapler is used to divide the stomach. A standard 60 mm Roux limb is fashioned by dividing the proximal jejunum with a 60 mm linear stapler. The limb is brought up in a retrocolic, retrogastric path to the small (15 ml) proximal gastric pouch. A circular stapler is used for the gastroje-junostomy. The anvil is inserted via the oral cavity by endoscopic approach and using a percutaneous pull wire technique. An anastomosis is fashioned by connecting the anvil to the stapler introduced through the 18 mm port. A stapled side-to-side entero-enterostomy is then done to restore gastrointestinal continuity.

Laparoscopic Adjustable Gastric Banding

An alternative gastric restrictive operation is the adjustable silicone gastric banding (ASGB) procedure. It was first introduced for placement through laparotomy by Kuzmak in 1986. This operation has the advantage of being the least invasive operation as it is completely reversible and allows for adjustment of the gastric pouch outlet.

The main steps of laparoscopic adjustable silicone gastric banding are as follows (Fig. 43.2).

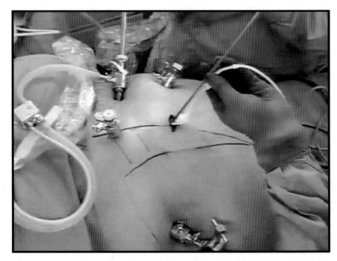

Fig. 43.2: Port position of laparoscopic gastric banding

The patient is placed in a lithotomy position and in reverse Trendelenburg's as for most gastric operations. A total of six ports are placed. The liver retractor is placed through a right subcostal one, the telescope is inserted through a subxiphoid positioned port. The main operating ports are in the right and left paramedian positions. The assistant uses a left subcostal and an epigastric port. The left paramedian port is 15 mm for introduction of the band device. All of the other ports are 10 mm.

A gastric calibration tube is placed via the mouth into the stomach. The balloon is inflated to 15 cc and pulled up through the gastroesophageal junction.

A site on the lesser curve is chosen to begin dissection that corresponds to the widest circumference of the balloon inside stomach. The balloon is deflated

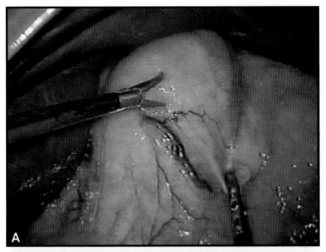

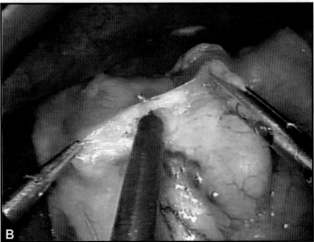

Figs 43.3A and B: Lesser curvature a site choosen to start dissection

and the tube is withdrawn back into the esophagus (Figs 43.3A and B).

A retrogastric tunnel is then created using blunt dissection, staying close to the gastric wall. The posterior gastric wall should be easily recognized to prevent injury. A small opening in the phrenicogastric ligament is made with electrocautery (Figs 43.4A and B).

A grasping instrument is then placed through the retrogastric tunnel. The band is then introduced into the abdomen and grasped with the instrument. The

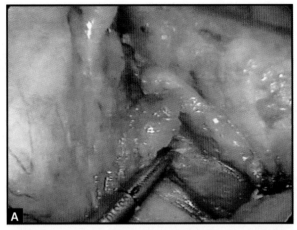
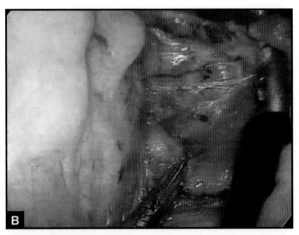

Figs 43.4A and B: Creation of a retrogastric tunnel

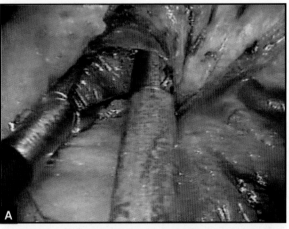
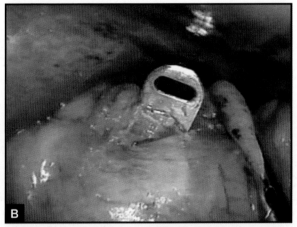

Figs 43.5A and B: Grasping instrument coming from behind through retrogastric tunnel

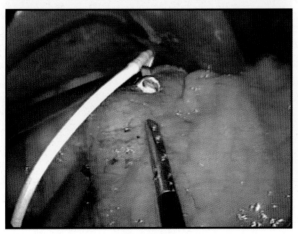
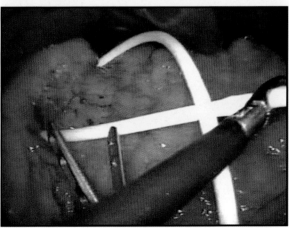

Fig. 43.6AFig. 43.6B

Section Six

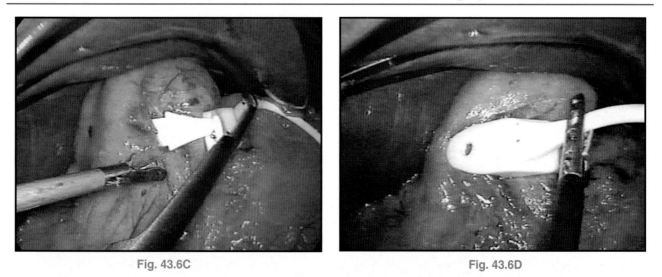

Fig. 43.6C   Fig. 43.6D

Figs 43.6A to D: Band is pulled from below the stomach through retrogastric tunnel and is tightened leaving 15 ml volume of stomach above

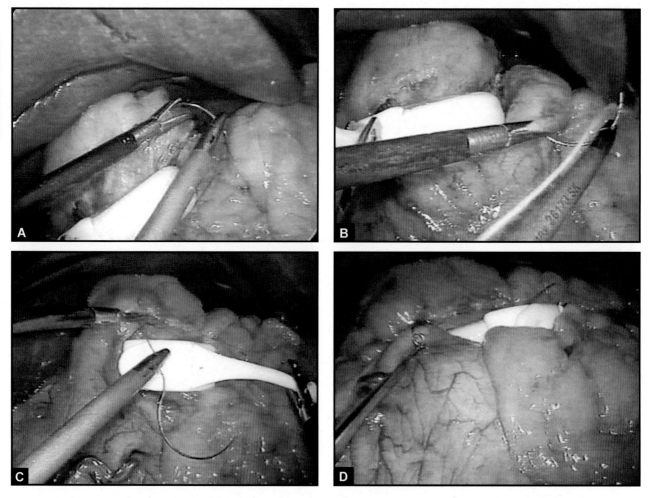

Figs 43.7A to D: Suture is placed to fix the band in position

band is pulled into position around the stomach (Figs 43.5A and B).

The calibration tube is then reinserted into the proper position and the band closed around the tube. The calibration tube allows for proper stoma calibration (Figs 43.6A to D).

At least four sutures are then placed in the seromuscular layer of the stomach just proximal and distal to the band to keep it in the proper position otherwise the chances of displacements are there. The injection port is then connected to the band tubing and implanted into the left rectus sheath at the paramedian port site (Figs 43.7A to D) .

CONCLUSION

In developed world obesity is a major national health problem. It is clear that morbidly obese patients suffer from significant comorbidity and die at younger age than healthy weight individuals. Weight loss to, and maintenance of normal weight corrects the majority of weight-related morbidity and returns life expectancy to that of the general population. All the laparoscopic surgeons should remember that morbidly obese patients are at an increased risk of significant morbidity and mortality with laparoscopic surgery. However, strict attention to detail allows for proper selection of patients for surgery with reduction in the perioperative risk.

BIBLIOGRAPHY

1. 24 Tsai AG, Wadden TA. Systematic review: an evaluation of major commercial weight loss programs in the United States. Ann Int Med 2005;142:56–66.
2. Adams T, Gress RE, Smith SC, et al. Long-term mortality after gastric bypass surgery. N Engl J Med 2007;357:753–61.
3. Alexander CI, Liston WA. Operating on the obese woman – a review. BJOG 2006;113:1167–72.
4. Amorim AR, Ro¨ssner S, Neovius M, Lourenco PM, Linne´ Y. Does excess pregnancy weight gain constitute a major risk for increasing long-term BMI? Obesity 2007;15:1278–86.
5. Angrisani L, Favretti F, Furbetta F, et al. Italian Group for Lap-Band System: results of multi-center study on patients with BMI , or ¼ 35 kg/m2. Obes Surg 2004;14:415–8.
6. Angrisani L, Lorenzo M, Borrelli V. Laparoscopic adjustable gastric banding versus Roux-en-Y gastric bypass: 5-year results of a prospective randomized trial. Surg Obes Relat Dis 2007;3:127–32.
7. Baughcum AE, Burklow KA, Deeks CM, Powers SW, Whitaker RC. Maternal feeding practices and childhood obesity: a focus group study of low-income mothers. Arch Pediatr Adolesc Med 1998;152:1010–4.
8. Baughcum AE, Powers SW, Johnson SB, et al. Maternal feeding practices and beliefs and their relationships to overweight in early childhood. J Dev Behav Pediatr 2001;22:391–408.
9. Baxter J. Obesity surgery – another unmet need. BMJ 2000;321:523–4.
10. Baxter J. Obesity surgery. Lancet 2008;371:557.
11. Bessesen DH. Update on obesity. J Clin EndoMetab 2008;93:2027–34.
12. Buchwald H, Avidor Y, Braunwald E, et al. Bariatric surgery: a systematic review and meta-analysis. JAMA 2004;292:1724–37.
13. Buchwald H, Varco RL, Matts JP, et al. Effect of partial ileal bypass surgery on mortality and morbidity from coronary heart disease in patients with hypercholesterolemia. Report of the Program on the Surgical Control of the Hyperlipidemias (POSCH). N Engl J Med 1990;323:946–55.
14. Busetto L, Angrisani L, Basso N, et al. Safety and efficacy of laparoscopic adjustable gastric banding in the elderly. Obesity 2008;16:334–8.
15. Cannizzo Jr F, Kral JG. Obesity surgery: a model of programmed undernutrition. Curr Opin Clin Nutr Metab Care 1998;1:363–8. ME Miller and JG Kral Surgery for obesity in older women Menopause International 2008;14(4):161.
16. Chapman IM. Obesity in old age. Front Horm Res 2008;36:97–106.
17. Chart 'Obesity' pp 197, OECD Factbook 2005: Economic, Environmental and Social Statistics. OECD, 2005. www.sourceoecd.org/factbook.
18. Christou NV, Sampalis JS, Liberman M, et al. Surgery decreases long-term mortality, morbidity, and health care use in morbidly obese patients. Ann Surg 2004;240:416–23.
19. Cohen RV, Schiavon CA, Pinheiro JS, Correa JL, Rubino F. Duodenal-jejunal bypass for the treatment of type 2 diabetes in patients with body mass index of 22–34 kg/m2: a report of 2 cases. Surg Obes Relat Dis 2007;3:195–7.
20. DeMaria EJ. Bariatric surgery for morbid obesity. N Engl J Med 2007;356:2176–83.
21. Dennis KE. Postmenopausal women and the health consequences of obesity. J Obstet Gynecol Neonatal Nurs 2007;36:511–9.
22. Dixon JB, O'Brien PE, Playfair J, et al. Adjustable gastric banding and conventional therapy for type 2 diabetes. JAMA 2008;299:316–23.
23. Eckel RH. Clinical practice. Nonsurgical management of obesity in adults. N Engl J Med 2008;358:1941–50.
24. Fatima J, Houghton SG, Iqbal CW, et al. Bariatric surgery at the extremes of age. J Gastrointest Surg 2006;10:1392–6.
25. Favretti F, Sagato G, Ashtor D, et al. Laparoscopic adjustable gastric banding in 1,791 consecutive obese patients: 12-year results. Obes Surg 2007;17:168–75.

26. Fernandez AZ, Demaria EJ, Tichansky DS, et al. Multivariate analysis of risk factors for death following gastric bypass for treatment of morbid obesity. Ann Surg 2004;239:698–702.

27. Ferro-Luzzi A, Toth MJ, Elia M, Schurch B. Report of the ODECG Working Group on body weight and body composition of the elderly. Eur J Clin Nutr 2000;54 (suppl. 3):S160–1.

28. Finkelstein EA, Fiebelkorn IC, Wang G. State-level estimates of annual medical expenditures attributable to obesity. Obes Res 2004;12:18–24.

29. Flum DR, Salem L, Elrod JAB, et al. Early mortality among Medicare beneficiaries undergoing bariatric surgical procedures. JAMA 2005;294:1903–8.

30. Folsom AR, Kushi LH, Anderson KE, et al. Associations of general and abdominal obesity with multiple health outcomes in older women. Arch Intern Med 2000;160:2117–28.

31. Fontaine KR, Barofsky I. Obesity and health related quality of life. Obes Rev 2001;2:173–82.

32. Fontaine KR, Redden DT, Wang C, Westfall AO, Allison DB. Years of life lost due to obesity. JAMA 2003;289:187–93.

33. Fried M, Hainer V, Basdevant A, et al. Inter-disciplinary European guidelines on surgery of severe obesity. Int J Obes 2007;31:569–77.

34. Gagner M, Milone L, Yung E, Broseus A, Gumbs AA. Causes of early mortality after laparoscopic adjustable gastric banding. J Am Coll Surg 2008;206:664–9.

35. Gastrointestinal surgery for severe obesity: NIH Consensus Development Conference. Consensus Statement 1991 (March 25–27);9(1):1–20.

36. Greendale GA, Unger JB, Rowe JW, Seeman TE. The relation between cortisol excretion and fractures in healthy older people: results from the MacArthur studies – Mac. J Am Geriatr Soc 1999;47:799–803.

37. Hallowell PT, Stellato TA, Schuster M, Graf K, Robinson A, Jasper JJ. Avoidance of complications in older patients and Medicare recipients undergoing gastric bypass. Arch Surg 2007;142:506–10 (discussion 510–2).

38. Harris TB, Launer LJ, Madans J, Feldman JJ. Cohort study of effect of being overweight and change in weight on risk of coronary heart disease in old age. Br Med J 1997;314:1792–4.

39. Hawkes K. The grandmother effect. Nature 2004;428:128–9.

40. Holmes E, Loo RL, Stamler J, et al. Human metabolic phenotype diversity and its association with diet and blood pressure. Nature 2008;453:396–400.

41. Joon Cho G, Hyun Lee J, Tae Park H, et al. Postmenopausal status according to years since menopause as an independent risk factor for the metabolic syndrome. Menopause 2008;15:524–9.

42. Kral JG, Biron S, Simard S, et al. Large maternal weight loss from obesity surgery prevents transmission of obesity to children followed 2–18 years. Pediatrics 2006;118:e1644–9.

43. Kral JG, Sjo¨stro¨m L, Gustafson A. Effects of jejuno-ileal bypass on serum lipoproteins and glucose tolerance in severely obese patients. Eur J Clin Invest 1980;10:363–7.

44. Kral JG. A stitch in time versus a life in misery. Surg Obes Relat Disord 2007;3:2–5.

45. Kral JG. ABC of obesity. Management: Part III – surgery. Br Med J 2006;333:900–3.

46. Kral JG. Effects of truncal vagotomy on body weight and hyperinsulinemia in morbid obesity. Am J Clin Nutr 1980;33:416–9.

47. Kral JG. Morbid obesity and related health risks. Ann Int Med 1985;103:1043–7.

48. Kral JG. Morbidity of severe obesity. Surg Clin North Am 2001;81:1039–61. M E Miller and J G Kral Surgery for obesity in older women 160 Menopause International 2008;14(4).

49. Kral JG. Preventing and treating obesity in girls and young women to curb the epidemic. Obes Res 2004;12:1539–46.

50. Lahdenpera¨ M, Lummaa V, Helle S, Tremblay M, Russell AF. Fitness benefits of prolonged post-reproductive lifespan in women. Nature 2004;428:178–81.

51. Linne´ Y, Dye L, Barkeling B, Ro¨ssner S. Long-term weight development in women: a 15-year follow-up of the effects of pregnancy. Obes Res 2004;12:1166–78.

52. Livingston EH, Huerta S, Arthur D, et al. Male gender is a predictor of morbidity and age a predictor of mortality for patients undergoing gastric bypass surgery. Ann Surg 2002;236:576–82.

53. Loos RJ, Lindgren CM, Li S, et al. Common variants near MC4R are associated with fat mass, weight and risk of obesity. Nat Genet 2008;40:768–75.

54. M E Miller and J G Kral Surgery for obesity in older women 162 Menopause International 2008;4:14 .

55. Marceau P, Hould FS, Simard S, et al. Biliopancreatic diversion with duodenal switch. World J Surg 1998;22:947–54.

56. Mark A. Dietary therapy for obesity: an emperor with no clothes. Hypertension 2008;51:1426–34.

57. McLean JA, Barr SI, Prior JC. Cognitive dietary restraint is associated with higher urinary cortisol excretion in healthy premenopausal women. Am J Clin Nutr 2001;73:7–12.

58. McMahon MM, Sarr MG, Clark MM, et al. Clinical management after bariatric surgery: value of a multidisciplinary approach. Mayo Clin Proc 2006;81 (10 suppl.):S34–45.

59. McTigue K, Larson JC, Valoski A, et al. Mortality and cardiac and vascular outcomes in extremely obese women. JAMA 2006;296:79–86.

60. Moo TA, Rubino F. Gastrointestinal surgery as treatment for type 2 diabetes. Curr Opin Endocrinol Diabetes Obes 2008;15:153–8.

61. National Center for Health Statistics. Health, United States, 2004 with Chartbook on Trends in the Health of Americans. Hyattsville, MD: US Department of Health and Human Services, Centers for Disease Control and Prevention, 2004.

62. National Institute for Health and Clinical Excellence. Obesity: guidance on the prevention, identification, assessment and management of overweight and obesity in adults and children. London: NICE; 2007. See http://www.nice.org. uk/nicemedia/pdf/CG43NICEGuideline.pdf.

Section Six

63. Nguyen NT, Paya M, Stevens CM, et al. The relationship between hospital volume and outcome in bariatric surgery at academic medical centers. Ann Surg 2004;240:586–94.

64. Nguyen NT, Paya M, Stevens CM, Mavandadi S, Zainabadi K, Wilson SE. The relationship between hospital volume and outcome in bariatric surgery at academic medical centers. Ann Surg 2004;240:586–93.

65. O'Brien PE, Dixon JB. Laparoscopic adjustable gastric banding in the treatment of morbid obesity. Arch Surg 2003;138:376–82.

66. O'Brien PE, et al. Treatment for mild to moderate obesity with laparoscopic adjustable banding or an intensive medical program: a randomized trial. Ann Intern Med 2006;144:625–33.

67. Ogden CL, Carroll MD, Flegal KM. High body mass index for age among US children and adolescents, 2003–2006. JAMA 2008;299:2401–5.

68. Oster G, Thompson D, Edelsberg J, Bird AP, Colditz GA. Lifetime health and economic benefits of weight loss among obese persons. Am J Public Health 1999;89:1536–42.

69. Perry CD, Hutter MM, Smith DB, Newhouse JP, McNeil BJ. Survival and changes in comorbidities after bariatric surgery. Ann Surg 2008;247:21–7.

70. Pories WJ, MacDonald Jr KG, Morgan EJ, et al. Surgical treatment and its effect on diabetes: 10-year follow-up. Am J Clin Nutr 1992;55:(2):582S–5S.

71. Poulose BK, Griffin MR, Moore DE, et al. Risk factors for postoperative mortality in bariatric surgery. J Surg Res 2005;127:1–7.

72. Puhl R, Brownell KD. Bias, discrimination and obesity. Obes Res 2001;9:788–805.

73. Raftopoulos Y, Gatti GG, Luketich JD, Courcoulas AP. Advanced age and sex as predictors of adverse outcomes following gastric bypass surgery. JSLS 2005;9:272–6.

74. Rand CSW, Macgregor AMC. Successful weight loss following obesity surgery and the perceived liability of morbid obesity. Int J Obes 1991;15:577–9.

75. Reeves GK, Pirie K, Beral V, et al. Cancer incidence and mortality in relation to BMI in the million women study: cohort study. Br Med J 2007;335:1134–45.

76. Rehfeld JF, Juhl E, Quaade F. Effect of jejunoileostomy on glucose and insulin metabolism in ten obese patients. Metabolism 1970;19:529–38.

77. Reid IR. Glucocorticoid osteoporosis – mechanisms and management. Eur J Endocrinol 1997;137:209–17.

78. Rideout CA. High cognitive dietary restraint is associated with increased cortisol excretion in postmenopausal women. J Gerontol A Biol Sci Med Sci 2006;61:628–33.

79. Rooney BL, Schauberger CW. Excess pregnancy weight gain and long-term obesity: one decade later. Obstet Gynecol 2002;100:245–52.

80. Rubino F, Forgione A, Cummings DE, et al. The mechanism of diabetes control after gastrointestinal bypass surgery reveals a role of the proximal small intestine in the pathophysiology of type 2 diabetes. Ann Surg 2006;244:741–9.

81. Sabeti PC, Varilly P, Fry B, et al. Genome-wide detection and characterization of positive selection in human populations. Nature 2007;449:913–8.

82. Schauer P, Chand B, Brethauer S. New applications for endoscopy: the emerging field of endoluminal and transgastric bariatric surgery. Surg Endosc 2007;21:347–56.

83. Schilling PL, Davis MM, Albanese CT, Dutta S, Morton MD. National trends in adolescent bariatric surgical procedures and implications for surgical centers of excellence. J Am Coll Surg 2008;206:1–12.

84. Scopinaro N, Gianetta E, Adami GF, et al. Biliopancreatic diversion for obesity at eighteen years. Surgery 1996;119:261–8.

85. Seehra H, MacDermott N, Lascelles R, et al. Lesson of the week: Wernicke's encephalopathy after vertical banded gastroplasty for morbid obesity. Br Med J 1996;312:434.

86. Shanley DP, Sear R, Mace R, Kirkwood TBL. Testing evolutionary theories of menopause. Proc R Soc B 2007;274:2943–9.

87. Sjöström L, Lindroos AK, Peltonen M, et al. Lifestyle, diabetes, and cardiovascular risk factors 10 years after bariatric surgery. N Engl J Med 2004;351:2683–93.

88. Sjöström L, Narbro K, Sjöström CD, et al. Effects of bariatric surgery on mortality in Swedish obese subjects. N Engl J Med 2007;357:741–52.

89. Sjöström L, Narbro K, Sjöström CD, et al. Swedish Obese Subjects Study. Effects of bariatric surgery on mortality in Swedish obese subjects. N Engl J Med 2007;357:741–52.

90. Srinivasan M, Patel MS. Metabolic programming in the immediate postnatal period. Trends Endocrinol Metab 2007;19:146–52.

91. St Peter SD, Craft RO, Tiede JL, Swain JM. Impact of advanced age on weight loss and health benefits after laparoscopic gastric bypass. Arch Surg 2005;140:165–8.

92. Stettler N, Zemel BS, Kumanyika S, Stallings VA. Infant weight gain and childhood overweight status in a multicenter, cohort study. Pediatrics 2002;109:194–9.

93. Sugerman HJ, DeMaria EJ, Kellum JM, et al. Effects of bariatric surgery in older patients. Ann Surg 2004;240:243–7.

94. Taylor C, Layani L. Laparoscopic adjustable gastric banding in patients > or = 60 years old: is it worthwhile? Obes Surg. 2006;16:1579–83.

95. The NHS Information Centre. See http://www.ic.nhs.uk/.

96. van Baal PHM, Polder JJ, de Wit GA, et al. Lifetime medical costs of obesity: prevention no cure for increasing health expenditure. PloS Med 2008;5:e29.

97. Vincent RP, Ashrafian H, le Roux CW. Mechanisms of disease: the role of gastrointestinal hormones in appetite and obesity. Nat Clin Pract Gastroenterol Hepatol 2008;5:268–77.

98. Whitmer RA, Gustafson DR, Barrett-Connor E, et al. Central obesity and increased risk of dementia more than three decades later. Neurology 2008:Epub 26 March 2008 (doi:10.1212/01.wnl.0000306313.89165.ef)

99. Zaninotto P, Wardle H, Stamatakis E, et al. Forecasting Obesity to 2010. See http://www.dh.gov.uk/en/ Publicationsandstatistics/ Publications/PublicationsStatistics/ DH_4138630 (last accessed 3 June 2008).

Section Six

44 Complications of Minimal Access Surgery

INTRODUCTION

Initial development of "Minimal Access Surgery" began in the animal lab and was later studied in select academic centers. It was imported to the community hospitals only when its benefits and safety were established. The development of laparoscopic cholecystectomy was not designed to enhance the safety of the procedure, but rather to reduce the discomfort associated with the surgical incision. The fierce economical competition in medicine fueled by the managed care movement, led to the rapid adoption of laparoscopic surgery among surgeons and gynecologist in community hospitals who were not formally trained in this technique and acquired their knowledge by subscribing to short courses.

Low complication rates were reported by centers specializing in laparoscopic surgery, mostly in academic centers. These centers were able to reduce the complication rate to minimum by developing proficiency in this surgery. Regrettably many inexperienced surgeons perform this technique with insufficient training and are responsible for the majority of complications seen during the performance of laparoscopic surgery.

Physicians who performed less than 100 such procedures reported 14.7 complications per 1000 patients. In contrast experienced surgeon reported a complication rate of only 3.8 complications per 1000 procedures. The Southern Surgeons Club Survey reported that the incidence of bile duct injury was 2.2% when the surgeon had previously performed less than 13 procedures. As surgeons gained experience the incidence of bile duct injury dropped to 0.1% afterwards.

ANESTHETIC AND MEDICAL COMPLICATIONS IN LAPAROSCOPY

Although all types of anesthesia involve some risk, major side effects and complications from anesthesia in laparoscopy are uncommon. Anesthetic complications include those that are more common in association with laparoscopic surgery as well as those that can occur in any procedure requiring general anesthetics. One-third of the deaths associated, with minor laparoscopic procedures such as sterilization or diagnostic laparoscopy are secondary to complication of anesthesia.

Among the potential complications of all general anesthetics are:

- Hypoventilation
- Esophageal intubation
- Gastroesophageal reflux
- Bronchospasm
- Hypotension
- Narcotic overdose
- Cardiac arrhythmias
- Cardiac arrest.

Laparoscopy results in multiple postoperative benefits including fewer traumas, less pain, less pulmonary dysfunction quicker recovery and shorter hospital stay. These advantages are regularly emphasized and explained. With increasing success of laparoscopy, it is now proposed for many surgical procedures. Intraoperative cardiorespiratory changes occur during pneumoperitoneum $PaCO_2$ increases due to CO_2 absorption form peritoneal cavity. Laparoscopy poses a number of inherent features that can enhance some of these risks. For example, the Trendelenburg's position, in combination with the increased intraperitoneal pressure provided by pneumoperitoneum by CO_2, exerts greater pressure on the diaphragm, potentiating hypoventilation, resulting hypercarbia, and metabolic acidosis. This position, combined with anesthetic agents that act as muscle relaxant opens the esophageal sphincter, facilitates regurgitation of gastric content, which, in turn, often leads to aspiration and its attendant complications of bronchospasm, pneumonitis, and pneumonia. Intraoperative aspiration pneumonia is very common in Laparoscopy but postoperative pneumonia is common after open surgery.

Various parameters of cardiopulmonary function associated with CO_2 insufflation include reduced PaO_2, O_2 saturation, tidal volume and minute ventilation, as well as an increased respiratory rate. The use of intraperitoneal CO_2 as a distension medium is associated with an increase in $PaCO_2$ and a decrease in pH. Increased abdominal pressure and elevation of the diaphragm may be associated with basilar atelectasis, which can result into right-to-left shunt and a ventilation perfusion mismatch.

Although during laparoscopy the patient's anesthetic care is in the hands of the anesthesiologist, it is important for the laparoscopic surgeon to understand the prevention and management of anesthetic complications by proper knowledge of risk involved with pneumoperitoneum.

Carbon Dioxide Embolism

Several case reports and experimental data suggest that the first finding during a carbon dioxide embolism may be a rapid increase in end-tidal carbon dioxide tension as some of the carbon dioxide injected into the vascular system is excreted into the lungs. As more gas is injected a vapor lock is formed in portions of the lungs. Areas of the lung are ventilated but not perfused (i.e. become dead space), and the end-tidal carbon dioxide rapidly falls. In contrast, during an air embolism the end-tidal carbon dioxide tension falls immediately. Other findings of a massive carbon dioxide embolism include a harsh, mill wheel murmur, a marked decrease in blood pressure and a decrease in hemoglobin-oxygen saturation. In minimal access surgery the use of CO_2 was started just to minimize the risk of CO_2 embolism. Carbon dioxide is the most widely used peritoneal distension medium. Part of the reason for this selection is the ready

absorption of CO_2 in blood. It is 20 times more absorbable than room air; consequently, the vast majority of frequent microemboli that do occur are absorbed, usually by the splanchnic vascular system, quickly and without any incident. However, if large amounts of CO_2 gain access to the central venous circulation, if there is peripheral vasoconstriction, or if the splanchnic blood flow is decreased by excessively high intraperitoneal pressure, severe cardiorespiratory compromise may result. The reported incidence of death due to CO_2 embolism is not clearly and authentically mentioned in any of the published article but it is assumed to be 1:10,000.

Diagnosis of CO_2 Embolism

CO_2 embolism is difficult to diagnose clinically. Among the presenting signs of CO_2 embolus are sudden, otherwise unexplained hypotension, cardiac arrhythmia, cyanosis and the development of the classical "mill-wheel" or "water-wheel" heart murmur. The end tidal CO_2 may increase and findings consistent with pulmonary edema may manifest. Accelerating pulmonary hypertension may also occur, resulting in right- sided heart failure.

Prevention of CO_2 Embolism

Because gas embolism may occur as a result of direct intravascular injection via an insufflation needle, the surgeon should ensure that blood is not emanating from the needle prior to the initiation of insufflation. Gynecologic surgeons can uniformly reduce the risk of CO_2 embolus by operating in an environment where the intraperitoneal pressure is maintained at less than 20 mm Hg. In most instances, excepting the initial placement of trocar in an insufflated peritoneum, the surgeon should be able to function comfortably with the intraperitoneal pressure between 8 and 12 mm Hg, maximum 15 mm Hg. Such pressures may also provide protection from many of the other adverse cardiopulmonary events. The risk of CO_2 embolus is also reduced by the meticulous maintenance of hemostasis, and avoiding open venous channels which is the portal of entry for gas into the systemic circulation. Another option in high-risk patient is the use of "gasless" or "apneumic" laparoscopy, where extra or intraperitoneal abdominal lifting mechanisms are used to create a working space for the laparoscopic surgeon. However, limitations of these devices have, to date,

Section Six

precluded their wide acceptance by most of the surgeons.

The anesthesiologist should continuously monitor the patient's skin colors, blood pressure, heart sounds, electrocardiogram, and end-tidal CO_2 so that the signs of CO_2 embolus are recognized early and can be managed.

Management of CO_2 Embolism

If a carbon dioxide embolism should occur:
1. The patient should receive on 100 percent oxygen.
2. Insufflation should be stopped and the abdomen decompressed.
3. The patient should be placed with the right side elevated in the Trendelenburg's position to avoid further entrapment of carbon dioxide in the pulmonary vasculature.
4. A central venous catheter, if placed rapidly, may allow aspiration of carbon dioxide.
5. Full inotropic support should be instituted.

Cardiopulmonary bypass may be required to evacuate the gas lock and help remove the carbon dioxide.

If CO_2 embolus is suspected or diagnosed, the operating room team must act quickly. The surgeon must evacuate CO_2 from the peritoneal cavity and should place the patient in the Durant, or left lateral decubitus position, with the head below the level of the right atrium. A large bore central venous line should be immediately established to allow aspiration of gas from the heart. Because the findings are nonspecific, other causes of cardiovascular collapse should be considered.

Periodically gases other than carbon dioxide are investigated for use for laparoscopy. Argon, air, helium and nitrous oxide have all been used in an attempt to eliminate the problems associated with hypercarbia and peritoneal irritation seen with carbon dioxide. The lack of solubility of air, helium, and argon effectively prevents hypercarbia that occurs with insufflation with carbon dioxide, but increases the lethality many fold if gas embolism occurs. Deaths from argon gas embolism, when the argon beam coagulator has been used during laparoscopy, suggests that this concern is real. Nitrous oxide has solubility similar to that of carbon dioxide, but unfortunately it can support combustion. Explosions when electrocautery was used following insufflation with nitrous oxide have occurred. An intra-abdominal fire when carbon dioxide was intended to be used for insufflation has also been reported.

Cardiovascular Complications

Laparoscopic surgery requires the insufflation of CO_2 into the abdominal cavity. Complications associated with CO_2 insufflation include:
1. Escape of CO_2 into the heart or pleural cavity.
2. Effects of the resultant increased intra-abdominal pressure on cardiac, renal and liver physiology.
3. Effects of the absorbed CO_2 on cardiorespiratory function.

The fatal complication of CO_2 embolization to the heart and lung were discussed earlier. CO_2 is insufflated under 12-15 mm Hg pressure to elevate the abdominal wall and allow the camera the necessary distance to the organ operated on. Depending on the intra-abdominal pressure used and the position the patient is placed - head up or head down - several potential harmful physiologic derangements may occur.

Cardiac arrhythmias occur relatively frequently during the performance of laparoscopic surgery and are related to a number of factors, the most significant of which is hypercarbia and the resulting acidemia. Early reports of laparoscopy associated arrhythmia were in association with spontaneous respiration. Consequently, most anesthesiologists have adopted the universal practice of mechanical ventilation during laparoscopic surgery. There are also a number of pharmacological considerations that lead the anesthesiologist to select agents that limit the risk of cardiac arrhythmia. The surgeon may aid in reducing the incidence of hypercarbia by operating with intraperitoneal pressures that are less than 15 mm Hg.

The use of an alternate intraperitoneal gas is another method by which the risk of cardiac arrhythmia may be reduced. However, while nitrous oxide is associated with a decreased incidence of arrhythmia, it increases the severity of shoulder tip pain, and, more importantly, is insoluble in blood. External lifting systems (apneumic laparoscopy) are another option that can provide protection against cardiac arrhythmia.

Hypotension can also occur secondary to excessively increased intraperitoneal pressure resulting in decreased venous return, and resulting decreased cardiac output. This undesirable result may be potentiated if the patient is volume depleted. Hypotension secondary to cardiac arrhythmias may also be a consequence of vagal discharge in response to increased intraperitoneal pressure. All of these side effects will be more dangerous for the patient with pre-existing cardiovascular compromise.

Gastric Reflux During Laparoscopy

Patients undergoing laparoscopy are usually considered at high risk of acid aspiration syndrome due to gastric regurgitation which might occur due to the rise in intragastric pressure consequent to the increased IAP. However, during pneumoperitoneum, the lower esophageal sphincter tone far exceeds the intragastric pressure and the raised barrier pressure limits the incidence of regurgitation.

Many study aimed to evaluate whether or not the use of intermittent positive pressure ventilation via the laryngeal mask airway is associated with a higher risk of gastroesophageal reflux when compared with intermittent positive pressure ventilation via a tracheal tube in patients undergoing day case gynecological laparoscopy in the head-down position.

Generally gastric regurgitation and aspiration are complications potentiated by laparoscopic surgery. Some patients are at increased risk, including those with obesity, gastroparesis, hiatal hernia or any type of gastric outlet obstruction. In such patients, it is important to quickly secure the airway with a cuffed endotracheal tube and to routinely decompress the stomach with a nasogastric or orogastric tube. The surgeon can contribute to aspiration prophylaxis by operating at the lowest necessary intraperitoneal pressure. Patients should be taken out of the Trendelenburg's position prior to being extubated. The adverse effects of aspiration may be minimized with the routine preoperative administration of metclopramide, H2 blockers, and nonparticulate antacids.

Extraperitoneal Gas

During laparoscopic surgery a number of the complications associated with pneumoperitoneum or its achievement are described in the vascular, gastroenterologic, urologic, and anesthetic sections. However, the problem of extraperitoneal placement or extravasation of gas has not been considered. In some instances, this complication occurs as a result of deficient technique (incorrect placement of insufflation needles; excessive intraperitoneal pressure); while in others the extravasation is related to gas tracking around the ports or along the dissection planes themselves.

Subcutaneous emphysema may occur if the tip of the Veress needle does not penetrate the peritoneal cavity prior to insufflation of gas. The gas may accumulate in the subcutaneous tissue or between the fascia and the peritoneum. Extraperitoneal insufflation, which is associated with higher levels of CO_2 absorption than intraperitoneal insufflation, is reflected by a sudden rise in the EtCO$_2$, excessive changes in airway pressure and respiratory acidosis.

Subcutaneous emphysema most commonly results from preperitoneal placement of an insufflation needle or leakage of CO_2 around the cannula sites, the latter frequently because of excessive intraperitoneal pressure. The condition is usually mild and limited to the abdominal wall. However, subcutaneous emphysema can become extensive, involving the extremities, the neck, and the mediastinum. Another relatively common location for emphysema is the omentum or mesentery, a circumstance that the surgeon may mistake for preperitoneal insufflation.

Diagnosis

Usually the diagnosis will not be a surprise, for the surgeon will have had difficulty in positioning the primary cannula within the peritoneal cavity. Subcutaneous emphysema may be readily identified by the palpation of crepitus, usually in the abdominal wall. In some instances, it can extend along contiguous fascial planes to the neck, where it can be visualized directly. Such a finding may reflect the development of mediastinal emphysema. If mediastinal emphysema is severe, or if pneumothorax is developing, the anesthesiologist may report difficulty in maintaining a normal pCO$_2$, a feature that may indicate impending cardiovascular collapse.

Prevention

The risk of subcutaneous emphysema during laparoscopic surgery is reduced by proper positioning of an insufflation needle. Prior to insertion, it is important to check the insufflation needle for proper function and patency and to establish the baseline flow pressure by attaching it to the insufflation apparatus. The best position for insertion is at the base of the umbilicus, where the abdominal wall is the thinnest. The angle of insertion varies from 45° to near 90°, depending upon the patient's weight, the previous abdominal surgery and type of anesthesia as described in the section on prevention of vascular injuries. The insertion action should be smooth and firm until the surgeon, observing and listening to the device passing through the layers-two (fascia and peritoneum) in the umbilicus and three (two layers of fascia; one peritoneum) in the left upper quadrant feels that placement is intraperitoneal.

No one test is absolutely reliable at predicting intraperitoneal placement. Instead, a number of tests should be used. Of course, aspiration of the insufflation needle should precede all other evaluations. Two tests depend upon the preinflation intraperitoneal pressure. If a drop of water is placed on the open end of the insufflation needle, it should be drawn into the low-pressure intraperitoneal environment of the peritoneal cavity. Although some disagree, the elevation of the anterior abdominal wall is a reasonable way of creating a negative intraperitoneal pressure. Perhaps a more quantitative way of demonstrating the same principle is to attach the tubing to the needle after insertion but prior to initiating the flow of gas. Elevation of the abdominal wall should result in creation of a low or negative intraperitoneal pressure (1 to 4 mm Hg). Insufflation should be initiated at a low flow rate of about 1 liter per minute until the surgeon has confidence that proper placement has been achieved. Loss of liver dullness should occur when about 500 ml of gas has entered the peritoneal cavity. The measured intraperitoneal pressure should be below 10 mm Hg but up to14 mm Hg if the patient is obese. Abdominal distension should be symmetrical. If, at any time, the surgeon feels that, the needle is not located intraperitoneally, it should be withdrawn and reinserted. Once the peritoneal cavity has been insufflated with an adequate volume of gas, the primary trocar is introduced. The laparoscope is introduced, and, if the cannula is satisfactorily located the tubing is attached to the appropriate port.

The risk of subcutaneous emphysema may be reduced by maintaining a low intraperitoneal pressure following the placement of the desired cannulas Operate below 15 mm Hg and usually work at about 10 mm Hg. Although primary blind insertion of sharp trocar has been demonstrated to be as safe as secondary insertion following pneumoinsufflation, the relative incidence of subcutaneous emphysema is unknown.

Management

Subcutaneous emphysema often presents a management dilemma. Rarely, subcutaneous emphysema has pathophysiologic consequences. More often, it is extremely uncomfortable for the patient, and is often disfiguring and alarming for patients and family. When subcutaneous emphysema is severe, physicians may feel compelled to treat it, but the currently described techniques are often invasive or ineffective.

If the surgeon finds that the insufflation has occurred extraperitoneally, there exist a number of management options. While removing the laparoscope and repeating the insufflation is possible, it may be made more difficult because of the new configuration of the anterior peritoneum. Open laparoscopy or the use of an alternate sites such as the left upper quadrant should be considered. One attractive approach is to leave the laparoscope in the expanded preperitoneal space while the insufflation needle is reinserted through the peritoneal membrane, caudal to the tip of the laparoscope under direct vision.

For mild cases of subcutaneous emphysema, no specific intra-or postoperative therapy is required, as the findings, in at least mild cases, quickly resolves following evacuation of the pneumoperitoneum. When the extravasation extends to involve the neck, it is usually preferable to terminate the procedure, as pneumomediastinum, pneumothorax, hypercarbia and cardiovascular collapse may result. Following the end of the procedure it is prudent to obtain a chest X-ray. The patient should be managed expectantly unless a tension pneumothorax results, when immediate evacuation must be performed, using a chest tube or a wide bore needle (14-16 gauge) inserted in the second intercostal space in midclavicular line.

Electrosurgical Complications

Unlike open surgery where hemostasis (control of bleeding) is accomplished by pressure and careful application of fine clamps and ligatures, laparoscopic surgery must rely on electrosurgery to achieve hemostasis. Excessive use of energy can burn a hole in the wall of the organ involved. Current can also cause injury to adjacent organs, and even distant organs. Complications of electrosurgery occur secondary to thermal injury from one of three basic causes. The first is thermal trauma from unintended or inappropriate use of the active electrode(s). The second from current diverting to another, undesirable path, causing injury remote from the immediate operative field. Third is injury at the site of the "return" or dispersive electrode. Active electrode injury can occur with either unipolar or bipolar instruments, while trauma secondary to current diversion or dispersive electrode accidents only occurs with the unipolar technique. Complications of electrosurgery are reduced with strict adherence to safety protocols coupled with a sound understanding of the circumstances that can lead to undesirable effects on tissue.

Active Electrode Trauma

Unintended activation in open space without touching the tissue is one of the more common mechanisms by which the active electrode causes complications. Such a complication frequently occurs when an electrode, left untended within the peritoneal cavity, is inadvertently activated by compression of the hand switch or depression of the foot pedal. Control of the electrosurgical unit or generator (ESU) by someone other than the operating surgeon is also a source of accidental activation of the electrode.

Direct extension is another mechanism by which the active electrode(s) cause complications. The zone of vaporization or coagulation may extend to involve large blood vessels or vital structures such as the bladder, ureter, or bowel. Bipolar current reduces, but does not eliminate, the risk of thermal injury to adjacent tissue. Consequently, care must be taken to isolate blood vessels prior to desiccation, especially when near vital structures, and to apply appropriate amounts of energy in a fashion that allows an adequate margin of non-injured tissue.

Diagnosis

During minimal access surgery the diagnosis of direct thermal visceral injury may be suspected or confirmed intraoperatively. Careful evaluation of nearby intraperitoneal structures should be made if unintended activation of the electrode occurs. The visual appearance will depend upon a number of factors including the type of the electrode, its proximity to tissue, the output of the generator, and the duration of its activation. High power density activations will often result in vaporization injury, and will be more easily recognized than lower power density lesions that result in desiccation and coagulation.

The diagnosis of visceral thermal injury is often delayed until the signs and symptoms of fistula or peritonitis present. This will be particularly true with desiccation injury. Because these complications may not present until two to at least ten days following surgery, long after discharge, both the patient and the physician must be made aware of the possible consequences. Consequently, patients should be advised to report any fever or increasing abdominal pain experienced postoperatively.

Prevention

Electrosurgical injuries are largely prevented if, (a) the surgeon is always in direct control of electrode activation, and (b) all electrosurgical hand instruments are removed from the peritoneal cavity when not in use. When removed from the peritoneal cavity, the instruments should be detached from the electrosurgical generator or they should be stored in an insulated pouch near to the operative field. These measures prevent damage to the patient's skin if the foot pedal is accidentally depressed.

Management

Once diagnosed thermal injury to bowel, bladder, or ureter, recognized at the time of laparoscopy, should immediately be managed appropriately, considering the potential extent of the zone of coagulative necrosis. The extent of thermal trauma will depend upon the characteristics of the energy transferred to tissue. An electrosurgical incision made with the focused energy from a pointed electrode will be associated with a minimal amount of surrounding thermal injury, and may be repaired in a fashion identical to one created mechanically. However, with desiccation injury created as a result of prolonged contact with a relatively large caliber electrode, the thermal necrosis may extend centimeters from the point of contact. In such instances, wide excision or resection will be necessary.

Remote Injury

Remote injury due to current diversion can occur when an electrical current finds a direct path out of the patient's body via grounded sites other than the dispersive electrode. Alternatively, the current can be diverted directly to other tissue before it reaches the tip of the active electrode. In either instance, if the power density becomes high enough, unintended and severe thermal injury can result. These injuries can only occur with ground-referenced ESUs because they lack an isolated circuit. In such generators, when the dispersive electrode becomes detached, unplugged, or otherwise ineffective, the current will seek any grounded conductor. If the conductor has a small surface area, the current or power density may become high enough to cause thermal injury. Examples include electrocardiograph patch electrodes or the conductive metal components of the operating table.

Modem ESUs are designed and built with isolated circuits and impedance monitoring systems or active electrode monitoring system. Consequently, if any part of the circuit is broken, an alarm sounds, and/or the machine "shuts down," thereby preventing electrode activation. Since the widespread introduction of such generators, the incidence of burns to alternate sites has become largely confined to cases involving the few remaining ground referenced machines.

Insulation Failure

Failure in the insulation coating the shaft of a laparoscopic electrosurgical electrode can allow current diversion to adjacent tissue. The high power density resulting from such small points of contact fosters the creation of a significant injury. During laparoscopic surgery, bowel is frequently the tissue near to, or in contact with, the shaft of the electrode, making it the organ most susceptible to this type of electrosurgical injury. The fact that the whole shaft of the electrode is frequently not encompassed by the surgeon's visual field at laparoscopy makes it possible that such an injury can occur unaware to the operator.

Prevention of complication of insulation failure starts with the selection and care of electrosurgical hand instruments. Loose instrument bins should be replaced with containers designed to keep the instruments from damaging each other. The instruments should be examined prior to each case, searching for worn or obviously defective insulation. When found, the damaged instrument should be removed and repaired or replaced. Despite all efforts, unobserved breaks in insulation may rarely occur. While the use of disposable instruments is often claimed as a way of reducing the incidence of insulation failure, there is no guarantee that this is the case, as invisible defects may occur in the manufacturing process. Furthermore, the insulation on disposable electrodes is thinner and more susceptible to trauma. Consequently, when applying unipolar electrical energy, the shaft of the instrument should be kept free of vital structures and, if possible, totally visible in the operative field.

Direct Coupling

During minimal access surgery direct coupling occurs when an activated electrode touches and energizes another metal conductor such as a laparoscope, cannula or other instrument. If the conductor is near to, or in contact with, other tissue, a thermal injury can result. Such accidents often happen following unintentional activation of an electrode. Prevention of direct coupling is facilitated by removal of the electrodes when not in use and visually- confirming that the electrode is not in inappropriate contact with other conductive instruments prior to activation.

Capacitive Coupling

Many capacitive coupling of diathermy current have been reported as causes of occult injury during surgical laparoscopy. Capacitance reflects the ability of a conductor to establish an electrical current in an unconnected but nearby circuit. An electrical field is established around the shaft of any activated laparoscopic unipolar electrode, a circumstance that makes the electrode a capacitor. This field is harmless if the circuit is completed via a dispersive, low power density pathway. If capacitive coupling occurs between the laparoscopic electrode and a metal cannula positioned in the abdominal wall, the current without any complication returns to the abdominal wall where it traverses to the dispersive electrode. However, if the metal cannula is anchored to the skin by a nonconductive plastic retaining sleeve, or anchor (a hybrid system), the current will not return to the abdominal wall because the sleeve acts as an insulator. Instead, the capacitor will have to search elsewhere to complete the circuit. Consequently, bowel; or any other nearby conductor, can become the target of a relatively high power density discharge. The risk is greater with high voltage currents, such as the coagulation output on an electrosurgical generator. This mechanism is also more likely to occur when a unipolar electrode is inserted through an operating laparoscope that, in turn, is passed through a plastic laparoscopic port. In this configuration, the plastic port acts as the insulator. If the electrode capacitively couples with the metal laparoscope, nearby bowel will be at risk for significant thermal injury.

During minimal access surgery prevention of capacitive coupling can largely be accomplished by avoiding the use of hybrid laparoscope cannula systems that contain a mixture of conductive and nonconductive elements. Instead, it is preferred that all plastic or all-metal cannula systems be used. When and if operating laparoscopes are employed, all metal cannula systems should be the rule unless there is no intent to perform unipolar electrosurgical procedures through the operating channel.

Risk of this injury is very much minimized if low voltage radio-frequency current (cutting) is used, and when the high voltage outputs are avoided.

Dispersive Electrode Burns

The use of isolated circuit generators with return electrode monitors has all but eliminated dispersive electrode related thermal injury. Return electrode monitoring (REM) is actually accomplished by measuring the impedance (sometimes called resistance) in the dispersive electrode, which should always be low because of the large surface area. To accomplish this, most return electrode monitors, actually are divided into two electrodes, allowing the generator to compare the impedance from the two sides of the pad. If the overall impedance is high, or if there is a significant difference between the two sides, as is the case with partial detachment, the active electrode cannot be activated. Without such devices, partial detachment of the patient pad could result in a thermal injury because reducing the surface area of the electrode raises the current density. It is important for the surgeon to establish what type of ESU is being used in each case. Absence of a REM system is a reason for increased scrutiny of the positioning of the dispersive electrode, both before the surgery begins, and as the operation progresses.

Electrode Shields and Monitors

A United States-based company, (Electroscope Inc.) markets a system that helps to reduce further the chance of direct or capacitive coupling. A reusable shield is passed over the shaft of the laparoscopic electrode prior to its insertion into the peritoneal cavity. This shield protects against insulation failure and detects the presence of significant capacitance. Should an insulation break occur, or when capacitance becomes threatening, the integrated monitoring system automatically shuts down the generator. The shield enlarges the effective diameter of the electrode by about 2 mm, making it necessary to use larger caliber laparoscopic ports.

Despite perceptions to the contrary, electrosurgery has been rendered a safe modality for use in surgical procedures. However, safe and effective application of electrical energy requires an adequate understanding and implementation of basic principles as well as the availability of modern electrosurgical generators and appropriate education of medical and support staff. Care and prudence must be exercised when utilizing electricity within the peritoneal cavity. The zone of significant thermal injury usually extends beyond that of the visible injury, a feature that must be borne in mind when operating in close proximity to vital structures such as bowel bladder, ureter, and large and important blood vessels. It is equally important to impart the minimal amount of thermal injury (if any) necessary to accomplish the task at hand, even around nonvital structures, by using the ideal power output and the appropriate active electrodes.

HEMORRHAGIC COMPLICATIONS

Hemorrhagic complications may occur as a consequence of entry into the peritoneal cavity or as a result of trauma incurred to blood vessels encountered during the course of the procedure.

Hemorrhage Associated with Access Technique

Great Vessel Injury

During access the most dangerous hemorrhagic complications of entry are to the great vessels, including the aorta and vena cava as well as the common iliac vessels and their branches, the internal and external iliac arteries and veins. The incidence of major vascular injury is probably under reported, but has been estimated to range widely from 0.93 to 9 per 10,000 cases. The trauma most often occurs secondary to insertion of an insufflation needle, but may be created by the tip of the trocar. However, not uncommonly, the injury is associated with the insertion of ancillary laparoscopic ports into the lower quadrants. The vessels most frequently damaged are the aorta and the right common iliac artery, which branches from the aorta in the midline. The anatomically more posterior location of the vena cava and the iliac veins provides relative protection, but not immunity, from injury. While most of these injuries are small amenable to repair with suture, some have been larger, requiring ligation with or without the insertion of a vascular graft. Not surprisingly, death has been reported in a number of instances.

Diagnosis

If great vessels are injured most often the problem presents as profound hypotension with or without the appearance of a significant volume of blood within the peritoneal cavity. In some instances, the surgeon aspirates blood via the insufflation needle, prior to introduction of distension gas. Frequently, the bleeding may be contained in the retroperitoneal space, a feature that usually delays the diagnosis. Consequently, the development of hypovolemic shock in the recovery room may well be secondary to otherwise unrecognized laceration to a great vessel. To avoid the late recognition, it is important to evaluate the course of each great vessel prior to completing the procedure.

Prevention

There are a number of ways by which the incidence of large vessel trauma can be minimized. Certainly it is essential that the positioning of ancillary or secondary trocar in the lower quadrants be performed under direct vision. This is more difficult for the primary cannula. It has been suggested that the use of "open laparoscopy" for the initial port entirely avoids the issue of great vessel injury secondary to insufflation needles and trocars. However, open laparoscopy has its own potential drawbacks such as increased operating time, the need for larger incisions, and a greater chance of wound infection, all without eliminating the incidence of bowel injury at entry.

The risk of large vessel injury should be reduced if careful attention is paid to access technique and equipments used. If used, both insufflation needles and the trocar should be kept sharp and surgeon should use same instrument each time. The safety sheath of the insufflation needle should be checked to ensure that both the spring and the sliding mechanism are functioning normally. Many disposable trocar-cannula systems are constructed with a safety mechanism that covers or retracts the trocar following passage through the fascia and peritoneum. However, there are currently no available data that demonstrate a reduction in the incidence of major vessel injury with the use of these devices.

The application of appropriate technique is based upon a sound understanding of the normal anatomic relationships between the commonly used entry points and the great vessels. A "safety zone" exists inferior to the sacral promontory in the area bounded superiorly by the bifurcation of the aorta, posteriorly by the sacral curve, and laterally by the iliac vessels. Safe insertion of the insufflation needle mandates that the instrument be maintained in a midline, sagittal plane while the operator directs the tip between the iliac vessels, anterior to the sacrum but inferior to the bifurcation of the aorta and the proximal aspect of the vena cava. Such positioning requires elevation of the abdominal wall while angling the insufflation needle about 45° to horizontal. The tactile and visual feedback created when the needle passes through the fascial and peritoneal layers of the abdominal wall, if recognized and heeded, may prevent overaggressive insertion attempts. Such proprioceptive feedback is diminished with disposable needles as compared to the classic Veress model. Instead, the surgeon must listen to the "clicks" as the needle obturator retracts when it passes through the rectus fascia and the peritoneum. The needle should never be forced.

It is critical to note that these anatomic relationships may vary with body type and with the orientation of the patient to the horizontal position. In women of normal weight and body habitus, in the horizontal recumbent position, the bifurcation of the aorta is located immediately beneath the umbilicus. However, in obese individuals the umbilicus may be positioned up to 2 or more cm below bifurcation. Fortunately, this circumstance allows the insufflation needle to be directed in a more vertical position-those between 160 to 200 pounds between 45° and 90°, while those women over 200 pounds at nearly 90°. Women placed in a head down position (Trendelenburg's position); will shift their great vessel more superiorly and anteriorly in a fashion that may make them more vulnerable to an entry injury. Consequently, positioning of the insufflation needle, and at least the initial trocar and cannula, should be accomplished with the patient in a horizontal position. This approach additionally facilitates the evaluation of the upper abdomen, an exercise that is limited if the intraperitoneal content is shifted cephalad by the patient's head down position.

The risk of great vessel injury is likely reduced by insufflating the peritoneal cavity to adequate pressure. An intraperitoneal pressure of 20 mm Hg, while not desirable for prolonged periods of time, can aid in separating the abdominal wall from the great vessels during the process of insertion of a sharp trocar.

Management

If blood is withdrawn from the insufflation needle, it should be left in place while immediate preparations are made to obtain blood products and perform laparotomy. If the diagnosis of hemoperitoneum is made upon initial visualization of the peritoneal cavity, a grasping instrument may be used, if possible, to temporarily occlude the vessel. While it is unlikely that significant injury can predictably be repaired by laparoscopically directed technique, if temporary hemostasis can be obtained, and the laceration visualized, selected, localized lesions can be repaired, with suture, under laparoscopic guidance. Such an attempt should not be made by any other than experienced and technically adept surgeons. Even if such an instance exists, fine judgment should be used so as not to delay the institution of life-saving, open surgical repair.

Most surgeons should gain immediate entry into the peritoneal cavity, and immediately compress the aorta and vena cava just below the level of the renal vessels, gaining at least temporary control of blood loss. At that juncture, the most appropriate course of action, including the need for vascular surgical consultation, will become more apparent.

Abdominal Wall Vessels

Most commonly injured abdominal wall vessels are the inferior epigastrics and superior epigastric vessel. They are invariably damaged by the initial passage of an ancillary trocar, or when a wider device is introduced later in the procedure. The problem may be recognized immediately by the observation of blood dripping along the cannula or out through the incision. However, it is not uncommon for the cannula itself to obstruct the bleeding until withdrawal at the end of the case.

More sinister, are injuries to the deep inferior epigastric vessels, branches of the external iliac artery and vein that also course cephalad but are deep to the rectus fascia and often deep to the muscles themselves. More laterally located are the deep circumflex iliac vessels that are uncommonly encountered in laparoscopic surgery. Laceration of these vessels may cause profound blood loss, particularly when the trauma is unrecognized and causes extraperitoneal bleeding.

Diagnosis

Diagnosis of abdominal wall vasculature injury is by visualization of the blood dripping down the cannula, or by the postoperative appearance of shock, abdominal wall discoloration, and/or a hematoma located near to the incision. In some instances, the blood may track to a more distant site, presenting as a pararectal or vulvar mass. Delayed diagnosis may be prevented at the end of the procedure by laparoscopically evaluating each peritoneal incision following removal of the cannula.

Prevention

With the help of telescope transillumination of the abdominal wall from within will, at least in most thin women, allow for identification of the superficial inferior epigastric vessels. However, the deep inferior epigastric vessels cannot be identified by this mechanism because of their location deep to the rectus sheath. Consequently, prevention of deep inferior epigastric vessel injury requires that the surgeon understand the anatomic course of these vessels.

The most consistent landmarks are the median umbilical ligaments (obliterated umbilical arteries) and the entry point of the round ligament into the inguinal canal. At the pubic crest, the deep inferior epigastric vessels begin their course cephalad between the medially located medial umbilical ligament and the laterally positioned exit point of the round ligament. The trocar should be inserted medial or lateral to the vessels, if they are visualized. If the vessels cannot be seen, and it is necessary to position the trocar laterally, it should be positioned 3-4 cm lateral to the median umbilical ligament, or lateral to the lateral margin of the rectus abdominis muscle. Too lateral an insertion will endanger the deep circumflex epigastric artery. The operator may further limit risk of injury by placing a No: 22 spinal needle though the skin at the desired location, directly observing the entry via the laparoscope. This not only provides more reassurance that a safe location has been identified, but the easily visualized peritoneal needle hole gives the surgeon a target for inserting the trocar with greater precision.

A common mistake is to fashion the incision appropriately, only to direct the trocar medially in its course through the abdominal wall, thereby injuring the vessels. Another factor that may contribute to the risk of injury is the use of large diameter trocar. Consequently, for this and other reasons, the surgeon should use the smallest trocar necessary for performance of the procedure.

Management

Superficial inferior epigastric artery lacerations usually respond to expectant management. Rotation of the cannula to a position where compression is possible is also helpful. Rarely is a suture necessary.

We have found that the use of a straight suture passer, is most useful for the ligation of lacerated deep inferior epigastric vessels. A number of other devices and techniques have been introduced that facilitate the accomplishment of this task. To summarize, the trocar and cannula are removed. Then, under laparoscopic visualization, and using a ligature carrier, a ligature is placed through the incision and directed laterally and inferiorly, where it is held by a grasping forceps. The ligature carrier is removed and subsequently passed through the incision again, without a suture, but this time medial and inferior to the lacerated vessels. The suture is threaded into the carrier from within the peritoneal cavity, and is then externalized and tied. For small incisions, narrower than the diameter of the surgeon's finger, the knot may be tightened with a knot manipulator.

There are other, less uniformly successful methods for attaining hemostasis from a lacerated deep inferior epigastric vessel. The most obvious is the placement of large, through-and-through mattress sutures. These are usually removed about 48 hours later. Electrodesiccation may be successful. Either a unipolar or bipolar grasping forceps is passed through another ancillary cannula taking care to identify, grasp, and adequately desiccate the vessel. Either continuous or "blended" current is used at appropriate power outputs for the machine and the electrode. Another method that has enjoyed some success is temporary

compression with the balloon of a Foley's catheter, passed through the incision into the peritoneal cavity, then secured and tightened externally with a clamp. While some suggest that the balloon should be left in place for 24 hours, the delicate channel may be damaged by the clamp, making it impossible to deflate the balloon. For this reason, we not recommend this option.

Intraperitoneal Vessel Injury

The bleeding may result from inadvertent entry into a vessel failure of a specific occlusive technique, or human error in the application of the selected technique. Furthermore, in addition to the problem of delayed hemorrhage inherent in transection of arteries, there may be further delay in diagnosis at laparoscopy because of the restricted visual field and the temporary occlusive pressure exerted by the CO_2 within the peritoneal cavity.

Diagnosis

During laparoscopy inadvertent division of an artery or vein will usually become immediately self-evident. However, in some instances, transected arteries will go into spasm only to begin bleeding minutes to hours later, an event that may temporarily go unnoticed due to the limited field of view presented by the laparoscope. Consequently, at the end of the procedure, all areas of dissection should be carefully examined. In addition, the CO_2 should be vented, decreasing the intraperitoneal pressure to about 5 mm Hg, allowing recognition of vessels occluded by the higher pressure.

Prevention

Attention to meticulous technique is at least as important in laparoscopically directed surgery as it is for open or vaginal cases. During dissection, vessels should be identified and occluded prior to division, a task made simpler by the magnification afforded by the laparoscope. If suture is used to occlude a vessel it must be, of the appropriate caliber, positioned with an adequate pedicle, and tied snugly with a secure knot. Electrosurgery if used should be applied in the appropriate waveform and power density and for a time adequate to allow for sufficient tissue desiccation. Clips should be of a size appropriate for the vessel and they must be applied in a secure fashion, also with an adequate pedicle of tissue. Care should be exercised to avoid manipulation of pedicles secured with clips or suture; as such trauma could adversely affect the security of the closure. When linear stapling devices are employed, the appropriate staple size should be selected and the tissue encompassed in the staple line should be of uniform thickness. Failure to maintain relatively uniform tissue thickness may result in inadequate compression of blood vessels that course through the thinner areas of the pedicle.

Management

Transected vessels should be secured immediately. If electrosurgical desiccation is used to maintain or achieve hemostasis, the use of a serial ammeter is useful to demonstrate the endpoint of energy application. There is evidence that artery larger in diameter than 3 mm are less reliably occluded with desiccation than are those 3 mm or less. Care must be exerted to avoid blind clamping and electrosurgical desiccation, even with bipolar instruments, especially when less than 1 cm from ureter or bowel. When a vessel is in such a location, it is usually preferable to secure it with a clip.

Identification of small vessel bleeding and ooze is often facilitated by the use of copious irrigation and even underwater examination. Capillary ooze may be managed with higher voltage fulguration currents using electrodes with a bulbous tip. When using electrosurgery for this purpose, the use of electrolyte-containing solutions should be avoided, as they disperse current, rendering the technique ineffective. Instead the low viscosity fluids like glycine are recommended as, in addition to being nonconductive, they may facilitate localization of the vessels.

GASTROINTESTINAL COMPLICATIONS

Following laparoscopy, it is not uncommon for the patient to experience nausea. However, in some instances the problem becomes severe. Gastrointestinal viscera potentially injured during the performance of gynecologic laparoscopy include the stomach, the small bowel, and the colon.

Insufflation Needle Injuries

Needle entry into the stomach almost invariably happens in the presence of gastric distension. While this may occur secondary to aerophagia, the complication is frequently related to difficult or improper intubation or to the use of mask induction with an inhalation anesthetic. Mechanical entry into large or small bowel may occur in any instance, but is up to 10 times more common when laparoscopy is performed on patients with previous intraperitoneal inflammation or abdominal surgery. In such instances, loops of intestine can adhere to the abdominal wall under the insertion site. Perforation may also occur following an overly aggressive attempt to insert the insufflation needle.

Recognition

Recognition of gastric entry by the insufflation needle may follow identification of any or all of the signs of extraperitoneal entry, including increased filling pressure, asymmetric distension of the peritoneal cavity, or the aspiration of gastric particulate matter through the lumen of the needle. However, the hollow, capacious nature of the stomach may allow the initial insufflation pressure to remain normal. Unfortunately, in some instances, the problem is not identified until the trocar is inserted and the gastric mucosa identified by direct vision. Recognition of bowel entry usually follows observation of the signs described above for gastric injury, with the addition of feculent odor to the list of findings. Prevention of insufflation needle injury to the gastrointestinal tract is important because such measures largely eliminate the risk of more sinister trocar trauma. Gastric perforation can largely be eliminated with the selective use of preoperative oral or nasogastric suction. The surgeon should request that this be performed if there has been difficulty with intubation or when the needle is intentionally inserted near to the stomach in the left upper quadrant.

Many have suggested that open laparoscopy is the most appropriate and effective way to reduce the incidence of intestinal injury in a patient at risk because of previous lower abdominal surgery. However, there are no studies that prove this to be the case. Indeed, there exists evidence that open laparoscopy is itself associated with intestinal injury. Consequently, many surgeons have suggested the use of left upper quadrant insertion with a properly decompressed stomach.

Although not strictly a prophylactic measure, the routine use of preoperative mechanical bowel preparation, at least in selected, high-risk cases, will

Section Six

diminish the need for laparotomy and/ or colostomy if large bowel entry occurs.

Management

The management of any trauma to the gastrointestinal tract depends in part upon the nature of the injury and in part upon the organ(s) involved. In general, insufflation needle punctures that have not resulted in a defect significantly larger than their diameter may be handled expectantly. Larger defects should be repaired or resected, by laparoscopic or a laparotomy based technique, depending upon extent of the lesion.

If, following insertion of an insufflation needle, particulate debris are identified, the needle should be left in place and an alternate insertion site identified, such as the left upper quadrant. If the insufflation needle possesses a removable obturator, a narrow caliber optical fiber or laparoscope may be passed to evaluate the location of the tip and to aid in later identification of the puncture site. Immediately following successful entry into the peritoneal cavity, the site of injury is identified. Unless significant injury or bleeding is identified, the situation may be handled expectantly. If there is unexpected extension of the laceration, it should be managed similarly to a trocar injury.

Trocar Injuries

During access technique damage caused by sharp trocar penetration is usually more serious than when needle injury occurs. Most often, the injury is created by the primary trocar because of its blind insertion. However, inadequate attention paid to the insertion of ancillary cannulas may also result in visceral injury.

Diagnosis

If a primary trocar penetrates bowel, the diagnosis is usually made when the surgeon visualizes the mucosal lining of the gastrointestinal structure following insertion of the laparoscope. If large bowel is entered, feculent odor may be noted. However, in some instances, the injury may not immediately be recognized as the cannula may not stay within, or it may pass through, the lumen and out the other side of the viscus. Such injuries usually occur when a single loop of bowel is adhered to the anterior abdominal wall near to the entry point. Consequently, it is important at the end of the procedure to directly view the removal of the

primary cannula, either through the cannula itself or via an ancillary port. Routine direct visualization of primary port incisional closure will facilitate the accomplishment of this task. Unfortunately, the injury may go unrecognized until it presents postoperatively as peritonitis, abscess, enterocutaneous fistula, or death.

Management

The following measures were reported to reduce the incidence of trocar injuries:

1. Disposable laparoscopes are usually sharper. They require less force to insert and thus there is less chance of compressing the trocar against the bowel or blood vessels.
2. Some manufacturers provide a plastic sheath which springs and cover the sharp edge of the trocar after insertion. Safety shields will not prevent injury, however, in case of bowel adhesions.
3. The use of ultrasound to "map" the abdominal wall for safe entry area is recommended especially when adhesions are present.
4. The smaller - 5 mm cannula - is safer as it requires less pressure to insert. Equipped with a camera it allows safe placement of the larger cannula under vision.
5. Hasson described an open surgical approach to placement of the cannula thus reducing the risk of perforation by the blind closed technique.
6. Before the conclusion of surgery, a thorough search for bowel injuries must be performed as delay in recognition of such injury can be catastrophic. Thus review of the video tapes can ascertain if safety measures were taken during this critical part of the procedure.

Despite the widespread use of retractable trocars or safety sheaths, injury to bowel or other structures may occur. As stated above, many employ, routinely or selectively, the concept of "open" laparoscopy, where the peritoneal cavity is entered directly via an intra-or intraumbilical incision. Despite the apparent virtues of this approach, bowel entry may still occur. An alternative approach, especially when entering an abdomen with previous laparotomy scars, is the insertion of a narrow caliber cannula in the left upper quadrant following decompression of the stomach. It is unusual for a patient to have had previous surgery in this location. Following placement of the cannula, usually just below the costal margin in the midclavicular line, a narrow diameter laparoscope may be passed, allowing a direct view of the abdominal wall under the umbilicus or other planned site of insertion. If necessary, the small laparoscope may be used to direct the dissection of intestine from under the insertion site. This approach gains additional value with the introduction of a fiber laparoscope small enough to fit through the lumen of an insufflation needle.

Stomach injuries most frequently occur when there has been difficulty in intubation, and may be more common following left upper quadrant insertion if the stomach has not previously been decompressed. Consequently, liberal use of oral or nasogastric decompression will likely reduce the incidence of trocar injury to the stomach.

Most common cause of bowel injuries usually is when the intestine is adherent to the abdominal wall under the site of trocar insertion. Adherence is usually secondary to previous surgery. Consequently, in such patients open laparoscopy or left upper quadrant entry may be used. Preoperative mechanical bowel preparation should be employed in high-risk patients to facilitate repair of colonic defects without the need to perform a laparotomy.

Management

Trocar injuries to bowel require repair. If it can be ascertained that the injury is isolated, and if the operator is capable, the lesion may be sutured under laparoscopic guidance with a double layer of running 2-0 or 3-0 synthetic absorbable suture. Extensive lesions may require resection and reanastomosis. In well trained and experienced hand, this may be performed under laparoscopic direction. However, in most instances, laparotomy will be required. Regardless of the method of repair, copious irrigation should be employed and the patient admitted for postoperative observation. The patient is kept without oral intake and nasogastric decompression should be liberally used at the discretion of the surgeon. If the injury is to the sigmoid colon, primary repair may be attempted if the bowel has been mechanically prepared preoperatively. Otherwise, colostomy should be considered, with the possible exception of ascending colon lesions. If uncertainty exists regarding the extent of injury, laparotomy is always indicated.

INJURY TO BLADDER

Laparoscopy associated damage to the bladder or ureter may occur secondary to mechanical or thermal trauma. Vesical injury is often secondary to a trocar entering the undrained bladder, but may also occur during dissection of the bladder, either from other adhered structures or from the anterior aspect of the uterus. The proliferation of laparoscopically directed retropubic suspension for urinary incontinence will likely be associated with bladder injury. Ureteric injury is more commonly encountered secondary to thermal damage. However, more recently; there have been descriptions of ureteric trauma secondary to other causes, such as mechanical dissection or the use of linear stapling devices.

Diagnosis

If urinary bladder is injures intraoperative identification of the injury is the most important aspect of management. The surgeon may be cognizant of entering a hollow viscus or may note the presence of urine in the operative field. If an indwelling catheter is in place, hematuria or pneumaturia (CO_2 in the indwelling drainage system) may be noted. Existence of a bladder laceration may be confirmed with the injection of sterile milk or a dilute methylene blue solution via a catheter. Thermal injury to the bladder may not be initially apparent, presenting later in the patient's postoperative course.

Unfortunately, although intraoperative recognition of ureteric injury has been described, diagnosis is usually delayed until some time following the procedure. Ureteric lacerations may be proven intraoperatively with the injection of indigo carmine. Thermal injury will present, 24 hours to 14 days following surgery with one or a combination of fever, abdominal or flank pain, and the clinical findings of peritonitis. A leukocytosis may be present and an intravenous pyelogram (IVP) will demonstrate extravasation of urine or urinoma. Intraoperative recognition of mechanical obstruction, with staples or a suture, will be made only by direct visualization. Not surprisingly, cases of laparoscopy associated ureteric obstruction seem to present at a time similar to those that follow laparotomy based procedures a few days to a week following the operation. These patients present with flank pain and may have fever. The

Section Six

diagnosis may be suggested by abdominal ultrasound, but an IVP can be more precise at identifying the site and completeness of the obstruction.

Uretero or vesicovaginal fistula will present in a delayed fashion with incontinence or discharge. Confirmation of bladder fistula will be by direct visualization and/ or the leakage of instilled methylene blue onto a tampon. Ureterovaginal fistula will not pass the methylene blue from the bladder, but will be demonstrated with the intravenous injection of indigo carmine.

Prevention

Before start of surgery patient should void urine. Trocar-related cystotomies are generally preventable with routine preoperative bladder drainage. Additional caution must be exercised in the patient previously exposed to abdominal or pelvic surgery, where there is a tendency for the bladder to be pulled above the level of the symphysis pubis. The urachus, although rarely present, should be avoided if possible. It is likely that the placement of an indwelling catheter, at least for prolonged or difficult cases, will reduce the incidence of injury resulting from dissection. Surgical separation of the bladder from the uterus or other adherent structures requires good visualization, appropriate retraction, and excellent surgical technique. Sharp mechanical dissection is preferred, particularly when relatively dense adhesions are present.

If the surgeon cannot, with assurance, steer a wide path from its course, the ureter must be directly visualized. This is especially true when laser, electrosurgical, or stapling techniques are employed. Frequently, the ureter can be seen through the peritoneum of the pelvic sidewall between the pelvic brim and the attachment of the broad ligament. However, because of patient variation, or the presence of pathology, the location of the ureter can become obscured. In such instances, the ureter can usually be visualized through the peritoneum at the pelvic brim, although the maneuver is slightly more difficult on the left because of the location of the sigmoid mesentery. If CO_2 laser energy is to be employed, fluid injected at an appropriate location between the peritoneal surface and the ureter can provide a degree of protection from thermal injury.

If entry into the retroperitoneal space is required for exposure, there should be no hesitation to undertake such dissection. The surface of the peritoneum should be breached with scissors at the closest level proximal, and anterior, to the most distal site of planned dissection where the location of the ureter is known or anticipated. If the ureter is seen through the peritoneum, it may be grasped with a Babcock forceps to minimize trauma while the peritoneum is incised. Careful sharp and blunt dissection then may be applied to provide adequate exposure in the operative field. If the ureter cannot be seen through the peritoneal surface, a fine, toothed forceps should be employed to grasp and elevate the peritoneum allowing careful entry into the retroperitoneal space.

The techniques used for retroperitoneal dissection are also important in reducing the risk of ureteric injury. Blunt dissection can be facilitated with the instillation of fluid into the retroperitoneal space under pressure. Others have advocated the selective preoperative placement of ureteric stents including those that are illuminated, to provide additional safety. We prefer instead the use of mechanical (sharp or blunt) dissection with sharp-curved scissors and a narrow, pointed grasping forceps attached to an electrosurgical generator. The assistant is provided with a narrow, pointed, and toothed grasping forceps as well as a suction irrigation system to use, as requested, through an ancillary cannula. Dissection proceeds, respecting the blood supply of the ureter by minimizing direct manipulation and by preserving the integrity of its sheath. If electrical energy is used, it must be applied judiciously, at safe distances from the ureter and its blood supply. The narrow, pointed grasping forceps facilitates precise and safe desiccation of small caliber blood vessels.

Treatment

Most of the injury of the bladder can be managed conservatively. Small caliber injuries to the bladder (1-2 mm) may be treated expectantly, with prolonged catheterization for 7 to 14 days. However, in such cases the duration of catheterization can be reduced or eliminated if repair is undertaken intraoperatively. When a more significant injury to the bladder is identified, it may often be repaired under laparoscopic direction, provided the presence of adequate surgical skill and a location that is amenable to laparoscopic technique. Further evaluation of the location and extent of the laceration may be provided by direct laparoscopic examination of the mucosal surface of the bladder. Should the laceration be near to or involve the trigone, open repair may be preferable. In making this evaluation, the mechanism of injury should be considered, as desiccation resulting from electrical energy may extend beyond the visible limits of the lesion.

A purse string closure may be fashioned using any of a number of synthetic absorbable sutures of 2-0 to 3-0 caliber, tying the knot either intra-or extracorporeally. For linear lacerations, the defect is preferably closed in two layers. If there is significant thermal injury, it may be valuable to excise the coagulated segment. Postoperative catheterization with either a large caliber urethral or suprapubic catheter should be maintained for 5-7 days for simple fundal lacerations, and for two weeks for those closer to the trigone, the vaginal vault, or those that may be associated with significant thermal injury.

During minimal access surgery intraoperative diagnosis of ureteric injury provides the opportunity for intraoperative management. If damage is less it may respond adequately to the passage of a ureteric stent for about 10 to 20 days. However, in most instances, repair is indicated. The principles should follow those previously established for open cases. While laparoscopically directed repair of ureteric lacerations and transections have been described, such maneuvers should be practiced only by those with exceptional surgical skill and experience. Even in these cases it is advisable to consult intraoperatively with a specialist in urology.

When the diagnosis of ureteral injury is delayed until following surgery, the imperative is to establish drainage. Some obstructions or lacerations, if incomplete or small, may be successfully treated with either the retrograde or anterograde passage of a ureteral stent. Urinomas may be drained percutaneously. If a stent cannot be successfully manipulated across the lesion, a percutaneous nephrostomy should be created and plans should be made for operative repair.

NEUROLOGIC INJURY

The incidence of nerve injury associated with laparoscopy is more common in obese patient, but has been estimated at 0.5 per 1000 cases. Peripheral neurologic injury is usually related either to inappropriate positioning of the patient or occurs secondary to pressure exerted by the surgeon or assistants. During laparoscopy, nerve injury may happen rarely as a result of the surgical dissection.

In the lower extremity, the trauma may be direct, such as compression of the perineal nerve against stirrups. Alternatively, the femoral nerve or the sciatic nerve or its branches may be overstretched and damaged by inappropriate positioning of the hip or the knee joint.

Brachial plexus injuries may occur secondary to the surgeon or assistants leaning against the abducted arm during the procedure. Alternatively, if the patient is placed in steep Trendelenburg's position, the brachial plexus may be damaged because of the pressure exerted on the shoulder joint.

Diagnosis

If nerve is damaged in most instances, the patient is found to have sensory and/ or motor deficit as they emerge from the effects of the anaesthesia. The diagnosis can usually be suspected by clinical examination. Injuries to the perineal nerve will be reflected by loss of sensation in the lateral aspect of the leg and foot together with a foot drop. Brachial plexus injuries may be variable, but usually involve damage to the C-5, 6 roots manifesting in loss of flexion of the elbow and adduction of the shoulder. Electromyography can be used to further define the extent and location of the lesion by testing nerve conduction and recording the electrical potential for various muscles. This evaluation should be delayed for three weeks to allow for complete degeneration of injured nerves.

Prevention

During laparoscopic procedure if nerve injury has to be prevented then surgeon should must achieve a good ergonomics of patient. The incidence of brachial plexus injury can be reduced by placing the arms in an adducted position, which also facilitates the performance of pelvic surgery by allowing the surgeon to stand in a more comfortable position. Should it be necessary to leave the arm in an abducted position, adequate padding and support of the arms and shoulders are necessary and can be facilitated with the use of shoulder supports, preventing the slippage of the patient up the table when placed in Trendelenburg's position. Furthermore, in such a position, the surgeon may not lean on the patient's arm.

Sciatic and perineal nerve injury is minimized with the use of appropriate stirrups and careful positioning protocols. Those stirrups that combine both knee and foot support are probably best. Additional measures include simultaneous raising and lowering of the legs, flexion of the knees before flexion of the hips, and limitation of external rotation of the hip. Assistants should be admonished to avoid placing undue pressure on the inner thighs.

Injury to the obturator and genitofemoral nerves is uncommon but will likely increase as greater numbers of retroperitoneal dissections are performed. In such cases, it will be important to clearly understand the anatomy, maintain hemostasis, and to exert the utmost care in performing the dissections, carefully identifying the neural structures as they are encountered.

Management

Most injuries to peripheral nerves recover spontaneously. The time to recovery depends upon the site and severity of the lesion. For most peripheral injuries, full sensorineural recovery occurs in three to six months. Recovery may be facilitated with physical therapy, appropriate braces, and electrical stimulation of the affected muscles. Transection of major intrapelvic nerves will require open microsurgical repair.

Dissection and Thermal Injury Recognition

Diagnosis of injury to the bowel incurred during the course of dissection may be more straightforward. Any length of dissected bowel should be carefully examined prior to proceeding further with the procedure. This is, if anything, more important during laparoscopic operations in comparison to those performed via laparotomy, for comprehensive "running" of the bowel near the end of the case is far more difficult under endoscopic guidance.

There has been confusion in the past regarding the frequency of thermal injury to bowel following the use of electrical energy. Formerly, many injuries actually caused by mechanical trauma were erroneously attributed to electrosurgical accidents.

Thermal injury to bowel may be more difficult to diagnose intraoperatively, particularly if created with electrical or laser energy, a feature that makes careful adherence to safety protocols a surgeon's imperative. Even if thermal injury is recognized, it is difficult to estimate the extent of the damage by visual inspection, as the zone of desiccation may exceed the area of visual damage. An understanding of the differing impacts of the various types of electrical current is essential for estimation of the extent of injury. In some instances, diagnosis is delayed until the development of peritonitis and fever, usually a few days later, but occasionally not for several weeks.

Prevention

Total prevention of dissection or thermal injury is impossible, but the incidence of penetrating or energy based enteric complications may be reduced with patience, prudence, and meticulous technique. A sound understanding of the principles of electrosurgery is critical to reducing the incidence of electrical trauma.

When dissecting, exposure of the operative field must be accomplished with a combination of good visualization and adequate traction and, if necessary, countertraction applied by forceps. In many instances, it will be necessary to enlist the aid of a competent assistant. Dissection close to bowel should be performed mechanically, using sharp scissors, not with electrical or laser energy sources. Occlusion of blood vessels near to bowel is preferably accomplished with clips, but may be performed with bipolar current provided that there is an adequate margin of tissue, a circumstance that usually requires skeletonization of the vessel.

There is no certainty about the proper distance to maintain between the electrode and the bowel serosa. Animal histological studies, using the rather large caliber Kleppinger forceps, have demonstrated that desiccation injury begins to affect bowel serosa and muscularis between 5 and 10 mm away. It is likely that the zone of safety is less for instruments that compress tissue well or that use electrodes with a smaller surface area. Regardless, if the difficulty of the dissection makes the surgeon uncomfortable, alternative methods for hemostasis should be used. If this is not feasible, the aid of more experienced colleagues should be sought the procedure abandoned, or converted into an open case.

Management

The treatment of mechanical bowel trauma recognized during the dissection follows the principles described above for trocar injury. If the diagnosis is delayed until the postoperative recognition of peritonitis, surgical consultation should be obtained and laparotomy arranged.

Thermal injury may be handled expectantly, if the lesion is superficial and confined. It is possible to estimate the degree of tissue injury if the nature of the current and other parameters is known, such as the wattage, current density, and duration of contact with tissue. For example, fulguration current, arcing to bowel, is unlikely to cause thermal injury more than 1 mm deep, even with rather prolonged exposure. On the other hand, the high power density provided by a sharp electrode will quickly cause penetrating injury of the bowel. Such lesions will have relatively little collateral thermal injury and may be repaired as if they were created by mechanical means. This is a circumstance vastly different from that occurring when there is direct, and even relatively short, duration of contact (seconds) with a low power density electrode. The significant thermal injury that results will often mandate wide excision of the lesion or local resection of the injured segment of bowel.

INCISIONAL HERNIA

It is not that the incidence of laparoscopic incisional hernia is unknown, it is clear that the complication has been underreported. Recent reports of incisional hernia after laparoscopy have stressed the relationship of this complication with the use of ports 10 mm in diameter or larger. In our opinion, this can probably be attributed to increased operating times which result in excessive manipulation of the port site, thereby widening the fascial and peritoneal defects.

While no incision is immune to the risk of herniation, those defects that are 10 mm or more in diameter are particularly vulnerable. The increasing number and size of the incisions, ID combination with the surgeon's variable propensity to close them, will likely further contribute to the increasing incidence. Another important contributing factor may be the use of cannula anchoring devices that effectively increase the diameter of the incision by 2 to 3 mm.

Diagnosis

After laparoscopy the most common hernia appears to occur in the immediate postoperative period where bowel or omentum passes through the unopposed or inadequately repaired defect. The patient may be symptomatic or can present with any or a combination of pain, fever, periumbilical mass, obvious evisceration, and the symptoms and signs of mechanical bowel obstruction, often within hours and usually within the first postoperative week. Consequently, the surgeon should take care not to casually disregard the patients who talk about symptoms consistent with herniation.

Because Richter's hernias contain only a portion of the circumference of the bowel wall in the defect, the diagnosis is often delayed. It is likely that such lesions most commonly occur in incisions that are made away from the midline. The initial presenting symptom is usually pain, since the incomplete obstruction and still allows the passage of intestinal content. Fever can present if incarceration occurs, and peritonitis may result from the subsequent perforation. The diagnosis is difficult to make and requires a high index of suspicion. Ultrasound or CT scanning may be useful in confirming the diagnosis.

While many defects likely remain asymptomatic, late presentation may occur if bowel or omentum becomes trapped. The symptoms and findings are similar to that described for earlier presentations.

Prevention

The underlying fascia and peritoneum should be closed not only when using trocars of 10 mm and larger as previously suggested but also when extensive manipulation is performed thorough a 5 mm trocar port, causing extension of the incision.

There are a number of unproven but seemingly logical pre-emptive strategies. First, it is desirable to use the smallest possible cannula whenever possible recognizing that hernia has even been reported in conjunction with the use of 5 mm trocars. Second, the "Z-track" insertion method, particularly applied, in the umbilicus, may be of value. This approach offsets the skin and fascial incisions by entering the subcutaneous tissue, then sliding the conically-tipped trocar along the fascia for a short distance prior to penetrating it. Such a track is purported to close like a curtain, reducing the incidence of hernia. Third, all ancillary cannula should be removed under direct vision to ensure that bowel is not drawn into the incision. Insertion of an obturator (or a laparoscope) into the cannula may further prevent suction from drawing bowel or omentum into the incision. Fourth, at least those incisions 10 mm or greater in diameter should undergo fascial closure under direct laparoscopic vision, thereby preventing incorporation of bowel. This may be accomplished by using a small caliber diameter laparoscope through one of the narrow cannula to direct incisional closure. A narrow diameter, three-quarter round, needle (Ethicon UR-6) facilitates such a closure, as does the use of one of the newer devices. Finally, the laparoscope cannula should be removed with the laparoscope in position, preventing accidental incorporation of bowel.

If the final incision is of sufficiently large diameter to require closure, blind insertion of needles may be avoided by prepositioning sutures. They are placed when the laparoscope is in another location and tied following removal of the final cannula. The sutures should be used to elevate the abdominal wall as the laparoscope and cannula are simultaneously removed, looking down the endoscope to ensure that bowel or omentum are not inadvertently drawn into the wound.

Management

Management of postoperative development of incisional hernia after laparoscopy is same as that of open surgery. Management of laparoscopic incisional defects depends upon the timing of the presentation and the presence or absence of entrapped bowel and its condition. Evisceration will always require surgical intervention. If the diagnosis is made in the recovery room, the patient may be returned to the operating room, the bowel or omentum replaced in the peritoneal cavity (provided there is no evidence of necrosis or suture incorporation), and the incision repaired, usually under laparoscopic guidance. However, if the diagnosis is delayed it is likely that the bowel is incarcerated and at risk for perforation. In such circumstances, resection will likely be necessary, usually via laparotomy. Most gynecologic surgeons should request general surgical consultation.

INFECTION

Wound infection following laparoscopy is less but not rare. Even a case of postoperative wound infection due to *Mycobacterium chelonae* also been reported. A 35-year-old woman presented with multiple erythematous nodules, plaques and discharging sinuses over the abdomen, 45 days after she had undergone laparoscopic ovarian cystectomy. The seropurulent discharge from the wound showed acid-fast bacilli on Ziehl-Neelsen stain and culture yielded *Mycobacterium chelonae*. The patient responded to clarithromycin and doxycycline. The source of infection was probably contaminated water or disinfectant solution used for sterilization of laparoscopic instruments. In the urologic and general surgical wound infection rates seem to range from 5 to 6 per 1000 cases. While the vast majority of wound infections are handled successfully with expectant management, drainage, or antibiotics, severe necrotizing fascitis has been reported.

Many other types of post-laparoscopy infection have been reported including bladder infection, pelvic cellulitis, and pelvic abscess. While bacteremia has been described, there have been no reports of disseminated infection following laparoscopic surgery.

This is true that the risk of infection associated with laparoscopy is low; much lower than that associated with open abdominal or vaginal surgery. Nevertheless, until clinical studies dictate otherwise, it is prudent to continue to practice strict sterile technique and to offer appropriate prophylactic antibiotics to selected patients. These could include those with enhanced risk for bacterial endocarditis, as well as those who are to undergo procedures (e.g. laparoscopic hysterectomy), suspected of increasing, the chance of wound or vault infection. Patients should be instructed to routinely take their temperature following discharge and to immediately report fever of 38 °C or more.

BIBLIOGRAPHY

1. Azagra JS, Goergen M, Gilbart E, Jacobs D. Laparoscopic anatomical (hepatic) left lateral segmentectomy—technical aspects. Surg Endosc 1996;10:758–61.
2. Belli G, Fantini C, D Agostino A, Belli A, Cioffi L, Russolillo N. Laparoscopic left lateral hepatic lobectomy: a safer and faster technique. J Hepatobiliary Pancreat Surg 2006;13:149–54.
3. Berci G, Cuschieri A. Creation of pneumoperitoneum and trocar insertion. In Practical Laparoscopy, G Berci, A Cuschieri, editors. London, Bailli~re Tindall, 1986;44-64.

4. Berci G, Cuschieri A. Practical Laparoscopy, Chs. 5-7. London, Bailli~re Tindall, 1986.

5. Berci G, Dunkelman D, Michel SL, Sanders G, Wahlstrom E, Morgenstern L. Emergency minilaparoscopy in abdominal trauma: an update. Am J Surg 1983;146:261.

6. Berci G, Sackier J, Paz-Partlow M. Emergency laparoscopy. Am J Surg 1991;161:332.

7. Berci G, Wahlstorm E. Emergency laparoscopy. In Surgical Endoscopy, L Dent, editor. Chicago, Year Book, 1985;478-83.

8. Berci G. Complications of laparoscopy. In Practical Laparoscopy, G Berci, A Cuschieri, editors. London, Bailli~re Tindall, 1986;165-77.

9. Berci G. Laparoscopy for oncology. In Textbook of Oncology, AR Moosa, St. C Schimpff, MC Robson, editors. Baltimore, Williams & Wilkins, 1991;210-19.

10. Berci G. Laparoscopy in general surgery. In Endoscopy, G Berci, editor. Norwalk, CT, Appleton-Century-Crofts, 1976;382-400.

11. Boyce WN, Cammerer RC, Anderson DL. Laparoscopy and hepatology. In Endoscopy, G Berci, editor. Norwalk, CT, Appleton- Century-Crofts, 1976;401-11.

12. Cadeddu JA, Wolfe JS Jr, Nakada S, Chen R, Shalhav A, Bishoff JT. Complications of laparoscopic procedures after concentrated training in urological laparoscopy. J Urol 2001;166:2109.

13. Cadiere GB, Torres R, Dapri G, Capelluto E, Himpens J. Multimedia article: laparoscopic left lateral hepatic lobectomy for metastatic colorectal tumor. Surg Endosc 2005;19:152.

14. Caione P, Micali S, Rinaldi S, Capozza N, Lais A, Matarazzo E, Maturo G, Micali F. Retroperitoneal laparoscopy for renal biopsy in children. J Urol 2000;164:1080-85.

15. Carnevale N, Baron N, Delaney HM. Peritoneoscopy as an aid in the diagnosis of abdominal trauma: a preliminary report. J. Trauma 1977;17:634.

16. Castilho LN, Castillo OA, Denes FT, Mitre A1, Arap S. Laparoscopic adrenal surgery in children. J Urol 2002; 168:221-4.

17. Chee-Awai Chandhoke RA, Chandhoke PS, Koyle MA. Laparoscopic nephrectomy in children. Semin Laparosc Surg 1998;5:47.

18. Chen HW, Lin GJ, Lai CH, Chu SH, Chuang CK. Minimally invasive extravesical ureteral reimplantation for vesicoureteral reflux. J Urol 2002;167:1821-3.

19. Cherqui D, Husson E, Hammoud R, Malassagne B, Stephan F, Bensaid S, Rotman N, Fagniez PL. Laparoscopic liver resections: a feasibility study in 30 patients. Ann Surg 2000;232:753-62.

20. Colodny AH. Laparoscopy in pediatric urology: too much of a good thing? Semin Pediatr Surg 1996;5:23.

21. Critchley LA, Critchley JA, Gin T. Haemodynamic changes in patients undergoing laparoscopic cholecystectomy: measurement by transthoracic electrical bioimpedance. Br J Anaesth 1993;70:681-3.

22. Cuschieri A, Berci G. Laparoscopic Biliary Surgery. London, Blackwell, 1990.

23. Cuschieri A. Value of laparoscopy in hepatobiliary disease. Ann R Coll Surg 1975;57:33.

24. Delarue A, Guys JM, Louis Borrione C, Simeoni J, Esposito C. Pediatric endoscopy surgery: pride and prejudice. Eur J Ped Surg 1994;4:323.

25. DeSouza G, Lewis MC, TerRiet MF. Severe bradycardia after remifentanil. Anesthesiology 1997;87:1019–20.

26. Dexter SP, Vucevic M, Gibson J, et al. Hemodynamic consequences of high- and low-pressure capnoperitoneum during laparoscopic cholecystectomy. Surg Endosc 1999;13:376–81.

27. Docimo SG, Moore RG, Adams J, Kavoussi LR. Laparoscopic bladder augmentation using stomach. Urology 1995;46: 565-9.

28. Dorsay DA, Greene FL, Baysinger CL. Hemodynamic changes during laparoscopic cholecystectomy monitored with transesophageal echocardiography. Surg Endosc 1995;9:128–33.

29. Duckett JW. Pediatric laparoscopy: prudence please [editorial]. J Urol 1994;151:742.

30. Eguchi D, Nishizaki T, Ohta M, Ishizaki Y, Hanaki N, Okita K, Ohga T, Takahashi I, Ojima Y, Wada H, Tsutsui S. Laparoscopy- assisted right hepatic lobectomy using a wall-lifting procedure. Surg Endosc 200;20:1326–8.

31. El-Ghoneimi A, Valla JS, Steyaert H, Aigrain Y (1998) Laparoscopic renal surgery via a retroperitoneal approach in children. J Urol 1998;160:1138-41.

32. Esposito C, Ascione G, Garipoli V, De Bernardo G, Esposito G. Complications of pediatric laparoscopic surgery. Surg Endosc 1997;ll:665.

33. Esposito C, Damiano R, Gonzalez-Sabin MA, Savanelli A, Centone A, Settimi A, Sacco R. Laparoscopy-assisted orchidopexy: an ideal treatment for children with intraabdominal testes. J Endourol 2002;9:16.

34. Esposito C, Garipoli V, Di Matteo G, De Pasquale M. Laparoscopic management of ovarian cysts in newborns. Surg Endosc 1998;12:1152-4.

35. Esposito C, Monguzzi G, Gonzalez-Sabin MA, Rubino R, Mantinaro L, Papparella A, Amici G. Laparoscopic treatment of pediatric varicocele: a multicenter study of the italian society of video surgery in infancy. J Urol 2000;163:1944-6.

36. Esposito C, Monguzzi G, Gonzalez-Sabin MA, Rubino R, Montinaro L, Papparella A, Esposito G, Settimi A, Mastroianni L, Zamparelli M, Sacco R, Amici G, Damiano R, Innaro N. Results and complication of laparoscopic surgery for pediatric varicocele. J Pediatr Surg 2001;36:767-9.

37. Gaisford W. Peritonoscopy: a valuable technique for surgeons. Am. J. Surg. 130:671, 1975.

38. Galizia G, Prizio G, Lieto E, et al. Hemodynamic and pulmonary changes during open, carbon dioxide pneumoperitoneum and abdominal wall-lifting cholecystectomy. A prospective, randomized study. Surg Endosc 2001;15:477–83.

39. Gaur DD, Agarwal DK, Purohit KC. Retroperitoneal laparoscopic nephrectomy initial case report. J Urol 1993;149:403.

40. Gazzaniga AB, Slanton WW, Barlett RH. Laparoscopy in the diagnosis of blunt and penetrating injuries to the abdomen. Am J Surg 1976;131:315.

Section Six

41. Gettman MT, Peschel R, Neururer R, Bartsch G. A comparison of laparoscopic pyeloplasty performed whit the daVinci robotic system versus standard laparoscopic techniques: initial clinical results. Eur Urol 2002;42:453-8.

42. Gill SI, Kavoussi RL, Clayman RV. Complications of laparoscopic nephrectomy in 185 patients: a multi-institutional review. J Urol 1995;154:479.

43. Godje O, Friedl R, Hannekum A. Accuracy of beat-to-beat cardiac output monitoring by pulse contour analysis in hemodynamical unstable patients. Med Sci Monit 2001;7:1344–50.

44. Grady RW, Mitchell ME, Carr MC. Laparoscopic and histologic condition of the inguinal vanishing testis. Urology 1998;52:866-9.

45. Guilloneau B, Ballanger P, Lugagne PM, Valla JS, Vallancien G. Laparoscopic versus lumboscopic nephrectomy. Eur Urol 1996;29:288-91.

46. Henning H, Look D. Complications. In Laparoscopy H, Henning D. Look, editors. Stuttgart, Thieme, 1985.

47. Henning H, Look D. Laparoskopie. Stuttgart, Thieme, 1985.

48. Hirvonen EA, Nuutinen LS, Kauko M. Hemodynamic changes due to Trendelenburg positioning and pneumoperitoneum during laparoscopic hysterectomy. Acta Anaesthesiol Scand 1995;39:949–55.

49. Hofer CK, Zalunardo MP, Klaghofer R, et al. Changes in intrathoracic blood volume associated with pneumoperitoneum and positioning. Acta Anaesthesiol Scand 2002;46:303–8.

50. Hopkins HH. Optical principles of the endoscopies. In Endoscopy G. Berci, editor. Norwalk, CT, Appleton-Century-Crofts, 1976;3-26.

51. Jacobeus HC. Kurze Obersicht uber meine Erfahrungen mit der Laparosckopie. Munch. Med. Wochenschr. 58:2017, 1911.

52. Joris JL, Noirot DP, Legrand MJ, et al. Hemodynamic changes during laparoscopic cholecystectomy. Anesth Analg 1993;76:1067–71.

53. Kalk H, Bruhl W. Leitfaden der Laparoskopie. Stuttgart, Theime, 1951.

54. Kallipolitis GK, Milingos SD, Creatsas GK, Deligeoroglou EK, Michalas SP. Laparoscopic gonadectomy in a patient with testicular feminization syndrome. J Pediatr Adolesc Gynecol 2000;13:23-26.

55. Kaneko H. Laparoscopic hepatectomy: indications and outcomes. J Hepatobiliary Pancreat Surg 2005;12:438–43.

56. Kaneko H, Takagi S, Shiba T. Laparoscopic partial hepatectomy and left lateral segmentectomy: technique and results of a clinical series. Surgery 1996;120:468–75.

57. Kelling G. Verhandlung deutscher Naturforscher und Aerzte. Leipzig, Vogel, 1902.

58. Khurana S, Borzi PA. Laparoscopic management of complicated urachal disease in children. J Urol 2002;168:1526-8.

59. Machado MA, Makdissi FF, Bacchella T, Machado MC. Hemihepatic ischemia for laparoscopic liver resection. Surg Laparosc Endosc Percutan Tech 2005;15:180–83.

60. McCallum RW, Berci G. Laparoscopy in hepatic disease. Gastroint. Endosc 1976;23:20-24.

61. Meininger D, Byhahn C, Bueck M, et al. Effects of prolonged pneumoperitoneum on hemodynamics and acid-base balance during totally endoscopic robot-assisted radical prostatectomies. World J Surg 2002;26:1423–7.

62. Meininger D, Byhahn C, Mierdl S, et al. Positive endexpiratory pressure improves arterial oxygenation during prolonged pneumoperitoneum. Acta Anaesthesiol Scand 2005;49:778–83.

63. Merrot T, Ordorica-Flores R, Steyeart H, Ginier C, Valla JS. Is diffuse xanthogranulomatous pyelonephritis a contraindication to retroperitoneoscopic nephroureterectomy? A case report. Surg Laparosc Endosc 1998;8:366-9.

64. Meynol F, Steyaert H, Valla JS. Adnexa torsion in children: earlier diagnosis and treatment by laparoscopy. Arch Pediatr 1997;4:416-9.

65. Miller OF, Bloom TL, Smith L J, McAleer IM, Kaplan GW, Kolon TF. Early hospital discharge for intravesical ureteroneocystostomy. J Urol 2002;167:2556-9.

66. Millward-Sadler GH, Whorwell PJ. Liver biopsy. In Liver and Biliary Disease, R. Wright et al. editors. London, Bailli~re Tindall 1985;496-514.

67. Morgenstern L, Shapiro SJ. Techniques of splenic conservation. Arch Surg 1979;14:449.

68. Nyirady P, Kiss A, Pirot L, Sarkozy S, Bognar Z, Csontai A, Merksz M. Evaluation of 100 laparoscopic varicocele operations with preservation of testicular artery and ligation of collateral vein in children and adolescent. Eur Urol 2002;42:594-7.

69. O Rourke N, Fielding G. Laparoscopic right hepatectomy: surgical technique. J Gastrointest Surg 2004;8:213–6.

70. Odeberg S, Ljungqvist O, Svenberg T, et al. Haemodynamic. effects of pneumoperitoneum and the influence of posture during anaesthesia for laparoscopic surgery. Acta Anaesthesiol Scand 1994;38:276–83.

71. Pauli C, Fakler U, Genz T, et al. Cardiac output determination in children: equivalence of the transpulmonary thermo-dilution method to the direct Fick principle. Intensive Care Med 2002;28:947–52.

72. Paz-Partlow M. Documentation of laparoscopy. In Practical Laparoscopy G, Berci A, Cuschieri, editors. London, Bailli~re Tindall, 1986;1%32.

73. Peters CA. Complications in pediatric urological]aparoscopy: results of a survey. J Urol 1996;155:1070.

74. Peters CA. Laparoendoscopy renal surgery in children. J Endourol 2000;14:841.

75. Reid JE, Mirakhur RK. Bradycardia after administration of remifentanil. Br J Anaesth 2000;84:422-3.

76. Robinson BC, Snow BW, Cartwright PC, De vries CR, Hamilton BD, Anderson JB. Comparison of laparoscopic versus open partial nephrectomy in a pediatric series. J Urol 2003;169:638-40.

77. Root HO, Hauser CW, McKinley CR, La Fave JW, Mendiola RP. Diagnostic peritoneal lavage. Surgery 1965;57:633.

78. Ruddock C. Peritoneoscopy. Surg. Gynecol. Obstet 1937;65:523.

79. Sakka SG, Reinhart K, Meier-Hellmann A. Comparison of pulmonary artery and arterial thermodilution cardiac output in critically ill patients. Intensive Care Med 1999;25:843–6.

80. Sandham JD, Hull RD, Brant RF, et al. A randomized, controlled trial of the use of pulmonary-artery catheters in highrisk surgical patients. N Engl J Med 2003;348:5–14.

81. Sherwood R, Berci G, Austin E, Morgenstern L. Mini laparoscopy for blunt abdominal trauma. Arch Surg 1980;115:672.

82. Sherwood R, Berci G, Austin E, Morgenstern L. Minilaparoscopy for blunt abdominal trauma. Arch Surg 1980;115:672.

83. Stubbe H, Schmidt C, Hinder F. [Invasive cardiovascular monitoring—four methods compared]. Anaesthesiol Intensivmed Notfallmed Schmerzther 2006;41:550–55.

84. Takasaki K. Glissonean pedicle transection method for hepatic resection: a new concept of liver segmentation. J Hepatobiliary Pancreat Surg 1998;5:286–91.

85. Takasaki K, Kobayashi S, Tanaka S, Saito A, Yamamoto M, Hanyu F. Highly anatomically systematized hepatic resection with Glissonean sheath code transection at the hepatic hilus. Int Surg 1990;75:73–7.

86. Veress J. Neues Instrument zur ausfurung von brust oder Bauchpunktionen. Dtsch. Med. Wochenschr 1938;41:1480-81.

87. Vibert E, Perniceni T, Levard H, Denet C, Shahri NK, Gayet B. Laparoscopic liver resection. Br J Surg 2006;93:67–72.

88. Von ST, Wietasch G, Bursch J, et al. [Cardiac output determination with transpulmonary thermodilution. An alternative to pulmonary catheterization?]. Anaesthesist 1996;45:1045–50.

89. Wittgen CM, Andrus CH, Fitzgerald SD, et al. Analysis of the hemodynamic and ventilatory effects of laparoscopic cholecystectomy. Arch Surg 1991;126:997–1000.

90. Wood RAB, Cuschieri A. Laparoscopy for chronic abdominal pain. Br J Surg 1979;60:900-02.

91. Yamanaka N, Tanaka T, Tanaka W, Yamanaka J, Yasui C, Ando T, Takada M, Maeda S, Okamoto E. Laparoscopic partial hepatectomy. Hepatogastroenterology 1998;45:29–33.

92. Zoeckler SJ. Peritoneoscopy: a reevaluation. Gastroenterology 1958;34:969.

93. Zuckerman R, Gold M, Jenkins P, et al. The effects of pneumoperitoneum and patient position on hemodynamics during laparoscopic cholecystectomy. Surg Endosc 2001;15:562–5.

Section Six

Role of Training in Minimal Access Surgery

The popularity of laparoscopic techniques has led to a new domain in surgical training, with a move away from the apprenticeship model, toward structured programs of teaching new skills outside the operating room. Hands-on courses enables young surgeons to practice techniques on synthetic, porcine or more recently virtual-reality models, are now commonplace. The aim has been to ensure trainees are armed with basic laparoscopic skills, such as hand-eye coordination and depth perception prior to entering the operating room (Fig. 45.1). The success of these initial courses led to the development of similar courses for the advanced laparoscopic skills required for gastric and colonic surgery.

Compared to aviation, where virtual reality (VR) training has been standardized and simulators have proven their definite benefit in increasing skill, the objectives, needs, and means of VR training in minimal access surgery (MIS) is established (Fig. 45.2).

Rasmussen distinguishes three levels of human behavior:
1. Skill-based level
2. Rule-based level
3. Knowledge-based behavior

Skill-based Behavior

This represents surgeon's behavior that takes place without conscious control. Task execution is highly automated at this level of behavior and is based on fast selection of motor programs which control the appropriate muscles. The motor programs are based on an accurate internal representation of the task, the system dynamics, and the environment at hand (e.g. learned by training and experience). An example of an everyday skill is walking. Many tasks in surgery can be considered as a sequence of skilled acts. For example, an experienced surgeon performs a suture task smoothly, without conscious control over his or her movements.

In MIS, suturing can also be considered as skill-based behavior. However, because of the indirect access to the tissue, it is a much more complicated skill because of reduced depth perception and difficult handeye coordination (Fig. 45.3).

Rule-based Behavior

At the next level of human behavior, rule-based behavior is applied. During rule-based behavior task

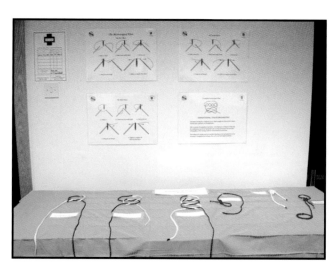

Fig. 45.1: Demonstration of different types of knot to keep them in memory

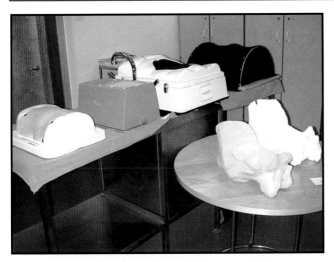

Fig. 45.2: Different types of simple pelvitrainers

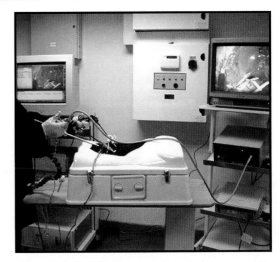

Fig. 45.3: Pelvitrainer exercises to improve skill

execution is controlled by stored rules or procedures. These may have been derived empirically from previous occasions or communicated from other persons' expertise as instructions or as a cookbook recipe. Appropriate rules are selected according to their "success" in previous experiences. For example, procedural steps and the recognition of anatomy and pathology in MIS require rule-based behavior. At the rule-based level, the information is typically perceived as discrete signs . A sign serves to activate or to trigger a stored rule. Stopping your car in front of a red light is a good example of a sign (red light) that triggers a stored rule (stop car). In laparoscopic cholecystectomy, having fully established the critical view of safety is the sign that triggers the rule that the appropriate structures may be clipped next.

Knowledge-based Behavior

In unfamiliar situations, faced with a task for which no rules are available from previous encounters, human behavior is knowledge based. During knowledge-based behavior the goal is explicitly formulated, based on an analysis of the overall aim. Different plans are developed, and their effects mentally tested against the goal. Finally a plan is selected. Serious complications that occasionally occur during surgery demand a great deal of knowledge-based behavior from the surgeon. He or she has to analyze the complication and the aim of the surgical procedure in order to develop strategies to counter the complication. Then he or she has to select the best strategy and consequently take the appropriate actions.

At the knowledge-based level, information is perceived as symbols. Symbols refer to chunks of conceptual information, which are the basis for reasoning and planning. Pathological symptoms are a good example of symbols in medical practice.

Training in laparoscopic surgery is beginning to evolve into a stepwise, curricular approach that is not organ or procedure-specific. Instead, it is necessary to learn manipulative skills, which are then combined to achieve proficiency in tasks such as laparoscopic suturing or division of a vessel. The constituent parts can then be combined with anatomical knowledge to enable completion of a specific procedure. Basic psychomotor skills can be learnt with a simple, cheap version of a video-box trainer. Higher level skills such as dissection and use of high-energy instruments will necessitate the use of more realistic tissues, which can be achieved on porcine or human cadaveric models. Recent advances in virtual reality simulation are also beginning to produce realistic simulations of complete procedures, for example, laparoscopic cholecystectomy.

It would be rational to assume that a high-fidelity simulation model, such as anesthetized animal tissue, would be superior in terms of training outcome to a synthetic plastic model (Fig. 45.4).

In fact, a study comparing two groups learning to perform microanastomotic repair of a transected spermatic cord on either the animal or synthetic model found no difference in eventual outcome of the two groups. The synthetic model is obviously cheaper and does not require specialized storage facilities. It can be

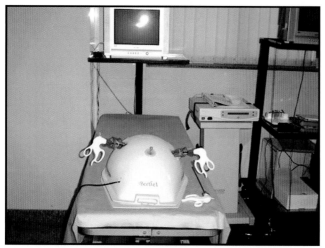

Fig. 45.4: The simple pelvitrainer can be used for improving suturing skill

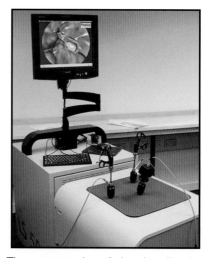

Fig. 45.5: The programming of virtual reality simulator will increase rule base level

assumed that as the subjects were using real sutures and instruments, the nature of the task was learnt regardless of the fidelity of the simulated tissue.

Training-Objectives, Needs, and Means

To enable the design and evaluation of an effective and efficient training method it is of utmost importance to determine the training objectives, needs, and means, since they provide an answer to the questions:
1. What is the end goal of the training?
2. What should be trained?
3. How can we train it?

The objectives represent the level of competence that is expected of the trainee after he or she has completed the training. Training needs are the difference between the initial level of competence of the trainees and the required level of competence after successful completion of the training defined in the objectives. Ultimately, demands for effectivity and efficiency on the one hand, and the state-of-the-art in technology on the other hand, determine the tools and methods for training, i.e. the training means. Effective training ensures that all training objectives are met. Efficient training ensures that the training means are cost effective and that the required training time is minimized. Since safety and patient outcome are the most important criteria in surgery, training effectivity should be of primary importance (Fig. 45.5).

The complexity and the costs of the training means are largely determined by the training objectives that

have been set. Fulfilling all training needs of laparoscopic residents with only one training method will require a highly complex and probably very expensive trainer in which all three levels of behavior can be trained. Such a trainer is not yet available. The complexity and the cost of a training means are relatively low if the training objectives comprise skill-based behavior only, since this can be trained with simple models such as pelvitrainers (Fig. 45.6). Evidently, the cost and complexity of a training means increase when the training objectives advance from the training of skill-based behavior to the training of knowledge-based behavior. Fortunately, the overall effectivity of training increases as well when higher levels of behavior, such as knowledge-based behavior, are incorporated in the training objectives.

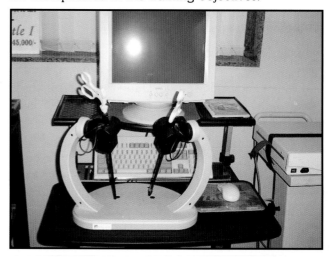

Fig. 45.6: Prototype virtual reality pelvitrainers

Present Training in Laparoscopy

A closer look at the training program of laparoscopic residents provides an indication of the training needs that are addressed and the training means that are available today. Much as in conventional surgery, the laparoscopic surgeon must effectively combine the three levels of behavior. Instrument handling and dissection techniques require skill-based behavior, whereas the recognition of surgical anatomy requires a great deal of rule-based behavior. Complications such as uncontrollable bleeding or unsuspected situations such as the encountering of aberrant anatomy require problem solving on a knowledge-based level.

Obviously, training of skill-based behavior in laparoscopic surgery is highly desired as laparoscopy combines unusual hand–eye coordination with the use of complex instruments. Surgical residents are usually trained in laparoscopic surgery during a 2 days introduction course. Basic skill-based behavior such as instrument tissue handling and minimally invasive suturing are trained. Additionally, rule-based behavior is trained through lectures, textbooks, and video instructions. After the resident has successfully completed this course, he or she will receive training in the operating room. It is only in operating room that most knowledge- based behavior necessary to deal with complications and emergencies is acquired. Currently, a living animal model provides the only way to effectively train rule- and knowledge-based behavior outside the operating room. Training on living animal models is very useful in the training curriculum of resident surgeons. However, at the same time the use of laboratory animals for training is discouraged by many government policies. Technological innovations, such as virtual reality simulation, will change the way laparoscopic surgery is trained. Current accomplishments in surgical simulation envision the dawning of the next-generation surgical education. In this respect, aviation industry provides excellent examples of the effectiveness and efficiency of virtual reality simulators as a means of training.

Simulator training in aviation in contrast to surgery, the training needs in aviation has explicitly been defined by regulatory authorities like Federal Aviation Administration (FAA) and the training means are certified accordingly. The training objectives, needs, and means in pilot training have been investigated in

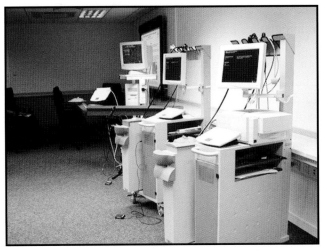

Fig. 45.7: Different types of virtual reality systems for endoscopy

depth, and models of pilot behavior have been developed as a tool to design, to evaluate, and to optimize training methods. Half a century of extensive research has resulted in many training tools, from basic flight training devices to the high-tech full flight simulator (FFS) (Figs 45.7 and 45.8).

After the introduction of VR training methods in the 1990s, the training of surgeons has often been compared to the training of pilots. The training of laparoscopic residents can best be compared to type conversion training of pilots. During type conversion training, young pilots who have finished flight training at the academies and have recently joined an airline are trained to fly a particular type of aircraft. The general objective of type conversion training is to teach the trainee how to safely control, navigate, and manage a particular operational aircraft. Since the trainees have already acquired much of the skill-based behavior required to fly a multiengine aircraft, the training needs mainly consist of acquiring additional rule- and knowledge-based behavior. The trainees have to learn the new checklists and the specific procedures during takeoff and landing, and they have to become familiar with all the aircraft systems like electronics, hydraulics. Furthermore, they have to train all sorts of emergency scenarios that may occur during actual flight. Training of this knowledge-based behavior is very important since it significantly improves flight safety. This training provides an excellent training tool to accomplish all the specified training needs. The high level of realism during training of a pilot have even made zero flight

Section Six

time training possible, during which type conversion training takes place completely outside a real aircraft.

For the sake of proper training and for the safety of our patients, the objectives, needs, and means in laparoscopy training should be defined. Along this guideline, VR simulators should be developed. An explicit formulation of the training objectives facilitates the development and certification of a simulator since it determines what the simulator should be capable of. For example, pilots spend many hours training on low-cost simulator (Fig. 45.9).

The laparoscopy simulators that have been developed during the past decade can all be considered as laparoscopy training devices. Most of these simulators specifically aim at training skill-based behavior, such as endoscopic manipulation and

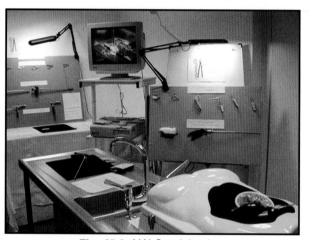

Fig. 45.8: HALS training box

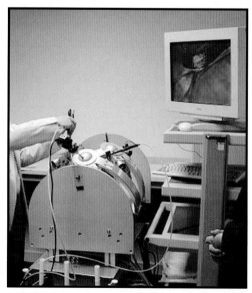

Fig. 45.9: Virtual reality trainer with programmable circuit

endoscopic camera navigation. However, performing safe laparoscopy also requires a professional level of rule- and knowledge-based behavior from the surgeon. Ideally these should also be trained outside the operation theatre. Currently, the training of rule- and knowledge based behavior outside the operation theatre is only possible on living animal models. However, technological innovations like increasing computing power, detailed anatomical models, soft tissue modeling, force feedback will enable the integration of all levels of behavior in a VR training simulator for laparoscopy. In the future, this might result in a full-scale laparoscopy simulator (FLS), comparable to the FFS in pilot training. Perhaps a FLS even introduces zero operating time training as the ultimate objective.

The medical society should establish detailed objectives of training. Recently, experts have begun to investigate what level of professional behavior is required to perform safe laparoscopy. In addition, they are establishing the training needs of laparoscopic residents by determining what should be trained to accomplish the training objective. The question of which aspects of skill, rule, and knowledge-based behavior should be trained is addressed. Currently, there is no such standard available. Once the training objectives have been standardized and the training needs at the different levels of behavior have been identified, the simulator society will have clear guidelines as to what their training devices should be capable of.

One of the most obvious training needs of laparoscopic residents is the training of manual skills. The manual skills required during laparoscopy are rather different from those in conventional surgery. Training of skill-based behavior is feasible with basic trainers such as a pelvitrainer. The VR basic skill trainers that are commercially available usually simulate a generic abdomen and endoscopic instruments on a computer monitor. Basic tasks, such as pick and place tasks, are implemented to train endoscopic manipulation. The training of skill-based behavior does not require a highly realistic anatomical environment, e.g. the organs do not necessarily have to be simulated realistically. For example, the virtual reality trainer simulates basic manipulation tasks in a highly simplified environment similar to the pelvi trainer box. Several studies have reported that training on the virtual reality

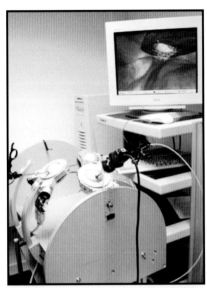

Fig. 45.10: Virtual reality trainer with software control

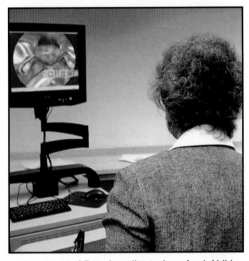

Fig. 45.11: Virtual reality trainer for LAVH

facilitated the learning of skill-based behavior (Fig. 45.10).

An advantage of virtual reality simulators over simple Pelvitrainers is the capability to easily extend the training to the rule-based level of behavior, since textbook theory, instructions, and training videos can easily be integrated in the simulator software. Much textbook material and many training videos that provide rule-based behavior training have been made available on the internet. Laparoscopy simulators are capable of training skill and rule-based behavior. To train knowledge-based behavior, a laparoscopy simulator should be capable of accurately imitating the surgical environment encountered during laparoscopic surgery (Fig. 45.11).

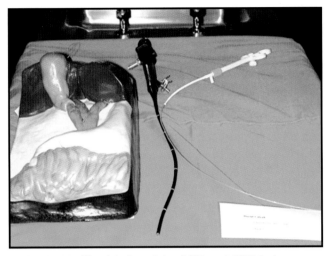

Fig. 45.12: Simulated models of GB and CBD to improve choledochoscopic skill

The perceived information from the environment should be simulated accurately to ensure effective training. The training of knowledge-based behavior on a simulator still poses a huge challenge. Two fundamental problems occur. Whereas the physics that determine the behavior of an aircraft is fairly well known and described mathematically, the physics that describes the behavior of soft-tissue organs is highly complicated and many parameters are simply still missing. Additionally, each aircraft roughly has the same flight characteristics and cockpit layout, but each new patient has a different anatomical layout than the previous one. Laparoscopy simulators have to be able to generate "random" patients (Fig. 45.12).

The integration of knowledge-based behavior training in a future simulator would enhance safety levels in laparoscopy, since then every possible surgical complication could be trained beforehand. As in aviation, intensive training can reduce a situation that at first required improvising at a knowledge-based behavior level from the trainee, to a situation that can be solved by applying trained rules.

LEARNING CURVE IN LAPAROSCOPY

TP Wright originally introduced the concept of a learning curve in aircraft manufacturing in 1936. He described a basic theory for costing the repetitive production of airplane assemblies. The term was introduced to medicine in the 1980s after the advent of minimal access surgery. It also caught the attention of the public and the legal profession when a surgeon

Section Six

told a public enquiry in Britain that a high death rate was inevitable while surgeons were on a learning curve. Recently, it has been labeled as a dangerous curve with a morbidity, mortality and unproven outcomes. Yet there is no standardization of what the term means. In an endeavor to help laparoscopic surgeons towards evidence based practices, this commentary will define and describe the learning curve, its drawing followed by a discussion of the factors affecting it, statistical evaluation, effect on randomized controlled trials and clinical implications for both practice and training, the limitations and pitfalls, ethical dilemmas and some thoughts to pave the way ahead.

DEFINITION AND DESCRIPTION

For the Wright learning curve, the underlying hypothesis is that the direct man-hours necessary to complete a unit of production will decrease by a constant percentage each time the production quantity is doubled. In manufacturing, the learning curve applies to the time and cost of production. Can a surgeon's learning curve be described on similar lines? A simple definition would be: The time taken and / or the number of procedures an average surgeon needs to be able to perform a procedure independently with a reasonable outcome. But then who is an average surgeon? Another definition may be that a learning curve is a graphic representation of the relationship between experience with a new procedure or technique and an outcome variable such as operation time, complication rate, hospital stay or mortality. A learning curve may also be operationally defined as an improvement in performance over time. Although learning theorists often disagree about what learning is, they agree that whatever the process is, its affects are clearly cumulative and may therefore be plotted as a curve. By cumulative it is meant that somehow the effects of experience carry over to aid later performance. This property is fundamental to the construction of learning curves. The improvement tends to be most rapid at first and then tails off. Hence, there are three main features of a learning curve. First, the initial or starting point defines where the performance of an individual surgeon begins. Secondly, the rate of learning measures how quickly the surgeon will reach a certain level of performance and thirdly the asymptote or expert level measures

where the surgeon's performance stabilizes. This has implications for the laparoscopic surgeon – it suggests that practice always help improve performance but the most dramatic improvement happens first. Also, with sufficient practice, surgeons can achieve comparable levels of performance.

THE DRAWING OF LEARNING CURVES

There are a variety of methods of constructing learning curves. They all assume that successive exposures in a learning series may be plotted on the X-axis, response characteristics on Y-axis and the data points distributed in the XY plane may be legitimately connected by a curve. This is the Cartesian method. More recently, the cumulative sum method has been applied for the construction of these curves for basic skills in anesthetic procedures – the method consists of relatively simple calculations that can be easily performed on an electronic spreadsheet. Statistical inferences can be made from observed success and failure. The method also provides both numerical and graphical representation of the learning process.

The multimode learning curve is useful because several factors can be put into one graph. The earlier used method of the performance analysis with it's on the spot appraisals at certain time intervals have been replaced by continuous assessment. For continuous data like operation time the moving average method is useful.

FACTORS AFFECTING LEARNING CURVES

Complex hierarchies of factors are involved here (Fig. 45.13). Factors like guidelines, protocols and standards for clinical governance agreed upon by the medical fraternity are vital. Next, the institutional policies and cost effectiveness are contributory. Needless to say the surgical team, the case mix and public awareness are relevant. The final level in the hierarchy that can influence individual learning is the characteristics of the surgeon such as attitude, capacity for acquiring new skills and previous experience.

Amongst the latter, that is the characteristics of the surgeon, the learning curve may depend on the manual dexterity of the individual surgeon and the background knowledge of surgical anatomy. The type of training the surgeon has received is also important as training on inanimate trainers and animal tissue has

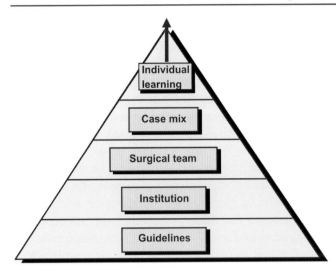

Fig. 45.13: Hierarchy of factors affecting learning curve

been shown to facilitate the process of learning. The slope of the curve depends on the nature of the procedure and frequency of procedures performed in specific time period. Many studies suggest that complication rates are inversely proportional to the volume of the surgical workload. However, rapidity of learning is not significantly related to the surgeon's age, size of practice or hospital setting. Another important factor that affects the learning curve is the supporting surgical team. A recent observational study to investigate the incidence of technical equipment problems during laparoscopic procedures reported that in 87% of procedures one or more incidents with technical equipment or instruments occurred. Hence, improvement and standardization of equipment combined with incorporation of check lists to be used before surgery has been recommended.

STATISTICAL EVALUATION OF LEARNING CURVES

Various statistical methods have been reported in the assessment of the learning curve. Commonly data are split into arbitrary groups and the means compared by chi-squared test or ANOVA. Some studies had data displayed graphically with no statistical analysis. Others used univariate analysis of experience versus outcome. Some studies used multivariate analysis techniques such as logistic regression and multiple regression to adjust for confounding factors. A systematic review concluded that the statistical methods used for assessing learning curves have been crude and the reporting of

studies poor. Recognizing that better methods may be developed in other non-clinical fields where learning curves are present (psychology and manufacturing) a systematic search was made of the non clinical literature to identify novel statistical methods for modeling learning curves. A number of techniques were identified including generalized estimating equations and multilevel models. The main recommendation was that given the hierarchical nature of the learning curve data and the need to adjust for covariant, hierarchical statistical models should be used.

EFFECT OF LEARNING CURVE ON RANDOMIZED CONTROLLED TRIALS

The learning curve can cause difficulties in the interpretation of RCTs by distorting comparisons. The usual approaches to designing trials of new surgical techniques has been either to provide intensive training and supervision or require participating surgeons to perform a fixed number of procedures prior to participation in a trial. Surgeons have been reluctant to randomize until they are proficient in a technique but once convinced of its worth, argue that it is too late to randomize. However, the best way to address the problem is to have a statistical description of the learning curve effect within a trial and various methods can then be used example Bayesian hierarchical model.

IMPLICATIONS FOR PRACTICE AND TRAINING

In the current era of evidence based medicine enthusiasm for laparoscopic surgery is rapidly gaining momentum. There is an immense amount of literature showing advantages of minimal access surgery and acceptance by the public. The learning curve for many procedures has been documented. As far as training is concerned, the introduction of laparoscopic techniques in surgery led to many unnecessary complications. This led to the development of skills laboratories involving use of box trainers with either innate or animal tissues but lacks objective assessment of skill acquisition. Virtual reality simulators have the ability to teach psychomotor skills. However, it is a training tool and needs to be thoughtfully introduced into the surgical training curriculum. A recent prospective randomized controlled trial showed that virtual simulator combined with inanimate box training

Section Six

leads to better laparoscopic skill acquisition. An interesting finding reported is that in skills training every task should be repeated at least 30 to 35 times for maximum benefit. The distribution of training over several days has also been shown to be superior to training in one day. Other factors enhancing training are fellowship programmer, or playing video games. One can also obtain feedback for improvement of training program. In one such study, the deficiency factors identified were lack of knowledge, lack of synchronized movement of the non dominant hand and easy physical fatigue. Incorporation of intensive, well planned *in vitro* training into the curriculum was made and the programmed reassessed.

WHAT ARE THE LIMITATIONS OR PITFALLS ?

"Steep" learning curves are usually used to describe procedures that are difficult to learn. However, this is a misnomer as it implies that large gains in proficiency are achieved over a small number of cases. Instead the curve for a procedure that requires a lot of cases to reach proficiency should be described as "flattened".

As long as no valid scoring system concerning the complexity of a surgical intervention exists, the learning curve cannot be used as benchmarks to compare different surgeons or clinics as legitimate instruments to rank surgeons or different hospitals. Limitations of long learning curves, facilities for training, mistakes of pioneers, surgical techniques not being described in books are some of the limitations. There are other limitations due to the nature of laparoscopic surgery like the lack of 3D vision and of tactile sensations, difficult hand eye co-ordination and long instruments.

ETHICAL DILEMMAS

Many dilemmas exist and many questions will always be with us – who bears the burden of the learning curve? Are the patients aware of the risks? Many reports validate the impression that a patient operated upon during the learning curve takes greater risks and incurs more adverse circumstances than the patient operated upon later. The issue of how informed the informed consent should be needs to be addressed. Is the integrity and conscience of a surgeon measurable? Should the forces of marketing be curtailed or regulated?

THE WAY FORWARD

Laparoscopic surgery is here to stay and success in it is determined by how quickly and effectively we learn. However, certain measures may be taken to lessen some of the adverse effects of the learning curve and others to help laparoscopic surgeons ease into the specialist. Setting up of minimal standards and credentialing is a must. Current guidelines in many countries are vague and general. The evidence for training is well documented. The message for individual surgeons is to identify their deficiencies, and chart a way forward for their personal graph of progress. Evaluation and monitoring in a systematic scientific manner will benefit the surgeon with a satisfactory learning curve that will ensure that patient welfare is not compromised.

CONCLUSION

In this article it has been pointed out that it is important to establish the training objectives, needs, and means, since they provide an answer to the questions What is the end goal of the training?, What should be trained?, and How can we train it? Rasmussen's model of human behavior provides a practical framework for the definition of the training objectives, needs, and means in MIS, and the evaluation thereof.

IMPORTANT RESOURCES

http://www.bjssoc.com
http://www.laparoscopyhospital.com
www.obgyn.net
http://www.laparoscopy.net
http://www.medscape.com
http://www.websurg.com
http://www.ivf.com/laprscpy.html
http://www.sages.org
http://www.edu.rcsed.ac.uk
http://www.webmd.com

BIBLIOGRAPHY

1. Aggarwal R, Grantcharov T, Moorthy K, Hance J, Darzi A. A competency-based virtual reality training curriculum for the acquisition of laparoscopic psychomotor skill. Am J Surg 2006;191(1):128–33.
2. Aggarwal R, Grantcharov TP, Eriksen JR, Blirup D, Kristiansen VB, Funch-Jensen P, Darzi A. An evidence-based virtual reality training program for novice laparoscopic surgeons. Ann Surg 2006;244(2):310–14.

3. Baldwin PJ, Paisley AM, Brown SP. Consultant surgeons' opinion of the skills required of basic surgical trainees. Br J Surg 1999;86(8):1078–82.

4. Bridges M, Diamond DL. The financial impact of teaching surgical residents in the operating room. Am J Surg 1989;210:118–21.

5. Broe D, Ridgway PF, Johnson S, Tierney S, Conlon KC. Construct validation of a novel hybrid surgical simulator. Surg Endosc 2006;20(6):900–04.

6. Brunner WC, Korndorffer JR Jr, Sierra R, Dunne JB, Yau CL, Corsetti RL, Slakey DP, Townsend MC, Scott DJ. Determining standards for laparoscopic proficiency using virtual reality. Am Surg 2005;71(1):29–35.

7. Brunner WC, Korndorffer JR Jr, Sierra R, Massarweh NN, Dunne JB, Yau CL, Scott DJ. Laparoscopic virtual reality training: are 30 repetitions enough? J Surg Res 2004; 122(2):150–56.

8. Carter FJ, Schijven MP, Aggarwal R, Grantcharov T, Francis NK, Hanna GB, Jakimowicz JJ. Consensus guidelines for validation of virtual reality surgical simulators. Surg Endosc 2005;19(12):1523–32.

9. Carter FJ, Schijven MP, Aggarwal R, Grantcharov T, Francis NK, Hanna GB, Jakimowicz JJ. Consensus guidelines for validation of virtual reality surgical simulators. Surg Endosc 2005;19:1523–32.

10. Champion HR, Gallagher AG. Surgical simulation—a 'good idea whose time has come'. Br J Surg 2003;90(7):767–8. 3. Grantcharov TP, Kristiansen VB, Bendix J, Bardram L, Rosenberg J, Funch-Jensen P. Randomized clinical trial of virtual reality simulation for laparoscopic skills training. Br J Surg 2004;91(2):146–50.

11. Chang L, Petros J, Hess DT, Rotondi C, Babineau TJ (16-12-2006) Integrating simulation into a surgical residency program: Is voluntary participation effective? Surg Endosc (in press).

12. Cuschieri A, Francis N, Crosby J, Hanna GB. What do master surgeons think of surgical competence and revalidation? Am J Surg 2001;182(2):110–16.

13. Dent TL. Training, credentialling and granting of clinical privileges for laparoscopic general surgery. Am J Surg 1991;161:399–403.

14. Deziel D, Millikan KW, Economou SG, Doolas A, Ko ST, Airan MC. Complications of laparoscopic cholecystectomy: a national survey of 4,292 hospitals and an analysis of 77,604 cases. Am J Surg 1993;165:9–14.

15. Eriksen JR, Grantcharov T. Objective assessment of laparoscopic skills using a virtual reality stimulator. Surg Endosc 2005;19:1216–9.

16. European Community. Directive 2000/34/EC of the European Parliament and of the Council of 22 June 2000 amending Council Directive 93/104/EC concerning certain aspects of the organisation of working time to cover sectors and activities excluded from that Directive. Official Journal of the European Communities, No. L 195, 1 August 2000;41–5.

17. Figert PL, Park AE, Witzke DB, Schwartz RW. Transfer of training in acquiring laparoscopic skills. J Am Coll Surg 2001;193(5):533–7.

18. Gallagher AG, McClure N, McGuigan J, Ritchie K, Sheehy NP. An ergonomic analysis of the fulcrum effect in the acquisition of endoscopic skills. Endoscopy 1998;30:617–20.

19. Gallagher AG, Ritter EM, Satava RM. Fundamental principles of validation, and reliability: rigorous science for the assessment of surgical education and training. Surg Endosc 2003;17(10):1525-9-1648.

20. Grantcharov TP, Kristiansen VB, Bendix J, Bardram L, Rosenberg J, Funch-Jensen P. Randomized clinical trial of virtual reality simulation for laparoscopic skills training. Br J Surg 2004;91:146–50.

21. Grantcharov TP, Rosenberg J, Pahle E, Funch-Jensen P. Virtual reality computer simulation: an objective method for the evaluation of laparoscopic surgical skills. Surg Endosc 2001;15:242–4.

22. Hackethal A, Immenroth M, Burger T. Evaluation of target scores and benchmarks for the traversal task scenario of the Minimally Invasive Surgical Trainer-Virtual Reality (MIST-VR) laparoscopy simulator. Surg Endosc 2006;20(4):645–50.

23. Hanna GB, Cuschieri A. Influence of the optical axis-totarget view angle on endoscopic task performance. Surg Endosc 1999;13:371–5.

24. Hanna GB, Shimi SM, Cuschieri A. Randomised study of influence of two-dimensional versus three-dimensional imaging on performance of laparoscopic cholecystectomy. Lancet 1998;351:248–51.

25. Hyltander A, Liljegren E, Rhodin PH, Lonroth H. The transfer of basic skills learned in a laparoscopic simulator to the operating room. Surg Endosc 2002;16(9):1324–8.

26. Hyltander A, Liljegren E, Rhodin PH, Lonroth H. The transfer of basic skills learned in a laparoscopic simulator to the operating room. Surg Endosc 2002;16(9):1324–8.

27. Hyltander A, Liljegren E, Rhodin PH, Lonroth H. The transfer of basic skills learned in a laparoscopic simulator to the operating room. Surg Endosc 2002;16:1324–8.

28. Jakimowicz JJ, Cuschieri A. Time for evidence-based minimal access surgery training—simulate or sink. Surg Endosc 2005;19(12):1521–2.

29. Kolkman W, Wolterbeek R, Jansen FW. Gynecological laparoscopy in residency training program: Dutch perspectives. Surg Endosc 2005;19:1498–1502.

30. Korndorffer JR Jr, Dunne JB, Sierra R, Stefanidis D, Touchard CL, Scott DJ. Simulator training for laparoscopic suturing using performance goals translates to the operating room. J Am Coll Surg 2005;201(1):23–9.

31. Korndorffer JR Jr, Scott DJ, Sierra R, Brunner WC, Dunne JB, Slakey DP, Townsend MC, Hewitt RL. Developing and testing competency levels for laparoscopic skills training. Arch Surg 2005;140(1):80–84.

32. Moore MJ, Bennett CL. The learning curve for laparoscopic cholecystectomy. The Southern Surgeons Club. Am J Surg 1995;170:55–9.

33. Rosser JC, Rosser LE, Savalgi RS. Skill acquisition and assessment for laparoscopic surgery. Arch Surg 1997;132(2):200–4.

34. Sakorafas GH, Tsiotos GG. New legislative regulations, problems, and future perspectives, with a particular emphasis on surgical education. J Postgrad Med 2004;50:274–7.

35. Schijven M, Jakimowicz J. Face-, expert, and referent validity of the Xitact LS500 laparoscopy simulator. Surg Endosc 2002;16(12):1764–70.

36. Schijven M, Jakimowicz J. Construct validity: experts and residents performing on the Xitact LS500 laparoscopy simulator. Surg Endosc 2003;17:803–10.

37. Schijven M, Jakimowicz J. Virtual reality surgical laparoscopic simulators: how to choose. Surg Endosc 2003;17:1943–50.

38. Schijven MP, Berlage JT, Jakimowicz JJ. Minimal-access surgery training in the Netherlands: a survey among residents-in-training for general surgery. Surg Endosc 2004;18(12):1805–14.

39. Schijven MP, Berlage JT, Jakimowicz JJ. Minimal-access surgery training in the Netherlands: a survey among residents-intraining for general surgery. Surg Endosc 2004;18:1805–14.

40. Schijven MP, Jakimowicz J. The learning curve on the Xitact LS 500 laparoscopy simulator: profiles of performance. Surg Endosc 2004;18:121–7.

41. Schijven MP, Jakimowicz JJ. Introducing the Xitact LS500 Laparoscopy Simulator: toward a revolution in surgical education. Surg Technol Int 2003;11:32–6.

42. Schijven MP, Jakimowicz JJ, Broeders IA, Tseng LN. The Eindhoven laparoscopic cholecystectomy training course—improving operating room performance using virtual reality training: results from the first E.A.E.S. accredited virtual reality trainings curriculum. Surg Endosc 2005;19:1220–26.

43. Schijven MP, Jakimowicz JJ, Carter FJ. How to select aspirant laparoscopic surgical trainees: establishing concurrent validity comparing Xitact LS500 index performance scores with standardized psychomotor aptitude test battery scores. J Surg Res 2004;121(1):112–9.

44. Scott DJ, Bergen PC, Rege RV, Laycock R, Tesfay ST, Valentine RJ, Euhus DM, Jeyarajah DR, Thompson WM, Jones DB. Laparoscopic training on bench models: better and more cost effective than operating room experience? J Am Coll Surg 2000;191(3):272–83.

45. Seymour NE, Gallagher AG, Roman SA, O'Brien MK, Bansal VK, Andersen DK, Satava RM. Virtual reality training improves operating room performance: results of a randomized, double-blinded study. Ann Surg 2002;236:458–63.

46. Taffinder NJ, Sutton C, Fishwick RJ, McManus IC, Darzi A. An objective assessment of surgeons psychomotor skills: validation of the MIST-VR laparoscopic simulator. Br J Surg 1998;85(Suppl 1):75.

47. Torkington J, Smith SG, Rees B, Darzi A. The role of the Basic Surgical Skills course in the aquisition and retention of laparoscopic skill. Surg Endosc 2001;15:1071–5.

48. Van Sickle KR, McClusky DA 3rd, Gallagher AG, Smith CD. Construct validation of the ProMIS simulator using a novel laparoscopic suturing task. Surg Endosc 2005;19(9):1227–31.

49. Verdaasdonk EG, Stassen LP, Monteny LJ, Dankelman J. Validation of a new basic virtual reality simulator for training of basic endoscopic skills: the SIMENDO. Surg Endosc 2006;20(3):511–8.

50. Verdaasdonk EG, Stassen LP, Schijven MP, Dankelman J. Construct validity and assessment of the learning curve for the SIMENDO endoscopic simulator. Surg Endosc 2007;21(8):1406–12.

51. Wilson MS, Middlebrook A, Sutton C, Stone R, McCloy RF. MIST VR: a virtual reality trainer for laparoscopic surgery assesses performance. Ann R Coll Surg Engl 1997;79:403–4.

52. Woodrum DT, Andreatta PB, Yellamanchilli RK, Feryus L, Gauger PG, Minter RM. Construct validity of the LapSim laparoscopic surgical simulator. Am J Surg 2006;191(1):28–32:1649.

46

Minimal Access Robotic Surgery

On July 11, 2000, FDA approved the first completely robotic surgery device, the daVinci surgical system from Intuitive Surgical (Mountain View, CA). The system enables surgeons to remove gallbladders and perform other general surgical procedures while seated at a computer console and 3-D video imaging system across the room from the patient. The surgeons operate controls with their hands and fingers to direct a robotically controlled laparoscope (Fig. 46.1).

This system and other robotic devices developed or under development by companies such as Computer Motion (Santa Barbara, CA) and Integrated Surgical Systems (Davis, CA) have the potential to revolutionize surgery and the operating room. They provide surgeons with the precision and dexterity necessary to perform complex, minimally invasive surgical (MIS) procedures, such as beating-heart single- or double-vessel bypass and neurological, orthopedic, and plastic surgery, among many other future applications.

Manufacturers believe that their products will broaden the scope and increase the effectiveness of MIS; improve patient outcomes; and create a safer, more efficient, and more cost-effective operating room. It is the vision of these companies that robotic systems will one day be applicable to all surgical specialties, although it is too early to tell the full extent to which they'll be used.

The first generation of surgical robots are already being installed in a number of operating rooms around the world. These aren't true autonomous robots that can perform surgical tasks on their own, but they are lending a mechanical helping hand to surgeons. These machines still require a human surgeon to operate them and input instructions. Remote control and voice activation are the methods by which these surgical robots are controlled. Robotics are being introduced to minimal access surgery because they allow for unprecedented control and precision of surgical instruments. So far, these machines have been used to position an endoscope, perform gallbladder surgery and correct gastroesophgeal reflux and heartburn. The ultimate goal of the robotic surgery field is to design a robot that can be used to perform closed-chest, beating-heart surgery.

Recently trans-atlantic surgery between USA and Strasbourg is a revolution in transatlantic minimal access surgery. In this surgery there was slight delay (66 millisecond) delay in transfer of data but in future this delay can easily minimized. In the future remote handling technology will overcome the manipulative restriction in the current instruments. There is no doubt

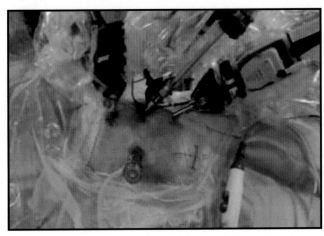

Fig. 46.1: Robotic surgery port placement for nephrectomy

10 years from now some surgeons will be operating exclusively via a computer interface controlling a masterslave manipulation. *If computer-controlled machinery can mimic the awareness, adaptability and knowledge of a human surgeon, such a takeover in the operating theater is actually realistic.*

In the operating room of the future, physicians will use tiny high-tech tools to travel inside the body with dexterity and precision beyond imagining. The future of any new technology depends upon the training.

Three surgical robots that have been recently developed are:
- daVinci Surgical System
- ZEUS Robotic Surgical System
- AESOP Robotic System.

The "da Vinci" system has seven degree of freedom movement so it can perform more complex task. The "daVinci" system has been used to perform a number of general surgical procedures like cholecystectomy and fundoplication. Robotic fundoplication allows easier passage around and behind the esophagus during its dissection and easier mobilization of the curvature of the stomach. Suturing the wrap and the crural approximation are also easier with the help of these robots.

The $1 million daVinci system consists of two primary components:
- A viewing and control console
- A surgical arm unit (Figs 46.2A to C).

In using daVinci for gallbladder surgery, three incisions, no larger than the diameter of a pencil are made in the patient's abdomen, which allows for three stainless-steel rods to be inserted. The rods are held in place by three robotic arms. One of the rods is equipped with a camera, while the other two are fitted with surgical instruments that are able to dissect and suture the tissue of the gallbladder. Unlike in conventional surgery, these instruments are not directly touched by the doctor's hands.

Effector tips of the daVinci surgical system incorporate miniature wrists that allow them to mimic any movement made by the surgeon at the control console. Sitting at the control console, a few feet from the operating table, the surgeon looks into a viewfinder to examine the 3-D images being sent by the camera inside the patient. The images show the surgical site and the two surgical instruments mounted on the tips

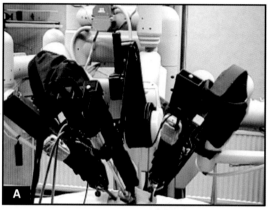

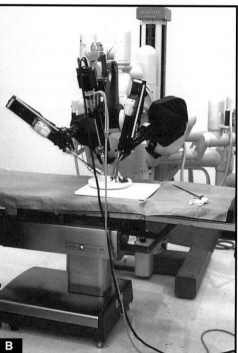

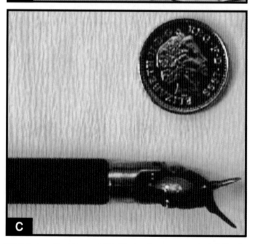

Figs 46.2A to C: (A and B) Robotic arms of daVinci surgical system, (C) Effector tips of the daVinci surgical system

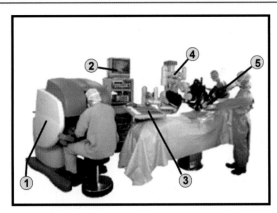

Fig. 46.3: Robotic surgery (1) Surgeon console, (2) Image processing equipment, (3) Endowrist instruments, (4) Surgical arm cart, (5) Hi-resolution 3-D endoscope

of two of the rods. Joystick-like controls, located just underneath the screen, are used by the surgeon to manipulate the surgical instruments. Each time one of the joysticks is moved, a computer sends an electronic signal to one of the instruments, which moves in sync with the movements of the surgeon's hands.

Another robotic system is the ZEUS System, made by computer motion, which is already available in Europe. However, both the daVinci and ZEUS systems must receive governmental approval for each procedure that a surgeon plans to use it for. The $750,000 ZEUS has a similar setup to that of the daVinci. It has a computer workstation, a video display, and hand controls that are used to move the table-mounted surgical instruments. While the ZEUS system has not yet been cleared for American use beyond clinical trials, German doctors have already used the system to perform coronary bypass surgery.

The ZEUS system employs the assistance of the Automated Endoscopic System for Optimal Positioning (AESOP) robotic system. Released by computer motion in 1994, AESOP was the first robot to be cleared by the FDA for assisting surgery in the operating room. AESOP is much simpler than the daVinci and ZEUS systems. It's basically just one mechanical arm, used by the physician to position the laparoscope. Foot pedals or voice-activated software allow the surgeon to position the camera, leaving his or her hands free to continue operating on the patient (Fig. 46.3).

The use of a computer console to perform operations from a distance opens up the idea of telesurgery, which would involve a doctor performing

delicate surgery thousands of miles away from the patient. If it were possible to use the computer console to move the robotic arms in real-time, then it would be possible for a doctor in New Delhi to operate on a patient in New York. A major obstacle in tele-surgery has been the time delay between the doctor moving his or her hands to the robotic arms responding to those movements. Currently, the doctor must be in the room with the patient for robotic systems to react instantly to the doctor's hand movements.

Having fewer personnel in the operating room and allowing doctors the ability to operate on a patient long-distance could lower the cost of health care. In addition to cost efficiency, robotic surgery has several other advantages over conventional surgery, including enhanced precision and reduced trauma to the patient. For instance, heart bypass surgery now requires that the patient's chest 30.48 cm long incision. However, with the daVinci or ZEUS systems, it is possible to operate on the heart by making three small incisions in the chest, each only 10 mm in diameter. The patient would experience less pain and less bleeding, which means a faster recovery.

Robotics also decreases the fatigue that doctors experience during surgeries that can last several hours. Surgeons can become exhausted during those long surgeries, and can experience hand tremors as a result. Even the steadiest of human hands cannot match those of a surgical robot. The da Vinci system has been programmed to compensate for tremors, so if the doctor's hand shakes the computer ignores it and keeps the mechanical arm steady.

While surgical robots offer some advantages over the human hand, we are still a long way from the day when autonomous robots will operate on people without human interaction. But, with advances in computer power and artificial intelligence, it could be that in this century a robot will be designed that can locate abnormalities in the human body, analyze them and operate to correct those abnormalities without any human guidance.

The fallopian tube reconnection procedure, referred to as tubal reanastomosis, was performed by Dr Tommaso Falcone, who is head of the Reproductive Endocrinology and Infertility Section at the Cleveland Clinic. Dr Falcone used Computer Motion's ZEUS robotic surgical system as part of a clinical trial,

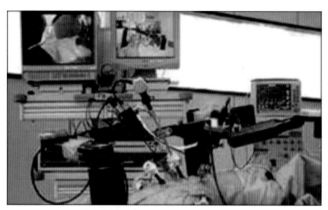

Fig. 46.4: Robotic surgery via master slave manipulator

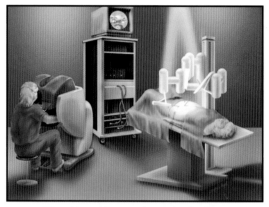

Fig. 46.5: Master slave manipulator

approved by the United States Food and Drug Administration (FDA).

The patient, a 38-year-old woman, and her healthy 10-day-old son are both in excellent condition and have returned to their Cleveland-area home. The mother had originally undergone a tubal ligation sterilization operation in her twenties. She and her partner later wished to have a child together and began preparing for a reversal operation. The patient saw an advertisement for the ZEUS study and consulted with trial leader Dr Falcone. The lady was informed in detail of the investigational protocol and agreed to have the robotically assisted procedure.

In addition to the ZEUS System, Computer Motion markets the AESOP 3000, a voice-controlled endoscope positioning system, and the HERMES Control Center, a centralized system which enables the surgeon to voice control a network of "smart" medical devices. Currently, the ZEUS system is under an FDA-approved investigational device exemption and is also CE marked for commercial sale in Europe.

Robotics is rapidly developing in surgery, although the word is slightly misused in this connection. None of the systems under development involves a machine acting autonomously. Instead, the machine acts as a remote extension of the surgeon. The correct term for such a system is a "master slave manipulator," although it seems unlikely that this term will gain general currency.

Minimal invasive surgery is itself a form of tele-manipulation because the surgeon is physically separated from the workspace. Tele-robotics is an obvious tool to extend the surgeons capabilities. The goal is to restore the tactile cues and intuitive dexterity

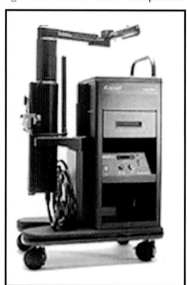

Fig. 46.6: Robotic console

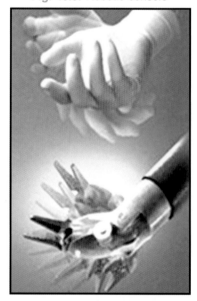

Fig. 46.7: Robotic arm

Section Six

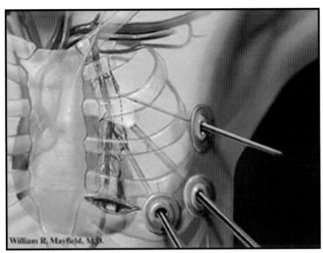

Fig. 46.8: Ports in cardiac minimal access surgery

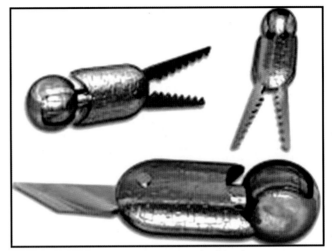

Fig. 46.9: Instruments used by the daVinci surgical system

of the surgeon, which are diminished by minimal invasive surgery. A slave manipulator, controlled through a spatially consistent and intuitive master with a force feedback system, could replace the tactile sensibilities and restore dexterity (Fig. 46.4).

Although the potential of robotic surgery is just beginning but progress may come quickly. Laparoscopic gallbladder surgery was first done in 1987, but it became standard within five years. Just think about a surgeon! He picks up this black box and waves it over your body, and you're fixed. How's that going to happen? One day a surgeon may use robotic devices to enter the body through its own orifices. They could carry medical instruments inside the body, where they would be manipulated by simple computer commands (Figs 46.5 to 46.7).

The robotic arm after addition of wrists permits the surgeon to mimic his own movements, rather than experience limitations of the rigid long cylindrical laparoscopic instrument and has obvious advantages in terms of dexterity and complexity of instrument (Fig. 46.9).

Four ports are used and robotic arm is introduced. One of the arms contains telescope which sends 12 to 15 times magnified clear image on the monitor. Another arm is for a stabilizer which is used to hold the diseased coronary artery in place while bypass is performed. The other two remaining right and left instrument is used to perform microvascular anastomosis. Currently robotic coronary bypass surgery should be considered only for the patient who have

single vessel disease but in near future we have hope to perform double or even triple bypass surgery (Fig. 46.8).

The attached instruments are controlled by the surgeon, who sits at an adjacent console. Several passive mechanical devices, primarily used to hold the telescope, have been developed as assistants for general laparoscopic surgery. They successfully reduce the stress on the surgeon by eliminating the inadvertent movements of a human assistant, which can be distracting and disorienting.

More and more surgeries from prostate to heart are being performed by doctors remotely guiding robotic arms. In such procedures, the surgeon's hands never enter the patient. After the initial incisions are made, robotic arms wielding a tiny camera and surgical tools make the snips, stanch the blood flow, and sew up inside when all is done. The surgeon sits at a console usually in the operating room, although the technology would allow a doctor to operate on a patient on the other side of the world peering into binocular like lenses at views provided by the camera inside the patient. The doctor guides the robot's work by twisting his wrists in stirrup-like handles, moving his thumb and forefinger in scissor-like loops, or tapping foot pedals to focus the camera or move a robotic arm.

The most common robotic surgery is radical prostatectomy. Its use has grown from just 1,500 procedures in 2000 to an estimated 20,000 last year. More than 8,000 prostate glands were removed robotically last year, up from 36 in 2000. The procedure

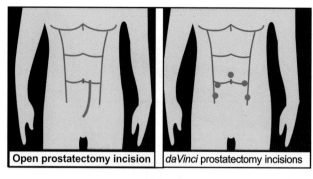

| Open prostatectomy incision | *daVinci* prostatectomy incisions |

Fig. 46.10: Comparison between open and daVinci prostatectomy

accounted for more than 10% of the 75,000 prostatectomies done in 2004. Busy professionals like the fact that they can be out of the hospital in a day, vs. two or three for open surgery, and resume normal activities in one week rather than six. Cutting nerves around the prostate can lead to incontinence or impotence, so precision is important. Between 25% and 60% of conventional prostatectomy patients suffer from postoperative impotence. Small studies of robotic surgery have shown at least a short-term benefit in terms of impotence and incontinence.

Not every patient is a candidate. Complicated cases when the patient is very sick, needs multiple procedures, or has had previous chest surgery are not suited to robotics. Nor can a heart transplant or artificial heart implant be done this way. If the complication arises, the patient may wind up being opened. So patients who want robotics smaller scars and quicker recovery times will need to ask hard questions. Find out how many times, the procedure you need has been done robotically and what the advantages and disadvantages are. Just as important, ask how many robotic surgeries, the doctor who will do yours has performed. In real life, you want the force of experience to be with you.

For qualified candidates, the robotic prostatectomy offers numerous potential benefits over the traditional open prostatectomy, including (Fig. 46.10):
- Shorter hospital stay
- Less pain
- Less risk of infection
- Less blood loss and transfusions
- Less scarring

- Faster recovery
- Quicker return to normal activities.

While still a technology that is in its infancy, the use of robots to assist in surgery is becoming more and more widespread. There are now large case series reported in the literature that show possible benefits to the patient in terms of recovery from such surgeries as prostate and cardiac procedures. Additionally, as these systems continue to develop, improved technology and software provide the surgeon with "assistance" that improves precision and accuracy (Figs 46.11A to D).

Robotic technology requires a tremendous financial investment, so you might not see it at every community hospital in the near future. However, as with all technology, the price will likely fall quickly as the applications are expanded, as more widespread adoption occurs, and as the field of robotics experiences additional breakthroughs. For now, many major academic institutions are beginning to purchase and deploy these systems.

Technology allows amazing things to be accomplished. Robotic surgery is a new and expensive tool that is beginning to see adoption. Minimally invasive surgery with a robot and without bypass is the next logical step in the development of cardiac surgery. It is beginning to show clear benefits for patients and this means that it will likely become more and more popular with time and as the price falls.

Robotic Versus Laparoscopic Prostatectomy

In laparoscopy, the surgeon uses long instruments through small openings and maneuvers them with direct hand contact. Robotic systems use even more delicate instruments that possess two additional degrees of movement excursion (for a total of six, as with a human hand). Comfortably seated at the robot console, the surgeon can maneuver the instruments via a computer interface.

Laparoscopic radical prostatectomy is associated with a steep learning curve. Even in the hands of expert surgeons, laparoscopic radical prostatectomy requires extensive learning; approximately 40 cases are needed to master this technique. In contrast, the learning of robotic prostatectomy seems to be more intuitive and less demanding.

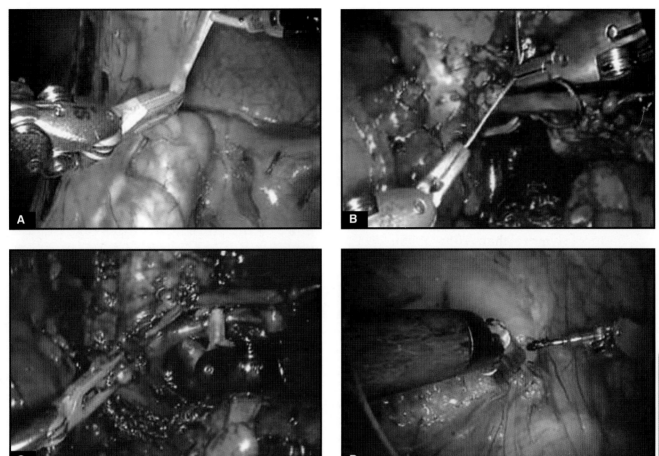

Figs 46.11A to D: Robotic assisted nephrectomy

CONCLUSION

Robotic prostatectomy is a safe, effective and reproducible technique for removing the prostate. In most patients, it can be performed within one and a half to two hours with minimal blood loss and few complications. The procedure incorporates principles of both laparoscopic and open radical prostatectomy. The patients enjoy benefits of surgical treatment in the setting of less invasion, minimal pain, limited blood loss and early functional and overall recovery.

BIBLIOGRAPHY

1. Berguer R. Surgery and ergonomics. Arch Surg 1999;134: 1011-6.
2. Berguer R, Rab GT, Abu-Ghaida H, Alarcon A, Chung J. A comparison of surgeons' posture during laparoscopic and open surgical procedures. Surg. Endosc. 1997;11:2139.
3. Beurger R, Rember M, Beckley D. Laparoscopic instruments cause increased forearm fatigue: a subjective and objective comparison of open and laparoscopic techniques. Min Invasive Ther Allied 1997;6:36-40.
4. Buess GF, Schurr MO, Fischer SC. Robotics and allied technologies in endoscopic surgery. Arch Surg 2000;132: 229-35.
5. Cadière GB, Himpens J, Bruyns J. How to avoid esophageal perforation while performing laparoscopic dissection of the hiatus. Surg. Endosc 1995;9:450.
6. Cadière GB, Himpens J, Vertruyen M, Favretti F. The world's first obesity surgery performed by a surgeon at a distance. Obes. Surg 1999;9:206.
7. Cadière GB, Houben JJ, Bruyns J, Himpens J, Panzer JM, Gelin M. Laparoscopic Nissen fundoplication technique and preliminary results. Br J Surg 1994;81:400.
8. Chan A, Chung S, Yim A, Lau J, Ng E, Li A. Comparison of two-dimensional vs three-dimensional camera systems in laparoscopic surgery. Surg Endosc 1997;11:438-40.

9. Cheah WK, Lenzi JE, So J, Dong F, Kum CK, Goh P. Evaluation of a head-mounted display (HMD) in the performance of a simulated laparoscopic task. Surg Endosc 2001;15:990–91.

10. Davies B. A review of robotics in surgery. Proc Inst Mech Eng 2000;214:129–40.

11. Dion YM, Gaillard F. Visual integration of data and basic motor skills under laparoscopy. Influence of 2-D and 3-D video-camera systems. Surg. Endosc. 1997;11:995.

12. Dosis A, Bello F, Rockall T, Munz Y, Moorthy K, Martin S, Darzi A. (200x) ROVIMAS: a software package for assessing surgical skills using the da Vinci telemanipulator system.

13. Felger JE, Nifong LW, Chitwood WR Jr. The evolution of and early experience with robot-assisted mitral valve surgery. Surg Laparosc Endosc Percutan Technol 2002;12:58–63.

14. Gallagher AG, Satava RM. Virtual reality as a metric for the assessment of laparoscopic psychomotor skills. Learning curves and reliability measures. Surg Endosc 2002;16: 1746–52.

15. Garcia-Ruiz A, Gagner M, Miller JH, Steiner CP, Hahn JF. Manual vs robotically assisted laparoscopic surgery in the performance of basic manipulation and suturing tasks. Arch. Surg 1998;133:9957.

16. Garcia-Ruiz A, Gagner M, Miller JH, Steiner CP, Hahn JF. Manual vs. robotically assisted laparoscopic surgery in the performance of basic manipulation and suturing tasks. Arch. Surg. 1998;133:957.

17. Garcia-Ruiz A, Smedira NG, Loop FD, Hahn JF, Miller JH, Steiner CP, Gagner M. Robotic surgical instruments for dexterity enhancement in thoracoscopic coronary artery bypass graft. J Laparoendosc. Adv. Surg. Tech. A. 1997;7: 5277.

18. Hanna GB, Cuschieri A. Influence of two-dimensional and three-dimensional imaging on endoscopic bowel suturing. World J Surg 2000;24:444–9.

19. Hernandez JD, Bann SD, Munz Y, Moorthy K, Datta V, Martin S, Dosis A, Bello F, Darzi A, Rockall T. The learning curve of a simulated surgical task using the da Vinci telemanipulator system. Br J Surg 2002;89(suppl):17–18.

20. Himpens J, Leman G, Cadière GB. Telesurgical laparoscopic cholecystectomy. Surg. Endosc 1998;12:81091.

21. Johns DB, Brewer JD, Soper NJ. The influence of three-dimensional video systems on laparoscopic task performance. Surg Laparosc Endosc 1996;6:191–7.

22. Kim VB, Chapman WHH, Albrecht RJ, et al. Early experience with Telemanipulative Robot-assisted laparoscopic cholecystectomy using da Vinci. Surg Laparosc Endosc Percutan Technol 2002;12:33–40.

23. McDougall EM, Soble JJ, Wolf JS Jr, Nakada S-Y, Elashry OM, Clayman RV. Comparison of three-dimensional and two-dimensional laparoscopic video systems. J. Endoural. 1996;10:371.

24. Mentges B, Buess G, Schafer D, Mancke K, Becker HD. Local therapy of rectal tumor. Dis. Colon Rectum 1996;39:8886. Cadière et al. Robotic Laparoscopic Surgery 1477.

25. Mueller MD, Camartin C, Dreher E, Hanggi W. Threedimensional laparoscopy: Gadget or progress? A randomized trial on the efficacy of three-dimensional laparoscopy. Surg Endosc 1999;13:469–72.

26. Munz Y, Hernandez H, Bann S, Bello F, Dosis A, Martin S, Moorthy K, Rockall T, Darzi A. The advantages of 3D visualization in surgical performance with the Da-Vinci telemanipulation system. J Soc Laparosc Surg 2002;6:264-794.

27. Satava RM. Emerging technologies for surgery in the 21st century. Arch. Surg. 1999;134:1197.

28. Shea JA, Healey MJ, Berlin JA, Clarke JR, Malet PF, Staroscik RN, Schwartz JS, Williams SV. Mortality and complications associated with laparoscopic cholecystectomy: A meta-analysis. Ann Surg 1996;224:609–20.

29. Taffinder N, Smith S, Mair J, et al. Can a computer measure surgical precision? Reliability, validity and feasibility of the ICSAD. Surg Endosc 1999;13(suppl 1): 81.

30. Voorhorst FA, Overbeeke CJ, Smets GJ. Spatial perception during laparoscopy: implementing action-perception coupling. Stud. Health Technol. Inform 1997;39:379.

31. Wappler M. Medical manipulators: a realistic concept? Minim. Invasive Ther. 1995;4:261.

32. Williams LF, Chapman WC, Bonau RA, McGee EC, Boyd RW, Jacobs JK. Comparison of laparoscopic cholecystectomy with open cholecystectomy in a single center. Am J Surg 1993;165:459–65.

33. Yohannes P, Rotariu P, Pinto P, Smith AD, Lee BR. Comparison of robotic versus laparoscopic skills: is there a difference in the learning curve? Urology 2002;60:39–45.

47 Transanal Endoscopic Microsurgery

Transanal endoscopic microsurgery (TEM) was developed by Professor Gerhard Buess from Tuebingen, Germany and it became available for widespread use in 1983 (Fig. 47.1). A surgeon's ability to remove rectal lesions transanally is limited by access and exposure, with conventional instruments usually restricting the surgeon to the distal six to seven centimeters of rectum. When transanal excision is not possible, the traditional transabdominal approach, a major surgical procedure is necessary. Transanal endoscopic microsurgery (TEM), with its longer reach and enhanced visibility of the entire rectum, extends the boundaries of transanal surgery, giving appropriately selected patients a minimally invasive surgical option with a faster and virtually pain-free recovery.

Transanal endoscopic microsurgery (TEM) allows for local excision of rectal neoplasm with greater exposure than transanal excision and less morbidity than transabdominal approaches. Supporters of the TEM technique praise the excellent exposure of the rectum and the minimal invasiveness, as opposed to conventional surgical techniques. The arrival of TEM was associated with an increase in the number of operations for rectal cancer; however, the use of TEM remained constant relative to radical resections. Use of TEM resection alone is appropriate for all adenomas and cancers staged Tis and T1. Use of TEM alone is not an appropriate treatment for T2 cancers.

Local excision of rectal neoplasms is an accepted method of treating selected lesions and can be accomplished through either a transanal approach or a posterior proctotomy. The former is hindered by poor

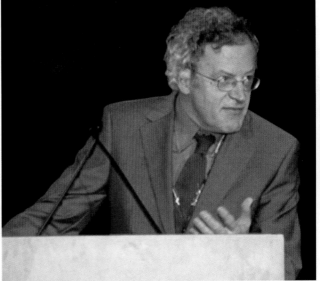

Fig. 47.1: Inventor of TEM technology

exposure and visibility of lesions in the middle and upper rectum. While the latter approach does give somewhat improved exposure of these more cephalad tumors, it may be complicated by fecal fistulae or sphincter impairment. Transanal endoscopic microsurgery (TEM) has emerged as a better technique for removing lesions in the middle and upper rectum, and it obviates the need for a posterior proctotomy. Furthermore, the transanal rectoscope extends the boundaries of transanal surgery by providing access to lesions previously inaccessible with conventional means. The net result is an operative approach to rectal lesions that is not hindered by the poor exposure and limited reach associated with conventional retractors.

Virtually any adenoma of any size or degree of circumferential involvement can be removed with TEM. Adenomas are removed with a 5 mm margin of normal mucosa, and dissection is undertaken in the submucosal plane. For large adenomas or those that have firm areas within them or previous histological evidence of atypia or dysplasia, the risk of harboring an occult cancer is increased; for such lesions, it is generally recommended that a fullthickness excision be performed. Other benign indications for TEM include transrectal rectopexy for prolapse, for which there has been limited experience to date, and correction of anastomotic strictures by stricturoplasty.

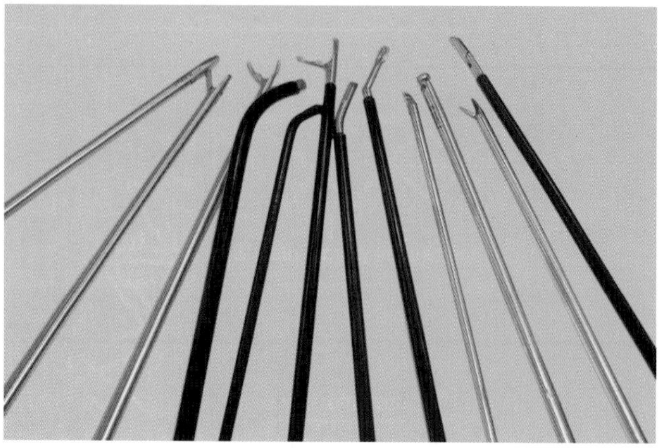

Indications of TEM

Benign

- Rectal polyps
- Carcinoid tumors
- Retrorectal masses
- Anastomotic strictures
- Extrasphincteric fistulae
- Pelvic abscesses

Malignant

- Malignant rectal polyps
- T1-T2 rectal cancer
- Palliative excision of T3 cancer

Instruments

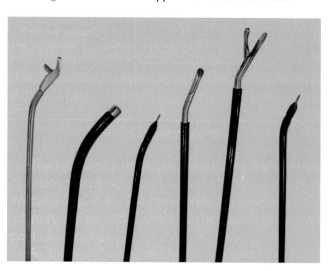

Fig. 47.3: Fine curve tipped instruments for TEM

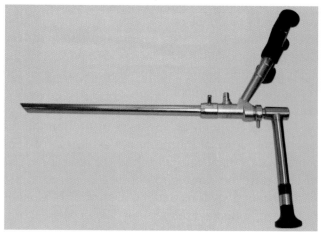

Fig. 47.4: Needle holders and electrosurgical instruments used in TEM

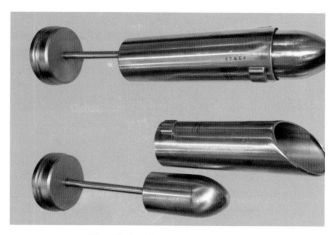

Fig. 47.2: 40 mm proctoscope

Fig. 47.5A

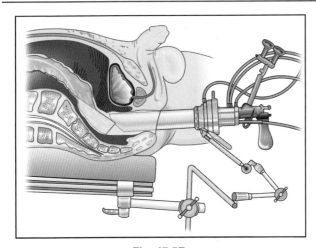

Fig. 47.5B

Figs 47.5 A and B: Stereoscope used in TEM

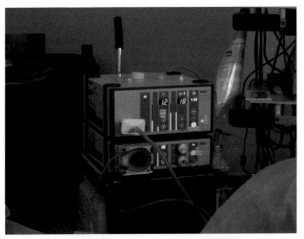

Fig. 47.6: Insufflator used in TEM

The basic TEM instrumentation includes the combined endosurgical unit, which regulates carbon dioxide insufflation, saline irrigation, and suction. The rectoscope is 40 mm in diameter and is available in lengths of 12 and 20 cm (Fig. 47.2). Once the rectoscope is inserted to the desired location within the rectum, it is secured to the operating room table with a double ball-and-socket supporting arm (Figs 47.5A and B). During the dissection, the supporting arm is moved frequently to maintain direct visibility of the lesion. The end of the rectoscope is sealed with an airtight face piece that has 5 entry ports. These ports, in turn, are sealed by rubber caps and sleeves so that the various instruments necessary for the dissection can be inserted. One of the big advantages of TEM is binocular vision (Figs 47.7 and 47.8). The binocular

stereoscopic eyepiece is inserted through one of the ports, and it has an accessory scope for video hook-up. The various instruments needed are suction catheter, a needle-tipped high-frequency electrical knife, tissue graspers that are oriented to either the right or left, scissors, and a needle holder. The suction catheter, tissue graspers, and needle-tipped knife can all be connected to the cautery unit, which greatly facilitates control of hemorrhage and coagulation of bleeding vessels (Figs 47.3, 47.4 and 47.6).

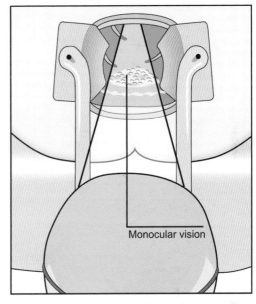

Monocular vision

Fig. 47.7: Monocular vision in laparoscopy

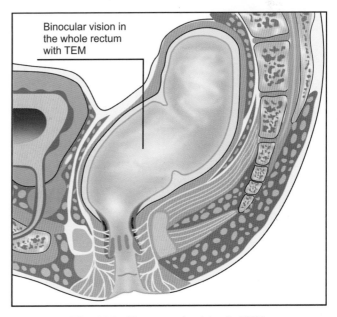

Binocular vision in the whole rectum with TEM

Fig. 47.8: Stereoscopic vision in TEM

Section Six

Patient Positioning in TEM

Position of lesion determines positioning of patient on the operating room table (Fig. 47.9). The patient should be positioned in such a way that the lesion should be made to be in the 6 o'clock position for the operator (Fig. 47.10). The position of the patient in the opera- ting room is dependent on tumor location. Since the bevel of the rectoscope must face downward, patients with anterior lesions are placed in the prone position, whereas patients with posterior lesions are placed in the lithotomy position. Patients with lateral lesions are placed accordingly into the appropriate decubitus position.

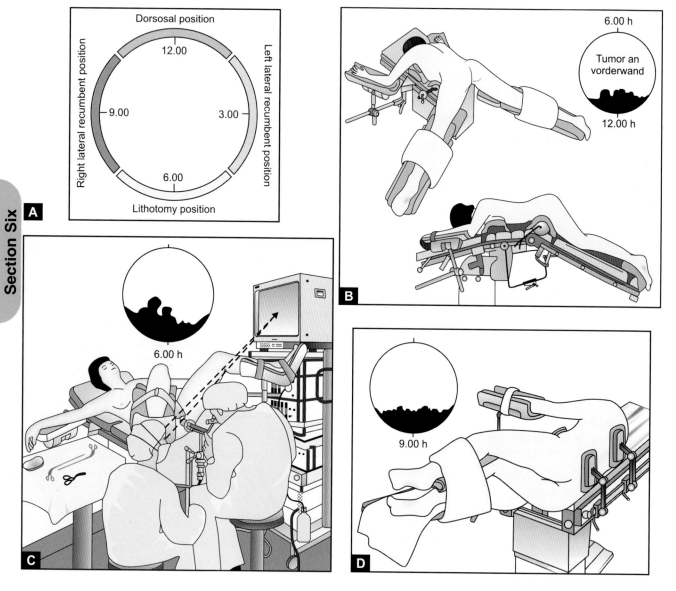

Figs 47.9A to D: Positioning of patient for TEM

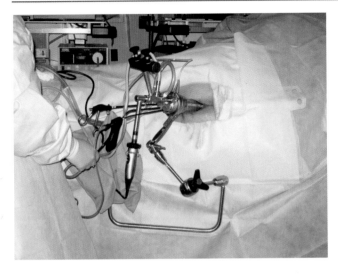

Fig. 47.10: Patient position for lesion at right lateral position

Properly selected rectal cancers can also be removed with TEM; for such lesions, a 1 cm margin of normal tissue surrounding the lesion should be obtained. A full-thickness excision is mandatory to accurately stage the depth of penetration and unpredictable in its location. Transanal endoscopic microsurgery is a safe technique, and having low number of complications; however, this procedure is not a license to disregard established criteria for local excision of cancers. The exceptions to this may be tumor size and location. With its superior optics, constant rectal distention, and longer instrument casing, TEM is not limited to small, distally located lesions. Because of the magnification capabilities of the TEM equipment - about 30 times greater than normal - we are better able to visualize the lesion and

TEM Procedures (Figs 47.11 to 47.15)

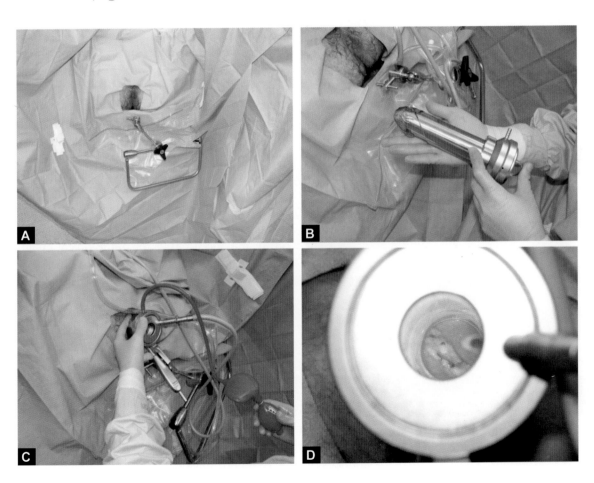

Figs 47.11A to D: Setting us instruments in TEM to start procedure

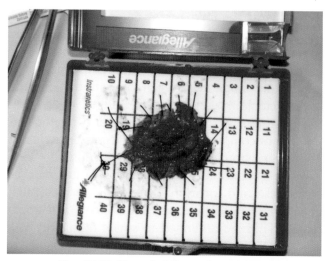

Fig. 47.12: Resected tissue through TEM

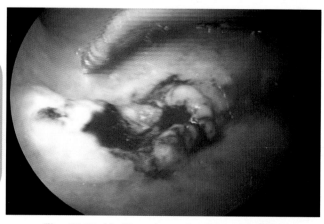

Fig. 47.13: Marking of margin of tissue in TEM

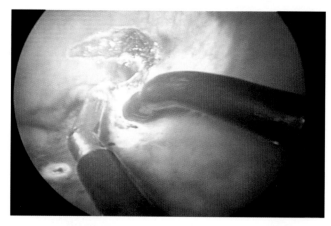

Fig. 47.14: Excision of Malignant tissue in TEM

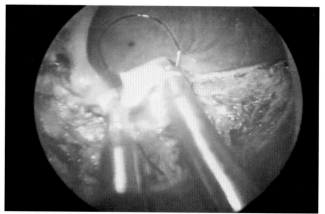

Fig. 47.15: Suturing in TEM

may argue that cancers within the middle and upper rectum should all be treated with low shrinking tumors, or even inducing a complete remission, TEM may have an increased role. However, this remains to be seen and can only be answered with further studies.

Data presented at the annual meeting of the American Society of Colon and Rectal Surgeons last July also suggests that TEM offers certain advantages over the more standard procedure. In a retrospective study that compared transanal excision with TEM for both benign and malignant rectal masses, the TEM procedure was much more likely to result in a complete resection and yield negative margins compared with transanal excision (88% vs 71%). This was true whether the lesion was benign or malignant. It was also more likely to produce an intact, non-fragmented specimen compared with transanal excision (94% vs 63%), making it easier for pathological evaluation.

The rate of recurrence, both local and distant, was also lower in patients who had undergone TEM compared with transanal excision (5% vs 25%). This was particularly true for rates of local recurrence, which were significantly lower for both benign and malignant lesions following TEM (4% vs 20%). The rate of complications was similar between both groups.

COMMON COMPLICATIONS

- Perforation of intraperitoneal rectal wall - unable to close using TEM in 3.9%
- Required LAR or diversion (1 patient)
- Early mild incontinence/soiling in 2.6% Resolved by 10 weeks

get very good margins. This minimizes the chances of the patient needing a colostomy, which can sometimes result with open surgery, even with benign lesions. One

CONCLUSION

The cost of the TEMS equipment must be mentioned. The capital outlay of more than $50,000 is considerable. However, this is offset by several factors. There is no doubt that some surgeons will argue about how many patients have rectal lesions that are definitely reachable only with the TEMS system. These patients are clearly saved a transabdominal rectal excision and realize a very significant cost saving. In addition, there are no disposable costs per case, and the equipment is robust, requiring minimal maintenance (our own system is now 10 years old). The imaging stack is compatible with the laparoscopic surgical system available in most operating suites. However, in view of the limited number of patients undergoing a TEMS in a tertiary referral center, we believe that this is not a suitable approach for every colorectal unit and suggest that only larger centers would have enough patients to justify the costs. TEM is appropriate for a very specific patient population that includes patients with rectal benign or early cancer with no lymph node involvement. However, in this setting, the benefits are such that this technique has a rightful place as part of the colorectal surgeon's operative armamentarium.

BIBLIOGRAPHY

1. Beuss G, Mentges B, Manncke K, Starlinger M, Becker HD. Technique and results of transanal microsurgery in early rectal cancer. Am J Surg 1992;163:63-9.
2. Beuss G. Review. Transanal endoscopic microsurgery (TEM). J R Coll Surg Edinb 1993;38:239-45.
3. Bleday R. Local excision of rectal cancer. World J Surg 1997;21: 706-14.
4. Bouvet M, Milas M, Giaceo GG, Cleary KR, Jnajan NA, Skibber JM. Predictors of recurrence after local excision and postoperative chemoradiotherapy of adenocarcinoma of the rectum. Ann Surg Oncol 1999;6:26-32.
5. Chakravarti A, Compton CC, Shellito PC, et al. Long-term follow-up of patients with rectal cancer managed by local excision with and without adjuvant irradiation. Ann Surg 1999;230:49-54.
6. Enker WE, Merchant N, Cohen AM, et al. Safety and efficacy of low anterior resection for rectal cancer. Ann Surg 1999;230:544-54.
7. Fielding LP, Philips RKS, Fry JS, Hittinger R. Prediction of outcome after curative surgery for large bowel cancer. Lancet 1986;2:904-6.
8. Fielding LP, Philips RKS, Hittinger R. Factors influencing mortality after curative resection for large bowel cancer in elderly patients. Lancet 1989;1:595-7.
9. Geraghty JM, Williams CB, Talbot IC. Malignant colorectal polyps, venous invasion and successful treatment by endoscopic polypectomy. Gut 1991;32:774-8.
10. Guillem JG, Paty PB, Cohen AM. Surgical treatment of colorectal cancer. CA Cancer J Clin 1997;47:113-28.
11. Hermanek P. A pathologist's point of view on endoscopically removed polyps of the colon and rectum. Acta Hepatogastroenterol 1978;25:169-70.
12. Hurst PA, Proust WG, Kelly JM, Bannister JJ, Walker RT. Local recurrence after low anterior resection using the staple gun. Br J Surg 1982;69:275-6.
13. Isbister WH. Colorectal cancer surgery in the elderly: an audit of surgery in octogenarians. Aust N Z J Surg 1997;67:557-61.
14. Jehle EC, Haehnael T, Starlinger MJ, Becker HD. Alterations of anal sphincter functions following transanal endoscopic microsurgery (TEM) for rectal tumours. Gastroenterology 1992;102:365.
15. Karanjia ND, Schache DJ, North WRS, Heald RJ. 'Close shave' in anterior resection. Br J Surg 1990;77:510-2.
16. Killingback M. Local excision of carcinoma of the rectum: indications. World J Surg 1992;16:437-46.
17. Matheson NA, McIntosh CA, Krukowski ZH. Continuing experience with single layer appositional anastomosis in the large bowel. Br J Surg 1985;70:S104-6.
18. McArdle CS, Hole D, Hansell D, Blumgart LH, Wood CB. Prospective study of colorectal cancer in the west of Scotland: ten year follow-up. Br J Surg 1990;77:280-2.
19. Mella J, Biffin A, Radcliffe AG, Stamatakis JD, Steele RJC. Population based audit of colorectal cancer management in two UK health regions. Br J Surg 1997;84:1731-6.
20. Mellow M. Neoplasms. In: Raskin J, Nord HJ, eds. Colonoscopy: Principles and Techniques. New York: Igaku-Shoin, 1995:345-56.
21. Mentges B, Buess G, Effinger G, Manncke K, Becker HD. Indications and results of local treatment of rectal cancer. Br J Surg 1997;84:348-51.
22. Mentges B, Buess G, Schafer D, Manncke K, Becker HD. Local therapy for rectal tumours. Dis Colon Rectum 1996;39:886-92.
23. Minsky BD, Enker WE, Cohen AM, Lauwers G. Clinicopathological features in rectal cancer treated by local excision and postoperative radiation therapy. Radiat Med 1995;13:235-41.
24. Muldoon JP. Treatment of benign tumours of the rectum. Clin Gastroenterol 1975;4:563-70.
25. Ota DM, Skibber J, Rich TA MD. Anderson Cancer Center experience with local excision and multimodality therapy for rectal cancer. Surg Oncol Clin North Am 1992;1:147-52.
26. Saclarides TJ. Transanal endoscopic microsurgery. Surg Clin North Am 1997;77:229-39.
27. Saclarides TJ. Transanal endoscopic microsurgery: a single surgeon's experience. Arch Surg 1998;133:595-8.
28. Taylor RH, Hay JH, Larsson SN. Transanal local excision of selected low rectal cancers. Am J Surg 1998;175:360-3.
29. Willett CG, Compton CC, Shelito PC, Efird JT. Selection factors for local excision or abdominoperineal resection of early stage rectal cancer. Cancer 1994;73:2716-20.
30. Winde G, Nottberg H, Keller R, Schmid KW, Bunte H. Surgical cure for early rectal carcinomas (T1). Transanal endoscopic microsurgery vs. anterior resection. Dis Colon Rectum 1996;39:969-76.

Section Six

48 Future of Minimal Access Surgery

MINIMAL ACCESS TECHNIQUES

Established

- Laparoscopic cholecystectomy
- Diagnostic laparoscopy
- Laparoscopic appendicectomy
- Laparoscopic Nissen fundoplication
- Laparoscopic (or thoracoscopic) Heller's myotomy
- Laparoscopic adrenalectomy
- Laparoscopic splenectomy
- Thoracoscopic sympathectomy
- Laparoscopic rectopexy.

Under Evaluation

- Laparoscopic hernia repair
- Laparoscopic colectomy
- Laparoscopic nephrectomy for living related donor transplant
- Parathyroidectomy (guided with hand held gamma probe)
- Laparoscopic repair of duodenal perforation.

Prospects

- Sentinel node biopsy
- Hepatic resection
- Gastrectomy.

The future laparoscopic technology includes three-dimensional, virtual reality, and HDTV. HDTV expands the scanning rate from 525 lines of resolution to 1000

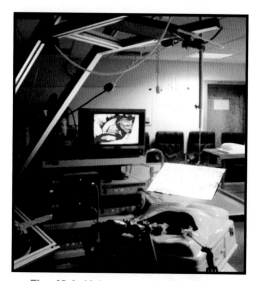

Fig. 48.1: Hologram projection system

or 1200 lines per frame and the quality of picture would be twice better than existing system.

With virtual reality, a three dimensional computer image is presented through liquid crystal glasses.

The future of three-dimensional images is not far away and many instrument companies have prototype in the field (Fig. 48.1).

Laparoscopic surgery is growing in such a speed that 3D image projection system is going to replace the conventional monitor in near future and surgeon will get a virtual image in air just above the body of patient. This new projection system will abolish all the limitation of current two dimensional images without depth perception.

NOTES

Over the past 10 years, the major drive in surgery has been the development and application of minimal access approaches to traditional operations. This philosophy has crossed all surgical specialties and has had a major impact on training, technological developments, and patient care.

In general surgery, the emphasis has been on laparoscopic techniques, which can now be applied to the majority of intra-abdominal procedures. Evidence suggests that the reduction in trauma to the abdominal wall and the physiology of the pneumoperitoneum has a positive impact on patients undergoing abdominal operations.

Although still not widely applied, these techniques have put surgeons on notice that flexible endoscopy may become an important component of their practice.

Surgeons have gone beyond the luminal confines of the gastrointestinal tract to perform intra-abdominal procedures. With existing flexible endoscopic instrumentation, the wall of the stomach is punctured and an endoscope is advanced into the peritoneal cavity to perform various procedures; thus far, the use of this technique for diagnostic exploration, liver biopsy, cholecystectomy, splenectomy, and tubal ligation has been reported in animal models. Recently Transvaginal endoscopic cholecystectomy is performed in France (Figs 48.3A to F).

After the intervention is finished, the scope is pulled back into the stomach and the puncture closed. Several videos have been shown at scientific meetings that suggest that at least transgastric appendectomy has been performed in humans. Other natural orifices, such as the anus or vagina, also allow access to the

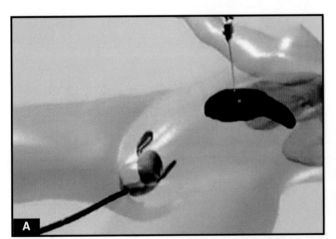
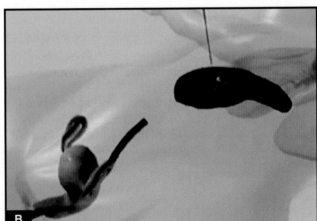
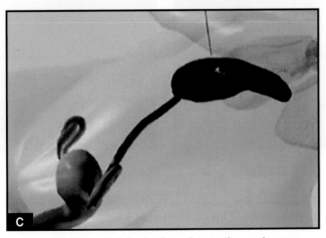

Figs 48.2A to C: Introduction of operative endoscope through the vaginal orifice

Section Six

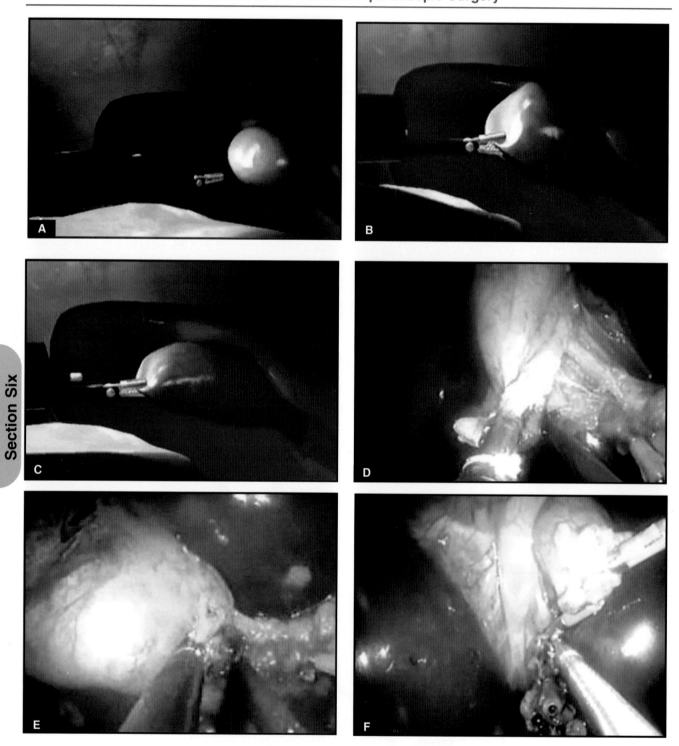

Figs 48.3A to F: Transvaginal cholecystectomy

peritoneal cavity (Figs 48.2A to C). Although in its infancy, the performance of NOTES (natural orifice transluminal endoscopic surgery) may thus further revolutionize the field of abdominal surgery.

Obvious questions are raised by the possibilities of NOTES:

1. Is there any clinical advantage to avoiding incisions in the abdominal wall? Can the visceral wall be closed safely and reliably?
2. Do the flora of the natural orifice lead more to peritoneal infection?
3. Who should perform these procedures, and how should the individuals be trained in NOTES?

Society of American Gastrointestinal and Endoscopic Surgeons (SAGES) and gastroenterologists from the American Society of Gastrointestinal Endoscopists (ASGE) held a summit meeting to build a conceptual framework for the initial safe application of NOTES procedures. It was acknowledged that the development of NOTES further blurred the lines between the traditional boundaries of GI surgeons and endoscopists. Several broad concepts and principles were agreed upon and will soon be published in detail in a white paper.

Safe Application of NOTES

The concepts included the following: Initially, NOTES should be performed by a team of experienced laparoscopic surgeons and interventional endoscopists in an operating room. Clinical procedures should be done under Institutional Review Board supervision and entered into a prospective outcomes database. Basic research is needed to assess the physiologic alterations caused by the visceral puncture and the bacteriology of the peritoneal cavity following transluminal interventions. Collaboration with industry is critical to the development of effective instruments allowing traction/countertraction and stable optical platforms, as well as the means to control hemostasis, securely close the visceral wall, and perform suturing functions and gastrointestinal anastomoses.

The roots of NOTES have been established but work is still needed to refine techniques, verify safety, and document efficacy. With continued research, NOTES may prove to be a sound method with clinical benefit to patients. Appropriate scientific scrutiny, collaboration among gastrointestinal interventionalists, and effective means of training for these techniques will be critical on emerging technologies.

Section Six

What would you do if the following situations occurred during a laparoscopic surgery?

a. The field turns pink or yellow.

1. White balancing may not have been done initially before inserting the telescope into the abdomen. White balance the camera should be done after withdrawing it.
2. There may be wrongly connected RGB cable. The RGB cable should be checked for proper connection.
3. Low voltage can sometimes alter the color.
4. Bile or blood spillage may turn the field pink or yellow due to staining of field. The inadvertent injury to bowel and spillage of bowel content may cause the field to turn yellow.

b. Sudden black out.

1. The cause of sudden black out may be due to fused bulb of light source. Switch of light source should be turn to use backup bulb.
2. There may be disconnected camera or monitor cable or the fuse of camera blown due to fluctuation in voltage. The fuse and connection of camera and monitor should be checked.
3. The tip of the telescope may be touching any object completely so there is no way for light to come out. The telescope should be repositioned.

c. Poor definition of picture.

1. The poor picture may be due to soiled lens with blood or other body fluids. It should be cleaned with warm water.

2. The camera may not be white balanced or focused properly. The fine tuning of camera should be tried. The proper white balance of camera is necessary to get a good quality picture. White balancing of camera should be done by placing the telescope 6 cm away from a complete white gauge piece or tissue paper.
3. Excessive blood in the operative field resulting in absorption of light and poor field is one of the causes of poor vision of operating field. Proper irrigation and suction should be tried to get a clear view.

What action would you take to control marked intra-abdominal bleeding from a trocar site?

a. For immediate control.

With inserted trocar, pressure should be applied on the bleeding site either from outside or using a pledget from within under vision.

A Foley's catheter can be inserted and the balloon can be inflated and pulled up creating a tamponade effect.

A purse string suture can be taken around the incision of trocar and tightened to check the bleeding.

A clamp can be applied to the port site till the bleeding is controlled.

b. For more permanent control.

1. The bleeding vessel can be sutured from within under vision or controlled with diathermy, or a full thickness bite can be taken externally at the region of the bleeding vessel.

2. The incision can be extended and the vessel can be found by proper debridement and then bleeding vessel should be ligated.

What action would you take if trocar injury to a large vessel occurs?

1. The trocar should be left in place. The adequate resuscitative measures should be taken (like blood should be at hand for the transfusion).
2. Urgent laparotomy should be performed and repair of the vessel with adequate exposure should be done.
3. The help of a vascular surgeon should be asked.

What would you do following a sudden collapse of the patient during an endoscopic procedure?

Possible causes for the collapse could be:
1. Vasovagal shock due to peritoneal irritation.
2. CO_2 embolism either by direct entry of gas into vessel or through absorption.
3. Hypercarbia due to systemic CO_2 absorption results in respiratory acidosis, pulmonary hypertension leading to cardiac dysrhythmia.
4. Arrhythmias – AV dissociation, junctional rhythm, sinus bradycardia and asystole due to vagal response to peritoneal stretching.

Insufflation should be stopped and abdomen should be deflated. The patient should be kept in a head-down and right up (steep left lateral Trendelenburg's position) and 100% O_2 should be administered. The blood gas levels should be analyzed and corrected accordingly. The gas in the right ventricle should be removed with a central venous catheter if possible. If there is any arrhythmia, atropine and anti-arrhythmic should be given. In case of ventricular fibrillation there may be need of DC defibrillator.

What pressure setting on the insufflator would you select at the start of a diagnostic laparoscopy in an adult healthy patient?

If general anesthesia is employed the starting flow rate is set at 1 L/minute, 12 mm Hg and volume- 2 to 3 L.

During diagnostic laparoscopy under local anesthesia insufflation is begun at a flow rate of 1 L/min. Initial low pressure- 2-3 mm Hg and volume not exceeding 2 L.

What would you do when?

a. High pressure is registered when CO_2 is insufflated in the VN before the needle has been placed in the body.

1. Veress needle may be blocked
2. The gas tap may not be opened
3. Gas tube may be kinked.

The tap should be checked for right direction and the needle should be flushed with saline to ensure that it is not blocked. The faulty Veress needle should be changed.

b. High pressures (10 or 15 mm Hg) are obtained during insufflation at 1 L/min.

1. The needle may be in the wrong plane and not in the peritoneal cavity.
2. Gas tap or needle may be partially blocked.

Right plane of insertion of needle should be checked by the saline drop test and negative aspiration test. If the problem continues than needle should be withdrawn and reinserted.

What would you do if after insufflation and on insertion of the telescope?

a. You saw gas in the greater omentum.

If there is gas in the grater omentum the probability is that either the Veress needle or the trocar has entered and insufflated gas into it. There is an increased risk of systemic absorption of CO_2 resulting in embolism. The necessary precautions to prevent this should be taken. Antithrombotics (Heparin) should be given, the patient should be tilted head down and left lateral and 100% O_2 should be given for inspiration.

b. Only fat is seen and there is no crepitance in the abdominal wall.

The telescope is probably in the omentum and should be withdrawn and any possible injury to the omental vessel should be checked.

What action would you take when?

a. You are unable to advance trocar into abdomen.

If the trocar is a disposable one confirm whether the blade tip is charged and reintroduce. Alternatively the tip may get discharged half way. The trocar should be removed recharged and inserted again. If it is a reusable trocar the tip may be blunt in which case it would be better to use a different sharp trocar.

b. The tip of the obturator is seen entering the abdominal cavity during insertion of a secondary trocar.

The skin incision may be small so the trocar has to be removed, the incision should be extended and the trocar should be reinserted.

List the safety mechanisms of different types of trocars.

a. Blunt (Hasson) trocar-blunt with insertion under direct vision. This type of trocar works on the safety of direct vision.

Some disposable trocar have a sharp blade with a spring loaded safety shield which cover the blade tip once the peritoneal cavity is entered. This spring loaded spring mechanism reduces the risk of injury to the underlying viscera by the blade tip.

Other disposable trocars require charging before insertion and when the tip enters the peritoneal cavity the blade tip retracts inside.

Reusable trocars have triangular and conical tips. The triangular tips are sharper and tend to cause more vascular injury.

Some disposable trocars have a screw shaped cannula, which has to be inserted like a screw, which enables the surgeon to have more control over the force with which he inserts the trocar. These have an additional advantage of not slipping out during the procedure.

Non-bladed obturator is used in some trocars for careful insertion where the problem of charging the blade tip and its potency does not arise.

Visiport is a mechanism in which the telescope is inserted into the cannula and the gun is fired through the abdominal wall visualizing each layer until the peritoneal cavity is reached. The trocars are thus inserted under vision layer by layer.

Radially dilating trocars are also available. It has the advantage of entry through a very small incision and then incision can be dilated with the serial dilator.

Ultrasonically activated trocar system is used in some high-risk patients. It consists of an ultrasonic generator and a transducer attached to the trocar spike.

The sharp pyramidal tip is activated with a frequency of 23.5 kHz and amplitude of 150 micrometers. The trocar fits a 5 mm plastic sheath that is introduced inside a 10 mm dilator whose tip is conical.

List the factors that contribute to increase the risk of complications with using Veress needle.

- Faulty needle – dysfunctional spring tip
- Wrong method of insertion
- Not guarding the needle and not inserting like a dart
- Uncontrolled forceful insertion of needle
- Wrong angle of insertion, i.e. directing straight down, instead of towards the pelvic cavity
- Excessive force from shoulder rather than wrist while inserting
- Previous abdominal surgery and scarred abdomen
- Thin scaphoid individual: Risk of deep entry
- Spinal deformities: Kyphoscoliosis
- Late pregnancy
- Morbid obesity
- Organomegaly
- Portal hypertension.

PROCEDURE CHECKLISTS: VERESS NEEDLE INSERTION

Check and Set the Insufflator

Pressure level and flow rate.

Initial flow rates should be set at around 1 liter/min. Optimal exposure is obtained with intra abdominal pressures of 12.0- 16.0 mm Hg. Lower pressures (e.g. 10 mm Hg) may give adequate visualization, especially in women with lax abdominal walls. This causes less stretching of the diaphragm, possibly reducing postoperative pain. Low pressure pneumoperitoneum may be used in conjunction with techniques to lift the abdominal wall in patients with impaired respiratory or cardiac states. An initial setting of 10.0 - 15.0 mm Hg is recommended for routine procedures.

- Connect gas supply to Veress needle.
- Check gas flow, needle patency and spring loaded central blunt stylet.
- Palpation test.
- Assessment of abdominal wall thickness by palpation with the fingers down to the aorta.

- Make a small skin incision.
- Tension abdominal wall and insert needle.

The safest technique is to hold the needle at a point along its shaft at a distance from the tip which equates with that estimated by palpation as the abdominal wall thickness. The other hand holds up the abdominal wall, providing counter tension as the needle is "threaded" in. You should be able to feel the needle puncture two distinct layers. Once the sharp tip enters the peritoneal cavity, the spring loaded blunt stylet is released with an audible (palpable) click.

Check that the Needle is in the Correct Position

A number of tests exist to confirm correct positioning of the needle tip.

- *Aspiration:* Uses a saline filled syringe
- *Saline drop test:* Uses a drop of saline in the Veress needle hub
- *Negative pressure test:* Retraction of the anterior abdominal wall
- Early insufflation pressures
- *Volume test:* Approximate 3 liters of gas are required to reach pressures of 10 mm Hg.

If an extraperitoneal position is suspected the needle can be withdrawn and repositioned. The number of passes required should be recorded. If a small amount of blood is aspirated, reinsertion is justified. If large amounts of blood escape up the needle, laparotomy is indicated. If bowel content is aspirated, the needle is withdrawn and reinserted in another location. Subsequent inspection and adequate treatment for bowel injury is mandatory.

Insufflate

After a minimum of 1 liter of gas has been insufflated and needle position has been confirmed, the rate may be increased for more rapid filling. Periodic checks should be made of symmetric distension and abdominal resonance. Once the desired pressure has been reached, close the gas tap on the needle and withdraw it.

Use of the Diathermy Hook

- Use a metal trocar.
- Pass the hook through an introducer tube or manually open the valve of the cannula to protect

the hook from damage. Trumpet type valves necessitate the use of the introducer.

- Select the tissue to be divided. You may require inserting the hooks tip parallel to the margin of the structure and then rotating it away to hook up tissue. You may need to use sweeping movements to separate the tissues. Do not lift too large an amount of tissue. Several small "bites" are more effective and safer. Work away from important structures.
- Inspect the tissue on the hook.
- Be aware of possible additional contact points.
- The camera operator may need to withdraw slightly to prevent the lens being splattered.
- Coagulate and/or cut the tissue on the hook.
- Control any possible overshoot.
- Continued dissection using this technique may require the hook to be cleaned of charred material Withdraw and clean with the supplied implement until clean. Smoke is generated if charring occurs, this can obscure the field. Open a tap on one of the cannula to allow gas to escape from the abdomen. This will automatically be replaced by fresh gas from the insufflator.
- When dissection is finished, watch the hook into the introducer tube as tissue may accidentally catch up and get damaged.
- Open the cannula valve if necessary to prevent damage to the hook.

Introduction of a Pledget into the Abdominal Cavity

- A traumatic, ratcheted grasper or a spiked biopsy forceps is passed through the introducer tube externally.
- The pledget is placed in the open jaws, making sure that enough pledget is placed between the jaws for a secure grip and enough pledget protrudes so that, in use, the grasper does not act on the tissues.
- The grip is secured by closing the jaws, doing up the racket and, as an added precaution against intra-abdominal loss, an elastic band is used to ensure closure is maintained.
- The pledget is then completely withdrawn into the introducer tube.
- The introducer tube is passed through a large cannula into the abdominal cavity.
- The pledget can now be extruded from the introducer and used.

Retrieval of a Pledget from the Abdominal Cavity

- When the pledget is no longer required it is withdrawn inside the introducer tube. It is extremely important that the camera follows the instrument and the pledget is seen to enter the tube.
- The tube can then be withdrawn from the cannula
- The pledget is extruded from the lower end and released from the grasper.

Application of Metal Clips

Is clip appropriate or would it be better to use a ligature?
- Load the clip applicator.
- Insert through an appropriate cannula.
- Place the jaws around the structure to be ligated
- Check for correct placement by observing from different angles or rotating the instrument.
- Partially close the instrument (This traps the tissue to be ligated and it can again be checked).
- Firmly close the jaws.
- Open and withdraw. Single clips should not be trusted for vessels of any size.

How to do laparoscopy on an abdomen with previous abdominal scar?

The patient with previous abdominal surgery is at high-risk for minimal access surgery. In these patients following techniques should be used:
1. The open insufflation technique
   - Hasson technique
   - Fielding technique.
2. Pneumoperitoneum should be created with a Veress needle by selecting an alternate site of insertion distant from the old abdominal incision.
3. Insufflations with a Veress needle inserted in posterior vaginal fornix or transuterus route
4. Insertion of optical trocar- primary port.

Hasson's Technique

This is a very safe technique to enter the abdomen, especially in patients with scarred abdomen from multiple previous surgeries.

This is an open technique where surgeon can see what he is doing. It is performed in an area of the abdomen distant from previous scars and likely to be free of adhesions. After the induction of anesthesia 1 cm horizontal incision is made. Blunt dissection is carried out until the underlying fascia is identified. The fascia is elevated with a pair of Kocher's clamps. Adherent subcutaneous tissue is gently dissected free. It is then incised to permit entry of trocar into the peritoneal cavity. Two heavy, absorbable sutures are placed on either side of the fascial incision just like repair of umbilical hernia. Care must be taken when applying these sutures not to injure the underlying viscera. The Kocher clamps are next removed, and 10 mm blunt trocar is advanced into the peritoneal cavity. The obturator is removed and the sleeve is secured in position with the previously placed two sutures. The sleeve of the trocar is wrapped with vaseline gauze to prevent leakage of insufflated gas around the trocar.

Open Fielding Technique

This technique developed by Fielding in 1992 involves a small incision over the averted umbilicus at a point where the skin and peritoneum are adjacent. Pneumoperitoneum can be created using Fielding technique in patients with abdominal incisions from previous surgery providing there is no midline incision, portal hypertension and re-canalized umbilical vein, and umbilical abnormalities such as urachal cyst, sinus or umbilical hernia present. A suture is not usually required to prevent gas leakage because the umbilicus has been everted (so the angle of insertion of the laparoscopic port becomes oblique) and the incision required is relatively small. However, one may be needed to stabilize the port. Thorough skin preparation of the umbilicus is carried out and the everted umbilicus (with toothed grasping forceps) is incised from the apex in a caudal direction. Two small retractors are inserted to expose the cylindrical umbilical tube running from the undersurface of the umbilical skin down to the linea alba. This tube is then cut from its apex downwards towards its junction with the linea alba. Further blunt dissection through this plane permits direct entry into the peritoneum. Once the peritoneal cavity is breached the laparoscopic port (without trocar) can then be inserted directly and insufflations started. A blunt internal trocar facilitates insertion of this port and an external grip that can be attached to the port to secure it in position.

The advantages of using the open technique are many:

1. The incidence of injury to adhesive although not eliminated is significantly reduced by entry into the peritoneal cavity under direct vision.
2. There is a decreased risk of injury to the retroperitoneal vessels. The obturator is blunt and the angle of entry allows the surgeon to maneuver the cannulas at an angle, which avoids viscera, while still assuring peritoneal placement.
3. The risk of extraperitoneal insufflations is eliminated. Placement under direct vision ensures that insufflation of gas is actually into the peritoneal cavity.
4. The likelihood of hernia formation is decreased because the fascia is closed as part of the technique.
5. In experience hands, the open technique is cost effective. The Hasson technique does not increase the operative time required, creating a pneumoperitoneum and may even lessen it.

Alternative Sites for Introducing Veress Needle

For avoiding the injury to the adhered portion of bowel in the patient with previous abdominal surgeries, the alternative site for the introduction of Veress needle can be chosen other than umbilicus.

For previous paparotomy with midline incision

For a previously operated abdomen with a midline incision, Veress needle should be placed in the upper left quadrant of the abdomen just lateral to the rectus sheath. The preperitoneal space in hypochondriac region is more easily insufflated than at the umbilicus. The Veress needle at hypochondriac region need to be passed more deeply into the abdomen in order to enter the peritoneal cavity because all the layers of abdomen are present here and there is a thick layer of muscle as well. The right upper quadrant should be avoided because of the size of the liver and the presence of the falciform ligament. There is some report of injury to liver if the liver is enlarged or the careless insertion of veress needle to right hypochondrium is performed.

For a previous laparotomy with upper midline incision

In patient with scar on the upper midline of abdomen the Veress needle should be placed in the right lower quadrant, the left lower quadrant should generally be avoided since in older patients there are usually sigmoid adhesions in the left lower quadrant.

For previously operated abdomen with a solitary incision in an upper or lower abdominal quadrant

In a patient with the scar in the upper or lower abdominal quadrant, the Veress needle should be passed in the opposite abdominal quadrant just lateral to the rectus muscle. The left lower and right upper quadrant should be avoided if it is possible.

For patient with previously operated abdomen in multiple quadrants

In these patients a Veress needle or open cannula in an area farthest from the existing abdominal scar should be used. When there is any confusion regarding the presence of adhesion inside the abdomen where Veress needle has to go, the opencannula technique should be used.

TRANSVAGINAL OR TRANSUTERINE INSUFFLATION

Some surgeons prefer to introduce Veress needle through the posterior fornix or though uterus in female with previous abdominal surgery. Although this method of pneumoperitoneum is now very popular the placement of a needle via the posterior fornix has been demonstrated to be safe. If this route of pneumoperitoneum has been chosen, than the needle must be placed in the midline about 1.75 cm behind the junction of the vaginal vault and smooth epithelium of external OS (Figs 49.1A and B).

Insufflation with an Optical Trocar (Visiport)

This is one of the techniques used for performing laparoscopic procedures in patient with previous scarred abdomen. An incision of 1 cm long is made in the area of the abdominal wall distant from the previous scars. The littlewood forceps is used to elevate the

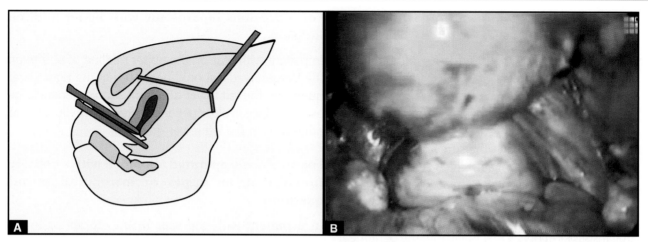

Figs 49.1A and B: Transvaginal route of insufflation

abdomen. The visiport optical trocar is introduced with telescope. The optical trocar is advanced slowly through the different planes of the abdominal wall. The blade at the tip of the visiport cuts the tissue which is visible also and there is very less chance of injury to intra-abdominal organ if the surgeon is experienced.

BIBLIOGRAPHY

1. Cataldo PA. Transanal endoscopic microsurgery. Surg Clin North Am 2006;86:915–25.
2. Fleshman J, Marcello P, Stamos MJ, Wexner SD. Focus Group on Laparoscopic Colectomy Education as endorsed by the American Society of Colon and Rectal Surgeons (ASCRS) and the Society of American Gastrointestinal and Endoscopic Surgeons (SAGES): guidelines for laparoscopic colectomy course. Surg Endosc 2006;20:1162–7.
3. Gavagan JA, Whiteford MH, Swanstrom LL. Full-thickness intraperitoneal excision by transanal endoscopic microsurgery does not increase short-term complications. Am J Surg 2004;187:630–4.
4. Heald RJ, Husband EM, Ryall RD. The mesorectum in rectal cancer surgery: the clue to pelvic recurrence? Br J Surg 1982;69:613–6.
5. Jagannath SB, Kantsevoy SV, Vaughn CA, Chung SS, Cotton PB, Gostout CJ, Hawes RH, Pasricha PJ, Scorpio DG, Magee CA, Pipitone LJ, Kalloo AN. Peroral transgastric endoscopic ligation of fallopian tubes with long-term survival in a porcine model. Gastrointest Endosc 2005;61:449–53.
6. Kantsevoy SV, Jagannath SB, Niiyama H, Chung SS, Cotton PB, Gostout CJ, Hawes RH, Pasricha PJ, Magee CA, Vaughn CA, Barlow D, Shimonaka H, Kalloo AN. Endoscopic gastrojejunostomy with survival in a porcine model. Gastrointest Endosc 2005;62:287–92.
7. Lezoche E, Guerrieri M, Paganini AM, D'Ambrosio G, Baldarelli M, Lezoche G, Feliciotti F, De SA. Transanal endoscopic versus total mesorectal laparoscopic resections of T2-N0 low rectal cancers after neoadjuvant treatment: a prospective randomized trial with a 3-years minimum follow-up period. Surg Endosc 2005;19:751–6.
8. Pai RD, Fong DG, Bundga ME, Odze RD, Rattner DW, Thompson CC. Transcolonic endoscopic cholecystectomy: a NOTES survival study in a porcine model (with video). Gastrointest Endosc 2006;64:428–34.
9. Park PO, Bergstrom M, Ikeda K, Fritscher-Ravens A, Swain P. Experimental studies of transgastric gallbladder surgery: cholecystectomy and cholecystogastric anastomosis (videos). Gastrointest Endosc 2005;61:601–6.
10. Rattner D Kalloo A. ASGE/SAGES Working Group on Natural Orifice Translumenal Endoscopic Surgery. October 2005. Surg Endosc 2006;20:329–33.
11. Swanstrom LL, Smiley P, Zelko J, Cagle L. Video endoscopic transanal-rectal tumor excision. Am J Surg 1997;173:383–5.
12. Wagh MS, Merrifield BF, Thompson CC. Survival studies after endoscopic transgastric oophorectomy and tubectomy in a porcine model. Gastrointest Endosc 2006;63:473–8.

Section Six

Index